AIDS UPDATE
2013

An Annual Overview of Acquired Immune Deficiency Syndrome

GERALD J. STINE, PH.D.

Department of Biology
University of North Florida, Jacksonville

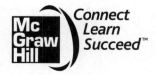

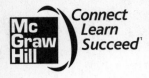

AIDS UPDATE 2013

Published by McGraw-Hill, a business unit of The McGraw-Hill Companies, Inc., 1221 Avenue of the
Americas, New York, NY 10020. Copyright © 2013 by The McGraw-Hill Companies, Inc. All rights
reserved. Printed in the United States of America. Previous edition(s) © 2012, 2011, and 2010. No
part of this publication may be reproduced or distributed in any form or by any means, or stored in a
database or retrieval system, without the prior written consent of The McGraw-Hill Companies, Inc.,
including, but not limited to, in any network or other electronic storage or transmission, or broadcast
for distance learning.

Some ancillaries, including electronic and print components, may not be available to customers outside the
United States.

This book is printed on acid-free paper.

This text is published by the **Contemporary Learning Series** group within the McGraw-Hill Higher
Education division.

1 2 3 4 5 6 7 8 9 0 DOC/DOC 1 0 9 8 7 6 5 4 3 2

MHID: 0-07-352766-1
ISBN: 978-0-07-352766-6
ISSN: 1081-5260

Managing Editor: *Larry Loeppke*
Marketing Director: *Adam Kloza*
Marketing Manager: *Nathan Edwards*
Developmental Editor: *Dave Welsh*
Lead Project Manager: *Jane Mohr*
Buyer: *Jennifer Pickel*
Design Coordinator: *Brenda A. Rolwes*
Cover Designer: *Rick Noel*
Senior Content Licensing Specialist: *Shirley Lanners*
Media Project Manager: *Sridevi Palani*

Compositor: *Laserwords Private Limited*
Cover Image: Reading about HIV and AIDS: © McGraw-Hill Companies Inc.; Truvada image courtesy of
Gilead Sciences, Inc.; The AIDS Memorial Quilt: © Courtesy of U.S. National Institutes of Health

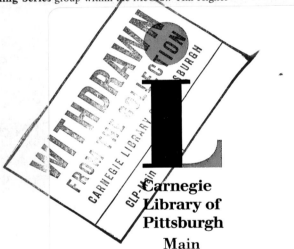

About the Author

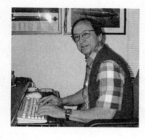

Gerald J. Stine is now a retired professor of the University of North Florida, Department of Biology, in Jacksonville, Florida. He received his B.S. degree from Southern Connecticut University, M.A. at Dartmouth, Ph.D. at the University of Delaware, and did a postdoctoral study in radiation genetics at Oak Ridge National Laboratory, Oak Ridge, Tennessee. He continued his research at the University of Tennessee, Knoxville, campus and published numerous scientific articles in recognized scientific journals. He then accepted a position at the University of North Florida. He has written 33 college-level textbooks, for example, *Laboratory Experiments in Genetics, Biosocial Genetics, Human Genetics, The Sexually Transmitted Diseases,* and the *AIDS UPDATE* series. Large segments of his work in genetics and the sexually transmitted diseases have been used in five special project publications used in a number of universities nationwide.

This edition of *AIDS UPDATE* is the 22nd. Dr. Stine's interest in AIDS began with the June 5, 1981, publication of reports by the CDC and others about a strange new disease that affected *only* gay males. Dr. Stine regarded this announcement as utter nonsense. Early in 1983, a high-level member of the CDC gave a presentation in Jacksonville to some 300 people about this new disease (the virus was not yet isolated). The speaker said, "if you are heterosexual, male, a woman, or a child, you have nothing to worry about, this is a gay male disease." At that very moment Dr. Stine knew of heterosexual males, hemophiliacs, and several women and children with this disease! Restraining himself, he left and began assembling his notes and learning about this new disease.

In 1988, he offered a new course called "Biological and Medical Aspects of AIDS." He began writing his first book on AIDS in 1991, published in 1993. This was the first formal general-purpose HIV/AIDS college-level textbook in the United States. He has continued to update for those needing the latest information on HIV/AIDS. The political and economic effects, pain, suffering, loss of life, and stigma due to HIV/AIDS continue.

Dr. Stine believes that AIDS, if it is not already, will soon be the worst transmittable viral or bacterial plague in human history. He has presented invited lectures on HIV/AIDS across the United States, in Canada, and in China. He received the Distinguished Alumni Award from his undergraduate college and presented the keynote address for the first Biotechnology Symposium held at Wuhan University, China. He was made an honorary professor of Wuhan University. He was a member of the First Sino-American HIV/AIDS management symposium, invited to China by the Chinese Medical Association. Dr. Stine is internationally recognized for numerous research publications and textbooks in the field of genetics, sexually transmitted diseases, and HIV/AIDS. In October 2008, Dr. Stine received the Leeann Porterfield achievement award for HIV/AIDS educator of the year. The award was made possible by the AIDS Community Alliance of South Central Pennsylvania. He has prepared and published four professional brochures for genetic counseling and prenatal diagnostic testing while directing a prenatal genetic diagnostic center at Memorial Hospital in Jacksonville, Fl and is sought after by publishers to review manuscripts on genetics and HIV/AIDS. He has been consultant to seven college textbook companies. He is listed in the *American Men & Women of Science, Students International Directory of Scientists,* and *Who's Who in Technology Today.*

Contents

3 Biological Characteristics of HIV   49

4 Anti-HIV Therapy   67

5 The Immunology of HIV Disease/AIDS   105

AIDS UPDATE 2013

WHY DO I WRITE ABOUT HIV/AIDS?

I began writing about a new disease, later called AIDS, in 1981, shortly after the Centers for Disease Control and Prevention issued the first of its reports. These writings were limited in scope because not much was known at the time. My writing then was for classroom use. Little did I know at the time the passion that I would develop about this disease. As the number of infected people and their deaths continued to rise, fear and discrimination reared their ugly heads because, in some cases, people are what they are, and, in other cases, because of the lack of available unbiased educational material. At the time, in the mid-1980s, I felt a need to write, to help educate people about this disease, hopefully to answer questions and reduce the blatant discrimination occurring against those who already had the overwhelming burden of HIV disease. So, I began—I created a college-level HIV/AIDS course and taught it for several years, constantly shaping and reshaping the information necessary to help others learn the facts about this pandemic, and to destroy destructive myths. After I felt I had set the record straight in my classroom, I began writing HIV/AIDS college-level textbooks so that information on this pandemic could be shared more broadly.

There are many reasons I have not stopped writing about HIV/AIDS. First, because as Yogi Berra supposedly said, "It ain't over til it's over," and it "ain't" near over yet! Second, AIDS summons up the greatest themes in literature, among them sex, faith, and death—themes that are universal and unexpectedly permanent. Anyone who has lost a loved one to death, untimely or by nature, can read about AIDS and understand the emotional forces involved. Anyone who has taken care of someone who has been ill understands the need for compassion. Anyone who has faced death from a prolonged or life-threatening illness should be able to identify with those who suffer with AIDS. Anyone interested in uncovering acts of human kindness or, conversely, acts of despicable behavior can find them in writings about this disease.

In many ways, HIV/AIDS is a sad and depressing story. Many lives have been lost and more are still at risk. There continues to be unjust inequities and impossible choices. Yet, HIV/AIDS is an inspirational story throughout this pandemic, there have been heroes-scientists, the infected and the impacted, whose actions, made a difference in lives and communities around them. It is a privilege and a responsibility to give voice to these people.

With this, the 22nd edition of the *AIDS UPDATE* series, I continue to write about AIDS because too many people have stopped talking and writing about it. But the need to continue the conversation about HIV/AIDS remains important because the virus, HIV, is still with us. HIV will remain with us until there is a vaccine or a cure for this terrible disease. In the meantime, there are still many untold stories that help define particular moments in the history of this disease.

But more than any of these reasons, my writing about AIDS is fueled by a need to do something, anything, to help. For the millions of people who are in pain and dying, I have little to offer except my writing. Although my only known risk factor was a blood transfusion in the mid-1970s, I cannot help but feel lucky that so far neither HIV/AIDS nor any other serious disease threatens my life or the lives of my wife and children. Is there a reason I have been spared to my present age when so many others have died? I write about AIDS, not just because I live but because it is part of our history. The AIDS pandemic has changed my feelings and attitudes toward people. I find myself more thoughtful and sensitive to others. AIDS has changed the world in some way for most everyone, and at least some of the information about this disease—its impact and repercussions—needs telling. So, I write about AIDS because someone needs to tell the story.

THIRTEEN YEARS INTO THE NEW MILLENNIUM

The war on HIV/AIDS, in my opinion, is approaching mid-way to the end. I have never been more positive about the future for those who are HIV infected in the United States and other developed and developing nations. The use of anti-HIV drugs and prevention techniques in combination has led to a dramatic reduction in HIV-infected babies and AIDS-related deaths, as well as to a significant reduction in new HIV infections and AIDS cases and reductions in opportunistic infections. These events, along with new insight into the biology and pathology of HIV, may lead to a preventive vaccine and provide a shining light against a stark history of the first 31 years of a pandemic first reported in the United States in 1981.

With the creation of the Global Fund for HIV/AIDS, Malaria, and Tuberculosis in 2001, the G8 (a group of eight industrial powers) founding of the International Global Fund for HIV/AIDS, and the decision by the world's largest antiretroviral manufacturers to dramatically lower drug costs to developing nations, there is now hope in those countries. However, the drugs are not yet free, and therefore are out of reach for millions of people living in poverty. But hope and help must begin somewhere—someone must first benefit before others can. **Let us pull together so that help, not just hope, will be available to all who need it!**
—Gerald Stine, Ph.D.

The information on HIV/AIDS within this text goes where the pandemic has taken us over the last 31 years (1981 through 2012) and into the future. This information is not designed to replace the relationship that exists between you and your doctor or other health adviser. For all medical events/needs, consult with an appropriate physician.

AIDS IS A WAR THAT NO ONE WANTS TO LOSE BUT NO ONE YET KNOWS HOW TO WIN

• • • • •

This book, as with my other twenty one HIV/AIDS college-level textbooks, is also dedicated to those who have died of AIDS, those who have HIV disease, those who care for them, and those who must prevent the spread of this plague—

EVERYONE, EVERYWHERE.

Thirty Two Years of HIV/AIDS and Counting: A Humanitarian Crisis

June 5, 1981–June 5, 2013

In the [31] years [1981 through 2012] since the first case was reported, AIDS has changed the world. It has killed 30 million people and infected [38] million more. It has become the world's leading cause of death among both women and men ages 15 to 59. It has inflicted the single greatest reversal in the history of human development. In other words, it has become the greatest challenge of our generation.

Kofi Annan
Former Secretary-General, United Nations

Those who cannot remember the past are condemned to repeat it.

George Santayana
Spanish Philosopher

Thirty-two years after the first AIDS cases were reported in the United States, the HIV epidemic continues to be heavily concentrated among men who have sex with men (MSM) in the United States. MSM are heavily impacted throughout most of the world and are the predominant risk group throughout the Americas and Western Europe; heterosexuals are the predominant risk group in sub-Saharan Africa; and injection-drug users predominate throughout Europe and Southeast Asia. In the United States, blacks and Latinos continue to be disproportionately affected, despite overall advances in HIV testing and care. The world continues to face the greatist public health threat in six centuries.

LOOKING BACK—
LOOKING FORWARD

Once upon a time, there was a world without HIV/AIDS. Surely this begins as many fairy tales do—"Once upon a time." But HIV/AIDS is no fairy tale! It is a horrible disease that has stripped naked the very soul of humankind. About 31 years ago the scourge of HIV/AIDS could have been the storyline in your favorite science-fiction comic book, or on the front page of some sensational tabloid: **"New germ threatens human survival on Planet Earth."** But, as we have all learned over time, truth is often stranger than or at least similar to fiction. Millions of lives have been lost, millions more will be lost, millions more damaged, and many millions more impacted in some way by HIV/AIDS.

In the beginning of HIV/AIDS on Planet Earth, humanity, in its ignorance to what this virus could do, quickly framed the battle against this virus with those against past viruses that we defeated. And as with other viruses that cause measles, polio, and smallpox, the battlefield against HIV quickly became global. It was global even before scientists knew they were dealing with a new and different virus. Clearly, like the discovery of electricity, the Second World War, penicillin, the dropping of the first atomic bomb, Watson and Crick's discovery of DNA's double helix, the introduction of satellites circling the earth for diverse reasons, computers in all their forms, and the Internet, HIV has permanently altered the world. There may never again be a world without HIV/AIDS! The HIV/AIDS pandemic is constantly evolving and continuously surprising! When HIV was emerging in the early 1980s, we clearly underestimated the global effect that the disease would have—that in only a few decades, tens of millions of people worldwide would become infected. This pandemic is the result of what 32 years ago was an unpredictable but tremendously potent combination of intimate personal behaviors such as unprotected sex, needle sharing, and socioeconomic factors, which include poverty, gender inequity, social exclusion, and migration, and have affected every country worldwide. We also underestimated the extent to which stigma and discrimination against people living with HIV and those most vulnerable to it would remain formidable obstacles to tackling HIV/AIDS. However, the introduction of antiretroviral treatment in developed countries about 18 years ago and its dissemination to developing countries in recent years has largely changed the perception that HIV/AIDS is a death sentence. But people living with HIV/AIDS in most countries continue to experience ostracism, violence, eviction, loss of employment, and restrictions on their ability to travel.

People with HIV/AIDS were/are considered the scourge of society—people didn't like them because they were either gay or injection drug users, and there was a fear of contagion, that if you were in the same room with someone with HIV/AIDS you might get HIV/AIDS. They had diarrhea, dementia, and wasting. It was an awful way to die. Can you imagine living to die that way?

HIV/AIDS IS DIFFERENT FROM OTHER STORIES

Think of the major interdisciplinary, complex stories of our time, stories that are worldwide, ongoing, and urgent. Perhaps you think of climate change, famine, or nuclear proliferation. None of these is like the HIV/AIDS pandemic.

HIV/AIDS is a story of great breadth and sharp contrasts; covering it requires knowledge and sensitivity around personal issues such as sexuality, addiction, and social vulnerability. At the same time, it is a global story requiring a broad understanding of international politics, economics, scientific facts, and diverse cultural traditions. Interwoven with these strands of the HIV/AIDS story are the scientific, medical, and healthcare stories that we, as authors, must be able to "translate" for you the student.

What complicates the presentations and explanations is the voluminous amount of difficult-to-interpret, tangled, intricate, complex, and perplexing information available during the 32 years of HIV/AIDS.

Socially, HIV/AIDS Is Different than Other Diseases?

The significant difference was spawned by the Public Health Service. For many scientists, physicians, epidemiologists, and sociologists, a major and disruptive difference separating HIV/AIDS from all other biological diseases and the sexually transmitted diseases in particular is that the U.S. Public Health Services has treated HIV/AIDS as being some type of special case-civil rights issue instead of a public health issue. It refused to use standard epidemiological methods to track the progression of the disease, such as identifying infected individuals and notifying those who came in contact with them, as is done for other communicable and venereal diseases, so those exposed could seek treatment. However, this method was not done with HIV/AIDS because the "privacy of those involved had to be protected." But, the privacy of those infected with syphilis and gonorrhea apparently does not meet the same high standard, even though they are essentially contracted in a very similar fashion. Because that is the case, the stigma attached to HIV/AIDS is due overwhelmingly (with the exception of in utero infections, blood transfusions, and infections on the job for health workers) to individuals who become infected by doing things they should probably not be doing, i.e., having sexual relations with strangers, engaging in various homosexual practices, utilizing the services of prostitutes, and using illicit injection drugs.

HUMANS AND HIV/AIDS

This is a political, medical, and social story about ourselves and the ways HIV/AIDS is moving through the world. HIV/AIDS is a deadly but preventable disease thriving in the human family, infecting or killing about 30 million of its members. It's a world in which HIV/AIDS has caused us to ask, what kind of people are we? How did we get to this point? Where are we going? Can we for once find ways of compassion, humanity, and dignity for all men and women? Many people still believe AIDS is an African or Latin American disease, and they blame the people from both these areas of the world for its spread. But they are not responsible for AIDS or HIV. The world is accountable, and until the world itself changes, HIV and AIDS will thrive in the human family for generations to come. There will be a very steep price to pay.

HOW DID IT ALL BEGIN?

June 5, 2006, was one of the most inauspicious anniversaries recognized in the United States. It marked the 25th anniversary of what would become the first case of AIDS in the United States. Michael S. Gottlieb didn't know it at the time, but when a 31-year-old man (also named Michael) was admitted to his hospital in 1981 with fever and weight loss, he was meeting the person who would become the first officially reported case in the global AIDS pandemic. Twenty-five years later, Michael or "Patient Zero" has long since died, but Gottlieb is still treating people with HIV. Since then, the United States has had the most severe HIV/AIDS epidemic of any developed country worldwide. The United States has the 10th largest HIV population. The other nine countries with higher HIV populations are in sub-Saharan Africa.

When this new disease was first recognized on June 5, 1981, the causative infectious agent was unknown. By 1983, AIDS cases had turned up in 28 nations. After it was determined in 1983 that the causative agent was a virus, the virus turned out to be unique even within its own classification of retroviruses. Since then, more has been learned about this retrovirus, the Human Immunodeficiency Virus (HIV), and in a shorter time span, than is known about any other virus in human history. Nonetheless, this anniversary in no way marked the end of the Age of AIDS, although it may have marked a new global beginning.

By the time HIV/AIDS emerged in the states of New York, California, Florida, Texas, and New Jersey, people were so terrified of this new disease that those afflicted by it were shunned by doctors, nurses, social workers, police officers, firefighters, and the public at large. This ugly scenario began with the first report in the Centers for Disease Control and Prevention (CDC) June 5, 1981, edition of *Morbidity and Mortality Weekly Report* (*MMWR*).

LOOKING BACK—LOOKING FORWARD

Pneumocystis pneumonia—Los Angeles

It all began on June 5, 1981, on paper, at least. That's the day that a medical publication reported an outbreak of Pneumocystis pneumonia among five young, gay men in Los Angeles, California. Nobody knew it at the time, but that nondescript, two-page article—simply entitled "Pneumocystis Pneumonia—Los Angeles" was the first published report on what is now known as AIDS and the virus that causes it,

HIV **(HIV/AIDS).** In 2013, we mark the 32nd anniversary of that report. Throughout the year, HIV/AIDS community members, public officials, and the rest of the world will write articles and blogs; will hold events, speeches, and vigils; and will reflect back on the past three decades, as well as what the future holds in store for the HIV/AIDS pandemic and the people who are part of it.

A FEW IMPORTANT THINGS LEARNED ABOUT HIV/AIDS

1. **HIV infection is no longer a death sentence.** A positive test result—even if your CD4 count is low—gives you the warning you need to take control of your health and stop the disease from getting worse. The majority of people who take HIV medications can plan on long and healthy lives.
2. **HIV infection or AIDS is not a punishment.** The virus causes this disease indiscriminately.
3. **HIV infection is not a reason for self-deprecation.** Taking responsibility for your health is important. Focus on the present, not the past. Learn new ways to heal yourself, not blame yourself.

Baffling Reports

In the June 1981 report, five young men, all active homosexuals, were treated for biopsy-confirmed *Pneumocystis pneumonia* (PCP, now referred to as *Pneumocystis jiroveci* pneumonia) at three different hospitals in Los Angeles, California. Two of the patients died. All five patients had laboratory-confirmed previous or concurrent Cytomegalovirus (CMV) infection and a candidal (fungal) mucosal infection. The authors of the report speculated that "some aspect of the homosexual lifestyle" or a "disease acquired through sexual contact" may have had a role in

these unusual cases of PCP and also postulated that "a cellular–immune dysfunction related to a common exposure" may have been involved.

In July 1981, one month after CDC's first report, doctors from New York and California reported in *MMWR* 26 cases of the rare skin cancer Kaposi's sarcoma in 26 gay males ages 15 to 49. Several of these men also had *Pneumocystis jiroveci* pneumonia (PCP) and Cytomegalovirus (CMV), and the authors cautioned, "Physicians should be alert for Kaposi's sarcoma, PCP, and other opportunistic infections associated with immunosuppression in homosexual men." Although the disease was yet to be called AIDS, and the infectious agent was not yet discovered, some 200,000 people in the United States were already HIV infected, and they began dying with increasing numbers yearly until AIDS deaths peaked in 1995 at 55,000! In some social groups, the dead outnumbered the living. For example, from the San Francisco Gay Men's Chorus, there were 210 singers and 257 obituaries. Now 32 years after the first reported case of AIDS and 30 years after the discovery of HIV as the cause of AIDS, effective control of the HIV/AIDS pandemic remains elusive. And the three words continuing to echo around the world are: **AIDS CRISIS WORSENS!**

In the modern world, 32 years seems a long time to be at war, but it is hardly surprising when the enemy is as elusive and pervasive as HIV. It has been 30 years since scientists first identified the cause of what was then a baffling new syndrome ravaging immune systems and destroying lives. Since then, AIDS has gone from being the scourge of relatively small groups, such as hemophiliacs, homosexuals, and intravenous-drug users in rich countries to arguably the biggest threat to life and prosperity in the developing world. And we now know that no single research group or discipline will solve the puzzles of how to conquer HIV/AIDS. It is now clear that scientists were naïve to believe there would be an easy path from the discovery of HIV to the development of a vaccine.

ANTIRETROVIRAL DRUGS (ARVD)

The slogan of the first 15 years of the HIV/AIDS pandemic was, "Until there is a cure!" Today it seems the global health leadership of the world is satisfied with "Until there is lifelong drug therapy for everybody." A dangerous sentiment is sweeping over the political/scientific HIV/AIDS establishment, calling for elimination of funding for HIV vaccine research and prevention programs, and shifting those dollars, euros, and yen to expanding HIV treatment. Yet, for every person who begins treatment for HIV infection, two to three others become newly infected. Treatment alone will not curtail the HIV/AIDS pandemic. To control and ultimately end this pandemic, we need a powerful array of proven HIV prevention tools that are widely accessible to all who would benefit from them.

FIVE OF THE GREATER ACHIEVEMENTS FROM THE USE OF ANTIRETROVIRAL THERAPY(ART) THROUGH 2012

- First, the mother-to-child (MTC) HIV infection rate in developed countries has, through the use of ART, fallen from 25% to 30% of newborns down to 1% to 2%, and it is now believed that MTC transmission can be eliminated by 2015.
- Second, in the 1980s, a young adult diagnosed with AIDS survived less than a year. Today a similar person can expect to live to age 70 or beyond if he or she is diagnosed early, has access to and receives ART, and can tolerate the drugs and their side effects.
- Third, preliminary studies released in early 2011 have shown that ART using Truvada

did prevent HIV infection among men having sex with men (MSM). But similar trials among women were not effective. The reason is not yet understood.

- Fourth, in May 2011 the National Institutes of Health released the results of HPTNO 52, an international study to determine if ART could reduce HIV transmission between heterosexual serodiscordant persons (one of the sexual partners is HIV positive, the other is HIV negative). The study began in 2005 and involved 1763 serodiscordant couples. It was stopped in 2011, four years before its scheduled completion in 2015. The reason for stopping the study was that the preliminary findings showed that the risk of transmitting HIV to the negative partner was reduced by 96% when the HIV-infected partner was placed on ART, these findings strongly indicate that in addition to the immediate benefits to the infected person, placing that person on ART immediately after diagnosis of infection, regardless of CD4 count, significantly reduces the transmission of HIV to a sexual partner.
- Fifth, prevention, care, and the use of ART has lowered the death rate by 20% over the last six years (2006–2012).

The Beginning of Antiretroviral Drugs: A Game Changer—Then a Life Changer

The first Food and Drug Administration (FDA)-approved antiretroviral drug (ARVD) was zidovudine (known as AZT) in 1987, but its toxic effect was almost as bad as the disease. It was, however, a beginning. In 1995, with about 350,000 people dead from AIDS, the first of the protease inhibitors and nucleoside reverse transcriptase inhibitors were FDA-approved, and the death rate from AIDS dropped dramatically. From 2001 through 2012, the death rate has held steady at between 14,000 and 17,000 AIDS deaths per year. Through the 32nd anniversary and counting, some 26 FDA ARVDs and seven combination drug therapies are being used to lengthen the lives of the HIV infected. Much has yet to be achieved concerning the arsenal of available ARVD because at least 20% to 40% of those infected cannot tolerate many of the drugs now available.

ORIGIN OF HIV

The best evidence entering 2013 states that a virus called Simian Immunodeficiency Virus (SIV), found in chimpanzees in Africa, crossed into humans and changed its form to become a lethal agent in humans. This crossover may have occurred in the late 1800s or early 1900s. It is speculated that HIV arrived in the United States around 1968 and spread undetected throughout the 1970s.

SOCIAL IMPACT OF THE NEW DISEASE

Over the past 32 years and counting, AIDS activists and their supporters have forced sweeping changes in how the U.S. blood supply is managed, the time frame used by the FDA for drug approval, and U.S. drug companies' search for new and improved antiretroviral drugs. They have also changed the rules on government-controlled marches and rallies. Socially, we have learned that antiretroviral drugs can prolong HIV/AIDS patients' lives; that cultural changes for HIV prevention are very difficult; that Africa is still poor and vulnerable to HIV infections; that Asia is still in denial that millions of HIV/AIDS orphans have nowhere to turn; that celebrities have chosen more glitzy causes; and that now black and gay communities bury their dead quietly. America is allowing HIV/AIDS to be normalized like homelessness and poverty. The global HIV/AIDS crisis is not over; it has just begun. The statistics over the last 32 years are numbing beyond comprehension. Who can understand the meaning of 38 million people (ending 2013) throughout the world living with the virus? Or that HIV infection continues to increase throughout the world? It is only when people realize that at the end of 2013, 30 million people will have died of AIDS, or that a 15-year-old in South Africa has a 50:50 chance of dying of AIDS before the age of 30, that the horror begins to take on a human scale. The American perception of HIV/AIDS has gone through a cycle of meanings over the last 32 years. In the early days, there was no name for the disease, and there was the white-knuckle scare when news reports displayed footage of emaciated people dying from HIV/AIDS. Today, there are no young people who have witnessed hospital wards overcrowded with people dying of HIV/AIDS. Today, we continue to ask how to cure it. In the early days there were major protests against the FDA and the medical and pharmaceutical companies. Today, there is quiet acceptance. The early demonstrators influenced basic research, the federal drug approval process, and the massive federal funding for a single disease. This disease as no other before it has changed the way people interact with their physicians, demand medical services, and take control of their own treatments regardless of illness. An entire generation has now been born that has never known an HIV/AIDS-free world. Children born with HIV have now themselves become mothers of newborns! The disease has changed the personal as well as the political— how we think and how we love, what we teach our children, and what words we say in public. More than anything else, HIV/AIDS has changed the way we view the threat of emerging diseases. Until HIV/AIDS, most of us thought of catastrophic plagues, such as the Black Death or the Spanish flu epidemic of 1918, as things of the past. We lost sight of the fact that every once in a while a new disease emerges. It happened with HIV/AIDS and it can happen again. Witness the current outbreaks of the Hanta, West Nile, SARS, monkeypox, avian, and H1N1 flu viruses. HIV/AIDS also changed what it means to be a patient. People with HIV/AIDS stormed scientific conferences, banded together in ways no other patients ever had, helped revolutionize the process of testing experimental drugs, and inspired others. There is no question that breast cancer activism started because of AIDS activism. Those with cancer saw AIDS activism's success and decided to emulate it, deploying thousands of people to lobby for increased research funding.

HIV/AIDS also changed what it means to be gay in America. The images of gay men dying of this disease rendered them objects of sympathy and opened the doors to compassion. In the eyes of straight America, death gave gay men a humanity they had long been denied. Homophobia and attacks on gays became less acceptable. Although some argue that HIV/AIDS divided gays—positives from negatives—it seems more likely that a united gay community was forged in the crucible of HIV/AIDS. People facing mortality responded courageously and seized the chance to proclaim their identity. And it forced society's institutions—from hospitals that barred gay men from seeing their dying lovers to employers who denied them bereavement leave—to recognize gay relationships.

Although HIV/AIDS is predominantly a disease of developing countries, cities like Washington, DC; Baltimore, Maryland; Newark, New Jersey; New York City; and cities in the Southeast have high rates of HIV infection in their black communities. In fact, in some sections of the United States, the incidences of HIV/AIDS are as high as those in developing nations. For example, Washington, DC, has a higher incidence of HIV/AIDS than any other city in the United States. Three percent of the population of D.C. is infected with HIV, and about two percent has AIDS! The Washington, DC, population is 60% black, and between 80% and 90% of new HIV infections each year are among the black population.

Over the last ten years, HIV/AIDS has increasingly become a disease of the black population in the United States. Of the approximately 1.62 million people living with HIV/AIDS in the United States, about half are black.

Given the above facts about this disease, how will history judge our actions?

STOPPING HIV/AIDS

HIV/AIDS will not be stopped until people are prevented from contracting the virus, which, in the absence of a vaccine, means forgoing risks including unprotected sex and injection drugs using contaminated needles. Thirty-one years after the emergence of HIV, many governments still have not grasped the idea that simple preventive measures, such as providing condoms, sterile needles, and education, have been shown to save lives and money. The greatest failure during this pandemic has been in prevention because many governments choose to ignore the subjects of sex and injection-drug use. Rumor, denial, and complacency remain the emotional cocktail that serves to numb people and their governments to the reality of HIV/AIDS. Half of all new HIV infections worldwide are occurring in those under age 25. HIV/AIDS cannot be stopped until young adults are protected and respected.

PREVENTION RESEARCH AND APPLICATION

The news—both good and bad—has come unceasingly. In 2005, a test-of-concept HIV vaccine trial began and in 2007 it was declared a failure. This is the third time a promising vaccine has failed. In December 2006, we learned that circumcision could reduce men's risk of HIV infection through vaginal sex. One month later, we learned that trials of the microbicide candidate cellulose sulfate would be halted because there appeared to be more infections in the active arm than in the placebo arm. And in July 2007, we learned that a major efficacy study of the diaphragm found no evidence that this particular cervical barrier reduced women's risk of infection.

We know that the field of HIV prevention research is getting closer to delivering a partially effective vaccine and microbicide. The response to male circumcision itself, which is only partially protective, reminds us that the good news of circumcision comes with concern, questions, and ambivalence. Today's proven prevention strategies and the materials to enact them are not reaching the people who need them. For example, males in sub-Saharan Africa have access to about three condoms a year, and female condoms are almost nonexistent. Global tallies of new infections versus expanded treatment access show that each year for every person who starts antiretroviral treatment, about three people are infected with HIV. This ratio places an incredible strain on the fragile infrastructure available for HIV treatment and care.

AND THE REALITY IS

Mitchell Warren, AIDS Vaccine Advocacy Coalition (AVAC) Executive Director, said the following with regard to prevention strategies to prevent HIV/AIDS: "The truth is this: if the cure for AIDS were a glass of clean water, the world would still be hard pressed to bring the epidemic to a halt today. This virus thrives in places where the most basic elements of subsistence—clean water, shelter, food—are in shamefully short supply. It thrives in places where basic human rights—to dignity, health care, protection by the law—are equally scarce." (AVAC Report (2007). *Resetting the Clock.* New York (AVAC), pages 1–64.)

And the reality is, through the first 32 years of HIV/AIDS, scientists have created a huge body of knowledge about HIV transmission and how to prevent it, yet every day, around the world, nearly 7000 people become infected with HIV. Although HIV prevention is complex, it ought not be mystifying. Local and national achievements in curbing the epidemic have been myriad, and have created a body of evidence about what works, but these successful approaches have not yet been fully applied. Essential programs and services have not had sufficient coverage; they have often lacked the funding to be applied with sufficient quality and intensity. Action and funding have not necessarily been directed to where the epidemic is or to what drives it. Few programs address vulnerability to HIV and structural determinants of the epidemic. A prevention constituency has not been adequately mobilized to stimulate the demand for HIV prevention. Confident and unified leadership has not emerged to assert what is needed in HIV prevention and how to overcome the political, sociocultural, and logistic barriers in getting there. Today, some 32 years after the emergence of the disease, it is startling to learn that facts about HIV/AIDS are still a guessing game for much of the world and that many are still in the dark about the reality that HIV/AIDS remains a top global killer.

Global AIDS-Related Deaths

According to the World Health Organization, the number of HIV/AIDS-related deaths worldwide is expected to peak in the next five years—from

2.2 million per year in 2008 to a maximum of 2.5 million in 2012—before declining to 1.2 million in 2030. But this assumes that 80% of the HIV infected are on antiretroviral drugs by 2012. This did not happen!

BY THE NUMBERS

Nearly everywhere, HIV/AIDS is now the leading killer of young people in their most sexually active years. Sex, after all, remains the recreation of the poor. At the first international conference on AIDS in Africa that was held in Brussels before it was clear that AIDS was definitely caused by HIV, a scientist warned that "if AIDS turns out to be a sexually transmitted disease [as it is], it would spread across the world like a prairie fire." And it has. But regardless of the large number of those who have died of AIDS and those infected, we still learn slowly. In 2013 in the United States, a significant number of people still believe that HIV is spread by kissing, by sharing a drinking glass, or from a toilet seat! In addition, the majority of people do not know that mother-to-child transmission is preventable and that other sexually transmitted diseases can increase your risk of becoming HIV infected.

On the 32nd anniversary of HIV/AIDS, there will be about 2.3 million HIV infections in the United States, and about 659,000 of those infected will have died of AIDS. Worldwide ending 2013, an estimated 30 million will have died of AIDS out of a total of 68 million HIV infected. About 50% are women. This disease will have orphaned some 15 million children worldwide. As we look back over the past 31 years of the HIV/AIDS pandemic there have been major changes since the early years when life after diagnosis largely amounted to a year or so of increasingly severe illness: frightful pneumonias, brain and eye infections, skin cancers, stark weight loss, and thrush, a fungal infection

frequently so flagrant it oozed out of a person's mouth. New drugs now thwart these infections in modernized nations, but the vast majority of people across the world with HIV/AIDS continue to suffer these awful physical conditions.

HELP IS ON THE WAY

Camus writes of epidemic-stricken Oran's calamity in *The Plague* being everybody's business. AIDS, to read the American narrative of the global pandemic, is not yet everybody's business.

The United Nations

In 2001, in a precedent-setting special session, the first ever devoted to a public health issue, the UN General Assembly met and wrote its "Declaration of Commitment to a Comprehensive Battle against HIV/AIDS." This session was called "Global Crisis—Global Action." Most of the goals set in this declaration, targeted for 2003 and 2005, never materialized, or programs were tried and failed. But this session of the General Assembly was an important turning point in the global response to HIV/AIDS. In June 2006, in acknowledgment of the 25th anniversary, a second special session of the UN General Assembly met to assess the progress made from the 2001 meeting and to determine what political statement must be made to further the global cause of combating AIDS. The 2006 Political Declaration called for $23 billion to be spent on HIV/AIDS in 2010. But about $50 billion was needed. The Declaration also promoted the protection of human rights, gender equality, and the education and empowerment of women and young people, especially girls, to reduce their vulnerability to HIV, access to essential life-saving commodities, including male and female condoms, harm reduction related to drug use, safe blood supplies, and early and effective treatment of sexually transmitted infections (STIs).

A third special session of the UN General Assembly was held in June 2011, the 30th anniversary of HIV/AIDS. This session called for zero new infections, zero stigma, zero AIDS-related deaths and to provide antiretroviral drugs to 15 million infected people by 2015. (See Point of Information 14.2, page 452.)

Clearly the road to success in reducing HIV infections globally lies in the success of HIV prevention and treatment (test and treat). To that end, recent advances in the production of an effective microbicide for vaginal and anal sex and the promise that circumcision holds for preventing the transmission of HIV are both positive steps for prevention. Even if the elusive vaccine can be found, its overall effect against HIV infections will be many years off, and because of global cultural views of handling a sexually transmitted disease, a vaccine may not be the final solution.

Each medical advance comes at a higher price and calls for more trained healthcare workers, and in the most intensely infected areas, both money and manpower are scarce.

Restarting the Conversation on HIV/AIDS—Let's Not Lose Another Generation

To bring HIV/AIDS under control in the coming years, government leaders are going to have to see the pandemic for what it is and will continue to be—the most confounding public health problem in the world—and at long last give it the priority it deserves.

An ongoing myth is that the problem of HIV/AIDS has somehow been solved. We have only just begun to see a return on the investments of the past decades in the form of falling rates of new infections and fewer deaths, indicating a new phase in HIV/AIDS responses; it by no means suggests that the problem is anywhere near solved. This new phase is characterized by a new set of challenges that could

well prove more difficult than any that we have encountered so far. We must not be led astray by the hope or promise of a technological fix to this pandemic, because one is not likely to be found anytime soon.

A Blueprint to Further the Conversation

Generic (generalized) responses to heterogeneous problems waste money. Policy-makers need to understand that not all HIV/AIDS epidemics are the same, in that they are not driven by the same underlying causes. So although treatment needs may be similar from place to place—an antiretroviral drug that works in sub-Saharan Africa is also going to work in Eastern Europe—that isn't true for prevention. The primary driver of the epidemic in the Ukraine—injecting drug use—is entirely unlike the main driver in Botswana, which is sexual contact between men and women. Efficient and effective prevention programs must be highly customized to the context—something that is only possible if you **know your epidemic**. Programs must anticipate where infections in a country are expected to occur (at what ages, in which cities, affecting which populations), so that they can focus on ensuring that interventions are focused on preventing those particular infections. Earmarks that require prevention funds to be used for specific interventions have handicapped program managers' ability to tailor programs to their local epidemics, unnecessarily wasting resources. Local program managers need more flexibility than such earmarks permit.

An emergency response, pretty much doing the same thing for everyone at a give time, may be appropriate for an earthquake, but wasteful and ineffective for an epidemic that has been with us for over thirty-two years. Policymakers grapple with this because every day thousands of people die of HIV/AIDS, making the epidemic simultaneously a daily emergency and a struggle that must be successful in the long term.

NOTE: There is no way to know just how the global economic downturn of 2009–2013 will affect the economies of global HIV/AIDS funding. In the United States, Americans may soon find themselves fed up with generosity. We will be servicing a national debt in the trillions of dollars while struggling with everything from global climate change to catastrophic disparities in access to food, energy, and water.

THE NEXT 32 YEARS

Just as no one was prepared for the holocaust of illness that was to come, no one can foresee what the full impact of 31 more years of this disease will entail, beyond knowing that the plight will be far worse, not better, as the nations with the largest populations, China and India, realize the full impact of HIV/AIDS.

Max Essex of the Harvard AIDS initiative said, "Just as the retrovirus that causes AIDS differs considerably today from the samples first studied 25 years ago, the virus will continue to change so much that 25 years from now it will bear virtually no resemblance to the HIV/AIDS virus types seen now. Its impact will change too." Will what we know about preventing current HIV infections be useless in 25 years?

PURSUING PREVENTION: A VACCINE?

Are There Missing Pieces?

Over the past year, the HIV vaccine field has intensified its focus on discovery and basic research. More scientific questions are being generated than answered, and it's not possible to put these sometimes disparate pieces of knowledge together to solve the AIDS vaccine puzzle. Just as with a real puzzle, the number of pieces gives us some idea of how big the big picture really is.

In late 2009, a low-impact (31% effective) HIV vaccine was developed. How or why this vaccine was effective at all remains a mystery. Regardless, this is a momentous first, and the results of these studies are new pieces to the ever-growing HIV vaccine puzzle.

How do we handle this pile of puzzle pieces, which keeps growing? First of all, by not discarding any piece prematurely. We learn as children that even if a piece doesn't look like it fits, it might later on, once more has been filled in. In the adult world, this means that the field must continue to balance funding decisions and scientific portfolios so that no single assumption—however cherished—gets a disproportionate investment of time, money, or human resources. For example, in the arena of T cell–mediated immunity, where there's ongoing work to define the qualities of an effective HIV-specific response, this means striking a balance between research on specificity and research on functionality.

On a larger scale, this means that work on understanding the mechanisms of virologic control must be balanced with research aimed at vaccine-induced prevention of infection. And on an even broader scale, it means making connections between HIV/AIDS vaccine research and research on pre-exposure prophylaxis (PrEP) and other proven and emerging strategies.

Seth Berkley said that an HIV vaccine is the Holy Grail in curbing this plague. Like the chalice of legend, it has proved elusive. Its urgency is underlined by the fact that AIDS is on its way to killing as many people as the Black Death, the plague in the Middle Ages. But even if there is a vaccine, eradication of HIV is unlikely—HIV has a firm grip on the world. Yet if a vaccine is not found, the increasing demands for antiretroviral drugs will be overwhelming and most likely will be available only to those who can afford them.

In the last decade, the international community has made great strides in expanding prevention, care, and treatment programs, and the results are promising. Deaths from HIV/AIDS has dropped by about 25% over the last six years (2006–2012). However, as HIV/AIDS marks its 32nd year, the disease continues to outpace our global response. The number of new HIV infections continues to climb globally.

Despite the advances in medical science against HIV/AIDS, the death toll over the next 25 to 50 years promises to far exceed the 30 to 40 million who died in the Black Plague of the 14th century or the 20 to 50 million who died during the 1918 Spanish flu pandemic.

WILL SUCCESS AGAINST HIV ALWAYS BE MARGINAL?

It is now possible to state—tentatively, and with conditions—that HIV is no longer a death sentence. In those areas and populations with access to antiretroviral therapy and related infrastructure, the life expectancy of a person living with HIV now exceeds the life expectancy of a person with diabetes. Considering the context of the time span in which this has occurred— 32 years—this is indeed cause for quiet celebration. However, should Truvada and other antiretroviral drugs prevent HIV infection, this is a single victory in a much larger war against the scourge of HIV/AIDS, and other battles have yet to be won. Indeed, it may be argued that scientists may be winning the war in treatment, but losing the larger war of prevention.

Does the next quarter century mark the endgame of this struggle between death and hope, or more repetitions of the cycle? Can treatment actually be delivered to all who need it? Will effective biological tools to prevent HIV infection be found? How will millions of deaths affect orphans, vulnerable youth, fragile cultures, and global security? It does not bode well that patients in many states within our own borders languish on waiting lists for HIV medication.

There is great hope that current ARVD might prevent high-risk people from becoming infected (PrEP—pre-exposure prophylaxis). Preliminary studies throughout mid-2012 have shown that the antiretroviral drug Truvada, used in an NIH-sponsored iPrEx study to treat HIV infection, did under a set of controlled conditions, prevent HIV infection in some but not all men who have sex with men (MSM). But similar trials using Truvada in women did not lower their risk of HIV infection. However, should Truvada and other antiretroviral drugs prevent HIV infection, there is the risk that treatment will create a resistant strain or, as some critics claim, cause people to lower their guard and have more unprotected sex. There are also postexposure drugs that appear to prevent HIV from successfully infecting the HIV-exposed person. And there is hope of having vaginal and anal microbicides to prevent HIV infection (see the CAPRISA trials discussed below).

Efforts to find an effective vaccine, thus far, have failed. The International AIDS Vaccine Initiative says 30 vaccines are being tested in small-scale trials. Will there be a successful HIV vaccine available in the next 25 years? It is anybody's guess. But one thing appears certain; the development of an HIV vaccine will not follow the same path to success as with earlier vaccines. As a preventive vaccine becomes less of a reality, more money and more efforts are being poured into prevention campaigns, but the efforts are uneven. Success varies widely from region to region and country to country.

HIV/AIDS 2010/2012

The years 2010 through 2012 were years of notable social and scientific achievements. To name some of the most important: Catholic Pope Benedict's landmark acknowledgment that condoms are sometimes morally justifiable to stop HIV/AIDS can apply to everyone—gays, heterosexuals, and transsexuals—if that is the only option to avoid transmitting HIV to others; lifting travel restrictions on HIV-infected people from migrating to the United States; the move away from federal funding of abstinence-only education programs; the finding by the Centers for Disease Control and Prevention (CDC) that there is a very strong linkage between low socioeconomic status and HIV infection—those living below the poverty line are twice as likely to become HIV infected as those living above it; and for the first time in 20 years of microbicide research there has been a real potential breakthrough—a gel containing 1% tenofovir (one of the antiretroviral drugs) provided a 34% reduction in HIV infections in the CAPRISA 004 microbicide trials. In addition, the tenofovir-based vaginal gel significantly reduced the risk of genital herpes (HSV-2) infection. This gel offers women, for the first time, a means of protecting themselves without the cooperation of their male partners. Also, results from the iPrEx studies mentioned above were first released in December 2010.

In 2011 there were the pre-exposure prophylaxis (PrEP) studies that demonstrated that the use of a variety of antiretroviral drugs would prevent the transmission of HIV. In particular the HPTNO52 trials that showed a 96% reduction in risk of HIV transmission between serodiscordant couples (one of the partners was HIV positive).

THE COMING YEARS MUST BE YEARS OF HEALING, HELP, HOPE, REDUCING STIGMA, AND SOLUTIONS

During the coming years, the spread of HIV/AIDS into the general populations of India and China will become a very frightening scenario. It has been estimated that by 2025, some 21 million people will die of AIDS in India and 15 to 18 million will die in China.

Tragically, the end of this global pandemic is nowhere in sight. We need a far more united coalition, united by a commitment to saving lives, even if we may have differences on tactics. We must spend our energy on fighting this pandemic, not on fighting each other. Surely one of the main lessons of these first 32 years is that when we are united we win; when we are divided, HIV wins. We must plan and act not just for today, but for the next generation. With every ounce of our intelligence, innovation, and determination, we must advance both social change and science in the fight against HIV/AIDS. The first decade of AIDS was defined by death and activism, the second by medicines and hope. The third decade was the unsuccessful search for a vaccine. The fourth decade must be one of better care, prevention, and access to ART. It must also be one of finding a successful vaccine and reducing stigma and discrimination against the HIV infected!

SUMMARY

On June 5, 1981, the U.S. Centers for Disease Control and Prevention reported the outbreak of an unusual form of pneumonia in Los Angeles. When, a few weeks later, its scientists noticed a similar cluster of rare cancer called Kaposi's sarcoma in San Francisco, they suspected that something strange and serious was afoot. That something was AIDS. Since then, 30 million people have died from AIDS and another 38 million are infected. The 32nd anniversary of the disease's discovery will once again be taken as a solemn occasion. Yet the war on HIV/AIDS is going far better than anyone dared hope. A decade ago, half of the people in several southern African countries were expected to die of AIDS. Now, the death rate is dropping. In 2005 the disease killed 2.1 million people. In 2009 the number was 1.8 million. In 2013 the estimated number is 1.5 million. Some five million lives have already been saved by drug treatment. In 33 of the worst affected countries, the rate of new infections is down by 25% or more from its peak. Even more hopeful are recent studies that suggest that the drugs used to treat HIV/AIDS can stop HIV transmission. These drugs could achieve much of what a vaccine would. Because of the 2011–2012 studies scientists now see treatment as prevention (T as P or T4P). The problem is how to get more drugs to more people in more countries including the United States. In the meantime, for too many people are becoming HIV infected and dying from AIDS and HIV/AIDS-related conditions. In December of 2011, Secretary of State Hillary Clinton and President Obama both suggested because T as P or T4P may work on a global scale, that there now exists the possibility of an **"AIDS–Free Generation."** At the moment, given the costs and problems involved, this possibility remains just that, a possibility. But, this is the first time this possibility has existed! We collectively wait for the day we can say R.I.P., HIV. We are still a long way from a cure, but, it's moved from the realms of science fiction to real science! The question for the world will no longer be whether it can provide universal access to these drugs to wipe out HIV/AIDS but whether it is prepared to pay the price.

WE CAN END THIS GLOBAL PANDEMIC; NOW WE MUST DO IT!

Preface

My hope is that this 2013 edition of *AIDS UPDATE* will help you gain a clearer perspective on HIV and AIDS and the ways in which the disease both fuels widespread controversy and suffers under a silence that restricts some of the most important information about it. HIV/AIDS is a slow, progressive, and permanent disease. With the disease, there is no loss of infectivity, no development of either individual or group immunity, and for too many, no recovery to a regular life. At present, there is no known biological mechanism that can stop the continuing expansion of the disease. The progressive increase in the pool of people carrying HIV, the virus that causes AIDS, will lead to an increase in the number of newly infected individuals. Until an effective vaccine can be developed or other interventions are at least moderately successful, the infection will continue to spread and will remain a crucial health issue. With the onset of this real human tragedy, we have been forced to learn about our social contradictions and examine our moral judgments. We have had some success in this venture, yet despite great improvements in our understanding of the scientific and social aspects of the disease, the HIV/AIDS crisis is not nearly over.

PURPOSE

While this volume is intended for use in college-level courses on HIV/AIDS and as a supplemental HIV/AIDS resource in medical and nursing schools, it is suitable for any situation in which information about the various aspects of HIV and AIDS is desired or required. This text reviews the most important information on all facets of HIV infection, HIV disease, and AIDS. It provides readers with a detailed background in the current biological, medical, social, economic, and legal aspects of this modern-day pandemic. Medical and social anecdotes bring a personal perspective to the worldwide HIV/AIDS tragedy, while other parts of the text detail the history and science of the pandemic. Special focus has been given to HIV transmission, including risk behaviors and means of prevention, and on the innumerable social issues surrounding this disease. Many of these issues are accompanied by open-ended questions to stimulate class discussions that help students reflect on what they have read.

IMPORTANCE

This book is important for at least two reasons. First, as educators, it is our job to expose our students to the new concepts in biology that are shaping humanity's future. To do that, we must expose them to new vocabulary, new methodologies, new information, and new ideas and promote appropriate discussion. It is my hope that this text will help in this endeavor. Second, because misinformation has increased the danger of the

HIV/AIDS pandemic, this text attempts to counter common distortions and myths by presenting the most current, consistent, and scientifically acceptable information possible. The text also provides students with a strong conceptual framework for the issues raised by the HIV/AIDS pandemic so they will be better able to deal with new information as it arises.

During the 31 years (1981 through 2012) since HIV/AIDS was defined as a new disease, more effort and money have been poured into research efforts surrounding HIV and AIDS than into any other disease in history. As a result, information on the virus that causes AIDS has accumulated at an unprecedented pace. The constant stream of new information about the changing social and scientific circumstances surrounding the disease makes it necessary to publish updated editions. The majority of references herein are dated between 1990 and 2012, with outdated information being replaced in each edition. What has been learned and what must still be learned to bring HIV infection, HIV disease, and AIDS under control is valuable information to all of us.

NEW TO THIS EDITION

This edition contains updated information and data in every chapter. Topics and content new to this edition include:

- Older data have been replaced by (a) estimated decreases in the global number of people living with HIV; (b) the number of people newly infected with HIV; and (c) the number of deaths from AIDS. This decrease in global numbers was reported in the "2007 AIDS Epidemic Update" published by the World Health Organization (WHO) and the United Nations Program on AIDS (UNAIDS). These data have been updated to reflect the estimated numbers

for 2009 through 2012 and 2013 presented in this edition of *AIDS UPDATE*.

- Older data from the Centers for Disease Control and Prevention (CDC) for the number of HIV infections in the United States have been replaced with data collected from 47 states and five dependent areas that used confidential name-based HIV infection reporting beginning 2002 through 2007. These data were published in the CDC's "HIV/AIDS Surveillance Report 2007" but were not published until February 2009. The estimated 2007 CDC data have been updated to reflect the estimated numbers for 2009 through 2012 and 2013 for all 50 states and presented in this edition of *AIDS UPDATE*.

SPECIAL FEATURES

- Each chapter begins with a **Chapter Highlights** section that allows students to preview the material and stay focused on key topics.

- A variety of **boxed essays** provide supplemental information on each chapter's topic. These features illustrate important events and information about HIV/AIDS, including stories (because everyone has a story of some kind about his or her experience with HIV/AIDS to bring to the table) from doctors and AIDS survivors, points of scientific note, and discussions of historical context that reveal how knowledge and perceptions of AIDS have evolved over time.

- **Discussion Questions** encourage students to think critically about difficult and controversial issues associated with HIV and provide a starting point for lively class discussions.

- **Further information** sources are listed at the end of relevant chapters. These Internet addresses and national hotline telephone numbers give students resources for additional information on prevention, therapy, healthcare providers, and specific focuses such as women, parents, children, and young adults.

- Chapter **Summaries** and **Review Questions** provide students with a quick review of the key concepts of the chapter and help students test their understanding of the chapter's material. Answers appear in an appendix.

- A list of all **References** allows students to see the sources of all scientific and social data within the book, as well as to engage in further research on their own.

- A **glossary** of the more significant scientific and medical terms can be found in the back of the book.

- A **multiple choice test bank** and a **DVD** on HIV replication and the use of antiretroviral drugs to prevent replication is available for the instructors. A source of HIV/AIDS films are available from the author. Contact: gstine@bellsouth.net.

IN APPRECIATION

The help of the following organizations and people is most deeply appreciated: The Centers for Disease Control and Prevention (CDC), Atlanta, for use of slides and literature produced in their *National Surveillance Report* and the *Morbidity and Mortality Weekly Report*; from the *Sun-Sentinel* of Ft. Lauderdale, Florida, Director of Photography Jerry Lower and Photo Archivist Britt Head for photographs out of the Caribbean; from the CDC, Richard Salik and Patricia Sweeney (Surveillance Branch); Robin Moseley, Patricia Fleming, Todd Webber (Division of HIV/AIDS Prevention); Berry Bennett, head of Retroviral Testing Services, for his permission and guidance on photographing HIV testing procedures at the Florida Health and Rehabilitation Office of Laboratories Services, Jacksonville, Florida; Denise Reddington, Department of Health and Human Services, Washington, DC; PANOS Institute for its help in obtaining data on the economics of HIV/AIDS worldwide; personnel of the National Institute for Allergy and Infectious Diseases, the National Center for Health Statistics, and the Brookwood Center for Children with AIDS in New York; the George Washington AIDS Policy Center in Washington, DC; the National Institutes of Health; Hoffman-LaRoche Co., Abbott Laboratories, the Pharmaceutical Manufacturing Association; the National Cancer Institute; Pan American Health Organization; the Office of Technological Assessment; the Physicians' Research Network; BIO-RAD Laboratories; Teresa M. St. John, University of North Florida, for illustrations; the individuals who have contributed photographs; the text reviewers whose work has been greatly appreciated; a special thank-you to Gilbertine Yadao, who word-processed the updated material; Guy Selander, M.D., and Jack Giddings, M.D., who, over the years, have shared their medical journals with me; James Alderman, Mary Davis, Signe Evans, Cynthia Jordan, Paul Mosley, and Barbara Tuck— reference/research librarians at the University of North Florida; a very special thank-you to Sarah Phillips, Director for Public Services librarian at the University of North Florida, for her diligent commitment to ensure the accuracy and timeliness of the information found throughout this book; to Michael Muyres for creating new photographic material used within this book; to Darwin Coy, Ph.D., who continues to make useful suggestions on improving this book; and to my wife, Delores, who demonstrated a great deal of patience and understanding and gave up family weekends so the text could be completed on time.

This book has benefited from the critical evaluation of the following reviewers:

Dale J. Erskine
Lebanon Valley College

Kyle Funderburgh
UT Southwestern Medical Center at Dallas

Susan W. Gaskins
University of Alabama
Capstone College of Nursing

Deborah Gritzmacher
Clayton State University

Jacquelyn K. Westfall
The Ohio State University

Calvin Odhiambo
University of South Carolina Upstate

Darwin Coy
University of North Florida

Bob Baugher
Highline Community College

Gerald J. Stine, Ph.D.
904-641-8979

gstine@bellsouth.net

**A set of HIV/AIDS films for use
with most chapters is available for
the cost of copying and shipping.
Contact the author via email.**

Introduction: Histories of Global Pandemics, AIDS, Its Place in History, Overview of HIV/AIDS, International AIDS Conferences, and Means of Remembering—the AIDS Quilt, Candlelight Memorial, and World AIDS Day

DO YOU REMEMBER WHERE YOU WERE AND WHAT YOU WERE DOING WHEN YOU FIRST HEARD THE WORD "AIDS" AND A FEW YEARS LATER–"HIV"? AS THE HIV/AIDS PANDEMIC ENTERS ITS FOURTH DECADE WRITING ABOUT IT CONTINUES TO BE CHALLENGE!

THIS TEXTBOOK TELLS THE STORY OF HIV/AIDS. IT IS TOLD WITH RESPECT TO THE SCIENTIFIC AND SOCIAL IMPLICATIONS OF THIS DISEASE. THE RESOURCES, SCIENTIFIC FACTS, AND SOCIAL REPERCUSSIONS REVEAL THE DIMENSION OF THIS PANDEMIC VISITED ON HUMANKIND.

MEDIA COVERAGE ABOUT HIV/AIDS HAS FALLEN BY 70% OVER THE LAST 21 YEARS IN THE UNITED STATES. MEDIA COVERAGE PEAKED IN 1991 AND THEN DROPPED. ONLY AREAS OF THE WORLD THAT ARE HARDEST HIT CONTINUE TO RECEIVE ATTENTION TO THEIR PROBLEMS. BUT EVEN IN THESE COUNTRIES THERE ARE FAR TOO FEW STORIES ABOUT HIV/AIDS PRESENT IN THE MEDIA FOR THEM. THAT SHIP ALSO SAILED IN THE EARLY 1990s AND PARTICULARLY WITH THE BEGINNING OF ANTIRETROVIRAL THERAPY AND INCREASE IN SURVIVAL RATES AND LIFE EXPECTANCIES. IN ADDITION TO THE DROP IN MEDIA COVERAGE, UNAIDS REPORTED IN 2011 THAT HIV INFECTIONS STABILIZED OR DECREASED BY ABOUT 20% OVER THE LAST 10 YEARS AND THAT HIV/AIDS DEATHS DROPPED ABOUT 21% OVER THE LAST FIVE YEARS IN 56 COUNTRIES. THESE DATA MAY IMPLY THAT HIV/AIDS IS LESS IMPORTANT THAN IT HAS BEEN. NOT TRUE— MILLIONS ARE LIVING AND DYING FROM THIS DISEASE, AND MILLIONS OF NEW INFECTIONS OCCUR ANNUALLY. THE MEDICAL, SOCIAL, ECONOMIC, AND POLITICAL IMPACT OF HIV/AIDS WILL CONTINUE FAR INTO OUR FUTURE! THUS, IT IS IMPORTANT THAT THIS TEXTBOOK CONTINUE TELLING STORIES AND PROVIDING UP-TO-DATE INFORMATION ABOUT HIV/AIDS OCCURRING IN OUR LIFETIME.

BECAUSE OF HIV/AIDS IN THE UNITED STATES, IN 1998 C. EVERETT KOOP, FORMER SURGEON GENERAL, SENT AN EIGHT-PAGE PAMPHLET TO EVERY AMERICAN HOUSEHOLD—ALL 108 MILLION OF THEM. THIS WAS THE FIRST TIME THE FEDERAL GOVERNMENT PROVIDED EXPLICIT SEX INFORMATION TO THE PUBLIC. IN 2011, KOOP SAID, "IF THERE IS A NEW FRONT IN OUR WAR AGAINST HIV/AIDS, IT IS IGNORANCE AND COMPLACENCY." HE DECLARED, "SIMPLY PUT, HIV IS NO

LONGER IN THE PUBLIC'S RADAR SCREEN, AND THE WAR AGAINST HIV/AIDS IS FAR FROM OVER."

HIV/AIDS USED TO BE ABOUT A WAY OF DYING AND DEATH; NOW IT'S ABOUT LIVING WITH HIV/AIDS. THIS CHANGE IN ATTITUDE WAS A GRADUAL TRANSITION THAT OCCURRED AS LIFE-SAVING ANTIRETROVIRAL DRUGS BECAME AVAILABLE STARTING IN 1995. HOWEVER, A MOMENT OF SILENCE IS IN ORDER FOR THOSE WHO HAVE DIED FROM THIS DISEASE—NOT BECAUSE OF WHO THEY WERE AS MUCH AS BECAUSE THEY WERE FELLOW HUMANS.

LIFE IS FULL OF MARKERS; ANNUALLY WE CELEBRATE THE DAY WE WERE BORN AND VARIOUS ANNIVERSARIES AND COMMEMORATE SPECIAL DAYS OF THOSE WHO HAVE PRECEDED US IN LIFE. THE END OF THE YEAR ALSO REPRESENTS A MARKER: ONE YEAR ENDING AND ANOTHER BEGINNING. FOR MANY, IT IS A TIME OF CELEBRATION; FOR OTHERS, A TIME OF SADNESS. MANY MEMORABLE DATES CAN BE FOUND WITHIN THE PAGES OF THIS BOOK.

HIV/AIDS BEGAN ONE PERSON AT A TIME AND WILL COME TO AN END ONE PERSON AT A TIME. AS A GLOBAL COMMUNITY, **WE ARE THE SOLUTION!**

The Author

Awareness **OR**
Ignorance
Death **OR**
Survival
It's your choice, get the facts!

The Author

HOW MUCH DO YOU REALLY KNOW ABOUT HIV/AIDS?

Following are eight questions about HIV/AIDS that go well beyond the basics of what HIV is, how it works, and who gets it. If you get all of these right, consider yourself an honorary member of the global fight against HIV. (The answers are given at the end of this exercise—do NOT look ahead.)

1. We have at least 27 FDA-approved anti-HIV drugs and they keep getting more effective at stopping the virus. Thanks largely to this treatment, how long can the average 20-year-old person with HIV expect to live if he or she is diagnosed today?

   a. Into his or her 30s and 40s

   b. Into his or her 50s

   c. Into his or her 60s

   d. Into his or her 70s

2. When Americans can't afford the huge cost of HIV treatment and the government can't afford to help them, they're placed on an AIDS Drug Assistance Program (ADAP) waiting list. What is the largest number of HIV-positive people who have been on these ADAP waiting lists at the same time?

   a. Over 671

   b. Over 2,348

   c. Over 6,773

   d. Over 9,217

3. We know that condoms are good at preventing HIV transmission. When used correctly, they reduce the risk of HIV transmission by as much as 94–97%. What about using two condoms by putting one on first, then putting a second one on over the first one?

   a. This doubles your protection.

   b. This increases protection by 50%.

   c. This doesn't change your protection.

   d. This reduces your protection.

4. In which of these groups are HIV infection rates rising the fastest within the United States?

   a. Men who have sex with men

   b. African Americans

   c. Injection drug users

   d. Heterosexual women

5. HIV/AIDS activists are frequently involved in efforts to get medical marijuana legalized in the United States What's the main reason?

   a. Marijuana alleviates symptoms of depression.

   b. Marijuana makes people with HIV eat more.

c. Marijuana makes it easier to put up with a lack of government attention to HIV.

d. Marijuana enhances the anti-HIV properties of some HIV medications.

6. Most folks know or may know that sub-Saharan Africa is home to the largest number of people living with HIV. But among the following four regions, which was home to the most living HIV-positive people as of 2012?

a. North America (United States, Canada, Mexico)

b. Central/South America (Argentina, Brazil, Colombia, etc.)

c. Western/Central Europe (France, Italy, Latvia, the United Kingdom, etc.)

d. Eastern/Central Asia (Armenia, Russia, Ukraine, etc.)

7. Question number 6 was about people living with HIV. Looking at those same four regions, which of them had the highest number of deaths related to HIV/AIDS in 2012?

a. North America (United States, Canada, Mexico)

b. Central/South America (Argentina, Brazil, Colombia, etc.)

c. Western/Central Europe (France, Italy, Latvia, the United Kingdom, etc.)

d. Eastern/Central Asia (Armenia, Russia, Ukraine, etc.)

8. In which of these regions did the number of adults newly infected with HIV raise the most from 2001 to 2012?

a. North America (United States, Canada, Mexico)

b. Central/South America (Argentina, Brazil, Colombia, etc.)

c. Western/Central Europe (France, Italy, Latvia, the United Kingdom, etc.)

d. Eastern/Central Asia (Armenia, Russia, Ukraine, etc.)

Answers: 1. C; 2. D; 3. D; 4. A; 5. B; 6. A; 7. D; 8. A

THREE WORDS ECHO AROUND THE WORLD: AIDS CRISIS WORSENS!

When Acquired Immune Deficiency Syndrome (AIDS) first emerged as a recognized disease 31 years ago (June 1981–June 2012) few people could have predicted how the epidemic would evolve, and fewer still could have described with any certainty the best ways of combating it. Now, in the year 2013, it is known from experience that HIV/AIDS can devastate whole regions, knock decades off national development, widen the gulf between rich and poor nations, and push already-stigmatized groups closer to the margins of society. Just as clearly, experience shows that the right approaches, applied quickly and with courage and resolve, can and do result in lower HIV infection rates and less suffering for those affected by the pandemic. An ever-growing HIV/AIDS pandemic is not inevitable; yet, unless action against the pandemic is scaled up drastically, the damage already done will seem minor compared with what lies ahead. This may sound dramatic, but it is hard to play down the effects of a disease that stands to kill more than half of the young adults in the countries where it has its firmest hold.

HISTORY OF GLOBAL PANDEMICS AND EPIDEMICS

There has never been a time in human history when disease did not exist. The history of epidemics dates at least as far back as 1157 B.C. to the death of the Egyptian pharaoh Ramses V from smallpox. Over the centuries, this extraordinarily contagious virus spread around the world, changing the course of history time and again. It killed 2000 Romans a day in the second century A.D., more than 3 million Aztecs during the 1520 conquest by Cortez, and some 600,000 Europeans a year from the 16th through the 18th centuries. Three out of four people who survived the high fever, convulsions, and painful rash were left deeply scarred and sometimes blind. Because victims' skin looked as if it had been scalded, smallpox was known as the "invisible fire." Even now, malaria in underdeveloped countries afflicts 350 to 500 million people, killing between 2 and 3 million each year. The problem is compounded by the development of drug-resistant malarial strains of protozoa. Thus epidemics and pandemics are not new to humankind, but the fear they impose on each generation is.

How Is This History Relevant?

First, it is important to place HIV (the immuno-deficiency virus that causes AIDS) and AIDS in a longer-term context: Human populations have been devastated by pandemics before, and have survived. Some populations have even evolved genetically as a result. **Second,** humankind's civil, emotional, and spiritual evolution appears linked to pandemics: Each and every one of the major pandemics (especially bubonic plague, or Black Death, and Spanish flu) followed major social upheaval and ended during periods when new social structures were established. Such social changes included new value systems and, of course, improved social conditions such as water, housing, and sanitation methods. **Third,** the evidence of history suggests that when these pandemics are over, the development of civilization takes a dramatically different turn. The bubonic plague accompanied the shift from force-as-law (military might—Roman Empire) to religious order (especially Catholicism), and also paralleled the breaking of the omnipotence of that same religious order, and the emergence of the Age of Reason (organized science and medicine). The Spanish flu accompanied the destruction of the all-pervasive class system and the emergence of communism, socialism, and capitalism as central global political and economic systems. An interesting speculation would be to consider whether these social evolutions would have occurred if these pandemics had not emerged.

The major recorded pandemics (global) and epidemics (regional) that have devastated large populations are described in Table I-1, page 5.

FEAR, IGNORANCE, AND CONDEMNATION: WHO IS TO BLAME?

Placing Blame: Déjà Vu All Over Again!

The history of epidemics teaches us, again and again, that blame is a central component of these events, whether it is cast upon socially ostracized groups of people, water supplies, politics, or religious or cultural beliefs. The sixteenth-century rise of Protestantism, especially Calvinism, increased public intolerance toward the ill. Victims of syphilis were condemned as targets of God's wrath and were ignored by many medical and charitable institutions. Religious artists often depicted Jesus striking down the unjust, raining murderous arrows down from heaven upon syphilis victims and those who suffered from bubonic plague. It was during this early modern period that the notion of "guilty" and "innocent" victims of disease arose.

The fear of HIV infection and AIDS and ignorance about this plague and its causes in our lifetime have also led to similar bizarre behavior and at times barbaric practices, strange rituals, and attempts to isolate those afflicted.

IMAGINE A WORLD WITHOUT AIDS

AIDS: Its Place in History

As the statistics on AIDS cases mounted, its identity as an inescapable plague seemed confirmed. It appeared to mimic the frightening pandemics of the past: cholera, yellow fever, leprosy, syphilis, and the plague. The history of AIDS—the history that seemed relevant to understanding the new pandemic—would be the history of the pandemics/epidemics of the past. Medical history suddenly gained new social relevance; policy analysts, lawyers, and journalists all wanted to know whether past pandemics/epidemics could provide some clues to the current crisis. How had societies attempted to deal with pandemics/epidemics in the past? The contemporary meaning of past plagues is read in the face of AIDS.

The AIDS pandemic is certainly one of the defining events of our time. There are stories to be told from it, stories of the people infected and affected by it—the well, the ill, the dying, and the survivors. There are the stories of scientific discovery, of HIV and viral mechanisms, and of genetic mysteries being understood. Then there are stories of scientific politics, claims and counterclaims, and the manipulating that goes on in the stratosphere of high-level science.

Table I-1 Plagues in History[1, 4, 5]

Disease	Dates	Place	Number Killed		Causative Organism	Time to Prevention/Cure (in years)
Measles	from 430 B.C.	Greece/Rome/World	Millions		Paramyxovirus	1712
Plague	542–1894	Europe/Asia/Africa	71 million		Yersinia pestis	580
Cholera	1826–1837	New Jersey	900,000		Vibrio cholerae	75
	1832	Paris	18 million			
	1849	United Kingdom	53,293			
	1947	Egypt	11,755			
Tuberculosis	1930–1949	United States	1,000,000		Mycobacterium tuberculosis	85
	1954–1970		150,000			
Malaria	1847–1875	Africa/India	20 million +		Plasmodia	100
Scarlet Fever	1861–1870	United Kingdom	972 per million people		Streptococcus pyogenes	45
Polio	1921–1970	North America	37,000		Polio viruses Types I, II, III	40
Typhus	1917–1921	Russia	2,500,000		Rickettsias	25
Influenza	1918–1919	Global	50 million		Influenza virus	57
Smallpox	from 1122 B.C.	Europe (Middle Ages)	Hundreds of millions		Smallpox virus	3050
	1926–1930	India	423,000			
	from 590 B.C.					
Gonorrhea	1921–1992	United States	57,477		Neisseria gonorrhoeae	71
HIV/AIDS[2]			*Deaths*	*HIV Infections*	Human Immunodeficiency Virus	Treatments but no cure
	1981–2011	United States (estimated)[3]	665,000	2,326,000		
	1981–2011	Global (estimated)	30,000,000	68,000,000		

1. Historical timeline on first suspected cases of the above diseases is: Plague, eleventh century B.C.; Cholera, 1781; Tuberculosis, 451 B.C.; Malaria, 1748; Scarlet Fever, 1735; Polio, 1894; Typhus, 1083; Influenza, 1580; Smallpox, 429 B.C.; Gonorrhea, 1768; Yellow Fever, 1647; HIV/AIDS, United States in the 1970s, in Africa, 1959.

2. Total AIDS data estimated through year 2013. Living in some state of HIV disease (11.5 million living with AIDS + 26.5 million people living with HIV infection + 30 million dead = 68 million total HIV infections worldwide).

3. United States: of the estimated number of people infected with HIV, about 28% or 665,000 will have died through 2013.

4. Since 1977, 30 new pathogens have appeared, and 20 of the older pathogens have reemerged in drug-resistant forms. Humankind and microbes are engaged in a war of survival wherein both adapt to each other's every move.

5. HIV/AIDS is now second only to the bubonic plague or Black Death as the largest plague or pandemic in history. AIDS, the more preventable of the two pandemics, is expected to surpass the historical statistics of the bubonic plague!

AIDS Is a "Weapon of Mass Destruction"!

America's former Secretary of State, Colin Powell, said in April 2004 that "HIV/AIDS is the greatest threat to mankind today, the greatest weapon of mass destruction on the earth."

OVERVIEW OF HIV/AIDS

AIDS: A Big Disease with a Little Name, an Earthquake in Slow Motion

The global numbers of people who are HIV-infected, along with those who have died from AIDS-related conditions, are seemingly too large to grasp, and the implications too terrifying to contemplate. (For the current numbers of HIV/AIDS cases and deaths, see Chapter 10.) At this time the future appears grim: First, there is no near-term prospect of a vaccine. Second, existing drug therapies, although relatively effective, are too expensive for the vast majority of those infected. Third, those preventive interventions that can be effective in reducing the numbers of people becoming infected annually are not in place in countries most in need because the majority of the infected are undereducated and their countries still lack the infrastructure to deal with many infectious diseases, including AIDS.

Landmark studies in 2011 have revealed that certain retroviral or anti-HIV drugs can be used to prevent HIV transmission and in the future may lead to an HIV/AIDS-free generation. The studies are presented in chapter 4, Sidebar 4.3, pages 85–89. Because of this information, Secretary of State Hillary Clinton in November 2011 called on the world to join the United States to achieve the goal of an "AIDS-free generation."

What Is AIDS?

AIDS is defined primarily by severe immune deficiency, and is distinguished from virtually every other disease in history by the fact that it has no constant, specific symptoms. Once the immune system has begun to malfunction, a broad spectrum of health complications can set in. AIDS is an umbrella term for any of at least 29 known diseases and symptoms. When a

person has any of these diseases or has a CD4 or T4 lymphocyte count of less than $200/\mu L$ (microliter) of blood and also tests positive for antibodies to HIV, an AIDS diagnosis is given. (See Chapter 1, Table 1-1, page 5 for a list of diseases.)

Key Terms (These terms are discussed more fully in chapter 5.)

T-Cells—The T stands for the thymus, the organ in which T cells mature. T cells include CD4 cells and the CD8 cells, which are both critical components of the body's immune system.

CD4 cells—A type of infection-fighting white blood cell. The number of CD4 cells in a sample of blood is an indicator of the health of the immune system. HIV infects and kills CD4 cells, which leads to a weakened immune system.

Cell counts (per microliter)—A measurement of the number of CD4 cells in a sample of blood. A CD4 cell count is used by health-care providers to determine when to begin, interrupt, or halt anti-HIV therapy; when to give preventive treatment for opportunistic infections; and to measure response to treatment. A normal CD4 cell count is between 500 and 1,200 cells/mm^3 of blood, but an individual's CD4 count can vary. In HIV-positive individuals, a CD4 count at or below 200 cells/mm^3 is considered an AIDS-defining condition.

AIDS: A Human Affair

The history of HIV/AIDS is a human affair and is partially a cultural process of attempting to come to terms with a new and often terrifying series of events—of young people dying before their time, of the intermingling of sex and death—in a period in which the world itself is changing before our eyes.

The social meaning of the history of HIV/AIDS intimately touches upon ideas about sexuality, social responsibility, individual privacy, health, and the prospect of living a normal life span. Understanding how to respond to HIV/AIDS and how to think about this pandemic is important not only for what it reveals about the ways in which health policy is created in the

United States and elsewhere, but also for what it implies about the human ability to meet the challenge of future emerging diseases and long-standing public health problems. The HIV/AIDS pandemic is a current and long-term public health problem worldwide.

HIV/AIDS is reversing decades of public health progress, lowering life expectancy, and significantly affecting international businesses. Lost productivity and profitability, the cost of sickness and death benefits, and the decline in a skilled workforce in the developing world have economic repercussions worldwide. HIV/AIDS is affecting the military capabilities of some countries as well as international peacekeeping forces.

Lessons Learned from Other Pandemics/Epidemics

From the lessons of history it is difficult to conceptualize how the AIDS pandemic will be halted, let alone reversed, in the absence of a cheap curative drug or a cheap and effective preventive vaccine. The syphilis epidemic at the early part of the twentieth century displayed a similar kind of epidemiology to the present-day AIDS epidemic in the United States. The campaigns that were initiated then closely parallel those in place at present for AIDS. There were vigorous educational programs to reduce high-risk sexual behavior, which were targeted at brothels and prostitutes as well as at military recruits to the U.S. Army. **Scare tactics** were spread through the use of posters, pamphlets, and radio—today it is television and many other kinds of electronic devices. Serological testing became mandatory before marriages could be licensed in certain states. However, these measures had little appreciable effect on the expansion of the syphilis epidemic. It was only the advent of a cheap, safe, and effective drug, penicillin, that eventually brought the epidemic under control.

One lesson learned from HIV/AIDS is that any disease that is occurring in a distant part of the globe may be in the United States, in your state, or in your town, tomorrow.

The advent of miracle drugs and vaccines that conquered the plagues of polio, smallpox, and measles led many people—including

scientists—to believe that the age of killer diseases was coming to an end. HIV/AIDS ended that misconception.

HIV/AIDS: A UNIQUE DISEASE

The impact of this pandemic is unique. Unlike malaria or polio, previous modern pandemics, it mostly affects young and middle-aged adults. This is not only the most sexually active time for individuals, but also their prime productive and reproductive years. Thus the impact of HIV/AIDS is demographic, economic, political, and social. HIV/AIDS is a disease of human groups in its demographic and social impacts. In the most HIV-affected areas of the world, infant, child, and adult mortality is rising and life expectancy is declining rapidly. The cost of medical care for each infected person overwhelms individuals and households.

HIV/AIDS: A CAUSE OF DEATH

Michel Sidibé (Figure I-1), executive director of the Joint United Nations Program on HIV/AIDS, speaking at the Thirty-Seventh Interscience Conference on Antimicrobial Agents and Chemotherapy, said "HIV has transformed the world, joining tuberculosis and malaria as a major cause of death worldwide. This epidemic won't be under control in any country until it is brought under control everywhere."

The facts on HIV infection, disease, and AIDS that are presented in the following chapters, when understood, clearly place the responsibility for avoiding HIV infection on *you*. You must assess your lifestyle; if you choose not to be abstinent, you must know about your sexual partner and you must practice safer sex. **Never think that you are immune to HIV infection.**

ANOTHER ANNIVERSARY

June 5, 2013, will mark the beginning of the 32nd year of the AIDS pandemic. No cure has been found and, although AIDS is now called a

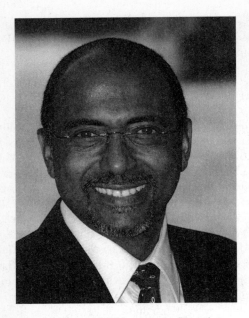

FIGURE I–1 Michel Sidibé became the Executive Director of the Joint United Nations Program on HIV/AIDS (UNAIDS) on January 1, 2009. He replaces Peter Piot, who led the agency since its inception in 1995. Sidibé, who is from Mali, has served as deputy executive director of UNAIDS for the past two years and began working for the organization in 2001 as a director of country and regional support. During his tenure as deputy executive director, Sidibé managed more than 70% of UNAIDS' budget and personnel, seven regional support teams, and 81 country offices. Before joining UNAIDS, Sidibé worked at UNICEF for 14 years, where he managed an immunization program for 30 million people in the Democratic Republic of the Congo and also worked in Burundi, Swaziland, and Uganda. (*Photo courtesy of UNAIDS.*)

"manageable illness," people who are sick must make endless compromises with this disease. The HIV/AIDS pandemic forces people to face their mortality daily, for months and years.

OTHER ANNIVERSARIES

March 21, 2013, marks the seventh annual National Native (American Indian, Alaska Native, and Native Hawaiian) HIV/AIDS Awareness Day.

National Native HIV/AIDS Awareness Day is an opportunity for Native people and others to create a greater awareness of the risk of HIV/AIDS to their communities; to remember those who have died; to acknowledge those who are infected and affected by HIV/AIDS; to call for increased resources for testing, early detection, and increased options for treatment; and to eventually decrease the occurrence of HIV/AIDS among Native people.

May 19, 2013, marks the Seventh Annual Asia and Pacific HIV/AIDS Awareness Day. This is a federally funded national anti-stigma social marketing campaign called the "Banyan Tree Project." In 2012, 20 cities held events celebrating this day. Asian/Pacific Islanders in the United States account for about 1% of total HIV/AIDS cases.

September 18 is National HIV/AIDS Aging Awareness Day. September 27 is National Gay Men's HIV/AIDS Awareness Day.

INTERNATIONAL AIDS CONFERENCES

The International AIDS Conference is believed to be the single most important meeting on HIV/AIDS. The International AIDS Conference has been the timepiece of the pandemic. The venue, content, style, and mood of each meeting temporarily freezes in time the state of the worldwide HIV/AIDS pandemic.

In 1983, there were so few groups involved with HIV/AIDS research that they could stay in contact by telephone. As the virus spread, many countries became involved in HIV/AIDS research and clinical care. International, national, and state meetings were formed as a way to exchange new information. Since the first International AIDS Conference in 1985, the conferences have grown in size to the point that scientists questioned their usefulness.

As of 1994, the International Conference on AIDS is held every two years (Table I-2). The 1996 Vancouver Conference will always be remembered because of the exciting breakthrough introduction of antiretroviral triple therapy and the use of protease inhibitors. The year 2000 Thirteenth International AIDS Conference was held in an underdeveloped nation for the first

Table I-2 International AIDS Conferences

Presented is a list of past International AIDS Conferences by month, year, and location. The number of *reported* AIDS cases and deaths are cumulative by year in the United States.

Number	Month	Year	Location	Total Deaths
1st	June	1985	Atlanta, Georgia	12,576
2nd	June	1986	Paris, France	24,686
3rd	June	1987	Washington, D.C.	41,088
4th	June	1988	Stockholm, Sweden	62,207
5th	June	1989	Montreal, Canada	90,000
6th	June	1990	San Francisco, California	121,536
7th	June	1991	Florence, Italy	157,000
8th	June	1992	Amsterdam, Netherlands	198,246
9th	June	1993	Berlin, Germany	243,627
10th	August	1994	Yokohama, Japan	298,496
11th	July	1996	Vancouver, Canada	381,896
12th	June	1998	Geneva, Switzerland	421,768
13th	July	2000	Durban, South Africa	463,905
14th	July	2002	Barcelona, Spain	497,630
15th	July	2004	Bangkok, Thailand	529,630
16th	August	2006	Toronto, Canada	561,630
17th	August	2008	Mexico City, Mexico	593,632
18th	July	2010	Vienna, Austria	625,000 Estimated
19th	July	2012	Washington, D.C.	655,000 Estimated
20th	July	2014	Melborne, Australia	———

Based on UNAIDS data, during the six days of the nineteenth conference, about 43,000 new HIV infections occurred and 35,000 people died of AIDS worldwide.

AIDS deaths are minimum estimates for the United States, based on data reported to the CDC, and updated. See Table 10-6 (page 314) for numbers of AIDS cases in each year.

Former UNAIDS Executive Director Peter Piot reported that between the Eleventh 1996 AIDS Conference and the Twelfth in 1998, 10 million people were infected with HIV! This, he said "represents a collective failure of the world." The rate of about 2 million new infections per year continues.

time. It was held in Durban, South Africa, a country where a significant proportion of the population has HIV/AIDS. Over 12,000 people attended this conference. The International AIDS Conferences are usually grim, but the Thirteenth International AIDS Conference was the grimmest yet, reporting death and infection rates that carried near-apocalyptic implications for the Third World, and particularly Africa.

The theme for this conference was "Breaking the Silence," but it is likely the conference will be remembered for the "Durban Declaration," a document signed by over 5000 physicians and scientists testifying to their belief that HIV causes AIDS. This declaration was created to convince the world that the experts in HIV research are certain that HIV causes AIDS. This document was to put those who, to this day, still do not believe HIV causes AIDS on notice that their beliefs are wrong. (More information on these HIV dissidents can be found in Chapter 2, pages 30–38.)

The 19th International AIDS Conference (IAC) was held in Washington, D.C., from July 22 to 27, 2012 (see Box 10.1, pages 290–292). The 20th IAC will be held in Melbourne, Australia, July 2014.

MEANS OF REMEMBERING: UNCOMMON THREADS

Nothing visually communicates to the world the magnitude and loss more than the giant patchwork of memories, the **AIDS Quilt.**

The quilt is "of the people, for the people and by the people." It is the most democratic memorial ever created and speaks to a global audience.

The Names Project

The AIDS Memorial Quilt Deemed a National Treasure by Congress in 2005—The quilt was the idea of Cleve Jones, of San Francisco, who in 1985 feared AIDS would become known just for the number of people it killed. He wanted a way of remembering the people, who were, in many cases, his friends.

During the eighth candlelight march in San Francisco, Jones asked fellow marchers to write on placards the names of friends and loved ones who died of AIDS. At the end of the march, Jones and others stood on ladders, above the sea of candlelight, taping these placards to the walls of the San Francisco Federal Building. The walls of names looked to Jones like a patchwork quilt.

Purpose and Dimensions of the Quilt

The purpose of the quilt is remembrance and education. The AIDS Quilt is made up of individual fabric panels, each the size of a grave, measuring three feet by six feet, stitched together into 12-foot by 12-foot sections. In October 1987, the entire AIDS Quilt was first put on display on the mall in Washington, D.C. At that time it contained 1920 panels and covered an area larger than two football fields. It took less than two hours to read all the names. In 1992 it took 60 hours. At the end of 2012 the quilt weighed about 60 tons, with about 53,000 panels containing about 95,000 names representing about 15% of those who have died of AIDS in the United States (Figure I-2). Displayed in its entirety, it would cover over 45 football fields. It is the largest piece of folk art in the world and continues to increase in size daily. If the 3-by-6 foot panels were laid end to end, the quilt would stretch over 50 miles. There are about 50 miles of seams and 26 miles of canvas edging. There are panels from each of the 50 states and Washington, D.C. Each day new panels arrive from across the United States and 37 foreign countries to be added to the quilt. For those left behind, the panels represent an expression of love and a sign of grief—a part of the healing process.

Portions of the quilt tour in major cities. Over 20 million people have visited the quilt at thousands

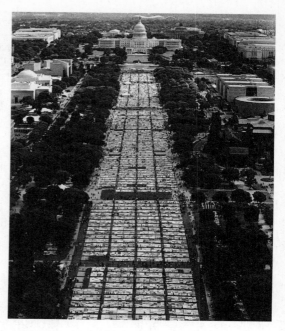

FIGURE I-2 The Quilt: Washington, D.C. 1996. This photograph shows the last time the quilt was displayed in its entirety on the capital mall, October 11–13. *(Photograph © AP/Wide World Photos.)*

of displays around the world. Donations made for viewing the quilt are being used to support local Names Project chapters and their staffs.

Each panel has its own story. The stories are told by those who make the panels for their lost friends, lovers, parents, and children. The complete quilt was displayed in Washington, D.C., October 11–13, 1996, for the last time—it is too large to view again as a whole. It took 10 boxcars to transport this work of art to the nation's capital.

By the end of 2013, about 665,000 Americans will have died from AIDS. If each of their names made up a separate panel, imagine the size of the quilt. If a name is read every 10 seconds, it would take over 62 days of calling names 24 hours a day!

Virtually Stitching the AIDS Memorial Quilt

The AIDS Memorial Quilt is being digitized so that it can be viewed in its entirety. Images of the quilt's panels have been sewn together virtually using

Microsoft Surface, an enhanced commercial computing platform. Viewers of the 60-inch-wide, interactive, touchscreen table can see the entire quilt. The first version of the table was on display during the Smithsonian Folklife Festival, June 27–July 8, 2012. The idea is that you use the table not as a substitute for looking at the textile panels. You still look at the physical panels—they're richer than any digital experience. But what the table allows you to do is search for a particular panel. Anne Balsamo, project director of the digitized quilt said, "Viewers also have the opportunity to add their own reflections, thanks to a mobile application. If you walk by a panel that really moves you, you can type in the panel number, go to the digital page, and leave a remembrance. We want to give people a way to get into the stories of the quilt."

A Reminder

People nationwide will celebrate the twenty-sixth anniversary of the AIDS Quilt on July 21, 2013. For more information about the Names Project's AIDS Memorial Quilt, call (404) 688-5500, ext. 223; www.aidsquilt.org.

THE 29TH CANDLELIGHT MEMORIAL

The first candlelight march for AIDS occurred simultaneously in New York City and San Francisco in May 1983. The memorial march is now international. The International AIDS Candlelight Memorial honors the memory of those lost to AIDS, shows support for those living with HIV and AIDS, raises community awareness of HIV/AIDS, and mobilizes community involvement in the fight against HIV/AIDS. In 2008, the opening ceremonies were held for the first time outside the United States, in Malawi. In 2012, the Candlelight Memorial was observed in about 3000 locations in 150 countries on every continent but Antarctica. The Candlelight march takes place on the third Sunday of May. (For additional information contact Sara Ann Friedman, email: candlelight@globalhealth.org or visit the website: http://www.globalhealth.org.)

WALKING TO CHANGE THE COURSE OF THE HIV/AIDS EPIDEMIC—UNITED STATES

The first **AIDS Walk** in America took place in Los Angeles, California, in 1985. The second AIDS Walk occurred in New York City in 1986. Since that time, HIV/AIDS volunteers in 43 other states have organized AIDS Walks (in at least 140 locations in numerous towns and cities within their borders) (Figures I-3, I-4, and I-5). The purpose of the AIDS Walk event is **people, all kinds of people, from all walks of life, helping people!** These walks, due to their popularity, size, and ability to raise large sums of money, gave large numbers of people who may not have otherwise become involved in the HIV/AIDS crisis a voice so loud and resourceful that it enabled them to get

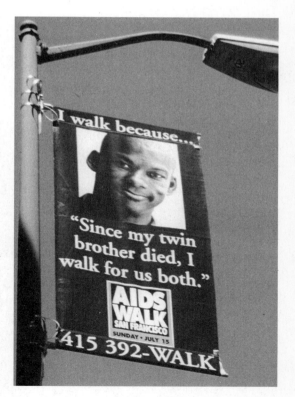

FIGURE I-3 A twin brother walks for HIV/AIDS because his brother, who died of AIDS, cannot. *(Photograph by Sarah Philips, with permission.)*

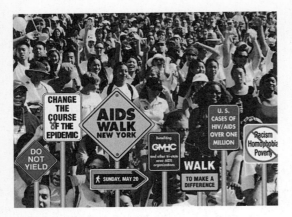

FIGURE I-4 AIDS Walk New York. In 2012, 45,000 people participated in the 27th annual Walk, and they raised over $6 million, the largest sum of money ever for an AIDS Walk. AIDS Walk San Francisco 2012 had 25,000 people participate and raised about $5.6 million (over $86 million since 1987). *(Photograph courtesy of Bert Champagne.)*

Canada have raised over $27 million since 1986, attracting over 500,000 people to walk.

The Beginning of AIDS Walks in America

When Craig Miller, Walkathon co-producer, first became involved in the 1985 AIDS Walk, it was still relatively early in terms of the public's awareness of the HIV/AIDS crisis. He said he was very nervous in organizing that first event. He and colleagues were concerned: Would the public really participate? Would they attract the thousands of people that they needed to make the event successful? Fortunately, the Los Angeles community did turn out in large numbers to support that first event. The event was hugely successful. Then, the Gay Men's Health Crisis of New York City asked if they would be willing to come to New York to help Gay Men's Health Crisis get an AIDS Walk off the ground. This was also a very successful event, and from there, AIDS Walks began across the United States. Through 2012, over 6.7 million people had participated in these walks, raising about $700 million! Dollar for dollar, AIDS Walk monies have been put to more effective use at the grassroots level, helping organizations and people

the government's attention and helped promote new and different types of legislation recognizing the impact HIV/AIDS was having in the United States. Annual walks in communities across

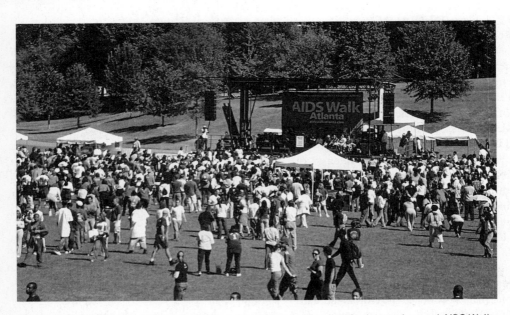

FIGURE I-5 AIDS Walk Atlanta. In 2012, over 10,000 people walked in the 22nd annual AIDS Walk, raising about $1,000,000. *(Photograph courtesy of Katerina Spasovska.)*

on the street, than any other form of money set aside to aid those infected with HIV.

China held its first ever AIDS walk on the Great Wall at Beijing, Oct 13, 2012. About 110 walkers and several groups donated $23,955 to their HIV/AIDS cause.

BICYCLE RIDING TO CHANGE THE COURSE OF THE HIV/AIDS EPIDEMIC—UNITED STATES

The goals of the AIDS Bike Rides Across the United States are the same goals listed for AIDS Walks. It was more difficult to obtain information on bike riding HIV/AIDS events than for AIDS Walks. In a number of cases, earlier records of bike riding events were not kept or were unavailable. Bike rides for HIV/AIDS go back to at least 1989. From 2007 through 2012, rides took place in 30 cities in 25 states, raising over $110 million. Together, AIDS Walks and bike rides raised about $725 million through 2012.

In addition to monies raised via these events, many millions of dollars have been raised by a large variety of social events, such as HIV/AIDS telethons, talk radio, gala balls, VIP dinners, and individual donations led by the stars of Hollywood (see Figure I-7 in Box I.1) and large foundations such as the MAC AIDS Fund. Their sales of lipstick and other cosmetics have raised, to date, over $200 million. Lady Gaga raised about $50 million in 2012. Sean Penn, Robert DeNiro, and Prince Albert of Monaco raised $10 million in one evening for HIV/AIDS research. Cindy and Howard Rachofsky have raised about $30 million, and Elton John's 2012 Oscar party raised $5.25 million. The Bill and Melinda Gates Foundation has given about $4 billion in grants to global HIV organizations.

THE AIDS OLYMPICS

The first-ever **AIDS Olympics** premiered in Washington, D.C., on March 18-19, 2011 (Figure I-6). The Olympics featured track and field events and live poetry. The Olympics was founded by Devin T. Robinson X, poet, actor, author, and HIV/AIDS activist. He is currently the president

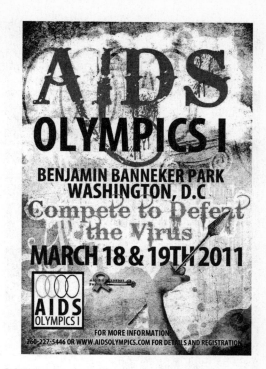

FIGURE I-6 One of the many posters displayed at the first AIDS Olympics held in Washington, D.C., March 18–19, 2011. *(Poster photo courtesy of Devin T. Robinson X and National AIDS Awareness Poets Inc.)*

of the National AIDS Awareness Poets Association. Robinson X said, "The Special Olympics was designed for individuals who are unable to compete in the Olympics due to disability. The AIDS Olympics was created to bring awareness to AIDS, the victims, the victors, and the victories surrounding this epidemic. This allows people to compete against the virus to bring awareness to a syndrome (virus) that has not slowed down one bit." When asked why this first AIDS Olympics was held in D.C., he responded, "No other place has such a mixture of irresponsible confusion than Washington, D.C. There is an overabundance of power that matches the sheer amount of powerless who walk the streets as sad zombies. Victims of bad decisions and poor leadership. Wealth is seen as you fly into the city but poverty is smelt and felt as you walk through it. Washington, D.C. has one of the highest HIV rates in the world. The next AIDS Olympics (renamed "The AIDS Games II") will be held in Ft. Lauderdale, Florida, in

BOX I.1

IN MEMORY OF DAME ELIZABETH TAYLOR, OSCAR–WINNING MOVIE STAR AND LONGTIME HIV/AIDS ACTIVIST (1932–2011)

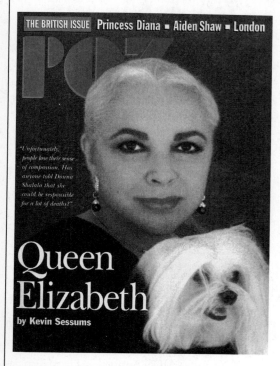

THE BRITISH ISSUE Princess Diana ▪ Aiden Shaw ▪ London

POZ

"Unfortunately, people lose their sense of compassion. Has anyone told Donna Shalala that she could be responsible for a lot of deaths?"

Queen Elizabeth

by Kevin Sessums

FIGURE I–7   ELIZABETH TAYLOR (1932–2011). She was a movie star and a humanitarian, a famous advocate for people with HIV/AIDS. "I will fight this disease and for the rights of people with AIDS until the day I die." And that is exactly what she did. *(From* POZ Magazine, *November 1997 cover photo. Copyright 1997 by* POZ Magazine. *Reprinted courtesy of Smart + Strong/POZ.)*

"Celebrity is not something that comes without responsibility. If I can help further a worthwhile cause simply by lending my voice, I feel that it is my place to do so." And lend her voice, she did: "I will not be silenced and I will not be ignored." Elizabeth Taylor lent her voice to the voiceless, her iconic image to those who had previously been invisible, and her compassion and determination to a cause many others have shunned: the fight against HIV/AIDS. Her willingness to speak out against apathy and silence in the early, frightening days of the epidemic and her instinctive sympathy for those in need earned her a place as one of the most influential advocates for people living with HIV in the United States and around the world. The Elizabeth Taylor AIDS Foundation rose to over $50 million! Dame Taylor was the first major Hollywood star to take up the fight against HIV/AIDS at a time when this cause was very unpopular. In 1984, Elizabeth Taylor organized the first AIDS fundraiser to benefit AIDS Project Los Angeles. This was the same year she learned her longtime friend Rock Hudson had contracted the virus. She helped to start the American Foundation for AIDS Research (amFAR) and befriended an Indiana teen named Ryan White who contracted AIDS from contaminated blood. Her friendship with White along with several others, including Sir Elton John and Michael Jackson, sparked enough action to create what is known today as the Ryan White Act (see Box 14.1, Figure 14–3, page 430 for information on the life of Ryan White). She earned numerous international awards and honors for the commitment she exhibited toward the fight against AIDS. Elizabeth Taylor will be remembered not just as an actress but as a champion in the HIV/AIDS community.

2013. (More information can be found at AIDSOlympics.com.)

WORLD AIDS DAY: AN INTERNATIONAL DAY OF COORDINATED ACTION: A TIME TO RECHARGE AND RECONNECT

World AIDS Day is every December 1st, a day set aside to pay tribute to those who have HIV/AIDS and to those who have died of HIV/AIDS. As in years past, rituals of candles and quilts coincide on World AIDS Day with the release of grave new statistics and heart-rending personal stories—not only from distant countries but also from our own backyards. While humanitarian concerns demand that developed nations take action in the developing world, a growing apathy about the HIV pandemic in America helps perpetuate a pandemic that has already claimed over 650,000 lives and counting.

The "Reading of Names" of Those Who Have Died of AIDS Is a World AIDS Day Vigil

Now well into the third decade since the recognition of AIDS, it is estimated that about 68 million people (by the end of 2013) will have been infected with HIV, clearly making this one of the worst pandemics of our time. Projections for 2005–2015 suggest that the situation will become even more serious as we may reach about 78 million infected individuals.

December 1, 2013, will be the 25th anniversary of WAD. For information on World AIDS Day, write 108 Leonard Street, 13th Floor, New York, NY 10013, or World AIDS Day Public Information Office, WHO-GPA, 1211 Geneva 27, Switzerland, or call (212) 513-0303.

First Global AIDS Week: May 18–24, 2006

Over 30 countries participated in 2012, the seventh annual event.

THE FUTURE

The history of HIV/AIDS is one of remarkable scientific achievement. Never in history has so much been learned about so complex an illness in so short a time. We moved into the new millennium, and the fourth decade of AIDS, with hope and the determination to find better therapies and a vaccine. The task is formidable, but it has to be done, and it will be accomplished. The evolving story of the HIV/AIDS epidemic has been one of the major medical news events of the past 31 years. It is getting hard to imagine medicine or society without HIV/AIDS.

HIV/AIDS is a truly persistent global pandemic and will require a proportionate response to bring it under control. It is the plague of our lifetimes—and probably that of our children's lives as well. We already have people age 31 and younger who don't know what an HIV-free world is. They were born into this recognized pandemic (1981). To survive this pandemic, society must prevent the face of AIDS from becoming faceless. The chapters on HIV infection, HIV disease, and AIDS in this book will help bring widespread information on the virus into focus. The information within these chapters should also help eliminate many of the myths and irrational fears, or FRAID **(fear of AIDS),** generated by this disease. There is much work to be done by both scientists and society.

Perhaps a borrowed anecdote says it best:

> As the old man walked the beach at dawn, he noticed a young woman ahead of him picking up starfish and flinging them into the sea. Finally catching up with the youth, he asked her why she was doing this. The answer was that the stranded starfish would die if left to the morning sun.
>
> "But the beach goes on for miles and there are millions of starfish," countered the old man. "How can your effort make any difference?"
>
> The young woman looked at the starfish in her hand and threw it to safety in the waves. "It makes a difference to this one," she said.

(Adapted from *The Unexpected Universe* by Loren Eiseley. Copyright 1969, Harcourt Brace, New York.)

Too easily we can become overwhelmed by the enormity of the AIDS pandemic. The numbers of the HIV infected and their constant needs have caused many to become paralyzed into inactivity and lulled into indifference. Like the old man, many ask "Why bother?"

For the sake of every individual living with HIV, we must focus on what each one of us can do. Each person can make a difference. Believing this, we are empowered to cope with the larger whole.

In June 2005, Peter Piot, head of the United Nations campaign to combat AIDS, said that "it is no longer realistic to hope that the world will meet its goal of halting and reversing the spread of HIV by year 2015." Robert Gallo, a leading HIV researcher and head of the University of Maryland's Institute of Human Virology, said "HIV/AIDS will be a problem for our children and our children's children." If by 2025, millions of people are still becoming infected with HIV each year, it will not be because there was no choice. It will not be because there is no understanding of the consequences of the decisions and actions being taken now, in the early years of the century. It will be because the lessons of the first 31 years of the epidemic were not learned, or were not applied effectively. It will be because, collectively, there was insufficient political will to change and/or halt the forces driving the HIV/AIDS pandemic. What politicians, institutions, communities, and individuals do today can change future, predictable scenarios of this pandemic. Such dire announcements actually increase the importance that everyone, everywhere become familiar with the various aspects of this global pandemic. For these reasons and many others each year, as this pandemic spreads across the globe, this book offers new insight into the many and varied aspects of HIV/AIDS. It provides much-needed information to students, their instructors, those that are HIV positive and negative, and the general public.

Valuable Stories

To aid in the understanding and acceptance of somewhat complex ideas and science in certain chapters, valuable **stories** provide first-hand testimony about the way research is done, its failures and successes, about the pain, suffering, and hardship endured by HIV-negative and -positive people as this disease impacts Planet Earth. Stories are mines of information, rich in memories and history, and this should be shared.

General Disclaimer

AIDS Update is designed for educational purposes only and is not engaged in rendering medical advice or professional services. The information provided through *AIDS Update* should not be used for diagnosing or treating a health problem or a disease. It is not a substitute for professional care. If you have or suspect you may have a health problem, consult your healthcare provider.

National AIDS Hotlines

- Centers for Disease Control and Prevention/National AIDS Clearing House, 1-800-458-5231.
- National AIDS, for the English-language service (open 24 hours a day, 7 days a week), call 1-800-232-AIDS (4636).

- The Spanish service (open from 8 A.M. to 2 A.M., 7 days a week) can be reached at 1-800-344-SIDA (7432).
- A TTY service for the hearing impaired is available from 10 A.M. to 10 P.M. Monday through Friday at 1-800-243-7889.
- National Prevention Information Network, 1-800-458-5231.
- National Herpes Hotline, 1-919-361-8488.
- National Native American AIDS Prevention, 1-510-444-2051.
- National Association of People with AIDS, 1-202-898-0414.
- National HIV Telephone Consultation Service for Health Care Professionals, 1-800-933-3413, San Francisco General Hospital, Bldg. 80, Ward 83, Room 314, San Francisco, CA 94110.
- HIV/AIDS Treatment Information Service, 1-800-HIV-0440 (448-0440), 9 A.M. to 7 P.M. Eastern time, Monday–Friday at 1-800-243-7012. Teletype number for the hearing-impaired, 9 A.M. to 5 P.M. Eastern time, Monday–Friday, Box 6303, Rockville, MD 20849-6303.
- AIDS Clinical Trials Information Service, 1-800-TRIALS-A (874-2572), 9 A.M. to 7 P.M. Eastern time, Monday–Friday. Information on clinical trials of AIDS therapies.
- National Gay and Lesbian Task Force AIDS Information Hotline, 1-888-843-4564.
- Gay Men's Health Crisis AIDS Hotline, 1-212-807-6655.
- National HIV/AIDS Education & Training Centers Program, 1-301-443-6364, Fax: 1-301-443-9887.
- AIDS National Interfaith Network, 1-202-546-0807, Fax: 1-202-546-5103, 110 Maryland Ave., NE, Room 504, Washington, D.C. 20002.
- National Hemophilia Foundation, 1-800-424-2634.
- Pediatric AIDS Foundation, 1-310-395-9051.
- National Pediatric HIV Resource Center, 1-800-362-0071.
- AIDSLINE via the National Library of Medicine. Free access via Grateful Med, obtained from NLM at 1-888-346-3656.
- National Institute on Drug Abuse Hotline, 1-800-662-HELP (4357).
- National Sexually Transmitted Diseases Hotline, 1-800-227-8922.
- American Civil Liberties Union Guide to local chapters, 1-202-544-1076.
- AIDS Policy and Law, 1-215-784-0860.
- National Conference of State Legislatures HIV, STD, and Adolescent Health Project, 1-303-830-2200.
- United States Conference of Mayors, 1-202-293-2352.
- Centers for Disease Control and Prevention, Public Inquiry, 1-404-639-3534.

- Food and Drug Administration, Office of Public Affairs, 1-301-443-3285.
- American Red Cross, Office of HIV/AIDS Education, 1-800-375-2040.
- World Health Organization, 1-202-861-4354.
- AIDS Treatment Data Network, 1-800-734-7104, 611 Broadway, Suite 613, New York, NY 10012. http://health.nyam.org:8000/public_html/network/index.html, email: AIDS-TreatD@aol.com. A home page on the Internet for people with AIDS and their caregivers, it provides information on approved and experimental treatments for AIDS-related conditions. It also publishes a quarterly directory of clinical trials on HIV and AIDS in English and Spanish.

Useful Internet Addresses

- AMA HIV/AIDS Information Center website (http://www.ama-assn.org) offers clinical updates, news, and information on social and policy questions. Cosponsored by Glaxo Wellcome Inc.
- Gay Men's Health Crisis (GMHC) website (http://www.gmhc.org) provides online forums hosted by GMHC representatives.

For additional help you may wish to consult with your college or community library. They may have access to the following AIDS-related databases:

- Centerforaids.org/rita.
- AEGIS (AIDS Education Global Information System): http://www.aegis.org or .com
- HIV Info Web: http://www.infoweb.org
- Kaiser Daily Global HIV/AIDS information: www.kaisernetwork.org
- Southern Africa AIDS Information Dissemination Service: www.safaids.org.zw
- Immunet: http://www.immunet.org
- Project Inform: http://www.projinf.org
- The Body: http://www.thebody.com/cgi/treatans.html
- HIVInSite: http://www.hivinsite.ucsf.edu/medical/tx-guidelines
- Search AIDSLINE, MEDLINE: http://www.igm.nim.nih.gov
- Vaccines: http://www.avi.org
- Women, children, healthcare workers, hemophiliacs, blind, deaf, and other affected groups: http://beaconclinic.org/website/groups
- Women's health: http://www.feminist.com/health
- Children with AIDS project: http://www.aidskids.org
- AIDS/HIV statistics: http://www.avert.org/statindx.htm

- http://www.healthcg.com/hiv/links.html (provides linkage to nine major U.S. Guidelines for HIV Testing, OIs, Treatment, etc.)
- The Centers for Disease Control and Prevention's (CDC) National Prevention Information Network (NPIN) Links: http://www.cdcnac.org/hivlink.html and http://www.cdcnac.org/daynews.html
- National Institute of Allergy and Infectious Diseases (NIAID) online at: http://www.niaid.nih.gov
- Critical Path AIDS Project, a Philadelphia organization for people with HIV disease, provides another online source for the latest news in HIV disease prevention, research, clinical trials, and treatments. The publication's hot link leads to a directory of AIDS-related publications: http://www.critpath.org
- UNAIDS Global HIV/AIDS information: www.unaids.org
- WHO HIV/STI Surveillance: http://www.who.int
- European Center for the Epidemiological Monitoring of AIDS: http://www.ceses.org
- United Kingdom (NAMlife): http://www.namlife.org
- HIV global molecular epidemiology: http://hivgenome.hjf.org
- AIDS MAP Global HIV/AIDS information: www.aidsmap.com
- Managing Desire: HIV Prevention Counseling for the 21st Century targets the HIV test counseling community as well as the general consumer. The site is produced by Nicholas Sheon, the prevention editor of the HIV Inside website of the UCSF Center for AIDS Prevention Studies (http://hivsinsite.ucsf.edu) and an HIV test counselor at the Berkeley Free Clinic: http://www.managingdesire.org
- AIDS offers abstracts from recent issues: http://www.aidsonline.com
- AIDS Weekly Plus contains more than 35,000 articles on health-related topics. Full access is available by subscription: http://www.newsfile.com
- AIDS Treatment News posts the contents of every issue since the publication began in 1986: http://www.immunet.org/immunet/atn.nsf/homepage
- AIDS WWW virtual library: http://planetq.com/aids
- The Bulletin of Experimental Treatment on AIDS (BETA) published by the San Francisco AIDS Foundation, is free online: http://www.sfaf.org/beta.html
- Treatment Issues, published by the Gay Men's Health Crisis, provides free access to issues dating back to 1995: http://www.gmhc.org/aidslib/ti/ti.html
- Project Inform email (info@projinf.org), website established in 1985 as a national, nonprofit, community-based HIV/AIDS treatment information and advocacy organization, serves HIV-infected individuals, their caregivers, and their healthcare and

service providers through its national, toll-free treatment hotline: http://www.projinf.org

♦ The Synergy APDIME ToolKit is a user-oriented, electronic one-stop shop of HIV/AIDS programming resources. Developed in collaboration with the University of Washington Center for Health Education and Research (CHER), the ToolKit contains five modules of the programming cycle covering Assessment, Planning, Design, Implementation Monitoring, and Evaluation: http://www.synergyaids .com/apdime/index.htm#

♦ The Centers for Disease Control and Prevention (CDC) National Center for HIV/AIDS, Viral Hepatitis, STD, and TB Prevention (NCHHSTP) released its Atlas, a new tool that will allow users to create maps, charts, and tables using HIV/AIDS, Viral Hepatitis, STD, and TB surveillance data.

The NCHHSTP Atlas currently includes options to:

  ♦ Create interactive maps, tables, pie charts, bar graphs

  ♦ Allow two-way HIV data stratifications and three-way STD data stratifications

  ♦ Display data trends over time and patterns across the United States or in specific communities

  ♦ Download and export data and graphics

  ♦ Access routinely reported surveillance data through a standardized user interface

  ♦ View, filter, explore and extract public health information

  ♦ Create detailed disease data reports and maps

  ♦ Submit ad hoc requests for customizable reports, and receive detailed and complete information on surveillance data footnotes and caveats.

♦ A video tutorial has been recorded and is available at www.cdc.gov/nchhstp/atlas. Please explore the NCHHSTP Atlas and check back for updates. There is also an email account NCHHSTPatlas@cdc.gov for you to send your questions and feedback.

The following is a sampling of general Internet resources for community research and HIV/AIDS information in Canada:

♦ Western Canada's largest AIDS group (in Vancouver, BC) has launched its redesigned website featuring online publications, a map of provincial resources, and links to over 100 AIDS websites. The website, published by the British Columbia Persons with AIDS Society, is one of the most popular sites in Canada and has operated for two years. The site carries information about:

  ♦ *Treatments:* http://www.bcpwa.org/treat.htm;

  ♦ *AIDS news:* http://www.bcpwa.org/news.htm;

  ♦ *Organizational activities:* http://www.bcpwa.org/AboutBCPWA/board.htm; and

  ♦ *Links:* http://www.bcpwa.org/Resources/links.htm

♦ For more information: Pierre Beaulne, Developer, Communications and Marketing, British Columbia Persons With AIDS Society, mail to: pierreb@pace.org

♦ The Community-Based HIV/AIDS Research Program National Health Research and Development Program, Health Canada: http://www.hc-sc.gr.ca/hppb/nhrdp/cdr.htm

♦ The HIV/AIDS Aboriginal Research Program National Health Research and Development Program, Health Canada: http://www.hc-sc.gr.ca/hppb/nhrdp/abrfp.htm

♦ Community-University Research Alliances (CURAs), Social Sciences and Humanities Research Council of Canada: http://www.sshrc.ca/english/programinfo/grantsguide/cura.html

♦ Canadian Strategy on HIV/AIDS: http://www.hc-sc .gc.ca/hppb/hiv_aids/

♦ Canadian HIV/AIDS Clearinghouse: http://www.cpha.ca/clearinghouse.htm

♦ Canadian AIDS Society: http://www.cdnaids.ca/

♦ Canadian Aboriginal AIDS Network: http://www.caan.ca/

♦ Community AIDS Treatment Information Exchange: http://www.catie.ca/

♦ Canadian HIV/AIDS Legal Network: http://www.aidslaw.ca/

♦ Bureau of HIV/AIDS, STD and TB, Health Canada: http://www.hc-sc.gc.ca/hpb/lcdc/bah/epi/epie.html

♦ Global Network of People Living with HIV/AIDS (GNP+), email: gnp@gn.apc.org

♦ AIDS.org is Google's #1 resource for AIDS information.

ACQUIRED IMMUNE DEFICIENCY SYNDROME (AIDS)

What do we know about AIDS? The next 14 chapters will present the many faces of the AIDS pandemic in the United States and other countries. Unlike people, the AIDS virus (HIV) does not discriminate; and it appears that most humans are susceptible to HIV infection, its suppression of the human immune system, and the consequences that follow. The viral infection that leads to AIDS is the most lethal, the most feared, and the most socially isolating of all the sexually transmitted diseases. We must, as a people, fight against HIV/AIDS, not against each other.

AIDS: Defining the Disease and Finding Its Cause

CHAPTER HIGHLIGHTS

- The letters A, I, D, S (AIDS) are an acronym for Acquired Immune Deficiency Syndrome.
- The Dark Era.
- The term "AIDS" was first used by the Centers for Disease Control and Prevention (CDC) in 1982.
- AIDS is a syndrome, not a single disease.
- Cases of severe immune deficiency (later confirmed as AIDS) were found in five women between 1975 and 1981.
- The first cases of AIDS-related *Pneumocystis carinii* pneumonia (PCP) were reported by the Centers for Disease Control and Prevention (CDC) in June 1981, the first case of Kaposi's sarcoma in July 1981.
- Luc Montagnier and Francoise Barre-Sinoussi discovered the AIDS virus (HIV-1) in 1983. They received the 2008 Nobel Prize in Medicine for their discovery.
- HIV-2 was discovered in 1985.
- The first CDC definition of AIDS was presented in 1982 and expanded in 1983, 1985, and 1987, and again on January 1, 1993.

A = Acquired = means not inherited, develops after birth by contact with the disease-causing agent; in the case of AIDS, a virus received from someone else

I = Immune = an individual's natural protection against disease-causing microorganisms and viruses

D = Deficiency = a deterioration of the immune system

S = Syndrome = a group of signs and symptoms that collectively characterize a disease, for example, together they define AIDS as a human disease

OR

A notable timeline	**H** human
In the history of human	**I** immunodeficiency
Death, Devastation,	**V** virus
Suffering and Sorrow caused by HIV	

DÉJÀ VU: A TIME OF AIDS

It was the best of times, it was the worst of times, it was the age of wisdom, it was the age of foolishness, it was the epoch of belief, it was the epoch of incredulity, it was the season of Light, it was the season of Darkness, it was the spring of hope, it was the winter of despair . . .

Charles Dickens, *A Tale of Two Cities*

THE NEW MILLENNIUM

Almost three decades since being discovered, HIV/AIDS remains a great challenge to public health, human rights, development, and national security. This is the first plague in the era of globalization. It has become the ultimate terrorist! The figures are truly alarming—through the last

13 years, 2000 through 2013, about 30 million people will have become infected with HIV, bringing the total number of infections to about 68 million since the outbreak of this pandemic. While 95% of the cases are concentrated in developing countries, industrialized countries are experiencing about 100,000 new infections each year. By the end of 2013 about 30 million people will have died from AIDS worldwide. HIV/AIDS is devastating for the individual who may be infected, and its impact on communities and society at large is enormous. This disease disproportionately affects those population groups that are already vulnerable: children, women, the poor, the destitute, and millions of others whose life situations are further degraded by the denial of basic human rights. The majority of those infected are unable to afford the cost of effective health care. Clearly, political and economic solutions must be found if millions of lives are to be saved. Of all the promises the new millennium holds, of all the secrets it will tell, a cure or a vaccine for HIV disease will surely unfold among them. Nothing in recent history has so challenged our reliance on modern science nor emphasized our vulnerability before nature. We live with the Acquired Immune Deficiency Syndrome (AIDS) pandemic, witnessing its paradoxes every day. People living with the Human Immunodeficiency Virus (HIV) live with fear, pain, and uncertainty about the disease; they also endure prejudice, scorn, rejection, and despair. **This must change!**

AIDS: A DISEASE OR A SYNDROME?

AIDS has been presented in journals, nonscience magazines, and newspaper articles and on television as a disease. However, a disease is a pathological condition with a single identifiable cause. As we learned from the days of Louis Pasteur and Robert Koch, there is a single identifiable organism or agent for each infectious disease.

AIDS patients may have many diseases—most AIDS patients have more than one disease at any given time. Each disease produces its own signs and symptoms. Collectively, the diseases that are expressed in an AIDS patient are referred to as

a **syndrome.** The number of different diseases an AIDS patient has and the severity of their expression reflects the functioning of that person's immune system (see Table 1.1, page 28).

AIDS Was First Officially Reported in the United States in 1981. However, AIDS Was in the U.S. Prior to the CDC Report of 1981

The first cases of AIDS in the United States were not in gay men. Five cases of extreme immune deficiencies were discovered between 1975 and 1981 in **heterosexual women.** (The term "AIDS" did not exist at this time. It was first used by the CDC in 1982.) The cases were reported by Henry Masur (1982), then of Cornell, now of the National Institutes of Health (NIH). For puzzling reasons this report was not published until October 1982. One can ask, if this information had been published before the June 1981 report on severe immunodeficiency in gay men or the July 1981 *New York Times* report of "Rare Cancer Seen in 41 Homosexuals," would AIDS have become known as a gay disease? Given the 10- to 11-year incubation period, it is likely that HIV was in the United States by 1965 or earlier.

In January 1981, while Ronald Reagan was taking his first oath of office as president, doctors around the country were just discovering the pattern of symptoms and infections in patients that was to become a very new disease.

Initially, AIDS was reported by the CDC among homosexual males, most frequently those who had many sexual partners. Further study of the gay population led to the conclusion that the agent responsible for AIDS was being transmitted through sexual activities. In July 1982, cases of AIDS were reported among hemophiliacs, people who had received blood transfusions, and injection drug users. These reports all had one thing in common—**an exchange of body fluids.** In particular, blood or semen was involved. In January 1983, according to the CDC, the first cases of AIDS in heterosexuals were documented. Two females, both sexual partners of injection-drug users (IDUs), became AIDS patients. This was clear evidence that the infectious agent could be transmitted from male to female as well as from male to male. Later in 1983, cases of AIDS were reported in Central Africa, but with a difference. The vast majority of African AIDS cases were not among gay men but among heterosexuals who did **not** use injection drugs. These data supported the earlier findings from the American homosexual population: that AIDS is primarily a sexually transmitted disease. Also, the risk for contracting AIDS increased with the number of sex partners one had and the sexual behaviors of those partners. Early empirical observations on which kinds of social behavior placed one at greatest risk of acquiring AIDS were later supported by surveillance surveys, testing, and analysis.

FIRST REACTION TO AIDS: DENIAL

When the disease that would eventually be called AIDS first emerged in 1981, a few officials within agencies like the Centers for Disease Control and Prevention realized that a new infectious agent was at work and that it could well be spreading rapidly. They most cautiously tried to sound the alarm, but the nation was not ready to talk about subjects like **anal sex, needles, and condoms.** Among those most heavily in denial were gay men, who were most at risk. They were still enjoying sexual liberation won in the 1970s, and nobody was in a mood to call the party off, even as close friends and sexual partners began dying.

New York playwright Larry Kramer attempted to break through this denial in early 1983 with an article in a widely read gay magazine. Headlined "1,112 and Counting," the article warned: "If this article doesn't rouse you to anger, fury, rage and action, gay men have no future on this Earth."

As they turned their fears into political engagement, the activists confronted a Washington that resisted action. Blood banks denied that any extra precautions were needed to prevent transmission. AIDS was buried deep inside newspapers and seldom mentioned on television. The death of movie star Rock Hudson in 1985 finally put AIDS on the front pages. But still, three young hemophiliacs, Ricky, Robert, and Randy Ray, were firebombed out of their Florida home when their neighbors learned they were HIV positive two years later.

Despite all of the evidence, over 10 years would pass before there was universal agreement that HIV caused AIDS and that HIV could not be transmitted by casual contact. People were, nevertheless, fired from their jobs across the country because of fears that they posed a threat to coworkers.

WHAT CAUSES AIDS?

In the Beginning: 1975, 1980, 1981, 1982

The appearance of AIDS in distinctly different populations, including women, young gay men, intravenous drug abusers, hemophiliacs, Haitians, infants, and blood transfusion recipients, argued for an infectious agent. But what kind of infectious agent would destroy the immune system of so many different groups of people?

THE BEGINNING, THEN SILENCE = DEATH: SILENCE AND STIGMA 1981 THROUGH 1987

June 1981—A report written by UCLA scientist Michael Gottlieb and published by the Centers for Disease Control and Prevention alerted physicians to an unusual constellation of fungal infection and pneumonia in otherwise healthy young gay men. The condition was later named Acquired Immune Deficiency Syndrome (AIDS). Activists took to the streets and convinced a skeptical public that AIDS was a deadly crisis.

In 1982, in San Francisco, the Bay Area Physicians for Human Rights (an association of gay and lesbian doctors) and several similar groups issued pamphlets with information about Kaposi's sarcoma—initially one of the most common symptoms of AIDS—including how to avoid infection with the as-yet-unidentified causal agent of AIDS. That year two publications that are now seen as having invented so-called safe sex and that laid the foundation for a new generation of prevention approaches were issued: the pamphlet *Play Fair!*, produced by the activist group Sisters of Perpetual Indulgence, and *How to Have Sex in an Epidemic: One Approach,* which advocated condom use and self-empowerment. By the end of 1982, a variety of informal efforts had coalesced into formal AIDS groups, including the Gay Men's Health Crisis in New York and the Terry Higgins Trust (later the Terrence Higgins Trust) in London.

By early 1987, 10,000 New Yorkers had already become sick with AIDS; half were dead. Along Christopher Street one could see dazed look of the doomed, skeletons and their caregivers alike. There was not even a false-hope pill for doctors to prescribe. Then the posters appeared. A small collective of artists had been working on a striking image they hoped would galvanize the community to act. Overnight, images bearing the radical truism **SILENCE = DEATH,** created by Arnam Finkelstein, appeared on walls and scaffolding all over Manhattan. The fuse was set—and then the writer and activist Larry Kramer struck a match. He'd been invited to be a last-minute substitute for a lecture series at the Lesbian and Gay Community Center. Kramer said, "If my speech tonight doesn't scare the shit out of you, we're in trouble. I sometimes think we have a death wish. I think we must want to die. I have never been able to understand why we have sat back and let ourselves literally be knocked off man by man without fighting back. I have heard of denial, but this is more than denial—it is a death wish." He concluded by saying, "It's your fault, boys and girls. It's our fault." Just like that new grassroots direct-action movement congealed. Within weeks it would adopt the name ACT UP (the AIDS Coalition to Unleash Power) and a deceptively simple demand: **Drugs into bodies.** That was twenty-six years ago and so much has happened since then, all stemming from that one electric moment. ACT UP revolutionized everything from the way drugs are researched to the way doctors interact with patients. Ultimately, it played a key role in catalyzing the development of the drugs that since 1996 have helped keep patients alive for a near-normal life span. ACT UP also redrew the blueprint for activism in media-saturated world.

Gay Men's Health Crisis, the nation's oldest AIDS service organization, marked its 30th anniversary in April 2012.

There were very few facts, but many plausible theories about the causes of AIDS. Perhaps the cytomegalovirus (sito-meg-ah-lo-virus) had mutated to cause a more severe illness. Maybe the illness was related to "poppers" (amyl and butyl nitrite) and other drugs popular among gay men for enhancing sexual pleasure. One theory linked the origin of HIV to the 1970s, when government-sponsored hepatitis B vaccine experiments used thousands of gay men as guinea pigs in New York, Los Angeles, and San Francisco—the same cities that were the first to report AIDS cases. Some researchers thought the other sexually transmitted infections that many gay men contracted somehow overwhelmed the immune system to cause the mysterious disease. Government researchers suggested that sperm in the male bowel caused the disease, a theory that made little sense because homosexuality is probably as old as society. Few doctors immediately considered the possibility of a new infectious agent. Prior to the outbreak of this strange disease, infectious disease scientists arrogantly believed that virtually all diseases were known. In fact, in the late 1960s, Surgeon General William H. Stewart stated it was "time to close the book on infectious diseases, declare the war against pestilence won, and shift national resources to such chronic problems as cancer and heart diseases." It was just that many things were unknown about the individual diseases. In fact, an editorial in *The New England Journal of Medicine* in December 1981 on possible causes of AIDS disregarded and omitted the whole idea that AIDS might be caused by an unknown infectious agent! And in 1982, this journal refused to publish Michael Gottlieb's work on the very first cases of this new disease that devastated the immune system. The article was said to have been rejected because the disease was considered unusual and not of much importance!

The Dark Era

During the time AIDS was first discovered, all of the people with this new disease died within a year or two after the onset of symptoms. During the earliest time, 1981 until early 1983, scientists did not know what caused this strange new disease. Then, after discovering that it was caused by a virus (see below) there followed a five-year period of no available treatments or antiviral drugs. The first drug tried was almost as lethal as the virus! It took some 13 years to find the first effective drug.

Discovery of the AIDS Virus (HIV)

Early in 1983, the agent that destroys an essential portion of the human immune system was identified by French scientists as a virus. From that point on there was a specific infectious agent associated with the cause of AIDS. The symptoms of viral-induced AIDS can begin *only* after one has been infected with a specific virus. This virus is now called the **Human Immunodeficiency Virus (HIV).** The viral-induced disease is referred to as HIV/AIDS because there are other reasons for a suppressed immune system, like congenital inherited immune deficiencies, exposure to radiation, alkylating agents, corticosteroids, certain forms of cancer, and cancer chemotherapy that also produce AIDS-like symptoms (Stadtmauer et al., 1997).

HIV/AIDS is a term used to refer to three categories of diagnoses collectively: (1) a diagnosis of HIV infection (not AIDS), (2) a diagnosis of HIV infection and a later diagnosis of AIDS, and (3) concurrent diagnoses of HIV infection and AIDS.

President Ronald Reagan on AIDS

On September 17, 1985, President Ronald Reagan held his first press conference since the public disclosure three months earlier that actor Rock Hudson had AIDS. Up to that point, Reagan had never spoken publicly about the epidemic, despite the fact that the first cases of AIDS had been reported more than four years earlier and more than 12,000 people had been diagnosed. But things changed with the disclosure of Hudson's diagnosis; Americans who had never given the epidemic any thought were now confronted with the chilling notion that anyone—a Hollywood actor or even a child—could get AIDS.

Reagan's staff, anticipating questions on the subject, prepared him to respond. Just as they expected, he was asked whether, if he had school-aged children, he would send them to school with a child who had AIDS. "I'm glad I'm not faced with that problem today," Reagan answered. He expressed his compassion for "the child that has this," while stating as a given that "he is now an outcast and can no longer associate with his playmates and schoolmates." Reagan continued, "it is true that some medical sources had said that this cannot be communicated in any way other than the ones we already know and which would not involve a child being in the school. And yet medicine has not come forth unequivocally and said, 'This we know for a fact, that it is safe.' And until they do, I think we just have to do the best we can with this problem."

Reagan's answer left many public health and AIDS experts aghast. He had directly contradicted an advisory issued less than three weeks earlier by the federal Centers for Disease Control and Prevention (CDC), stating that "casual person-to-person contact as would occur among schoolchildren appears to pose no risk." But among those who must have been delighted with the president's answer was a 30-year-old attorney in the Office of the White House Counsel.

Five days before the press conference, he reviewed the president's briefing materials and recommended the deletion of a sentence encapsulating the CDC's conclusion: "As far as our best scientists have been able to determine, AIDS virus is not transmitted through casual or routine contact." In a memorandum, the assistant counsel to the president explained, "I do not think we should have the president taking a position on a disputed scientific issue of this sort. There is much to commend the view that we should assume AIDS can be transmitted through casual or routine contact, as is true with many viruses, until it is demonstrated that it cannot be, and no scientist has said AIDS definitely cannot be transmitted." Exactly 20 years later, that lawyer, John G. Roberts, Jr., became the Chief Justice of the United States Supreme Court.

By the end of 1985, over 900,000 people in the United States were infected with HIV and about 13,000 had died from AIDS. In 1987, when the president gave his first speech on AIDS, over 1 million people were HIV infected, and 76,000 men, women, and children had been diagnosed with AIDS, of which 40,000 had died of AIDS.

It took just two and a half years to find the cause of AIDS, HIV. It took another two years for blood tests to detect HIV to become commercially available. Once that occurred, the transmission of HIV through blood transfusions fell to almost zero in developed countries.

Early Politics of AIDS

After years of insults and innuendos among scientists and in the press, President Ronald Reagan and French Prime Minister Jacques Chirac agreed to name as AIDS co-discoverers America's Robert Gallo and France's Luc Montagnier (mon-tan-yay). Naming co-discoverers was a political solution to end a dispute over patent rights covering the blood test for HIV.

Naming the Disease

Early in 1981, practically coincident with the report of the first cases of a new disease in the male homosexual community in the United States, there were reports of 34 cases of a new disease among Haitian immigrants to the United States and 12 cases of a disease previously unrecognized in Haiti—an aggressive form of **Kaposi's sarcoma** (kap-o-seez sar-ko-mah). Michael Gottlieb, who had identified the new disease that seemed to target gay men, found that although each of the cases was different, **all had one thing in common: Whatever was making the men sick had singled out the T lymphocyte cells for destruction.** Eventually the body's battered defenses couldn't shake off even the most harmless microbial intruder. The men were dying from what doctors termed opportunistic infections, such as *Pneumocystis* **pneumonia,** which attacks the lungs, and **toxoplasmosis,** which often ravages the brain.

THE CENTERS FOR DISEASE CONTROL AND PREVENTION REPORTS

The Centers for Disease Control and Prevention (CDC) began in 1948. Its mission is to improve the quality of health in the United States and globally. In June 1981, the CDC first reported on diseases occurring in gay men that previously had only been found to occur in people whose immune systems were suppressed by drugs or disease (*Morbidity and Mortality Weekly Report (MMWR),* 1981b).

The report stated that five young men in Los Angeles had been diagnosed with *Pneumocystis carinii* pneumonia (PCP) in three different hospitals. Because cases of PCP occurred almost exclusively in immune-suppressed patients, five new cases in one city at one time were considered unusual. The report also suggested "an association between some aspects of homosexual lifestyle or disease acquired through sexual contact and PCP in this population. Based on clinical examination of each of these cases, the possibility of a cellular immune dysfunction related to a common exposure might also be involved."

In July 1981, the CDC (*MMWR,* 1981b) reported that an uncommon cancer, Kaposi's sarcoma (KS), had been diagnosed in 26 gay men who lived in New York City and California. Between June 1, 1981, and May 28, 1982, the CDC received reports of 355 cases of Kaposi's sarcoma and/or serious opportunistic infection (OI), especially *Pneumocystis carinii* pneumonia (PCP), occurring in previously healthy persons between 15 and 60 years of age. Five states—California, Florida, New Jersey, New York, and Texas—accounted for 86% of the reported cases. The rest were reported by 15 other states. New York was reported as the state of residence for 51% of homosexual male patients, 49% of the heterosexual males, and 46% of the females. The median age at onset of symptoms was 36.0 years for homosexual men, 31.5 years for heterosexual men, and 29.0 years for women. Overall, 31% of all reported cases had onset before January 1, 1981 (*MMWR,* 1981a; Masur et al. 1981).

These were unusual findings because KS, when it occurred, was usually found in older men of Hebrew or Italian ancestry. The sudden and dramatic increase in pneumonia cases, all of which were caused by a widespread but generally harmless fungus, then called *P. carinii,* and KS cases indicated that an infectious form of immune deficiency was on the increase. At first, the new disease was referred to as the "4 H disease" or the "scarlet letter H disease" because the first cases of the disease were found among homosexuals, Haitians, heroin users, and hemophiliacs. Later this immunodeficiency disease was called **GRID** for **Gay-Related Immune Deficiency.** This new mysterious and lethal illness appeared to be associated with one's lifestyle. These early cases of immune deficiency heralded the beginning of an epidemic of a previously unknown illness. By 1982 and 1983, the disease was reported in adult heterosexuals and children. *Because a cellular deficiency of the human immune system* was found in every AIDS patient, along with an assortment of other signs and symptoms of disease, and because the infection was *acquired* from the action of some environmental agent, it was then named **AIDS** for **Acquired Immune Deficiency Syndrome.**

The events mentioned above occurred in the early 1980s, before the Internet and e-mail—and

they were happening across the United States. Early HIV/AIDS investigators did not have the advantage of instant communications. They used the telephone, wrote letters, or traveled to each others' research laboratories. To their great credit they overcame and moved forward!

DISCOVERY OF WHAT CAUSES AIDS

There was no shortage of ideas on what caused AIDS. It was believed by some to be an act of God, a religious curse or penalty against the homosexual for practicing a biblically unacceptable lifestyle that included drugs, alcohol, and sexual promiscuity. The Reverend Billy Graham said "AIDS is a judgment of God." Jerry Falwell stated that AIDS is God's punishment, the scripture is clear, "we do reap it in our flesh when we violate the laws of God." Some believed AIDS was due to sperm exposure to amyl nitrate, a stimulant used to heighten sexual pleasure (Gallo, 1987). Others believed there was no specific infectious agent. They believed that certain people who *excessively stressed their immune systems* experienced immune system failure, and before it could recover, other infections killed them. But many scientists who had expertise in analyzing the sudden onset of new human diseases thought the cause of this form of human immune deficiency was an infectious agent. They believed that the agent was transmitted through sexual intercourse, blood, or blood products, and from mother to fetus. They also believed that this agent, which led to the loss of T4 or CD4+ cells, was smaller than a bacterium or fungus because it passed through a filter normally used to remove those microorganisms. This agent fit the profile of a virus.

In January 1983, Luc Montagnier and colleagues at the Pasteur Institute in Paris isolated the virus that causes AIDS. In May of that year, they published the first report on a T cell retrovirus found in a patient with **lymphadenopathy** (lim-fad-eh-nop-ah-thee), or swollen lymph glands. Lymphadenopathy is one of the early signs in patients progressing toward AIDS. The French scientist (Figure 1-1) named this virus

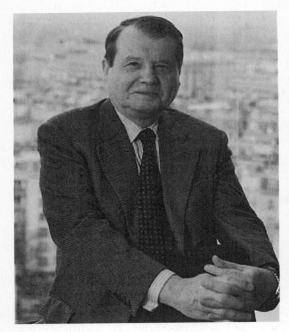

FIGURE 1-1 Luc Montagnier, President of the World Foundation for AIDS Research and Prevention.
He is the co-discoverer of the Human Immunodeficiency Virus (HIV), the cause of AIDS. He has co-founded two Centers for the Prevention, Treatment, Research, and Diagnosis of AIDS, one in the Ivory Coast and the other in Cameroon. His current studies are on the diagnosis and treatment of microbial and viral factors associated with cancers, and neuro-degenerative and articular diseases. In 2008, he and colleague Francoise Barre-Sinoussi received the Nobel Prize in Medicine for their discovery of HIV.

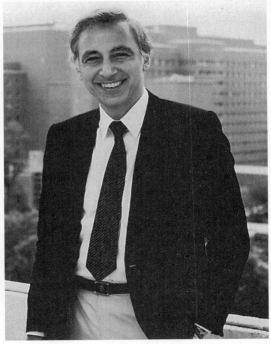

FIGURE 1-2 Robert Gallo, Director, Institute of Human Virology
Co-discoverer of the first human retrovirus and discoverer of HIV, developer of the first HIV blood test, director, Institute of Human Virology at the University of Maryland School of Medicine, he has received 27 honorary degrees and has twice won the Albert Lasker Award in Medicine, the most recognized award for biomedical science in the United States.

lymphadenopathy-associated virus (LAV) (Barre-Sinoussi et al., 1983).

Naming the Viruses That Cause AIDS: HIV-1, HIV-2

During the search for the AIDS virus, several investigators isolated the virus but gave it different names. For example, Robert Gallo (Figure 1-2) named the virus HTLV III (for the Third Human T Cell Lymphotropic Virus). Because the collection of names given this virus created some confusion, the Human Retrovirus Subcommittee of the Committee on the Taxonomy of Viruses reduced all the names to one: **Human Immunodeficiency Virus** or **HIV.** This term is now used worldwide.

In 1985, a second type of HIV was discovered in West African prostitutes. It was named HIV type 2 or **HIV-2.** The first confirmed case of HIV-2 infection in the United States was reported in late 1987 in a West African woman with AIDS. By December 1990, 16 additional cases of HIV-2 infection were reported to the CDC (*MMWR,* 1990; 2011). Beginning in 2013, at least 242 HIV-2 infections have been reported from 50 states of the United States and the District of Columbia.

First Reported Case of HIV-2 Infection

The earliest evidence of an individual exposed to HIV-2 comes from a case report on an infection most likely occurring in Guinea-Bissau in the 1960s. Anne-Mieke Vandamme of the Catholic University of Leuren in Belgium and colleagues believe that HIV-2 first moved into humans near the town of Canchungo in western Guinea-Bissau, since that is where the largest proportion of people carry it. The researchers calculate that HIV-2 jumped into humans in about 1940 for the A subtype and 1945 for the B subtype, a time when there were still mangabey monkeys around Canchungo. A local fondness for eating the primates could have both wiped them out and exposed people to mangabey viruses. In genetic terms, HIV-2 is much more closely related to the Simian Immunodeficiency Virus (SIV), a group of monkey viruses, than to HIV-1. Both HIV-2 and HIV-1 are said to have been derived from ancestral SIV variants that were from distinct regions and species and do not appear to be direct genetic descendants of each other (Marlink, 1996; Hahn et al., 2000). Clinically, what has been learned about HIV-1 appears to apply to HIV-2, except that HIV-2 appears to be less harmful (cytopathic) to the cells of the immune system, progressing to AIDS in only 20 percent of those infected, and it reproduces more slowly than HIV-1. Also, HIV-2 does not respond to some of the antiretroviral drugs that are effective against HIV-1. Cases of HIV-2 infection are most likely underreported.

UNLESS STATED OTHERWISE, ALL REFERENCES TO HIV IN THIS BOOK REFER TO HIV-1 OR HIV.

DEFINING THE ILLNESS: AIDS AND SURVEILLANCE

The CDC reported that through 1983 there were 3068 AIDS cases in the United States and 1478 of these had died (48%). All demonstrated a loss of CD4+ or T4 lymphocytes, and all died with severe opportunistic infections. Opportunistic infections (OI) are caused by organisms and viruses that are normally present but do *not* cause disease unless the immune system is damaged (see Chapter 6). Clearly there was an immediate need for a name and definition for this disease so that a national surveillance program could begin.

The First Definition of AIDS: 1982

In order to establish surveillance, a system for monitoring where and when AIDS cases occurred, a workable definition had to be developed. The definition had to be *sensitive* enough to detect every possible AIDS patient, while at the same time *specific* enough to exclude those who may have AIDS-like symptoms, but did not have AIDS.

In 1982, there was no *single characteristic* of AIDS that would allow for a useful definition for surveillance purposes. And so, the first AIDS surveillance definition was based on the clinical description of symptoms. The first of many criteria for the diagnosis of AIDS were (1) the presence of a reliably diagnosed disease at least moderately predictive of cellular immune deficiency; and (2) the absence of an underlying cause for the immune deficiency or for reduced resistance to the disease (*MMWR*, 1982). Because the symptoms varied greatly among individuals, this was a poor first definition.

AIDS Definition Modified: 1983, 1985, 1987

The initial definition of AIDS was thus an arbitrary one, reflecting the partial knowledge of the clinical consequences that prevailed at the time. Various systems for classifying HIV-related illnesses have been revised since 1982 to take into account increasing knowledge about the spectrum of those illnesses. Had the whole picture of HIV infection and its clinical consequences been known in 1982, the term **"AIDS"** would not have been used. Instead, it would have been called **"HIV disease"** (or perhaps, following an older tradition, "Gottlieb's disease," after Mike Gottlieb, who first described it).

The 1982 definition was modified in 1983 to include new diseases then found in AIDS patients. With this modification, AIDS became reportable to the Centers for Disease Control and Prevention (CDC) in every state. In 1985 and 1987 additional diseases were included in the AIDS case definition.

Broadly speaking, the term **AIDS** may be understood as referring to the onset of life-threatening illnesses as a result of HIV disease that results from an HIV infection. AIDS is the end stage of a disease process that may have been developing for 5, 10, 15, or more years, for most of which time the infected person will have been well and quite possibly unaware that he or she has been infected.

Thus the number of AIDS cases reported from 1987 through 1992 reflects the revisions of the initial surveillance case definitions.

Problems with AIDS Definitions, 1981–1992

One major drawback to all the CDC AIDS definitions is the fact that through 1992, the Social Security Administration (SSA) used the CDC AIDS definition to determine disability. But all the definitions were primarily based on symptoms and opportunistic infections in men. Therefore, about 65% of women with HIV/AIDS symptoms were excluded from Supplemental Security Income (SSI) benefits. They were excluded because of failure to be diagnosed with AIDS by the CDC AIDS definition (Sprecher, 1991).

AIDS Redefined in 1993, 1994, 2000

On January 1, 1993, the newest definition of AIDS was put into the surveillance network. The reason for the new CDC definition was that epidemiologists felt the 1987 definition failed to reflect the true magnitude of the pandemic. In particular, it failed to address AIDS in women. Thus, the CDC expanded the AIDS surveillance case definition to include all HIV-infected persons who have less than 200 CD4+ or T4 lymphocytes/μL (microliter) of blood, or a T4 lymphocyte percentage less than 14% of total lymphocytes. In addition to retaining the 23 clinical conditions in the 1987 AIDS

surveillance case definition, the expanded definition includes (1) pulmonary tuberculosis, (2) invasive cervical cancer, and (3) recurrent pneumonia (Table 1-1). The objectives of these

---

Table 1–1 List of 29 Conditions in the AIDS Surveillance Case Definition

- Candidiasis of bronchi, trachea, or lungs
- Candidiasis, esophageal
- Cervical cancer, invasive[1]
- Coccidioidomycosis, disseminated or extrapulmonary
- Cryptococcosis, extrapulmonary
- Cryptosporidiosis, chronic intestinal (>1 month duration)
- Cytomegalovirus disease (other than liver, spleen, or nodes)
- Cytomegalovirus retinitis (with loss of vision)
- HIV encephalopathy
- Herpes simplex: chronic ulcer(s) (>1 month duration); or bronchitis, pneumonitis, or esophagitis
- Hepatitis C (HepC)
- Histoplasmosis, disseminated or extrapulmonary
- Human papillomavirus (HPV)
- Isosporiasis, chronic intestinal (>1 month duration)
- Kaposi's sarcoma[2]
- Lymphoma, Burkitt's (or equivalent term)[2]
- Lymphoma, immunoblastic (or equivalent term)[2]
- Lymphoma, primary in brain[2]
- *Mycobacterium avium complex* or *M. kansasii*, disseminated or extrapulmonary
- *Mycobacterium tuberculosis*, disseminated or extrapulmonary
- *Mycobacterium tuberculosis*, any site (pulmonary[1] or extrapulmonary)
- *Mycobacterium*, other species or unidentified species, disseminated or extrapulmonary
- Oral hairy leukoplakia
- *Pneumocystis carinii* pneumonia
- Pneumonia, recurrent[1]
- Progressive multifocal leukoencephalopathy
- Salmonella septicemia, recurrent
- Toxoplasmosis of brain
- Wasting syndrome due to HIV

1. Added in the 1993 expansion of the AIDS surveillance case definition.
2. These are cancers.
(Adapted from the CDC, Atlanta.)

changes are to simplify the classification of HIV infection and the AIDS case reporting process, to be consistent with standards of medical care for HIV-infected persons, to better categorize HIV-related morbidity, and to reflect more accurately the number of persons with severe HIV-related immunosuppression who are at highest risk for severe HIV-related morbidity and most in need of close medical follow-up.

In 1994 pediatric case definitions were updated and in 2000, the surveillance case definition for HIV was revised to incorporate new laboratory tests.

Problems Stemming from Changing the AIDS Definition for Surveillance Purposes

Each time the definition of AIDS has been altered by the CDC, it has led to an increase in the number of AIDS cases. In 1985, the change in definition led to a 2% increase over what would have been diagnosed prior to the change. The 1987 change led to a 35% increase in new AIDS cases per year over that expected using the 1985 definition. The 1993 change resulted in a 52% increase in AIDS cases over that expected for 1993. Such rapid changes alter the baseline from which future predictions are made and make the interpretations of trends in incidence and characteristics of cases difficult to process. **For the first time because of the 1993 AIDS definition, one could be diagnosed with AIDS and remain symptom-free for years (become HIV positive and have a T4 or CD4+ cell count of less than 200).**

Summary

Much continues to be written about HIV/AIDS. Some of it, especially in lay articles, has been less than accurate and has led to public confusion and fear. **HIV infection is not AIDS. HIV infection is now referred to as HIV disease. AIDS is a syndrome of many diseases,** each resulting from an opportunistic agent or cancer cell that multiplies in humans who are immunosuppressed. The new 1993 CDC AIDS definition will allow, over the long term, earlier access to federal and state medical and social services for HIV-infected individuals.

Review Questions

(Answers to the Review Questions are on page 463.)

1. The letters A, I, D, and S are an acronym for?
2. The letters H, I, and V are an acronym for?
3. Is AIDS a single disease? Explain.
4. When was the AIDS virus discovered and by whom?
5. In what year did the CDC first report on a strange new disease that later was named AIDS?
6. Name one different acronym for HIV.
7. How many times has CDC changed and expanded the definition of AIDS? In what years?
8. What is one major advantage of the new CDC AIDS definition for the HIV-infected?

2
What Causes AIDS: Origin of the AIDS Virus

CHAPTER HIGHLIGHTS

- AIDS dissidents say AIDS is not caused by HIV infection.
- HIV/AIDS scientists say AIDS is caused by HIV infection.
- An unbroken chain of HIV transmission has been established between those infected and the newly infected.
- HIV is believed to have crossed into humans from chimpanzees.
- A viral precursor to HIV may have entered humans 300 years ago or in the early 1900s.
- A third new HIV strain has been found.
- The earliest AIDS case to date was reported in 1959.

THE CAUSE OF AIDS: THE HUMAN IMMUNODEFICIENCY VIRUS (HIV)

The unexpected appearance and accelerated spread of an unknown lethal disease soon raised two important questions: **What** is causing the disease? **Where** did it come from? These questions will be answered.

This section has a subtitle that states that AIDS is the result of HIV infection. However, 30 years after the identification of HIV as the cause of AIDS (1983–2013) there are still a relatively small number of scientists and nonscientists who claim that HIV does *not* cause AIDS. For a balanced HIV/AIDS presentation, this claim will be presented first.

HIV DOES NOT CAUSE AIDS: DISSIDENTS AND THEIR CULTS: A MINORITY POINT OF VIEW

Throughout the HIV/AIDS pandemic, there have been skeptics who have challenged or dissented from the most widely held beliefs of the world's best HIV/AIDS scientists. The scientists' belief, based on overwhelming scientific data, that HIV does cause AIDS is the conventionally accepted wisdom worldwide. Those who do not accept the scientific data about HIV/AIDS are referred to as "AIDS dissidents" or "AIDS denialists." They contend that there is no connection or link between HIV and AIDS. They contend that HIV/AIDS is the greatest medical hoax in history!

Dissidents/Denialists employ rhetorical tactics to give the appearance of argument or legitimate debate, when in actuality there is none. These false arguments are used when one has few or no facts to support one's viewpoint against a scientific consensus or against overwhelming evidence to the contrary. These arguments are effective in distracting from actual useful debate using emotionally appealing, but ultimately empty and illogical, assertions.

Fronted locally by ACT UP/San Francisco, a renegade chapter long ago disowned by the rest of the AIDS activist movement (and not to be confused with ACT UP/Golden Gate, which respects most conventional AIDS research), members have repeatedly plastered the Castro district with stickers reading, "AIDS Is Over" and "Don't Buy the HIV Lie" (Figure 2-1). In May and June 1999, the Los Angeles-based dissident group Alive & Well ran a series of full-page ads in several gay/lesbian and alternative papers, including the *Bay Area Reporter,*

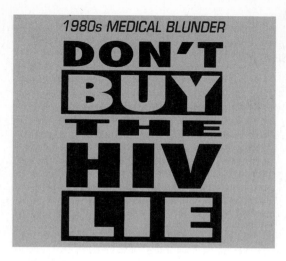

FIGURE 2-1 The image HIV/AIDS dissidents still support! *(Smith, T.C. and Novella, S.P. (2007) HIV Denial in the Internet Era. PLoS Med 4(8):e256.)*

Bay Times, and *Bay Guardian,* arguing that AIDS is not contagious, HIV is harmless, and that HIV/AIDS drugs are the real danger. The first of the ads states that "What we have experienced for 20 years is not a sexually transmitted epidemic but a tragic medical mistake. Contrary to popular beliefs, AIDS is not a new disease, AIDS is a new name given by the Centers for Disease Control (CDC) to a collection of 29 old illnesses and conditions. . . . These illnesses and conditions are called AIDS only when they occur in persons who also have certain protective, disease-fighting proteins called antibodies in their blood." In her book, *What If Everything You Thought You Knew About AIDS Was Wrong?,* Christine Maggiore, who died of pneumonia in December 2008, wrote, "None of these diseases appear exclusively in those who test [HIV] positive. . . . All 29 indicator diseases have established causes and treatments unrelated to HIV." AIDS, in other words, isn't an epidemic at all; it's a phony construct. Maggiore, who tested HIV positive in 1992, never took antiretroviral drugs. She believed that those who died of AIDS actually died from prescription or recreational drugs, or fear. Her explanations for the global AIDS pandemic: In Africa, people are dying at the same rate as before; in America, people are victims of the prescription drugs. (See Box 2.1, page 32 for more on Christine Maggiore.)

Who Was Christine Maggiore?

(The following information was abstracted from the *Los Angeles Times* article "A Mother's Denial, a Daughter's Death," by Charles Ornstein and Daniel Costello, September 2005.)

Her background commands attention. She was an engaging, articulate woman. She owned her own clothing company. She presented talks on HIV at local schools, and health fairs and has appeared on TV shows presenting her dissident or anti-HIV views about AIDS. Her disbelief that HIV causes AIDS was in line with the beliefs of University of California, Berkeley biology professor Peter Duesberg, whose well-publicized dissident views on AIDS (presented below) place him outside the mainstream of scientific beliefs that HIV does cause AIDS. She founded Alive & Well AIDS Alternatives, a nonprofit group that challenges common assumptions and scientific facts about HIV/AIDS. (See Box 2.1.)

Disbelieving Scientists (HIV/AIDS Dissidents)

Scientist Peter Duesberg is perhaps the most vocal in his concern that the scientific community is investigating the wrong causative agent. Duesberg is a molecular biologist at the University of California at Berkeley and a member of the National Academy of Sciences. Duesberg has advanced his anti-HIV/AIDS hypothesis at great expense to himself. He states that "I have been excommunicated by the retrovirus-AIDS community with noninvitations to meetings, noncitations in the literature and nonrenewals of my research grants, which is the highest price an experimental scientist can pay for his convictions."

In 1971 at age 33, Duesberg co-discovered cancer-causing genes in viruses. But he has done no clinical research on HIV. In the March 1987 issue of *Cancer Research,* he published "Retroviruses as Carcinogens and Pathogens: Expectations and Reality." The article provoked a great deal of scientific discussion and received a lot of popular press coverage. In the article Duesberg argues that there is *no evidence* that HIV causes AIDS. He has published additional articles in

— BOX 2.1 —

CHRISTINE MAGGIORE, PROMINENT HIV DISSIDENT, LOST DAUGHTER TO AIDS?
(SHE DIED THREE YEARS LATER—CAUSE IS, AT THE MOMENT, SPECULATIVE)

According to the literature (some references provided below), the events of 2005 put an entirely new spotlight on Christine Maggiore's beliefs on HIV/AIDS. In May, her three-year-old daughter, Eliza Jane Scovill, died from an apparently sudden and unexpected illness. Several weeks prior to Eliza Jane's death, Maggiore stated that her two children were in excellent health. Neither son Charles or daughter Eliza Jane were HIV tested to this point in time.

TIMELINE TO ELIZA JANE'S DEATH (EXTRACTED FROM THE *LA TIMES* ARTICLE)

- The first hint that Eliza Jane was ill came at the end of April 2005 when she developed a runny nose showing yellow mucus.
- On April 30, Maggiore took her daughter to a pediatrician. The doctor found the girl had clear lungs, no fever, and adequate oxygen levels.
- May 5, Maggiore sought a second opinion from another pediatrician. During an interview with this pediatrician, he said that he suspected there was an ear infection but believed it could be resolved without antibiotics. In a follow-up call, he said Eliza's parents told him that she was getting better. Some time after that, Maggiore asked a Denver physician, who was visiting Los Angeles, to examine her daughter. This physician said he found fluid in her right eardrum.
- May 14, the Denver physician examined her again and prescribed the antibiotic amoxicillin.
- May 15, Eliza Jane vomited several times and was pale. While Maggiore's husband was on the phone with the Denver physician, Eliza Jane stopped breathing and "crumpled like a paper doll."
- May 16, Eliza Jane died early in the morning at Van Nuys hospital. It was reported that neither hospital staff nor the coroner were told that the mother was HIV positive. Maggiore said that she was never asked about her HIV status.

According to interviews and records and after some time interval, the Los Angeles medical examiner declared the cause of death to be "AIDS related pneumonia."

On December 10, 2005, Christine Maggiore, whose daughter allegedly died of AIDS-related pneumonia, appeared on *ABC News Primetime* to share her reasons for not testing her children for HIV. She maintained that Eliza Jane died of an allergic reaction to antibiotics. Her son, Charles, tested HIV negative after

his sister's death. Maggiore continued to question the coroner's findings. In a November 2005 article in "The Body" (www.thebody.com), the question was asked, "Is it right, is it fair, for a child to pay with her life for this level of arrogance on the part of the parent? Surely, the word denial has seldom had a more clear definition than what is seen here. Ms. Maggiore and her partner face a terrible dilemma in their grief. They are faced with acknowledging the possibility they have been wrong. If they acknowledge error, they must accept responsibility for the loss of their daughter. A denialist dilemma indeed."

In the April 2006 edition of *POZ Magazine*, Bob Lederer stated in his article "Dead Certain?" that several months after Eliza Jane died, James K. Ribe, MD, senior deputy medical examiner at the Los Angeles County coroner's office, pronounced that her death had been caused by *Pneumocystis carinii* pneumonia (PCP), one of the most common and fatal opportunistic infections associated with HIV, and her death was declared to be AIDS-related. Slides of cells from Eliza Jane's lung showed microscopic evidence of colonies of *Pneumocystis carinii*. The autopsy report also described the presence of HIV core proteins in the brain, which was diagnosed as HIV encephalitis. **The coroner's office would not confirm to *POZ Magazine* whether it had actually tested her blood for HIV infection or HIV antibodies.** However, according to other published reports, Eliza Jane's T4 or CD4+ cell counts were in the normal range. It would appear that the blood test for HIV would be crucial to the coroner's statement that Eliza Jane died of AIDS. Entering 2013, the L.A. coroner's verdict remains the official verdict on the death of Eliza Jane.

Filing of Charges Against Christine Maggiore with Respect to Her Daughter's Death

Neither the Los Angeles Police Department nor the Los Angeles Department of Children and Family Services saw fit to file charges against Christine Maggiore, as both agencies found that Eliza Jane was taken to see physicians on several occasions. (From the *Los Angeles Times*, December 31, 2008.)

CHRISTINE MAGGIORE'S DEATH, THREE YEARS FOLLOWING HER DAUGHTER ELIZA JANE'S DEATH

Christine Maggiore died at her home in Van Nuys, California on December 27, 2008, at the age of 52. She is survived by her husband, Robin Scovill, and her son, Charles. The coroner's report indicated that Maggiore

BOX 2.1 (continued)

had been under treatment for bilateral pneumonia for about six months. Whether she died from pneumocystis pneumonia, from a more generic form of pneumonia, from another opportunistic infection, or from an unrelated cause may never be revealed. Unlike the case of her daughter, Eliza Jane Scovill, there will probably not be an autopsy by the coroner's office. Maggiore's supporters and her critics are left to speculate on the cause of her death. Christine Maggiore's legacy includes the nonprofit organization Rethinking AIDS: The Group for the Scientific Reappraisal of the HIV/AIDS Hypothesis, and the cadre of AIDS dissidents known as Alive & Well AIDS Alternatives. (For additional information on her death, see Edward Grabe's article at AIDSTruth.org.)

Loved by Some, Dismissed by Others

There is no question that Christine Maggiore had supporters. She had many moments among dear friends and followers. Some of her supporters have written glowing articles on her beliefs in motherhood and her questioning of science and other values that many people agree with. However, she chose to define herself as one against well-documented scientific information on HIV/AIDS. Thomas Coates, known as an HIV/AIDS expert at the University of California, Los Angeles School of Medicine, said, "There are always positions and counter-positions in science and legitimate differences of opinion. People have the right to disagree, but in the case of questioning the link between HIV and AIDS, one has to ask a bigger question: what are the consequences? In the case of HIV/AIDS denialism, the consequences are disability, suffering, and finally death."

Rest in Peace

Christine Maggiore was steadfast in her beliefs and faithful to her cause. According to published reports, Maggiore knew she was HIV positive, but she breastfed both children—despite the accepted, scientifically substantiated evidence that breastfeeding increases the risk of mother-to-child HIV transmission.

To many people, she will remain a misguided HIV/AIDS dissident who denied the scientific evidence linking HIV to AIDS and to her death. Many believe that her refusal to use antiretroviral drugs led to the early death of her daughter and to her own premature death. It is very likely that history will have to wait for the final words on Christine Maggiore's legacy. For those who wish to read an in-depth report on the death of Christine Maggiore and her daughter, see the 31-page treatise by David Gorski: "Christine Maggiore and Eliza Jane Scovill: Living and Dying with HIV/AIDS Denialism" (www.sciencebasedmedicine.org).

Some References for Information about Christine Maggiore and Daughter Eliza Jane's Death:

Lederer, Bob (2006). Dead Certain? *POZ Magazine,* April edition. pp. a18–23. www.poz.com.

Project Inform Perspective (2005). Project Inform: A Denialist Dilemma. November issue. www.thebody.com/pinf/nov05/aids_denialists.html?rn128h. pp. 1–6.

Ornstein, Charles, et al. (2005). A Mother's Denial, a Daughter's Death [Home Edition]. *Los Angeles Times.* Los Angeles, CA. September 24. p. A1.

For a transcript of the December 2005 *ABC Primetime* interview with Christine Maggiore, go to www.transcripts.tv. For a copy of ABC News Home Video call 1-800-505-6139 or go to ABCNews at datapakservices.com.

Farber, Celia (2006). A Daughter's Death, A Mother's Survival. Los Angeles City Beat. August 3. pp. 1–10. www.lacitybeat.com.

ABCNEWS (December 8, 2005). Did HIV-Positive Mom's Beliefs Put Her Children at Risk? Coroner says 3-year-old died of AIDS; her mother and another doctor dispute that. abcnews.go.com/primetime/print.

Science (1988) and in the *Proceedings of the National Academy of Sciences* (1989) stating that HIV is not the cause of AIDS: that HIV is a passenger virus, and that the use of anti-HIV drugs causes AIDS. In short, Duesberg suggests that there is no single causative agent, that the disease is due to one's "lifestyle." He marshals arguments to support his theory that, in the United States and probably in Europe, AIDS is a collection of noninfectious deficiencies predominantly associated with drug use, malnutrition, parasitic infections, and other specific risks. To read more on Duesberg, see the Wayt Gibbs article "Dissident or Don Quixote?" in the August 2001 *Scientific American.*

Duesberg believes the tests that detect HIV antibodies are useless. In the June 1988 issue of *Discovery* he said, "If somebody told me today that I was antibody positive, I wouldn't worry one second. I wouldn't take Valium. I wouldn't write my will. All I would say is that my immune system seems to work. I have antibodies to a virus. I am protected."

In June 1990, Robin Weiss and Harold Jaffe wrote a critical refutation of Duesberg's theory that HIV cannot be the cause of AIDS. Duesberg's response suggested that he was unaware of published data that clearly answer the questions he raises concerning HIV involvement in AIDS. For example, one of Duesberg's major points is that no one has yet shown that hemophiliacs infected with HIV progress to AIDS. The data on matched groups of homosexual males and hemophiliacs, which show that *only* those infected with HIV develop AIDS, have been available for a number of years (Weiss et al., 1990).

Duesberg's arguments and disagreements with the vast majority of prominent scientists who have researched the causal agent of AIDS are many. But they pale when placed next to the overwhelming evidence that leaves no doubt in the opinion of most scientists that HIV causes AIDS (see Andrews, 1995; Cohen, 1993; Moore, 1996).

Based on an August 1992 report in *Newsweek,* a father discussed his decision, based on Duesberg's claims, to counsel his infected hemophiliac son to avoid zidovudine (ZDV) treatment. This situation is similar to what happened when desperate cancer patients followed the advice of a credentialed academician who recommended vitamin therapy as the cure for cancer. Based on such advice, some people failed to undergo truly effective therapy.

DISCUSSION QUESTION: Is Duesberg's opinion on this issue inadvertently harmful to humans? To the scientific process? Will the use of his idea, that HIV does not cause AIDS, provide a course of action that will stop the Acquired Immune Deficiency Syndrome?

Others Join Duesberg's Belief That HIV Does Not Cause AIDS

In 1996, Duesberg's book, *Inventing the AIDS Virus,* was published and in 1998 he and David Rasnick published a paper, *"The AIDS Dilemma: drug diseases blamed on a passenger virus."* Through 2012, it appears that Duesberg still believes that HIV does not cause AIDS. He believes that HIV is just another opportunistic agent (Duesberg, 1993, 1995a, 1995b; Moore, 1996; Duesberg, et al., 2009;

Cartwright, 2010; Duesberg, 2011). With each new scientific report, it becomes more difficult for Duesberg to maintain his position. But he will not admit any error in his beliefs regardless of the reports that newborn infants with HIV got HIV *only* from HIV-infected mothers and progress to AIDS, while noninfected newborns from the same mothers do not progress to AIDS, and that some 50% of HIV-infected hemophiliacs have developed AIDS, *yet no* HIV-negative hemophiliac has ever developed AIDS (Darby et al., 1995; Levy, 1995; Sullivan et al., 1995). In addition, Duesberg claims that the drug ZVD (zidovudine) causes AIDS. What does he make of the AIDS Clinical Trials Group (ACTG) Protocol 076 that demonstrated ZVD treatment of women during pregnancy and delivery reduced transmission of HIV from mother to infant from 25% in the placebo-treated mothers to 8% in those who received ZVD (Connor et al., 1994)?

For those who wish to know more on the rebuttal of Duesberg's arguments, read the study reporting on the death rate among HIV-positive and HIV-negative British hemophilia patients (Baum, 1995; Darby et al., 1995; Editorial, 1995). For more by Duesberg see his Web page, www. duesberg.com. Also see www.garynull.com and www.aidsisover.com.

Impact of HIV/AIDS Dissident Thinkers on the Former President of South Africa

Peter Duesberg, Christine Maggiore, and David Rasnick, an American chemist, are considered to be three of the leaders of the HIV/AIDS dissidents in the United States. They are also the people who are thought to be, at least partially, responsible for South African President Mbeki's (Figure 2-2) belief that HIV does not cause AIDS. In February 2002, Rasnick and South African computer science professor Philip Machanick, who believes that HIV causes AIDS and that the antiretroviral drugs are not as toxic as Rasnick says, have agreed, after a heated exchange of letters, to a challenge. The date, at this time, has not been set. But should this bizarre game of chicken occur, the scenario will go something like this: Rasnick will intentionally infect himself with HIV to prove that it does not cause disease, and

SCIENCE TAKES BACKSEAT TO POLITICS: SOUTH AFRICAN PRESIDENT THABO MBEKI SAYS HIS GOVERNMENT HAS A RIGHT/OBLIGATION TO DOUBT WHETHER HIV CAUSES AIDS

Beginning in March 2000, two tragedies began unfolding simultaneously in South Africa. The first was epidemiological, with millions of men, women, and children infected with HIV destined to develop AIDS. The second was political, with then President Thabo Mbeki (Figure 2-2) seriously entertaining a discredited view that challenges the role of HIV as the cause of AIDS. Together, the tragedies may well increase the AIDS pandemic in South Africa. The outcome can only be measured in untold suffering, death, and orphans.

DENIAL THAT HIV CAUSES AIDS

President Thabo Mbeki and other HIV dissidents believe that if HIV exists, it does not cause AIDS. The disease AIDS does not exist. There is no epidemic nor are there deaths from AIDS. There is just mass hysteria caused by a conspiracy among pharmaceutical multinationals, aided and abetted by political and medical self-interest.

Orthodoxy—People who believe HIV causes AIDS have demonstrated a rapidly expanding foundation of scientific and medical understanding that rests upon a detectable virus. They have documented evidence of the impact of this virus on the human immune system. There is an impressive array of leading scientific names—the signatories to the Durban Declaration include many Nobel laureates.

Believing in the orthodox position suggests that things can be done to prevent people from becoming HIV-infected and dying of AIDS.

Belief in the dissident view tends to suggest that because HIV does not cause AIDS, there is no epidemic; nothing needs to be done. People are dying of diseases exacerbated by poverty, as they have always done. It is simply that these are being recorded more often. There is no infectious agent at work, in South Africa or in the world, causing a new and different disease!

IT'S TIME TO FISH OR CUT BAIT?

HIV either causes AIDS or it does not, and the answer must come from science—not politics! The reasons supporting HIV as the cause of AIDS are too numerous to list here, but many of those reasons are found in this chapter and in Chapter 10 (see HIV/AIDS statistics for Africa, pages 325–331).

In April 2002, President Mbeki began to distance himself from the AIDS dissidents. Mbeki decided to cut informal contact with them and communicate with them only when the advisory panel meets.

WHEN LIFE GIVES YOU LEMONS, THEY CAN'T BE USED TO TREAT AIDS!

In July 2003 the South African Cabinet instructed Health Minister Manto Tshabalala-Msimang, an AIDS dissident, to develop a plan to make antiretroviral drugs available to all HIV-infected people, and she did. But in 2005 the health minister told a National Conference on AIDS in South Africa that the nation should be focused on other diseases—cancer, diabetes, and other communicable diseases—not just AIDS. Also in 2005 she said, "Raw garlic and a skin of the lemon—not only do they give you a beautiful face and skin, but they also protect you from AIDS." In 2007 she repeated her stand that antiretroviral drugs are not the answer to treating people living with HIV or AIDS, nutrition is the answer. She advocates a diet of beetroot, garlic, lemon juice, and olive oil.

At the 2006 16th International AIDS Conference, 81 internationally renowned HIV/AIDS scientists petitioned President Mbeki for his health minister's resignation. His response was to appoint a committee to

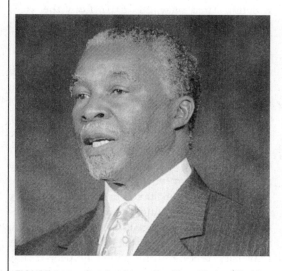

FIGURE 2-2 South African President Thabo Mbeki. In September 2003, Mbeki said he did not know anyone with HIV infection or AIDS. It is believed that members of his staff died of AIDS. In September 2008, Mbeki was forced to resign from his position and was replaced by Jacob Zuma as South Africa's fourth democratically elected president. *(Photograph © AP/World Photos.)*

oversee Tshabalala-Msimang's national HIV policy. And this committee set a five-year plan to prevent new HIV infections and the widespread use of anti-retroviral therapy. In August 2007 Mbeki fired his deputy health minister, Nozizwe Madlala-Routledge, who believes HIV causes AIDS.

In early 2008, after growing pressure from frustrated activists, the policy committee of the National Health Council ordered that South Africa's HIV-positive pregnant women would now have access to medication that could further reduce the risk of passing the virus to their babies. They are receiving the more effective dual therapy of zidovudine and nevirapine instead of a single antiretroviral treatment. In September 2008 along with Mbeki's resignation, his health minister Manto Tshabalala-Msimang was replaced by Barbara Hogan, who believes that HIV causes AIDS. Manto T-Msimang died in December 2009 from complications during a liver transplant. She was 69 years old.

A 2008 study by Harvard researchers estimates that Mbeki's South African government would have prevented the premature deaths of 365,000 people earlier in that decade if it had provided antiretroviral drugs to HIV/AIDS patients and widely administered drugs to help prevent pregnant women from infecting their babies. For a discussion/list of HIV/AIDS dissidents (denialists) who have died of AIDS, visit: AIDSTruth.org.

DISCUSSION QUESTION: What if you were president of a country in which 1 in 9 people were infected with a virus that you were told would kill them unless they were treated with exceptionally expensive medications that will always be outside the range of your healthcare system finances? Add to that a mandate from your country's constitution guaranteeing each citizen the right to health care. And, half its citizens, over 20 million, live below poverty level. And add to that the absolute need for clean water, decent highways, new schools, hospitals, fire departments, farming equipment, and many other services needed to run your country. What would you do? Might you search for a way to deny that HIV is a major factor in AIDS so that money saved could be better used elsewhere? Offer pro/con discussion.

Machanick will take drugs to prove they are not toxic. Under the agreement, Rasnick will inject himself with HIV on television and the two will meet annually to compare health status. It is doubtful that the action of this challenge will ever occur. Machanick is never going to get a doctor to prescribe him medication for a disease he doesn't have, and Rasnick stipulated that he be injected with a highly purified virus, a condition that is impossible to meet. Results, if any, will be offered after they occur.

NEWS FLASH 2010—LEADING HIV/AIDS DISSIDENT CLEARED OF MISCONDUCT FOLLOWING COMPLAINTS MADE AFTER HE AND OTHERS PUBLISHED A 2009 PAPER ARGUING THAT THERE IS "AS YET NO PROOF THAT HIV CAUSES AIDS"

Peter Duesberg escaped censure from the University of California, Berkeley, after an investigation upheld his academic freedom and found no clear evidence that he broke faculty rules in publishing the paper "HIV/AIDS hypothesis out of touch with South African AIDS—A new perspective." A letter dated May 28, 2010, from the vice-provost of academic affairs and faculty welfare to Duesberg effectively clears him of any wrongdoing. It states that there was "insufficient evidence" available to pursue any disciplinary action against him, although it stresses that the investigation was not concerned with the "accuracy or validity of the article." The publication of this paper led to a storm of protest from scientists. Retrospective peer review later led to its being permanently withdrawn. The journal's editor was fired and publisher Elsevier vowed to make changes to *Medical Hypothesis,* including peer review. Berkeley spokesman Robert Sanders said, "Academic freedom protects a professor's right to engage in scholarly research, even if it is controversial. The university relies on the scholarly peer-review process, rather than disciplinary procedures, for evaluating the value of scientific work."

UPDATE: In 2011, Duesberg's 2009 paper with minor adjustments was published in 2011 by the Italian *Journal of Anatomy and Embryology.* One member of the editorial board resigned and others said they would also resign because of this controversial publication in their journal.

DISSIDENTS' WEBSITES (AIDS DOESN'T EXIST OR HIV ISN'T THE CAUSE)

AIDS Denialists: How to Respond
www.aegis.org/pubs/atn/2000/atn34210.html
AIDS Dissident Web Ring (links to other websites)
http://e.webring.com/t/AIDS-MYTH-BUSTERS-WEBRING-Say-no-to-the-AIDS-lie
Alberta Reappraising AIDS Society
http://aras.ab.ca/index.php
Alive and Well—Alternative AIDS Information Network
www.aliveandwell.org
Answering the AIDS Denialists: CD4 (T-Cell) Counts, and Viral Load

www.aegis.com/pubs/atn/2000/ATN34102.html
Infectious AIDS: Have We Been Misled?
www.duesberg.com
Rethinking AIDS Website
www.virusmyth.net/aids/index.htm
The Scientific Evidence for HIV/AIDS
http://aidstruth.org
Survive AIDS!—ACT UP SF
http://actupsf.com

SUMMARY OF HIV/AIDS DISSIDENTS' VIEWPOINTS

People should be encouraged to question scientific orthodoxy. However, the views of AIDS dissidents, which have been well known for

---

SIDEBAR 2.1

SUPREME COURT OF SOUTH AUSTRALIA, JANUARY 2007

For the Defense

A medical physicist at Royal Perth Hospital, Eleni Papadopulos-Eleopulos, and emergency room doctor Val Turner gave testimony at the Supreme Court of South Australia during an appeal by a man convicted of exposing three women to HIV. Asked by the prosecutor whether "you would have unprotected vaginal sex with an HIV positive man," Ms. Papadopulos-Eleopulos replied "anytime." She and Val Turner were the lead expert witnesses for Andre Chad Parenzee, 35, who was convicted in February 2006 on three counts of having unprotected sex with three women despite knowing he was HIV positive. He infected one of them. His mother has spent $250,000 on her son's defense. Papadopulos-Eleopulos and Turner's key claim is that HIV has never been isolated and identified as a retrovirus, that HIV is the result of the misinterpretation of laboratory phenomena and experiment, and that HIV is not sexually transmitted or the cause of AIDS. Ms. Papadopulos-Eleopulos said AIDS is a disease that results from the oxidizing of the inside of the body and from repeated exposure to semen resulting from passive anal intercourse, and that HIV is not a virus and cannot be transmitted from one person to another during heterosexual sex.

The judge asked her to consider the good record of antiretroviral drugs in extending the lives of HIV/AIDS patients. He asked her, "Is it your evidence that it is a waste of resources to give antiretrovirals to pregnant women?" "Yes," she said.

For the Prosecution

The prosecutor asked seven eminent HIV/AIDS scientists to give rebuttal testimony. In short, all experts testified that the Perth group's testimony was wrong! One of the scientists who testified was Robert Gallo (Figure 1-2). Robert Gallo, along with Luc Montagnier (Figure 1-1), discovered HIV, and Gallo created a blood test for HIV in 1985. Robert Gallo said, "I can't believe that this case occupies the time of the court—it is absurd." He described the defense testimony as "beyond stupid, sad, deeply nonsensical, and extremely wrong." He suggested the defense witnesses, members of the HIV dissident study circle the Perth Group, were using the case as a ploy to advance their theories. He lost patience with defense lawyer Kevin Borick's provocative questioning of the accuracy of HIV tests. Gallo said, "You are driving me nuts with this . . . for God's sake." Gallo said, "No one knows more about HIV testing than me." Gallo said that his work had contributed to the cleansing of HIV from Australia's donor blood supply in the late 1980s. "I don't expect a thank you, but I don't expect to be provoked to that degree."

Conclusion:

The judge dismissed defense claims that HIV did not exist. Andre Chad Parenzee's appeal was dismissed. He was convicted on three counts of endangering life and was sentenced to nine years in prison.

many years and thoroughly debated in scientific journals, have failed to win support. The core arguments of the Perth Group (that HIV has not been isolated according to their own particular rules, and is therefore not conclusively [linked to/causative of] AIDS) and Dr. Duesberg (that no one fully understands how HIV causes AIDS) do not invalidate the wide range of evidence outlined in this section. The theory that HIV causes AIDS is compelling because it provides a simple, unique cause that consistently accounts for all of the observed phenomena.

EVIDENCE THAT HIV CAUSES AIDS

It has been firmly established that there is a high correlation between HIV infection and the development of AIDS. With respect to establishing HIV as the causative agent of AIDS, look at some of the evidence that concludes that HIV infection and AIDS are invariably linked in time, place, and population group.

1. The one common denominator is the presence of HIV within the entire range of people with this particular disease: individuals who are HIV positive over time will have symptoms of HIV disease. Individuals who are HIV negative will not.

2. The virus has been identified by electron microscopy inside and on the surface of T4 cells only in HIV-positive and AIDS patients.

3. Recent work by Bruce Patterson and Steven Wolinsky has shown that the genetic material of HIV (HIV DNA) can be found in as many as 1 in 10 blood lymphocytes of persons with HIV disease (Cohen, 1993).

4. Antibodies against the virus, viral antigens, and HIV-RNA are found only in HIV-positive and AIDS patients.

5. There is an absolute chronological association between the emergence of AIDS and the appearance of HIV in humans worldwide.

6. There is a chronological association of HIV-positive individuals who progress to AIDS. Significantly, in the years before AIDS, people with hemophilia had never been noted to be particularly susceptible to the more obvious fungal infections, such as candida esophagitis, common to AIDS patients and others with low-lymphocyte type immune deficiency. After 1984, this type of AIDS-associated opportunistic infection and immune failure rapidly became the single most common cause of death in people with hemophilia in America.

The rise in total mortality in people with hemophilia was sudden: Death in this population, which had been stable in 1982 and 1983, suddenly increased by a factor of approximately 900% in the first quarter of 1984. This increase was consistent with an epidemic, or some new very toxic contamination of the clotting factor supply. Mortality figures in hemophilia patients also showed something else important, that the new deaths of the late 1980s, by virtue of all being diagnosed with AIDS, demonstrated that most or all of them occurred in people with hemophilia who were HIV positive. Since these deaths accounted for almost the entire new increase in mortality, it could be inferred that the mortality rate for HIV-negative people with hemophilia did not increase much in the 1980s, if at all (Harris, 1995).

7. Hemophiliacs from low- and high-risk behavior groups were equally infected from HIV-contaminated blood factor VIII concentrates.

8. Studies of blood transfusion–acquired AIDS cases have repeatedly led to the discovery of HIV in the patient as well as in the blood donor.

9. With the exception of persons who had their immune systems suppressed due to genetic causes or by drug therapy, prior to the appearance of the virus, there were no known AIDS-like cases. The virus has been isolated worldwide—but only where there are HIV-positive people and AIDS patients.

10. An HIV-positive identical twin born to an HIV-positive mother developed AIDS, but the HIV-negative twin did not. (See *HIV and Molecular Immunity* by Omar Bagragra [1999].)

11. Only HIV-positive mothers transmit HIV into their fetuses and only these HIV-positive newborns progress to AIDS. HIV-negative newborns from HIV-positive mothers *do not get* AIDS!

12. Drugs developed specifically to inhibit the replication and/or maturation of HIV, thereby lowering the level of HIV found in HIV-infected people, have delayed the onset of HIV disease and, for HIV-infected pregnant women, have decreased the birth of HIV-infected infants in the USA by 90%.

13. In 2011, it was conclusively demonstrated that tha use of certain antiretroviral drugs would **prevent** the transmission of HIV in heterosexual couples where one of the pair was HIV positive!

14. If HIV does not cause AIDS, how do HIV dissenters explain the positive effects of drugs used to affect the early and late stages in the life cycle of HIV that have lowered viral load to unmeasurable levels in the blood? And what of those with HIV disease and AIDS who have been virtually restored to life and who are now back at work? Or, how do they explain the positive effects offered by HIV phenotype- and genotype-resistant drug testing?

15. The long list of denialists who have died from AIDS (posted on AIDStruth.org) contrasts with the fact that not one of the HIV-negative denialist leaders has died young, let alone with multiple strange infections that happen to be AIDS-defining.

16. Finally, there have been numerous reports in the literature on HIV-infected individuals (homosexual, bisexual, and heterosexual) transmitting the virus to their sexual partners and both eventually dying of AIDS. *The unbroken chain of HIV transmission between prostitutes and their customers, between injection-drug users sharing the same syringe, from infected mothers to their unborn fetuses, and so on all lead to the inescapable conclusion that HIV does cause AIDS.*

In short, Koch's postulates have been satisfied: HIV disease meets all four criteria.

1. The causative agent must be found in all cases of the disease. (It is.)

2. It must be isolated from the host and grown in pure culture. (It was.)

3. It must reproduce the original disease when introduced into a susceptible host. (It does.)

4. It must be found in the experimental host so infected. (It is.)

In summary, HIV is the singular common factor that is shared between AIDS cases in gay men in San Francisco, well-nourished young women in Uganda, hemophiliacs in Japan, and children in Romanian orphanages. The identification of HIV as the causative agent of AIDS is now firmly accepted by scientists worldwide.

The HIV/AIDS Surveillance Report, CDC, *MMWR* 1999; 48 (RR13): 1 provides abundant evidence that HIV causes AIDS. Questions and Answers at the end of this document address the specific claims of those who assert that HIV is not the cause of AIDS.

The Durban Declaration Admonishes HIV Dissidents—A statement signed by over 5000 HIV/AIDS scientists and physicians from 50 countries and five continents was released to the press on July 1, 2000 (www.nature.com). Their statement that HIV causes AIDS is their answer to those who believe otherwise. They believe the evidence that HIV causes AIDS is clear, concise, exhaustive, and unambiguous. To conquer AIDS, everyone must understand that HIV is the enemy. (The Durban Declaration can be found at www.eurakalert.org/releases/hte-uncc063000.html. The evidence that HIV causes AIDS can be found at www.thebody.com/niaid/hivcauseaids.html.)

In short, the dissidents' belief is an example of a myth masquerading as a topic for discussion. The vast majority of HIV/AIDS scientists and medical personnel may feel as George Orwell stated in his book *1984,* "What can you do against the lunatic . . . who gives your arguments a fair hearing and then simply persists in his lunacy?" *HIV DOES CAUSE AIDS!*

DISCUSSION QUESTION: You have just read some of the evidence for and against HIV being the cause of AIDS. Assuming you agree with the vast majority of HIV/AIDS investigators worldwide that HIV does cause AIDS, do you think there comes a time at which dissenters should forfeit their right to make claims on other people's time and trouble by the poverty of their arguments and by the wasted effort and exasperation they have caused?
NOW discuss the value of the dissenter.
NOW discuss the danger of the dissenter's information or claims.

ORIGIN OF HIV: THE AIDS VIRUS

Clarification of the Term "Origin of HIV"

Scientists are searching for the source of HIV or HIV-like ancestor. Finding this source will give us the origin of HIV as it pertains to where and in which animal the virus was housed prior to entering humans. But it does not mean the beginning of the virus per se—that will most likely never be known.

Tracking the origins and early history of a newly recognized disease is more than just an academic exercise. Unless we understand where HIV came from, we run the risk of new emergencies, and unless we understand the ecology that allowed it to spread, we will be unable to control newly identified diseases. A classic example of tracking a source of a disease and the local epidemic it caused is John Snow's investigation of the cholera epidemic in Golden Square, London, in 1854; his removal of the handle of the Board Street pump contained the outbreak.

Cholera is caused by a spiral-shaped microorganism called *vibrio cholerae,* which is carried in the cholera-infected person's feces and is transmitted to others via *vibrio cholerae*–contaminated water or food. Removing the handle from the pump stopped people from drinking or using the contaminated water.

More than virtually any other disease, HIV/AIDS has generated myths and far-fetched theories about its origin, its causes, and even its very existence. These are probably linked to fear and denial prompted by a virus that is fatal, incurable, and sexually transmitted—and can infect people for years before they show any signs of illness.

Why Do Scientists Want to Know Where HIV Originated?

The object of determining the origin of the AIDS virus is to gain insight into how the virus may have evolved the unique set of characteristics that enable it to destroy the human immune system. Such information will offer valuable clues as to how rapidly the virus is evolving and how to combat it and perhaps help prevent future viral plagues. Also, it has offered scientists new and novel insights into the functions of the human immune system.

In the modern era of diseases like the bird flu (avian influenza), Ebola (a hemorrhagic virus), SARS (severe acute respiratory syndrome), and the 2009 swine flu (H1N1 virus) outbreak, the question of what launches new epidemics and pandemics is extremely important. The somewhat shocking answer is that we actually know nothing about the factors that launch animal viruses into epidemics or pandemics. Equally important is the question of why most animal viruses fail to launch sustained human-to-human transmission. These are critically important questions that are being bypassed.

Is HIV a New or Old Virus?

The terms "new" and "old" are relative to time and age. Viruses known, say, less than 50 years are generally considered new. Whether a virus is considered new or old is of considerable importance.

If, for example, HIV is a new virus, say less than 40 years old, the many different varieties of HIV now infecting people worldwide probably evolved from a common ancestor sometime after World War II. New varieties can be expected to continue evolving at a frightening pace for several more decades, possibly producing new strains of the virus that are even more dangerous than those now infecting people. This could mean that vaccines now being developed based on current virus strains may not be useful in 10 to 20 years. But, should the known strains of the virus prove to be hundreds or thousands of years old, it might be possible that the current types of HIV are in a state of global balance, and most likely they would not offer scientists any shocking evolutionary surprises in the future.

Some Ideas on the Origin of HIV: UFOs, Biological Warfare, Cats, and Other Ideas

UFOs—Fear stimulates the imagination. Out of human fear have come some rather strange explanations for the origin of the HIV. Early reports had unidentified flying objects (UFOs) crashing to Earth and releasing a "new organism" that would wipe out humanity.

Biological Warfare—There were frequent reports in the Soviet press linking HIV and AIDS with American biological warfare research. The Soviets agreed in August 1987 to stop these reports (Holder, 1988).

Ethnic Cleansing: Conspiracy Beliefs—There are also reports of extremism, as in the case of Illinois State Representative Douglas Huff of Chicago who told the *Los Angeles Times* that he gave over $500 from his office allowance fund to a local official of the Black Hebrew sect to help the group investigate its claim that Israel and South Africa created HIV in a laboratory in South Africa. Huff said AIDS is "clearly an ethnic weapon, a biological weapon" designed specifically to attack nonwhites (*CDC Weekly,* 1988). Kenyan ecologist and 2004 Nobel Prize Winner Wangari Maathai said in 2004 that HIV was created by scientists "for the purpose of mass extermination. We know that developed nations are using biological warfare, leaving guns to primitive people. AIDS is not a curse from God to Africans or the black people. It is a tool to control them designed by some evil-minded scientists." A few days after this statement, in another interview, she said "HIV was deliberately devised to destroy black people."

In January 2005, according to results of a study released by the RAND Corporation and Oregon State University, nearly half of 500 black Americans ages 15 to 44 responding to a telephone survey said they believe that HIV is man-made, with approximately 12% saying they believe HIV was created and spread by the CIA and nearly 27% saying that AIDS was produced in a government laboratory. In addition, about 16% of respondents agreed that the government created HIV to control the black population, and about 15% agreed with a statement saying that AIDS is a form of genocide against African Americans. Over half, 53.4%, said they believed that there is a cure for AIDS but it is being withheld from the poor (Bogart et al., 2005).

Domestic Cats—Still another myth to surface is that the AIDS virus came from domestic cats. Because of its similarities to human AIDS, Feline Immunodeficiency Virus has been called "feline AIDS." The cat retrovirus may damage cats'

POINT OF INFORMATION 2.1

SCIENTISTS REPORT ON EARLIEST AIDS CASES: A DETECTIVE STORY IN THE MAKING. OLD SPECIMENS AND MODERN-DAY ANALYSIS

The first recorded AIDS case in America was that of a 15-year-old male prostitute who demonstrated Kaposi's sarcoma and died in 1969. Frozen tissue samples contained HIV antibodies. These findings were reported at the Eleventh International Congress of Virology in August 1999.

The first documented case of AIDS in Europe was seen in a Danish surgeon who had worked in Zaire. She died in 1976.

The first documented case of AIDS in Africa occurred in 1959. The second case was documented in 1960. Both people lived in the same city, Leopoldville, now known as Kinshasa.

Some Information on the Two African Cases

The scientists looked for signs of HIV in 1213 blood samples that were gathered in Africa between 1959 and 1982. They found clear signs of the virus in one taken from a Bantu man who lived in Leopoldville, Belgian Congo, Republic of Congo—in 1959. Scientists compared the genes from the 39-year-old sample of HIV with current versions of HIV. They realized that if they had an old sequence of HIV genes it would serve as

a yardstick to measure the evolution of the current HIV. HIV has mutated over the years to form 11 distinct subtypes, lettered A through K. One of these, subtype B, is the dominant strain in the United States and Europe, while subtype D is most common in Africa. The family tree of HIV looks like a bush with the various subtypes forming the limbs. Scientists believe the 1959 HIV is near the trunk, around the point where the subtypes B and D branch off, and that this virus is an ancestor to B and D. These data suggest that all HIV subtypes evolved from one introduction of HIV into people, rather than from many crossovers from animals to humans, as some have speculated. In 1960, a paraffin block containing lymph node tissue from a 28-year-old woman was found to contain HIV. The HIV samples taken from the man (1959) and the woman (1960) differed in their genetic material by 12%. That is very important information because it shows that these two people carried two different circulating subtypes of HIV! Scientists calculated that the virus took at least 50 years to evolve into these two different subtypes. These data clearly suggest that HIV was evolving in humans in the Congo for many years before 1959 and 1960.

immune systems, leaving the animals vulnerable to opportunistic infections *or* it may cause feline leukemia. However, the cat virus has never been shown to cause a disease in humans.

Other Ideas—The origin of HIV has been attributed to HIV-contaminated polio, smallpox, hepatitis, and tetanus vaccines; the African green monkey; African people; their cattle, pigs, and sheep—and the CIA. With respect to the use of HIV-contaminated vaccines, a number of articles suggest that early monkey kidney cultures used to produce the polio vaccine carried HIV. Review of the literature offers *no* evidence that this occurred. The argument for the safety of the polio vaccine lies in the absence of any AIDS-related diseases among the hundreds of millions of persons vaccinated worldwide (Hooper, 1999; Koprowski, 1992).

The Mystery Continues

The origin of HIV remains a mystery and may never be proven to everyone's satisfaction. Some of the scientific theories include the introduction of HIV into humans through (a) the use of HIV-contaminated polio vaccine from the late 1950s into the early 1960s, or (b) the worldwide introduction of disposable plastic syringes that were used and reused and reused until they were too short and blunt for sharpening. This means that serial passing of a precursor virus to HIV could change through the use of unsterilized needles and syringes into HIV. There is also (c) the cut hunter theory where the virus, e.g., SIVcpz (the theoretical precursor to HIV), would have a natural transfer via the handling of blood or chimpanzee tissue and body parts during the slaughter of these animals.

For many scientists, regardless of theory, there is still something missing, an explanation of how SIV (Simian Immunodeficiency Virus), a harmless infection in humans for perhaps thousands of years, suddenly becomes HIV and lethal. There is no evidence that people contract HIV or AIDS from monkeys (HIV-2) or chimpanzees (HIV-1). And SIV, in general, does not cause *an* AIDS-like illness in monkeys or chimpanzees. There is the possibility

that an SIV/HIV evolving hybrid remained in the human population for hundreds if not thousands of years until such time that the final genetic transformation or evolution of SIV into HIV occurred. After all, humans have hunted, handled, and eaten primates for thousands of years. Recent laboratory accidents have shown that SIV can infect humans. Even though at the moment no identifiable disease has been associated with the SIV/human infections, such accidents have demonstrated the potential for cross-species or zoonotic (acquired from a vertebrate animal) transmission of HIV-related viruses. Why not believe the same for the origin of HIV-1?

That being said, some of the current scientific ideas on the origin of HIV are presented. The answer to the origin of HIV is important because scientists have no idea what it takes to launch animal viruses into human epidemics or pandemics. And the occurrence of other viral human epidemics and pandemics is only a matter of time as the world waits for the next avian flu or SARS epidemic/pandemic.

Some Scientific Ideas on the Origin of HIV

Vanessa Hirsch and colleagues (1995) presented evidence that a virus isolated from a species of West African monkey, the sooty mangabey (an ash-colored monkey), may have infected humans 20 to 30 years ago. They believe this virus subsequently evolved into HIV-2. Hirsch et al. studied a virus known as the Simian Immunodeficiency Virus (SIV) that infects both wild and captive sooty mangabey monkeys (SIVsm). They molecularly cloned and sequenced the DNA of the virus and constructed an evolutionary tree of the several known primate immunodeficiency viruses. This tree showed SIVsm to be more closely related to HIV-2 than to HIV-1.

Gerald Myers of Los Alamos National Laboratory states that SIVsm and HIV are so closely related that when HIV-2 is found in a human, it may be the sooty mangabey virus. However, HIV-1 does not sufficiently resemble HIV-2 or SIVsm, thus HIV-1 probably did not evolve from SIVsm/HIV-2. The prevailing theory for

HIV-1 is that humans were first infected with HIV-1 through direct contact with precursor HIV-infected chimpanzees. The chimpanzee-to-human scenario is easier to accept than humans infecting chimpanzees.

Be a Virus, See the World

Albert Osterhaus of Erasmus University Rotterdam, The Netherlands, believes that *all* human viral infectious diseases ultimately have an animal origin, and natural transfer of these infections is a common event in animal populations.

The Current Theory on HIV Origin: A Chimpanzee (cpz)

Beatrice Hahn and colleagues (1999; 2000; 2003; 2006; 2011) from the University of Alabama at Birmingham say they have gathered sufficient evidence to believe the origin of HIV-1 in humans to be a cross-species transmission from a particular subspecies of chimpanzee— meaning that a simian virus closely related to HIV moved from chimpanzees to humans, and later mutated into its current form (Figure 2-3).

Hahn presented three lines of evidence in support of their thesis. First, the genes of **SIVcpz** isolates cluster on evolutionary trees according to their chimpanzee subspecies or origin, either *Pan troglodytes troglodytes* from West Africa or *Pan troglodytes schweinfurthii* in East Africa. By sequencing parts of the virus's genetic material, the scientists found that more segments of the simian and human virus overlapped than had been identified in three previous simian viruses isolated in recent years from other chimpanzees.

Second, all known HIV-1 strains, including the M group that accounts for about 99% of all HIV-1 infections, as well as the O group and the N group, form a genetic cluster with the West African chimpanzee viruses. This clustering is also geographic and consistent with the likely equatorial Central African origin of HIV-1 (Figure 2-4). Hahn said she had initially been equally ready to accept the idea that chimps had gotten HIV from humans, rather than vice versa. However, a third line of evidence convinced her that HIV-1

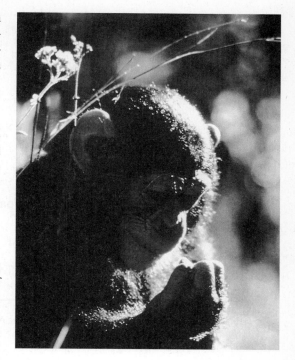

FIGURE 2-3 Photograph of *Pan troglodytes troglodytes.* This photograph was taken in the Gabon region of Africa where the sole species of *Pan troglodytes* is found. Their numbers are declining rapidly due to the "bush meat" trade—their slaughter and selling of their body parts. *(Photograph courtesy of Karl Ammann, wildlife photographer.)*

was introduced into the human population from at least three cross-species transmissions from chimpanzees—she found evidence of genetic recombination among the SIVcpz strains of the *troglodytes'* lineage.

In addition, scientists in the United States found evidence in chimpanzees that SIVcpz is found in East Africa as well as West Africa, suggesting that not only is the virus widely distributed in Africa, but continued hunting of the species for food and keeping the animals as pets could result in another outbreak of an AIDS-like disease. These data document, for the first time, that humans are continuously exposed to an unprecedented variety of SIVs through the consumption of bush meat (Santiago et al., 2002; Peeters et al., 2002; Kalish et al., 2005).

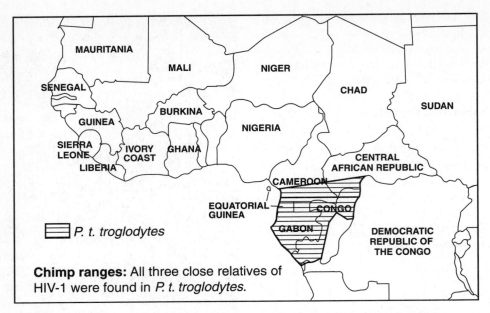

MAURITANIA
MALI
NIGER
SENEGAL
CHAD
SUDAN
BURKINA
GUINEA
NIGERIA
SIERRA LEONE
IVORY COAST
GHANA
LIBERIA
CENTRAL AFRICAN REPUBLIC
CAMEROON
EQUATORIAL GUINEA
CONGO
GABON
DEMOCRATIC REPUBLIC OF THE CONGO

P. t. troglodytes

Chimp ranges: All three close relatives of HIV-1 were found in *P. t. troglodytes*.

FIGURE 2–4 Geographic ranges of one subspecies of chimpanzee *Pan troglodytes*. (Adapted from Hahn, 1999.)

The question that remains is, where did SIVcpz come from?

In mid-2006, Hahn and colleagues reported on their detection of SIVcpz antibodies and nucleic acids in fecal samples from wild-living *P.t. troglodytes* apes in southern Cameroon, where prevalence rates in some *troglodytes* communities reached 29% to 35%. By sequence analysis of the endemic SIVcpz strains, they traced the origins of pandemic (group M) and non-pandemic (group N) HIV-1 to distinct, geographically isolated chimpanzee communities. These findings establish *P.t. troglodytes* as the natural reservoir of HIV. Hahn said, "Chimpanzees acquired their infections like humans did, by hunting and consuming naturally infected primates." The authors of the study also postulate that "given the extensive genetic diversity and phylogeographical clustering of SIVcpz now recognized, and the vast areas of west central Africa not yet sampled, it is quite possible that still other SIVcpz lineages exist that could pose risks for human infection and prove problematic

for HIV diagnostics and vaccines." This study, "Chimpanzee Reservoirs of Pandemic and Non-pandemic HIV-1," was published in the *Science* journal, website at Science Express (doi. 10.1126/ science. 1126531).

UPDATE 2012: Paul Sharp and Beatrice Hahn stated that acquired immunodeficiency syndrome (AIDS) of humans is caused by two lentiviruses, human immunodeficiency viruses types 1 and 2 (HIV-1 and HIV-2). They described the origins and evolution of these viruses, and the circumstances that led to the AIDS pandemic. They suggest that both HIVs are the results of multiple cross-species transmissions of simian immunodeficiency viruses (SIVs) naturally infecting African primates. And that these transfers resulted in viruses that spread in humans to only a limited extent. However, one transmission event, involving SIVcpz from chimpanzees in southeastern Cameroon, gave rise to HIV-1 group M—the principal cause of the AIDS pandemic. They discussed how host restriction factors have shaped the emergence of new HV zoonoses by imposing adaptive hurdles to cross-species transmission and/or secondary spread. They also show that AIDS has likely afflicted chimpanzees long before the emergence of HIV. Tracing the genetic changes that occurred as SIVs crossed from monkeys to apes and from apes to humans provides a new framework to examine the requirements of successful host switches and to gauge future zoonotic risk (Sharp and Hahn, 2012).

Is the Search for the Origin of HIV Over?

It is nice to think that the issue of HIV's origin has been solved. However, time will tell if Hahn's current effort will be the final word on the subject. Some questions still remain. Why, for example, does HIV-1 appear to be so benign in chimpanzees, as has been shown in numerous infection experiments over the years? For scientists, the new chimpanzee finding is just as much a beginning as an end. Although researchers may have the best evidence so far that HIV came from chimpanzees, no one can yet say how the virus became lethal to humans. Chimpanzees share over 98% of the genes that exist in humans, yet they don't generally express AIDS. So which of the remaining genes protect chimpanzees from an infection that has turned out to be almost universally fatal in people? Also, researchers are still investigating how, after taking root in just a few people, HIV gradually traveled all over the world.

How Often Did SIVcpz Cross Over into Humans?—Researchers now believe that AIDS-like viruses moved from chimp to human more than once, creating different strains of HIV. This means a vaccine against one strain of HIV may not control a new epidemic. As it turned out, *Pan troglodytes troglodytes* live in the region of Africa where HIV-1 was first recognized. Since there are four separate groups of HIV-1 (M, O, N and P), the scientists believe that HIV-1 crossed into people from chimps at least four times. Hahn said that SIV appears to have dwelled in primates for hundreds of thousands of years

before turning into the deadly human virus, HIV. Hahn believes hunting, which exposes people to excessive amounts of blood during slaughter, allowed precursor HIV to infect humans.

Why Do Chimpanzees Generally Resist HIV Infection?—With regard to the question of why chimpanzees resist HIV infection, in late 2002 Dutch investigators presented a theory that an AIDS-like epidemic killed large populations of chimps about 2 million years ago. The survivors of this viral (SIVcpz-like?) eradication were selected for survival because they carried the genes necessary to resist the viral infection. Over the years, this genetic selection gave rise to chimpanzees that are generally resistant to viruses closely related to HIV, for example SIVcpz and HIV itself.

DISCUSSION QUESTION: **If humans become infected with SIVcpz from chimpanzees, where or how did the chimpanzees get SIVcpz? Elizabeth Bailes and colleagues (2003) believe that SIV-infected monkeys gave rise to SIVcpz through monkey-to-monkey cross-species SIV transmission and recombination among slightly genetically different SIV to produce SIVcpz. Because chimpanzees feed on these monkeys, they become SIVcpz-infected, much like humans who consumed the SIVcpz-infected chimpanzees. Thus, chimpanzees and humans acquired their versions of the pre-HIV virus the same way—by killing and eating animals infected with similar viruses.**

Where Did HIV Begin to Circulate among Humans?—According to Nicole Vidal and colleagues (2000), because of the unprecedented degree of HIV-1 group M genetic diversity found in the Democratic Republic of Congo (9 of the 11 different group M subtypes), the HIV-1 pandemic must have originated in Central Africa.

Daniel Vangroenweghe (2001) states that the earliest cases of HIV infection and AIDS in the 1960s and 1970s occurred in Congo-Kinshasa (Zaire), Rwanda, and Burundi. These countries appear to be the source of the HIV group M epidemic, which then spread outward to

UPDATE ON THE ORIGIN OF HIV AND THE AIDS PANDEMIC ACCORDING TO PAUL SHARP AND BEATRICE HAHN, 2011

Acquired immunodeficiency syndrome (AIDS) of humans is caused by two lentiviruses, human immunodeficiency viruses types 1 and 2 (HIV-1 and HIV-2). Sharp and Hahn describe the origins and evolution of these viruses and the circumstances that led to the AIDS pandemic. Both HIVs are the result of multiple cross-species transmissions of simian immunodeficiency viruses (SIVs) naturally infecting African primates. Most of these transfers resulted in viruses that spread in humans to only a limited extent. However, one transmission event, involving SIVcpz from chimpanzees in southeastern Cameroon, gave rise to HIV-1 group M—the principal cause of the AIDS pandemic. Those authors discussed how host restriction factors have shaped the emergence of new SHIV zoonoses (an infection shared by humans and lower vertebrate animals) by imposing adaptive hurdles to cross-species transmission and/or secondary spread. They also show that AIDS has likely afflicted chimpanzees long before the emergence of HIV. Tracing the genetic changes that occurred as SIVs crossed from monkeys to apes and from apes to humans provides a new framework to examine the requirements of successful hot switches and to gauge future zoonotic risk. This genetic analysis helps explain the sudden emergence of HIV, its epidemic spread, and its uniqueness as a pathogen (this publication makes for fascinating reading). Lentiviruses cause chronic persistent infection in cats, horses, sheep, cows, and primates but only a few are endogenous, meaning transmitted vertically because they have infiltrated the host germ line. Simian immunodeficiency viruses

(SIV) are found in over 40 primate species, clustering within species. Some cross-species transmission occurs with chimpanzees likely infected through hunting and killing other mammals, including monkeys. A chimpanzee somehow infected a gorilla between 100 and 200 years ago, despite the fact that gorillas are vegetarians (herbivores), but it is not known if gorillas infected with HIVgor become ill as a result of the infection. As for humans, each of the 4 HIV-1 groups (M, N, O, and P) resulted from an independent cross-species transmission event, most likely through bush meat hunting. Group M is the pandemic from of HIV-1 that originated in southeastern Cameroon; Group O accounts for less than 1% and is found in Cameroon, Gabon, and neighboring countries; only 13 people with Group N have been identified (all from Cameroon); and only two people are known to have Group P (also from Cameroon). All four groups are all of chimpanzee origin originally, but P came to humans via gorillas, and O could be either chimp or gorilla in origin. Travel and commerce provided the link between the chimpanzee HIV-1 Group M reservoir in southeastern Cameroon and Loepoldville (current day Kinshasa) on the banks of the Congo River where early diversification of Group M in humans occurred. By 1959–1960 sub-types had appeared and today, in this region, there are nine sub-types (A-D, F-H, J, and K) and more than 40 circulating recombinant forms of HIV-1. Chronic immune activation, with increased HIV replication provides the stage for HIV's error-prone reverse transcriptase to accumulate mutations, which means that continued evolution of HIV is likely.

neighboring Tanzania and Uganda in the east, and Congo-Brazzaville in the west. Then it spread to Haiti. Hundreds of single men from Haiti participated in the UNESCO educational program in the Congo between 1960 and 1975, and it is believed that they returned to Haiti infected with HIV.

Do We Know How HIV Got into the United States?—Michael Worobey said at the March 2007 Fourteenth Conference on Retroviruses and Opportunistic Infections (CROI) that Haiti has the oldest HIV epidemic outside Africa and

provided the source for the strain of HIV seen in North America and Europe. Worobey said that an international team of researchers found that the type of HIV most prevalent in Haiti, the United States, and Europe—HIV-1 group M, subtype B—moved from Africa to Haiti around 1966. HIV spread around Haiti before a single migration of the virus took it out of Haiti to the United States by 1969 and then worldwide between 1969 and 1972. The research also suggests that HIV-1 group M originated comparatively recently, probably no earlier than the early 20th century (Worobey et al., 2007).

The exact circumstances surrounding the emergence of the strain of HIV in the United States and Europe have long been the subject of debate. Investigators from the United States, Denmark, and the United Kingdom recovered complete HIV-1 envelope (env) gene sequences from samples obtained from five Haitian AIDS patients between 1982 and 1983 who were recent migrants to the United States. To test the hypothesis that subtype B has a Haitian origin, they conducted phylogenetic analysis of samples obtained from these patients and of a further 117 samples obtained from patients in 19 different countries using the analysis of the group specific antigen (gag) gene sequence from the different viral samples. A U.S. or non–Haitian origin for subtype B was strongly rejected in favor of a Haitian origin.

When Did HIV Begin to Circulate among Humans?—Scientists do have some idea when the virus began to circulate among people. From looking at samples of HIV taken at different times and in different parts of the world, researchers have constructed a type of genetic clock for HIV-1. The speed of the clock is determined by how much the virus changes over time. A key to setting this clock came with the discovery of the two oldest known HIV infections, one found in 1959 in a man, the other in a woman in 1960 who lived in what is now Congo. After the AIDS epidemic began, both frozen samples were thawed and screened for the presence of HIV. In 2008 Michael Worobey and colleagues compared the genetic data from the older HIV with samples from newer HIV. They concluded that HIV has been circulating in humans since sometime between 1884 and 1924 (Worobey et al., 2008; Sharp et al., 2008)!

2010 information published by Michael Worobey and colleagues states that a common ancestor to all HIV strains existed between 32,000 and 78,000 years ago. But, that ancestor virus may have existed for millions of years!

Continued Evolution of HIV in Humans?—Possible *good* news (?) is that HIV would, after killing millions of humans, become a harmless

---

passenger as most likely its precursor SIV did thousands of years ago in chimpanzees. The bad news would be that HIV is evolving into a virus that is more easily spread and/or becomes more lethal. Time will tell.

SUMMARY ON THE ORIGIN OF HIV

In summary, there are at least three ideas on the possible origins of the AIDS virus: (1) It is a human-made virus, perhaps from a germ warfare laboratory; (2) it originated in the animal world and crossed over into humans; and (3) HIV has existed in small, isolated human populations for a long time and, given the right set of conditions, it escaped into the larger population. Computer modeling of DNA sequence in HIV and SIVsm and the recent work of Beatrice Hahn and colleagues suggests that HIV evolved within the last 100 to 300 years. So for now, the question remains: Is AIDS a new disease or an old disease that was late being recognized—so late that we will never know its true source, the origin of HIV? Continued investigations may answer these questions.

Has HIV Always Caused a Lethal Disease—AIDS?

An additional question to where HIV came from is whether it has always caused disease. From the study of human history, as it relates to human disease, scientists have numerous examples that show that as human habits change, new diseases emerge. Regardless of whether HIV is old or new, history will show that social changes, however small or sudden, have most likely hastened the spread of HIV. Increased rounds of HIV replication presented humans with new HIV mutations, some of which were to become lethal. In the 1960s, war, tourism, and commercial trucking forced the outside world on Africa's once isolated villages. At the same time, drought and industrialization prompted mass migrations from the countryside into newly teeming cities. Western monogamy had never been common in Africa, but as the French medical historian Mirko Grmek notes in his book, *History of AIDS* (1990), urbanization shattered social structures that had long contained sexual behavior. Prostitution exploded, and venereal diseases flourished. Hypodermic needles came into wide use during the same period, creating yet another mode of infection. Did these trends actually turn a chronic but relatively benign infection into a killer? The evidence is circumstantial, but it's hard to discount.

Summary

The AIDS virus was discovered and reported by Luc Montagnier and Francoise Barre-Sinoussi of France in 1983. Identifying the virus that caused the immuno-suppression that caused AIDS allowed for AIDS surveillance definitions that began in 1982. The recent recognition of non-HIV AIDS cases is not unexpected and can be explained. Presently, there is no new threat of another AIDS-causing biological agent.

The recent work of Beatrice Hahn and colleagues may have pinpointed the reservoir of a precursor HIV-like virus in the chimpanzee, *Pan troglodytes troglodytes.*

HIV was transported into the United States in the early 1970s by men who became HIV infected while working in the Congo.

Review Questions

(Answers to the Review Questions are on page 463.)

1. What may be the strongest evidence for saying that AIDS is caused by HIV?

2. Where did HIV originate and where did the first HIV infections appear?

3. Those who do not believe HIV causes AIDS are referred to as _____.

4. Name the woman (mother) who did not believe HIV causes AIDS, and name her 3-year-old daughter who is said to have died from AIDS.

5. Name the scientist who is the leading advocate of the idea that HIV does not cause AIDS.

6. The former president of South Africa who denied that HIV causes AIDS is _____.

7. Have Koch's postulates been satisfied in the laboratory under defined conditions that HIV is the causative agent of AIDS? Explain.

8. Is HIV a new or old virus?

9. Is it HIV or SIV that causes a disease in chimpanzees?

10. Name the scientist who appears to have the best evidence that HIV is a new virus and crossed from an animal into humans.

11. In what country was the first currently documented case of HIV infection found, and in what year?

Biological Characteristics of HIV

- HIV contains nine genes; its three major structural genes are GAG-POL-ENV.
- HIV contains 9,749 nucleotides, its genetic code.
- Six HIV genes regulate HIV reproduction, and at least one gene directly influences infection.
- HIV-RNA produces HIV DNA, which integrates into the host cell to become proviral DNA.
- Genome-wide scan reveals 273 human proteins that HIV uses to complete its life cycle.
- HIV undergoes rapid genetic changes in infected people.
- The reverse transcriptase enzyme is very error prone.
- HIV causes immunological suppression by destroying T4 helper or CD4+ cells.
- HIV is classified into major (M), outlier (O), and new (N) genetic subtypes. Type M is responsible for 99% of HIV infections worldwide.
- A fourth HIV group was identified in 2009, group P.

VIRUSES NEED A HOST CELL IN ORDER TO REPLICATE

Viruses are microscopic particles of biological material, so small they can be seen only with electron microscopes. A virus consists solely of a strip of genetic material (nucleic acid) within a protein coat.

Viral genomes (DNA and RNA that contain the genetic information to replicate) are very small and contain few genes compared to living cells. With their limited coding capacity, viruses must enter host cells and must borrow or hijack cellular proteins to complete their replication—to make more of themselves. In other words, a virus is *not* a self-sufficient living cell capable of cell division to reproduce like bacteria or other single-celled or multiple-celled organisms.

VIRUSES ARE PARASITES

Viruses are parasitic agents; they live inside the cells of their host animal or plant, and can reproduce themselves *only by forcing the host cell to make viral copies.* The new virus leaves the host cell and infects other similar cells. By damaging or killing these cells, some viruses cause diseases in the host animal or plant. Many viruses that infect humans are never eradicated. Examples of viruses that persist for the life of the individual include *herpes simplex* virus, cytomegalovirus, Epstein-Barr virus, and *varicella zoster* virus. These viruses typically do not cause progressive disease but are held in check by a protective immune response. Genetically, viruses are the simplest forms of "life-like agents"; the genetic blueprint for the structure of the **Human Immunodeficiency Virus (HIV)** is 100,000 times smaller than that contained in a human cell. The complete sequence of 9,749 nucleotides that form the genetic code for HIV have been identified and their arrangement sequenced—placed in their given order (mapped).

In 2009, Joseph Watts and colleagues reported on the entire HIV-RNA genome, or HIV's genetic code nucleotide by nucleotide—all 9,749 of them! This RNA single nucleotide resolution is key to unlocking the many roles of HIV-RNA in its life cycle and the life cycle of other RNA viruses. To understand the tricks of which

HIV-RNA is capable, such as how HIV escapes detection by the human immune system, scientists are asking the following question: If they cause mutations or changes in the HIV-RNA at a given nucleotide, what will happen? Will it be an important mutation, to slow or stop HIV replication and, if so, how? Answers to such questions will be important to new drug research as well as in the search for an effective vaccine.

Scientists have produced a great deal of information about HIV over a relatively short time. In the history of medical science, the immediate involvement of so many scientists followed by the rapid identification of the causative agent of AIDS is equaled only by the rapid identification of the SARS (severe acute respiratory syndrome) virus in 2003. More is known about

HIV than about the viruses that cause such long-standing human diseases as polio, measles, yellow fever, hepatitis, flu, and the common cold. Humankind is fortunate that HIV began spreading through the human population as a pathogen in the mid- to late-1970s. By then scientists had discovered and begun to exploit the molecular aspects of biology. Molecular methodologies necessary to begin the immediate molecular study of HIV were in place to define and refine our knowledge of viruses and, in particular, to learn about HIV. (See Figure 3-1.)

VIRUSES SPECIFIC TO CELL TYPE

1. Viruses are very specific with regard to the types of cells they can enter/reproduce.

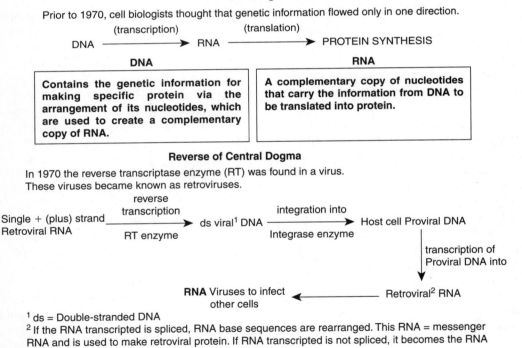

Central Dogma

Prior to 1970, cell biologists thought that genetic information flowed only in one direction.

$$\text{DNA} \xrightarrow{\text{(transcription)}} \text{RNA} \xrightarrow{\text{(translation)}} \text{PROTEIN SYNTHESIS}$$

DNA	**RNA**
Contains the genetic information for making specific protein via the arrangement of its nucleotides, which are used to create a complementary copy of RNA.	A complementary copy of nucleotides that carry the information from DNA to be translated into protein.

Reverse of Central Dogma

In 1970 the reverse transcriptase enzyme (RT) was found in a virus. These viruses became known as retroviruses.

Single + (plus) strand Retroviral RNA →(reverse transcription / RT enzyme)→ ds viral[1] DNA →(integration into / Integrase enzyme)→ Host cell Proviral DNA →(transcription of Proviral DNA into)→ Retroviral[2] RNA → **RNA** Viruses to infect other cells

[1] ds = Double-stranded DNA
[2] If the RNA transcripted is spliced, RNA base sequences are rearranged. This RNA = messenger RNA and is used to make retroviral protein. If RNA transcripted is not spliced, it becomes the RNA genome of the new virus.

FIGURE 3-1   Retroviral Flow of Genetic Information. The general directional flow of genetic information in all living species is from DNA, where the information is stored, into RNA, which serves as a messenger for the construction of proteins that are the cells' functional molecules. This unidirectional flow of genetic information has been referred to as the "central dogma" of molecular biology. In the 1960s, Howard Temin and colleagues discovered an enzyme that copied RNA into DNA, a reverse of what was normally expected, thus the name *reverse transcriptase*.

Not all viruses can attach to or enter all cells. Humans survive in a world full of viruses that *only* enter or reproduce in a variety of bacteria, protozoa, fungi, and higher forms of plant and animal life. It appears that most of these viruses are harmless to humans. If they enter the body they cannot reproduce in human cells and they do not cause human damage. For those viruses that do enter human bodies from animals such as pigs, chickens, rabbits, mice, cows, monkeys, etc. that cause a human disease, most are very specific as to which cells in a human body they can enter/reproduce and damage. For example, the flu virus enters the human respiratory tract cells. Epstein-Barr virus infects cells in the nose and throat. The hepatitis viruses enter liver cells, but each of the hepatitis viruses causes a different degree of human cell damage over time. Some cause a more immediate disease— for example, hepatitis A virus—while hepatitis B or hepatitis C may not cause significant cell damage for years. Polio virus enters cells of the human nervous system that are different from those cells of the nervous system that herpes virus invades. HIV enters and reproduces in cells of the human immune system.

2. **Why do different viruses enter specific cell types?** Each of the viruses that causes human disease does so by finding a cell type that carries a receptor molecule (a protein or a protein attached to a sugar molecule) that *fits* with a projection of a surface molecule of a given virus—much like the key to a lock. That's why specific viruses are known to be associated with certain types of human tissue. For example, there are viruses that attach only to the receptors of heart, gut, eyes, throat, liver, and other specific human cell tissues. Find a way to block either the human cell receptors (CD4, CXCKR-4, and CCKR-5—to which HIV attaches) without harming the cell or to block the given viral receptor (in HIV it's gp120), and one has a therapy for the given viral disease.

HOW DO HUMAN T4 OR CD4+ LYMPHOCYTES RELATE TO HIV INFECTION AND AIDS?

When HIV infects humans, the cells it infects most often are a specific kind of lymphocyte (white blood cell) carrying a specific protein called CD4 (Cluster Differentiating Protein or Antigen Number 4). These are referred to as T4 or CD4+ cells. The virus then becomes part of the cell's DNA and when the infected CD4+ cells multiply to fight an infection, they also make many copies of HIV. When a person is infected with HIV for a long time, the number of CD4+ cells they have (their CD4+ cell count) goes down. This is a sign that the immune system is being weakened. The lower the CD4+ cell count, the more likely the person will get sick. There are millions of different families of CD4+ cells. Each family is designed to neutralize or render a specific type of germ harmless. When HIV reduces the number of CD4+ cells, the body loses the ability to render HIV harmless and the result is AIDS. Thus, over time, HIV depletes a subset of lymphocytes called **T4 helper cells,** or **CD4+ cells,** that are essential in the production of cells necessary to promote immunity through the production of antibodies that neutralize HIV (Figure 3-2). Cell-mediated immunity (whole cells attack the virus) and antibodies (protein molecules that attack the virus) are critical components of the human immune system. Without the ability to produce a sufficient number of immune-specific cells and immune-specific antibodies, the body is vulnerable to a large variety of infections caused by organisms and viruses that normally do not cause human disease. These infections create the symptoms and progression of illnesses that eventually kill HIV-infected people. Because AIDS begins with HIV infection, technically it can be called **HIV disease, HIV T4 helper cell,** or **CD4+ cell disease,** but the popular press, scientists, and others still refer to HIV disease as AIDS. AIDS is the end stage of chronic HIV infection. **AIDS IS NOT TRANSMITTED, THE VIRUS IS.** People do not die of AIDS per se. They die of opportunistic infections, cancers, and organ failures brought on by the results of a failed immune system (see Chapters 5 and 6).

It is believed that eventually almost everyone who is **correctly** diagnosed with HIV/AIDS will die from AIDS. But not all who become HIV-infected will progress to AIDS. Estimates are that some 3% to 5% of the HIV-infected population

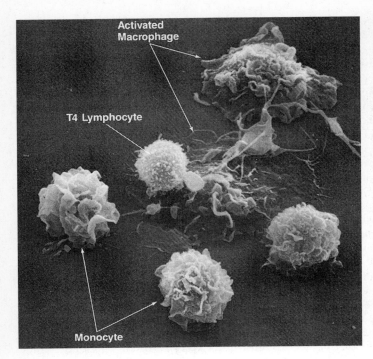

FIGURE 3-2 Normal Human T4 Lymphocytes, Monocytes, and Macrophages. Scanning electron micrograph of monocytes, macrophages, and a T4 or CD4+ lymphocyte, magnified 9000 times. These white blood cells are the targets of HIV infection. Note that the T4 lymphocyte (round cell, at the center) is adhered to a flattened macrophage. *(Photograph courtesy of Dr. M. A. Gonda.)*

will not progress to AIDS. This implies that there is a percentage of the population that is resistant to HIV-associated immune system suppression. Since mid-1996, several genes that offer resistance to HIV infection have been identified. (See Chapter 5, pages 120–123; see Chapter 7, "Possible explanation for Elite Controllers," pages 173–174.)

DESCRIPTION OF HIV; HOW IT ATTACHES TO A HOST CELL AND BUDS OUT OF THE CELL

As can be seen in Figure 3-3, the virus is a sphere measuring 1000 Å (angstroms) or 1/10,000 mm (millimeters) in diameter. The cone-shaped core in a spherical envelope is the dominant feature. Within the cone-shaped core there are two identical strands of viral RNA, each coupled to a molecule of transfer RNA (tRNA) that serves as a primer for reverse transcription of viral RNA into viral DNA. In order for HIV to replicate, it **must** make a DNA copy of its RNA. It is the DNA genes copied from HIV-RNA that allow HIV to replicate! Also present with the RNA are integrase,

protease, and ribonuclease enzymes. The new virus is processed internally by HIV protease to form the characteristic dense lentivirus core. Most HIV appear to have initiated DNA synthesis prior to completion of budding and maturation. Actual maturation of HIV takes place after it buds out of the cell (see Figures 4-1, page 72, and 4-4, page 79). The membrane of HIV is derived from the host cell. HIV gains the membrane while budding out or exiting the cell. The membrane, acquired from its host cell, consists of two lipid (fat) layers impregnated with some human proteins (Figure 3-4). The external viral membrane also contains molecules of viral glycoproteins (gp)—a sugar chain attached to protein. Each glycoprotein appears as a spike in the membrane. Each spike consists of two parts: one is **gp41,** which contains a coiled-up protein and extends through the membrane. On interaction between the HIV envelope and T4 cell coreceptors (CD4/chemokine receptors R4 and R5), the gp41 coiled protein is unsprung and like a harpoon, it pierces the cell membrane, initiating the first step in HIV infection. The

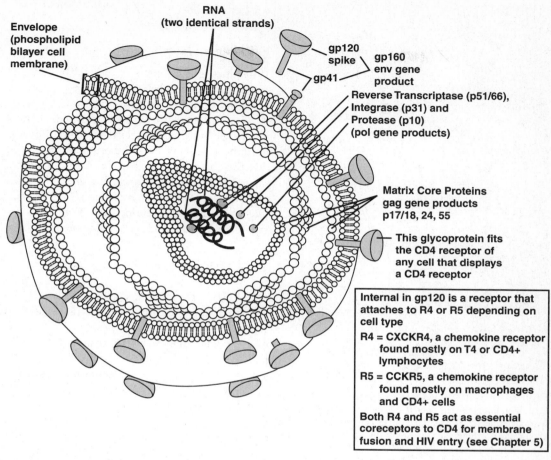

Envelope (phospholipid bilayer cell membrane)

RNA (two identical strands)

gp120 spike
gp41
gp160 env gene product

Reverse Transcriptase (p51/66), Integrase (p31) and Protease (p10) (pol gene products)

Matrix Core Proteins gag gene products p17/18, 24, 55

This glycoprotein fits the CD4 receptor of any cell that displays a CD4 receptor

Internal in gp120 is a receptor that attaches to R4 or R5 depending on cell type

R4 = CXCKR4, a chemokine receptor found mostly on T4 or CD4+ lymphocytes

R5 = CCKR5, a chemokine receptor found mostly on macrophages and CD4+ cells

Both R4 and R5 act as essential coreceptors to CD4 for membrane fusion and HIV entry (see Chapter 5)

FIGURE 3-3 Human Immunodeficiency Virus. It infects cells by a process of membrane fusion that is mediated by its envelope glycoproteins (gp120 gp41, or Env) and is generally triggered by the interaction of gp120 with at least two cellular components: CD4 and a coreceptor belonging to the chemokine receptor family (CXCKR-4 or R4 and CCKR-5 or R5). IN SUMMARY—HIV must reach a mucosal surface, whether it's on the surface of the penis or in the vagina or in the rectum. The virus must then penetrate through that mucosal surface and find an activated T4 cell or CD4 cell. Once that cell is infected, HIV replicates, progeny virus are produced, and HIV begins a cycle of repetitive infections in other CD4 cells and spreads to a point where HIV leaves the initial target tissue and establishes infection in the intestinal tract and in the lymph nodes of the body.

second part, **gp120,** extends from the end of gp41 to the outside and beyond the membrane (the numbers 41 and 120 represent the mass of the individual gps in thousands of daltons). As a complete unit, **gp41** plus **gp120** is called **gp160.** These two membranes or **envelope proteins** play a crucial role in binding HIV to CD4 protein molecules found in the membranes of several types of immune system cells. Full-length HIV-RNA

is complexed with capsid proteins, and the nucleocapsid is transferred to the cell surface membrane at envelope-containing sites.

HIV FITNESS

HIV fitness (or replication capacity) represents a measurement of a combination of events in HIV's life cycle, including cell entry, replication,

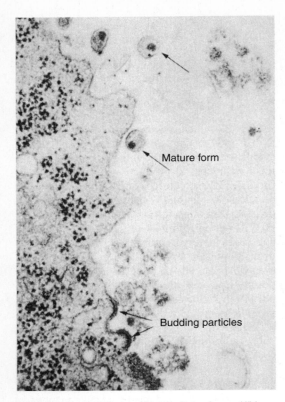

Mature form

Budding particles

FIGURE 3–4 Budding and Mature Retroviruses. HIV buds from infected cells only at special points on the cellular membrane known as "lipid rafts." The rafts are rich in cholesterol. Without the cholesterol HIV cannot fuse with new CD4+ or T4 cells (Hildreth, 2001). This is a photograph of HIV taken by electron microscopy. Note the difference between the free or mature HIV and those that are just budding out through the membrane of a T4 helper cell. This cell came from an HIV-infected hemophiliac. Closely observing the mature HIV, one can make out the core protein area surrounded by the cell's membrane (virus envelope). *(Courtesy of the Centers for Disease Control and Prevention, Atlanta.)*

and budding from the cell surface that together may influence the overall ability of HIV to replicate. Accumulating data from studies of antiretroviral drug selection pressure those HIV that continue to replicate in the presence of the drugs, indicate that drug-associated mutations impair HIV fitness and thus may influence viral load (some mutants replicate but do not reach high levels in the blood, while other mutants do reach high levels in the blood). Mutant HIV that reaches high levels regardless of the drugs used influence disease progression.

Functional Defects

Why does the immune system fail to contain replication, despite detection of huge numbers of HIV-specific immune cells? Increasing evidence suggests that the problem is not the quantity of these cells but their function. Most HIV-specific immune cells may be so functionally impaired that they have little effect on the virus. New data suggest that chronic or continuous antigenic stimulation can lead to exhaustion of CD4+ and CD8+ T cells by preventing them from progressing normally to become renewable memory cells.

THE HIV LIFE CYCLE

Once HIV gets inside a CD4+ cell, it basically hijacks it and transforms the cell into a factory whose mission is to create new copies of HIV. These copies then travel to other CD4+ cells, infect them, and turn them into HIV factories as well. These cellular factories can produce a billion or more copies of HIV per day. The specific number of HIV copies churned out each day will depend on how many CD4+ cells are infected and are producing virus. The level of production can be measured by the viral load (the number of copies of HIV in the blood)—the lower the viral load number, the fewer copies of HIV are being made. While HIV is busily creating copies of itself, it's also destroying the immune system.

UNDERSTANDING HOW HIV WORKS

Understanding how HIV works inside the human cell gives scientists important clues about how to attack it at its most vulnerable points. Knowing the secrets of how the virus functions and reproduces itself—a process called its life cycle—can help scientists design new drugs that are more effective at suppressing HIV replication and have fewer side effects. For people with HIV, knowing how HIV works can make it easier to understand the way drugs work in their bodies. Retroviruses have RNA as their genetic material—not DNA! In brief, retrovirus RNA is copied, using its reverse transcriptase enzyme, into a complementary single strand of DNA (Figures 3-1, page 50; 3-5). The single-strand retroviral DNA is then copied into double-stranded retroviral DNA (this replication occurs in the cell's cytoplasm). At this point the viral DNA has been made according to the instructions in the retroviral RNA. This retroviral DNA migrates into the host cell nucleus and becomes integrated (inserted) into the host cell DNA. A recent study indicates that the viral DNA integrates only into transcriptionally active genes. The integrated viral DNA is now a **provirus.** From this point on, the infection is irreversible—*the viral genes are now a part of the cell's genetic information and will be replicated whenever the cell replicates its DNA.* In this respect, HIV can be considered an acquired dominant genetic disease! A provirus, like the "mole" in a John le Carré spy novel, (*Tinker, Tailor, Soldier, Spy*), may hide for years before doing its specific job. But for HIV, there is evidence that in some human cells the provirus begins to produce new copies of HIV-RNA immediately after becoming a provirus or shortly thereafter.

Before the HIV provirus's genes can be expressed, RNA copies of them that can be read by the host cell's protein-making machinery must be produced. This is done by **transcription.** Transcription is accomplished by the cell's own enzymes. But the process cannot start until the cell's RNA polymerase is activated by various molecular switches located in two DNA regions near the ends of the provirus: the **long terminal repeats.** This requirement is reminiscent of the need of many genes in multicellular organisms to be "turned on" or "turned off" by proteins that bind specifically to controlling sequences.

Production of Viral RNA Strands or RNA Transcripts

Within the host cell nucleus, proviral DNA, when activated, produces new strands of HIV-RNA. Some of the RNA strands behave like messenger RNA (mRNA), producing proteins essential for the production of new HIV. Other

RNA strands become encased within the viral core proteins to become the new viruses. Whether the transcribed RNA strands become mRNA or RNA strands for new viruses depends on whether or not the newly synthesized RNA strands undergo complex processing. RNA processing means that after the RNA is produced, some of it is cut into segments by cellular enzymes and then reassociated or **spliced** into a length of RNA suitable for protein synthesis. The RNA strands that are spliced become the mRNA used in protein synthesis. The unspliced RNA strands serve as new viral strands that are encased in their protein coats (capsids) to become new viruses that bud out of the cell (Figure 3-5).

Two distinct phases of transcription follow the infection of an individual cell by HIV. In the first or early phase, RNA strands or transcripts produced in the cell's nucleus are snipped into multiple copies of shorter sequences by cellular splicing enzymes. When they reach the cytoplasm, they are only about 2000 nucleotides (chemical building blocks that are used in making up DNA or RNA) in length. These early-phase short transcripts encode only the virus's **regulatory proteins;** the structural genes that constitute the rest of the genome are among the parts that are left behind. In the second or late phase, two new size classes of RNA—long (unspliced) transcripts of 9749 nucleotides making up the new viral genome and medium-length (singly spliced) transcripts of some 4500 nucleotides—move out of the nucleus and into the cytoplasm. The 4500 nucleotide transcripts encode HIV's structural and enzymatic proteins (Greene, 1993).

Experimental results reported by Somasundaran et al. (1988) showed that when lymphoid cell lines or peripheral blood lymphocytes were infected with a laboratory strain of HIV, up to 2.5 million copies of the viral RNA were produced by cells; and within three days of infection, up to 40% of the total protein synthesized by the cells was viral protein. This is an unprecedented takeover for a retrovirus that typically makes only modest amounts of RNA and protein.

Much of what HIV does after entering the host cell or while integrated as a retroprovirus depends on the activity of its genes.

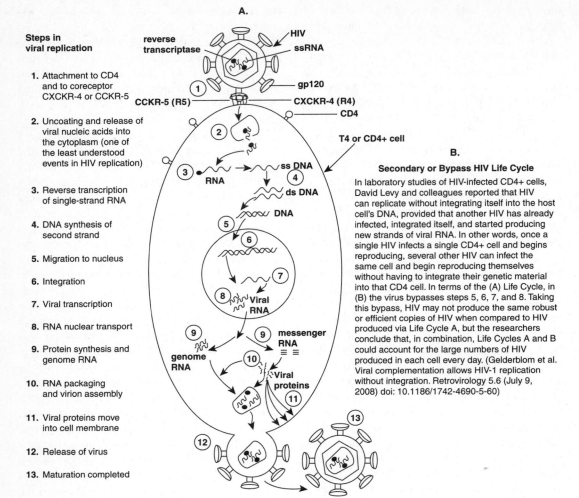

A.

Steps in viral replication

1. Attachment to CD4 and to coreceptor CXCKR-4 or CCKR-5
2. Uncoating and release of viral nucleic acids into the cytoplasm (one of the least understood events in HIV replication)
3. Reverse transcription of single-strand RNA
4. DNA synthesis of second strand
5. Migration to nucleus
6. Integration
7. Viral transcription
8. RNA nuclear transport
9. Protein synthesis and genome RNA
10. RNA packaging and virion assembly
11. Viral proteins move into cell membrane
12. Release of virus
13. Maturation completed

Diagram labels: reverse transcriptase, HIV, ssRNA, gp120, CCKR-5 (R5), CXCKR-4 (R4), CD4, T4 or CD4+ cell, ss DNA, RNA, ds DNA, DNA, Viral RNA, messenger RNA, genome RNA, Viral proteins

B.

Secondary or Bypass HIV Life Cycle

In laboratory studies of HIV-infected CD4+ cells, David Levy and colleagues reported that HIV can replicate without integrating itself into the host cell's DNA, provided that another HIV has already infected, integrated itself, and started producing new strands of viral RNA. In other words, once a single HIV infects a single CD4+ cell and begins reproducing, several other HIV can infect the same cell and begin reproducing themselves without having to integrate their genetic material into that CD4 cell. In terms of the (A) Life Cycle, in (B) the virus bypasses steps 5, 6, 7, and 8. Taking this bypass, HIV may not produce the same robust or efficient copies of HIV when compared to HIV produced via Life Cycle A, but the researchers conclude that, in combination, Life Cycles A and B could account for the large numbers of HIV produced in each cell every day. (Gelderblom et al. Viral complementation allows HIV-1 replication without integration. Retrovirology 5.6 (July 9, 2008) doi: 10.1186/1742-4690-5-60)

FIGURE 3–5 (A) Primary or Expected Life Cycle of HIV in a T4 or CD4+ Lymphocyte. On average, the life cycle of HIV in an infected T4 cell is about two days. This means that one HIV in one person in one year can produce about 180 generations of HIV. The lifetime of HIV in the blood is about six hours. After fusion of viral and cellular membranes, the inner part of HIV, called the **core**, is delivered into the cell cytoplasm. Uncoating of the core occurs, releasing two identical RNA strands, accompanying structural proteins and enzymes necessary for HIV replication. HIV-RNA is then copied into HIV DNA, which is then transported into the cell's nucleus for insertion or integration into the host cell's DNA. This feature of the virus life cycle is essential for the spread of HIV in vivo, because it allows infection of nondividing cells such as monocytes and terminally differentiated macrophages and dendritic cells. There is still some confusion as to whether HIV becomes a latent infection once HIV DNA becomes inserted or integrated into the host DNA. Evidence indicates that whether HIV is latent depends on the tissue that one is investigating. For example, in the T4 lymphocytes within the lymph nodes, HIV is constantly being replicated, while some T4 lymphocytes in the blood carry HIV in the latent state. (B) Secondary or Bypass HIV Life Cycle.

IN SUMMARY—Seven Broad Steps for the HIV Replication Cycle: 1. Fusion of the HIV cell to the host cell surface; 2. HIV RNA, reverse transcriptase, integrase, and other viral proteins enter the host cell; 3. Viral DNA is formed by reverse transcription; 4. Viral DNA is transported across the nucleus and integrates into the host DNA; 5. New viral RNA is used as genomic RNA and to make viral proteins; 6. New viral RNA and proteins move to cell surface and new, immature, HIV virus forms; 7. The virus matures by protease releasing individual HIV proteins.

PROTEINS THAT COULD BE USED TO HALT THE PRODUCTION OF HIV ARE IDENTIFIED

The life cycle of HIV is very complex; it has nine genes yet it only produces 15 recognized proteins. Clearly, HIV depends on multiple host-cell proteins to successfully complete its life cycle. This implies that there are many proteins that remain to be discovered. Finding these proteins may spotlight novel drug targets for use in antiretroviral therapy. In January 2008, Stephen Elledge and colleagues published an HIV research paper that Robert Gallo, head of the Institute of Human Virology in Baltimore, Maryland, and founder of the first HIV antibody test, said was "destined to become one of the key HIV papers of this decade, if not longer." Using cutting-edge molecular techniques, Stephen Elledge and colleagues found that HIV relies on 273 human proteins to do its work. Of these so-called HIV dependency factors (HDFs),

only 36 had been discovered to this time. Their discovery was made using a genome-wide scan of human DNA, specifically 21,000 human genes that encode proteins. The research team effectively short-circuited or blocked all 21,000 genes one at a time using small interfering RNAs as RNA interference screens (siRNA) and then asked if HIV could complete its life cycle. By a process of elimination, they isolated those genes that HIV uses to complete its life cycle. The most immediate challenge is to elucidate the molecular details of how these 273 HDFs interact with HIV. Because humans need some of these proteins, the challenge is to determine which proteins we can do without! Currently, the authors can only suggest possible connections. But what a great starting point (Cohen, 2008)!

HOW HIV ESCAPES THE INFECTED CELL

This is a primary example of how a virus, in this case HIV, uses living cells to achieve its mission—to infect, replicate, and exit a cell. In 2001, Jennifer Garrus and colleagues reported on how HIV takes over the human cell's normal processes in order to leave a cell. This discovery could lead to new drugs to control HIV disease in those who are HIV infected. In a key part of their study, scientists crippled the cells' machinery by silencing a gene that normally makes the protein (Tsg101) necessary for HIV to escape or bud out of the cell. Thus, clusters of connected HIV particles were stuck at the cell membrane and could not get out. The new study showed the Tsg101 protein within cells acts as a key link to the budding process. One part of the Tsg101 protein connects to an HIV protein while another part of the Tsg101 protein links to other proteins within a cell—proteins the virus uses to exit the cell. Shutting down the means by which HIV leaves the cell means that other susceptible cells will not become infected. Blocking Tsg101 protein after a person becomes infected could keep the virus from spreading to other cells. These scientists speculate that many other viruses may use the

same exit pathway. After over 30 years, scientists still do not know just how HIV kills cells bearing a CD4 protein, and scientists still do not know why T4 or CD4+ cells fall from about 1000 per microliter of blood to less than 100 per microliter of blood over a 10-year period while viral loads may remain constant or show an enormous increase over a short time interval. And in many people, the relationship of viral load to the rate of their disease progression is questionable at best.

Some of the animal retroviruses such as the Rous sarcoma virus contain an additional **oncogene** (onc) that, along with its LTRs, causes a rapid form of cancer in chickens that kills them in one to two weeks after infection. Without the **onc** gene the virus causes a slow, progressive cancer.

The Genes (Genome) of HIV

What sets the HIV genome apart from all other known retroviruses is the number of genes in HIV and the apparent complexity of their interactions in regulating the expression of the GAG-POL-ENV genes (Figure 3-6).

The Nine Genes of HIV—The HIV genome contains at least nine recognizable genes that produce at least 15 individual proteins. These proteins are divided into three classes: (1) GAG,

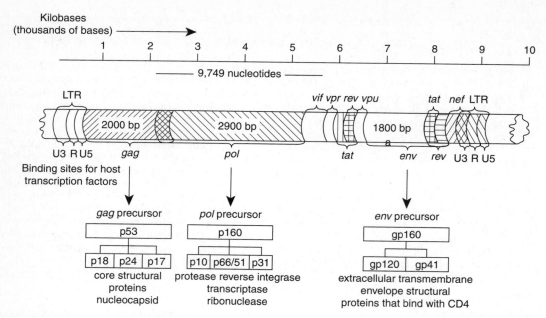

FIGURE 3–6 Genome of HIV. Nine of the genes making up the HIV genome have been identified. They are positioned as shown. Five are essential for HIV replication and six control reproduction (see text for details). The maxtrix protein, p17, forms the outer shell HIV, lining the inner surface of the viral membrane. Key functions of p17 protein are: orchestrating HIV assembly, directing GAG p55 protein to host cell membrane, interacting with transmembrane protein, gp41, retaining envelope-coded proteins within HIV, and containing a nuclear localization signal that directs HIV-RNA integration complex to the nucleus of infected cells.

POL, and ENV, the three major **structural** proteins; (2) Tat and Rev, the two **regulatory** proteins; and (3) Nef, Vif, Vpu, and Vpr, the four **accessory** proteins. Five of the nine genes are involved in regulating the expression of the GAG-POL-ENV genes.

The letters **GAG** stand for group-specific antigens (proteins) that make up the viral nucleocapsid. The GAG gene codes for internal structural proteins, the production of the dense cylindrical core proteins (**p24,** a nucleoid shell protein with a molecular weight of 24,000), and several internal proteins, which have been visualized by electron microscopy. The GAG gene has the ability to direct the formation of viruslike particles when all other major genes (POL and ENV) are absent. It is only when the GAG gene is nonfunctional that retroviruses (such as HIV) lose their capacity to bud out of a host cell. Because of these observations, the GAG

protein has been designated the virus particle-making machine (Wills et al., 1991).

The **POL** gene codes for HIV enzymes, protease (p10), the virus-associated polymerase (reverse transcriptase) that is active in two forms, and endonuclease (integrase) enzymes. The integrase enzyme cuts the cell's DNA and inserts the HIV DNA. Evidence from retroviral deletion studies shows that the loss of LTRs on the 3′ side of the POL gene stops viral DNA integration into the host genome. However, nonintegrated DNA, without its LTRs and integrase enzyme, can still produce new viruses. This clearly demonstrates that viral DNA integration is not essential for viral multiplication even though integration is the normal course of events (Dimmrock and Primrose, 1987).

The regulation of HIV transcription appears to be intimately related to the onset of HIV disease and AIDS. Thus interruption or inactivation of the POL gene would appear to have therapeutic effects.

The **ENV** gene codes for HIV surface proteins, two major envelope glycoproteins (gp120, located on the external "spikes" of HIV and gp41, the transmembrane protein that attaches gp120 to the surface of HIV) that become embedded throughout the host cell membrane, which ultimately becomes the **envelope** that surrounds the virus as it "buds" out. Studies on how HIV kills cells have revealed at least one way in which the envelope glycoproteins enhance T helper cell death. The envelope glycoproteins cause the formation of **syncytia;** that is, healthy T cells fuse to each other, forming a group around a single HIV-infected T4 or CD4+ cell. Individual T cells within these syncytia lose their immune function. Starting with a single HIV-infected T4 helper cell, as many as 500 *uninfected* T4 helper cells can fuse into a single syncytium. Continued creation of these syncytia could deplete a T4 cell population.

Several studies have demonstrated that the appearance of syncytium-inducing (SI) HIV strains during the chronic phase of HIV disease heralds an abrupt loss of T4 or CD4+ lymphocytes and a clinical progression of the disease (Torres et al., 1996).

The Six Genes of HIV That Control HIV Reproduction—Collectively, the six additional HIV genes tat and rev (regulatory genes), and nef, vif, vpu, and vpr (auxiliary genes) working together with the host cell's machinery actually control the reproductive retroviral cycle: adhesion of HIV to a cell, penetration of the cell, uncoating of the HIV genome, reverse transcription of the RNA genome producing proviral DNA and immediate production of new viral RNA, or the integration of the provirus and later viral multiplication. The six genes allow for the entire reproductive scenario—from infection to new HIV—to occur in 5 to 6 minutes in dividing cells. Currently there are no drugs that target a regulatory gene or its products.

Gene Sequence—The HIV proviral genome has been well characterized with regard to gene location and sequence, but the function of each

gene is not completely understood. The genes for producing regulatory proteins can be grouped into two classes: genes that produce proteins essential for HIV replication **(tat** and **rev)**, and genes that produce proteins that perform accessory functions that enhance replication and/or infectivity **(nef, vif, vpu,** and **vpr)** (Rosen, 1991).

Gene Function—Each end of the proviral genome contains an identical long sequence of nucleotides, the long terminal repeats. Although these LTRs are not considered to be genes of the HIV genome, they do contain regulatory nucleotide sequences that help the six regulatory/auxiliary genes control GAG-POL-ENV gene expression. For example, the **vif** gene is associated with the infectious activity of the virus. Currently, the predominant view is that vif acts at the late stages of infection to promote HIV processing or assembly (Potash et al., 1998).

The **tat** gene (transcription activator) is essential for HIV infection of T4 cells and HIV replication (Li, 1997; Stevenson, 1998). It is one of the first viral genes to be transcribed. The tat gene produces a transactivator protein, meaning that the gene produces a protein that exerts its effect on viral replication from a distance rather than interacting with genes adjacent to **tat** or their gene product. **Tat** contains two coding regions or exons—areas that contain genetic information for producing a diffusible protein—which, through the help of the LTR sequences, increases the expression of HIV genes, thereby increasing the production of new virus particles. The tat protein interacts with a short nucleotide sequence called TAR located within the 5' LTR region of HIV messenger RNA (mRNA) transcripts (Matsuya et al., 1990). Once that tat protein binds to the TAR sequence, transcription of the provirus by cellular RNA polymerase II accelerates at least one thousandfold.

The **rev** gene (regulator of expression of viral protein) selectively increases the synthesis of HIV structural proteins in the later stages of HIV disease, thereby maximizing the production of new viruses. It does this by regulating the splicing of the HIV-RNA transcript (cutting out nucleotide sequences that exist between exon-coding regions and bringing these regions together) and transporting spliced and unspliced RNAs from the nucleus to the cytoplasm (Patrusky, 1992; Fritz et al., 1995).

The **nef** (negative effector) gene produces a protein that is maintained in the cell cytoplasm next to the nuclear membrane. It is believed **nef** functions by protecting the cell from dying, allowing the cell to continue producing HIV. Several antigenic forms of nef protein have been found, which suggest multiple activities of nef within HIV-infected cells (Kohleisen et al., 1992; Sagg et al., 1995). Olivier Schwartz and coworkers (Cohen, 1997) showed that **nef** can prompt cells to yank down from their surfaces a molecule known as the major histocompatibility complex (MHC), which displays viral peptides to the immune system. The group predicted that this "down-regulation" of MHC would make HIV-infected cells resistant to cytotoxic T cell killing (Collins et al., 1998) (see Chapter 5).

In August 2001, Yuntao Wu and colleagues reported that after HIV-RNA manufactures a DNA copy, but prior to its integration into the cell's DNA, the HIV DNA stimulates the production of **tat** and **nef** viral proteins. These proteins awaken T4 cells out of their dormant state. Once the T4 cells are activated, they become vulnerable to nuclear invasion by HIV DNA, allowing the virus to integrate into the T4 cell DNA structure. Not only will the activated T4 cell allow HIV DNA to enter the nucleus and insert itself into human DNA, an activated T4 cell produces a higher rate of HIV-RNA replication (Wu et al., 2001). And last, HIV missing the **nef** gene will not replicate in CD4+ cells.

The functions of the **vpr** gene, which codes for a **v**iral **p**rotein **R,** is associated with the transport of cytoplasmic viral DNA into the nucleus. Vpr is also involved in steroid production that in turn helps produce HIV, is required for the efficient assembly or release of new HIV viruses, and stops T4 cell division. Although vpr protein is not needed for HIV to reproduce in T4 or CD4+ cell cultures, it appears to be very important for HIV to reproduce in macrophages. Vpr can induce CD4+

cell death even when the cells are not HIV-infected, and it is also poisonous to cell mitochondria, which may be important in killing cells that are HIV infected. It has recently been shown that HIV-infected people who are long-term nonprogressors to AIDS have a mutant or nonfunctional form of the vpr gene (Lum et al., 2003).

Vif, or the viral infectivity protein, is produced using one of the smallest and least understood of the nine genes that make up HIV. In 2002, scientists probing the secrets of Vif reported two startling developments. They found that human cells contain a powerful enzyme, a cytidine deaminase known as APOBEC3G (pronounced APPObeck) that can stop the production of HIV. Simultaneously, they discovered that HIV itself has overcome this natural defense by using Vif protein to neutralize that enzyme. It has been shown that as HIV buds out of a cell it carries the APOBEC enzyme, that is, the enzyme stows away inside the new virus. When HIV infects a new cell and begins making genetic copies of itself, APOBEC becomes active, causing HIV to mutate at such a rapid pace that resulting HIV copies are inactive. But HIV then produces Vif protein that destroys APOBEC—HIV's solution to survival! Some HIV/AIDS scientists believe that those findings are the most important new information in HIV/AIDS research since the identification of HIV in 1983. Once scientists gain an understanding of how Vif blocks this protective enzyme, they can devise tests to measure how well a potential new drug interferes with that process. Presumably a chemical that disables Vif from producing its protein or prevents it from attacking APOBEC could become a potent antiretroviral drug.

Vpu has two important functions in the life cycle of HIV. Vpu codes for a **v**iral **p**rotein **U** that destroys the CD4 protein within the T4 lymphocyte. This helps in the assembly and release of HIV from the cell. Vpu also has the important function of interfering with host cell proteins that cause new HIV to cluster on the cell's membrane surface. Cellular proteins called tetherins tether or hold the new virus on the membrane, stopping the release of that virus into the body. Vpu proteins block this tethering action. Vif, Vpr, and Vpu appear to be necessary for HIV to replicate.

Of the HIV proteins, tat, rev, and nef are termed *early* proteins because their production results from the cutting and splicing of full-length HIV mRNA; Vif, vpu, and vpr are termed *late* proteins because their production results from unspliced or single-spliced mRNA.

In summary, HIV/AIDS researchers have picked apart HIV, decoding its nine genes and isolating its 15 proteins. Now they are trying, piece by piece, to understand how these components work together to produce one of the most lethal microbes in history. As biologists learn what makes HIV tick, they get new ideas about how to destroy it.

How Genes Store Genetic Information and the Importance of Mutations or Change within Genes—Genes store the information necessary for creating living organisms and viruses. In sexually reproducing organisms, the information is stored in the form of DNA organized into structures called chromosomes. Apart from sex cells (eggs and sperm) and mature blood cells, every cell in the human body contains 23 pairs of chromosomes. One of each pair is inherited from the mother, the other from the father. Each chromosome is a packet of compressed and twisted DNA. Genes are sections of DNA containing the blueprint for the whole body, including such specific details as what kind of receptors cells will have, for example, CD4, CD8, R4, R5, and so on.

DNA is made up of a double-stranded helix held together by hydrogen bonds between specific pairs of bases. The four bases A, T, G, and C (adenine, thymine, guanine, and cytosine) bond to each other in fixed and complementary patterns that give humans and other species their individuality. If a gene is thought of as a sentence, and the nucleotides in DNA as letters, a change or mutation of only one letter can affect the entire sentence or the information the DNA gives the cell. To get an idea of how many mutations can occur in a cell, consider that humans have about 3.2 billion base pairs, in their haploid or 23 chromosomes, that make up just over 20,000

protein-coding genes or sentences that contain the information that makes a human. There are about a million differences between your 3.2 billion–letter DNA alphabet and that of another person. The kind, number, and sequence of nucleotides (bases) in human DNA and that of other species is much greater. Another way of saying this is that the closer a species resembles a human or vice versa, the closer will be the DNA base sequences.

For example, the DNA base sequence in a chimpanzee is about 98% identical to humans. That means the difference between human DNA and chimpanzee DNA is only a base sequence difference for about 60 million base pairs out of 3.2 billion human base pairs.

Importance of Genetic Stability to a Species— The individual or collective characteristics (phenotypes) of any virus, cell, or multicelled organism depend on the expression of their genes and the interaction of gene products within a given environment. From a biological point of view, changes in phenotype (observable characteristics) that are inheritable are by definition genetic changes. Such changes occur due to changes in the kind, number, and sequence of bases in DNA. Base changes may occur by addition, substitution, and deletion. These changes are referred to as **genetic mutations.** Genetic mutations provide biological heterogeneity and genetic diversity (similarity as a species but dissimilarity with regard to certain characteristics). Investigations on the rate at which genetic mutations occur in living species indicate that DNA is a stable molecule with relatively low mutation rates for any given gene. Because of low mutation rates within the DNA of a species's gene pool (all the genes that can be found in the DNA of a species) and selection pressures by a slowly changing environment, species evolution is constant but very slow.

Genetic mutations in the strain of an organism or virus produce genetic and phenotype **variants** (different members) of that strain. Regardless of the rate at which mutations occur, *they are genetic mistakes*—they are not intentional, they just happen by chance. Most mutations or genetic mistakes either make no difference to an organism or virus (silent mutations) or they cause a change. Few genetic mistakes within a stable environment improve the species. After all, the species arrived at this point in time via genetic and environmental selection pressures—those with the best constellation of genes survived to reproduce those genes. In species that produce large numbers of offspring, genetic mistakes that are lethal or lead to an early death are of little consequence to the species. A genetic mistake that improves the chance of survival and reproduction is retained.

Genetic Instability of HIV—A virus like HIV can produce hundreds of replicas within a single cell. Genetic mistakes during viral replication produce variant HIVs. In biological economic terms, HIV replicas are inexpensive to make. Even if most of these mutant HIV replicas are inactive or throwaway copies, it makes little if any difference to the HIV per se. However, if a few HIV replicas received environmentally advantageous mutant genes, these HIV mutants would survive as well as or better than the parent HIVs. Both parent HIV and mutant HIV can reproduce in the same cell and exchange genes. Over time, only the most fit mutant or variant HIVs are transmitted among people and undergo still further genetic changes. These variant HIVs could, with sufficient cumulative genetic changes, become a new type of HIV—for example, an HIV-3.

Investigations of some of the RNA viruses revealed relatively high mutation rates. Thus some of the RNA viruses are our best examples of evolution in "real" time. Because of their high error rate during replication they show, as expected, both high genetic diversity and biological heterogeneity in their host, and a rate of evolution about a million times faster than DNA-based organisms (Nowak, 1990). HIV, in particular, fits this category. Heterogeneity of HIV is reflected by (1) the difference in the kinds of cells variant HIV infects; (2) the way different HIV mutants replicate; and (3) the way different variants of HIV harm infected cells.

It is now known that HIV is capable of enormous genetic flexibility, which allows it to become resistant to drugs, to escape from immune responses, and to avoid potential HIV vaccines. What is not known are all the factors contributing to viral diversity in individual infections. Clearly the high error rate of the reverse transcriptase (because this enzyme lacks a 3' to 5' exonuclease proofreading ability, that is, it cannot correct mistakes once they are made) and the high turnover rate in infected cells generate vast numbers of different virus mutants. The diversity of newly produced variants, however, is shaped by a combination of mutation, recombinations of HIV-RNA, and selection forces. The main selective forces that have been proposed to drive HIV diversity are the immune response, cell tropism (cell types most likely to attract HIV), and random activation of infected cells. At the time of seroconversion a person may carry a homogeneous virus population, but then diversification occurs as HIV infects many different cell types and tissues in the body (Bonhoeffer et al., 1995).

For further information on HIV evolution, diversity, and HIV disease progression, see Chapter 7, Box 7.1, page 170.

Genetic Variability: HIV Subtypes or Clades

Michael Sagg and colleagues (1988) examined the generation of molecular variation of HIV by sequential HIV isolates from two chronically infected people. They found 39 distinguishable but highly related genomes (HIV variants). These results indicate that HIV heterogeneity occurs rapidly in infected individuals and that a large number of genetically distinguishable but related HIVs rapidly evolve in parallel and coexist during chronic infection. That is, whenever a drug or the immune response successfully attacks one variant, another arises in its place. Pools of genetically distinct variants that evolve from the initial HIV that begin the infection are often referred to as **quasispecies** (Delwart et al., 1993; Diaz et al., 1997). However, even though a person possesses diverse quasispecies of HIV, only a very narrow population (perhaps only one) of HIV is transmitted from mother to child or between sexual partners (Derdeyn et al., 2004).

Additional evidence indicates that some HIV genetic variants demonstrate a preference (tropism) as to the cell type they infect. This means that one genetic change may allow the virus to enter cells that were once immune to the virus. Also, a report by Helen Devereux and colleagues (2002) states that a wide variety of quasispecies circulate in each infected individual and that there may be HIV evolving independently in different body compartments. The rapid genetic change, which results in altered viral products, makes it very difficult to design a vaccine or drug that will be effective against all HIV variants. To date, HIV drug-resistant mutants have been found for all FDA-approved nucleoside and non-nucleoside analogs and protease inhibitors used in the treatment of HIV-infected people. (Chapter 4, pages 75–76 presents a discussion of currently used drug therapies for HIV/AIDS.)

DISTINCT GENOTYPES (SUBTYPES/CLADES) OF HIV-1 WORLDWIDE BASED ON ENV AND GAG PROTEINS

HIV is actually an umbrella term for two genetically distinct types of virus: HIV-1 and HIV-2. HIV-1 embraces three genetically distinct groups: M, N, and O. Of these, group M viruses, the ones that are perhaps most studied and are known to be most responsible for infections worldwide, have been subdivided into 11 genetically distinct subtypes, identified by letters A through K (Figure 3-7). Genetic analyses of HIV-2, the less virulent form of HIV, have yielded six subtypes, identified as A through F.

As stated previously, this book is about HIV-1, simply called HIV. In order to better understand globally circulating strains of HIV, HIV investigators have placed, based on genetic diversity, the various HIV strains into three

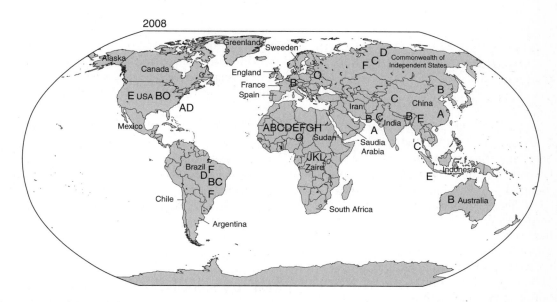

FIGURE 3-7 Global Distribution of the 11 M subtypes and O in 2008 in Areas of Highest Prevalence. Clearly this global map shows that HIV subtypes are no longer continent based—all subtypes are now present on all continents. No satisfactory explanation exists for the skewed worldwide distribution of HIV-1 subtypes. The worldwide spread of viral subtypes makes it clear that a world vaccine will be required, that is, one that is not subtype specific. None appears to be on the horizon, although large-scale trials with existing envelope vaccines are underway in some developing countries. *(Brodine et al., 1997 updated; Taylor et al., 2008.)*

major groups: **M,** for the **main** HIV genotypes or **clades** found in different populations, and groups **O** (outlier) and **N** (nonmajor, nonoutlier) for HIV genotypes or clades that are signif-icantly differ-ent from those in the **M** group.

Group M HIV causes over 99% of the world's HIV/AIDS. **Group O** and the more recently discovered **Group N** cause less than 1%.

In 2009, Jean-Christophe Planter and colleagues identified a new human immunodeficiency virus in a 62-year-old Cameroonian woman. It is closely related to Gorilla Simian Immunodeficiency Virus (SIVgor) and shows no evidence of recombination with other HIV-1 strains. This new virus seems to be the prototype of a new HIV-1 lineage that is distinct from HIV-1 groups M, N, and O. They propose to designate this new HIV as group P. This woman had no contact with gorillas or meat from wild animals and currently shows no signs of HIV/AIDS and remains untreated. How widespread this new virus is remains undetermined.

UNLESS SPECIFIED, THE INFORMATION ON HIV IN THIS BOOK RELATES ONLY TO HIV-1 GROUP M

Group M Subtypes or Clades

There are 11 subtypes or clades of group M: A, B, C, D, E, F, G, H, I, J, and K. The M subtypes have been analyzed with respect to the differences between them based on the variations found in their GAG and ENV proteins.

Within a subtype, envelope gene sequences vary from 7% to 12%. Between subtypes the genetic variation is up to 30%. There is the belief that a vaccine against one subtype won't offer protection against the rest. (For discussion of HIV vaccines, see Chapter 9 on prevention.) Subtypes B and E together make up about 14% of HIV infections worldwide. Subtypes A, C, and D make up about 84% of HIV infections.

The 11 different M subtypes or clades and O have been globally mapped (geographically located) in Figure 3-7 (Brix et al., 1996;

Workshop Report, 1997). This figure demonstrates the dissemination of the different subtypes from 1990 through 2008. Clearly, subtype B, closely related to subtype D, predominates in the Americas, although in Brazil, Argentina, and Uruguay substantial proportions of infections are caused by F subtype or BF recombinant viruses. Apart from these three countries, infections with non–B genetic forms are unusual; however, recently, it was reported that env subtypes A, C, and H had been identified in 5 of 11 samples in Cuba. The identification of diverse non-B subtypes in Cuba is not unexpected, considering that large numbers of Cuban military and civilian personnel had been stationed in the 1970s and 1980s in Angola, a country neighboring the Democratic Republic of Congo (DRC), where the highest group M diversity is found, and that many of the early cases of HIV infection in Cuba were detected among these individuals. The explosive epidemic in Southeast Asia is chiefly attributable to subtype E. There are ample documented introductions of subtypes C, E, and F from endemic areas into the United States and the Western Hemisphere. Subtype C now accounts for about 40% of *new* HIV infections worldwide—particularly in China and India. There is no one subtype that is representative of this global pandemic.

Global Predominant HIV-1 Subtypes

A. W. Africa, E. Africa, Central Africa, East Europe, Mideast
B. N. America, Europe, Mideast, E. Asia, Latin America
C. S. Africa, S. Asia, Ethiopia
D. E. Africa, Brazil
E. S.E. Asia

HIV-2 primarily West Africa.

Do HIV Subtypes or Clades Influence the Response to Antiretroviral Therapy?

This question is urgent, since only 12% of global infections are caused by the most studied subtype, B, and 50% of prevalent HIV infections and 47% of all new HIV infections are caused by subtype C. This discrepancy in the availability of clinical data for non-B subtype is exacerbated by the fact that, until the past few years, antiretroviral treatment has been largely unavailable in many countries with non-B subtypes of HIV.

Group O Subtypes

Group O contains at least 30 genetically different subtypes of HIV. Group O subtypes are referred to as **"outliers"** because their RNA base sequence is only 50% similar to the known genotypes of the M group. The O variants have been known since 1987 but have been found mainly in Cameroon, Gabon, and surrounding West African countries that, to date, have only been marginally affected by AIDS. Group O viruses were of concern primarily because their divergence from group M was sufficient to miss their detection by ELISA HIV testing. (The ELISA test is discussed in Chapter 13, pages 388–393.) Seven people in France were identified with group O HIV in 1994. The first documented case of group O HIV infection in the United States was found in April 1996 in Los Angeles. By the beginning of 2003, only three cases of HIV subtype O infection had been reported in the United States. This subtype was found in a Los Angeles County woman and a Maryland woman; both came into the United States from Africa. HIV subtype O is not routinely tested for in the United States.

New Group N Subtype?

In August 1998, Francois Simon and colleagues reported the discovery of a *new* HIV-1 isolate that *cannot* be placed in the M or O subtype category. The authors suggest that the new isolate be classified as group **N** for **"new"** or **"non-M non-O."** The new isolate, designated **YBF30**, was found in a small number of people in the West African nation of Cameroon. The first isolate was from a 40-year-old woman who died of AIDS. This virus is similar to SIV (cpz-gab), and it either branched with the SIV strain or between it and HIV-1 group M. The authors state that future strains of SIV (cpz) could be found, and strains that are closely related to YBF30 might circulate among Cameroonian chimpanzees.

SIV retroviruses are endemic in many species of primates but usually don't cause disease, which makes them natural hosts for what are

---

POINT OF INFORMATION 3.2

FIRST CONFIRMED CASES OF HIV GROUP O–CAUSED AIDS

A Norwegian sailor died of AIDS in 1976 at the age of 29. His wife and youngest daughter, born in 1967, also died of AIDS. The members of this Norwegian family represent the earliest confirmed cases of AIDS and the first case of HIV type O infection. The first symptoms appeared in 1966 in the sailor, in 1967 in his wife, and in 1969 in their daughter. Between 1961 and 1965 he traveled the world's oceans, calling at ports in all six inhabited continents. On his first voyage, which began in August 1961 just after his fifteenth birthday, he worked as a kitchen hand on a Norwegian vessel that sailed down the West African coastline, calling at ports in Senegal, Liberia, Cote d'Ivoire, Ghana, Nigeria, and Cameroon. A gonorrheal infection during this trip shows that he was sexually active. He returned home in May 1962, and never returned to Africa. No known evidence suggests that the sailor was bisexual, which means that sexual contact with a woman is the most straightforward explanation for his infection. This would suggest that HIV group O has been circulating in that part of Africa for at least 37 years.

Second Confirmed Cases of HIV Group O–Caused AIDS?

The second case of group O infection found in the literature is the second child of a French barmaid from Reims, who died in 1981. The child's clinical history is highly suggestive of neonatal AIDS. In 1992 a group O virus was isolated from the mother, who by then had AIDS.

known as lentiviruses, which have a long incubation period causing a slow clinical course of the disease. But when they cross the species barrier into a new host like humans, these viruses may become pathogenic, causing illness. Based on evolutionary studies, researchers think SIV has existed in sub-Saharan Africa for thousands of years, adapting to several species, including the African green monkey and sooty mangabey. There are six closely linked strains of SIV. Chimpanzees carry at least three different viral predecessors of HIV-1 that gave rise to groups M, O, and N. Sooty mangabeys carry an ancestor of HIV-2.

Simon's discovery of group N also raises other critical questions and challenges. Looking ahead, how many other SIV strains may have crossed the species barrier? Should we be mass screening for this new virus N or increasing surveillance of the other SIV strains? What about the human recombinant viruses? How well are we tracking them?

Summary

HIV is a retrovirus. It has RNA for its genetic material and carries reverse transcriptase enzyme for making DNA from its RNA. HIV, using its enzyme, copies its genetic information from RNA into DNA, which becomes integrated into host cell DNA and may remain silent for years, or until such time as it is activated into producing new HIV. HIV contains at least nine genes; three of them, GAG-POL-ENV, are basic to all animal retroviruses. The six additional genes are involved in the infection process and regulate the production of products from the three genes. HIV, because of its error-prone reverse transcriptase enzyme, mutates at an unusually high rate. With time, many mutant HIV variants can be found within a single HIV-infected person. A vaccine against one mutant HIV may not work against a second—like the vaccines made yearly against different mutant influenza viruses.

A new group of HIV has been identified, group N.

Review Questions

(Answers to the Review Questions are on page 463.)

1. Why is HIV called a retrovirus?

2. What are the three major genes common to all retroviruses? How many additional genes does HIV have?

3. Why are retroviruses, and HIV in particular, believed to be genetically unstable? Give two reasons for your answer.

4. What is believed to be the major reason for the high rate of genetic mutations in HIV production?

5. All of the following are HIV accessory genes except
   (a) tat   (b) env   (c) vpr
   (d) rev   (e) vpu

6. HIV contains _____ nucleotides and _____ genes.
   (a) 9/10,331   (b) 8/9746   (c) 6/9000
   (d) 3/8000   (e) 9749/9

7. Name the error-prone HIV enzyme that is a major cause of HIV mutants.
   (a) reverse holozyme   (b) reverse integrase
   (c) reverse transcriptase   (d) reverse spiral case
   (e) reverse nuclease

8. True or False: HIV is very specific with regard to the types of cells it can enter.

9. HIV attaches first to the following receptor on a T lymphocyte:
   (a) CD5+   (b) CD4+   (c) CD28+
   (d) CD8+   (e) CD9+

10. How many RNA strands does HIV contain?
    (a) 3   (b) 1   (c) 2   (d) 4   (e) 5

11. Name the three major genes of HIV.

12. In general, about how many CD4+ cells are in a microliter of blood?

13. What role does the vif gene play in HIV survival in an infected cell?

14. What two processes occur during the replication of HIV that gives HIV a chance to survive changing environmental conditions?

15. Group M has how many subtypes of clades and which subtypes cause most of the infections in the United States, China and India, and heterosexual South Africa?

Anti-HIV Therapy

- There may never be a cure for HIV disease/AIDS.
- The Dark Age of Anti-HIV Therapy (antiretroviral therapy—ART).
- Exciting times for ART. From March 1987 through early year 2013, 26 individual anti-HIV drugs and seven combination drug groups received FDA approval, and at least two other drugs have received expanded access approval.
- Current antiretroviral drugs work well regardless of HIV subtype.
- Is it time to revisit the question of an HIV cure: sterilizing versus functional cure?
- Timothy Brown, first person ever to be cured of HIV/AIDS is presented.
- There are no anti-HIV drugs free of clinical side effects.
- Drug interactions; drugs taken with/without food.
- All nucleoside analogs and non-nucleosides work by inhibiting the HIV reverse transcriptase enzyme, which functions *early* in the HIV life cycle.
- All protease inhibitors work by inhibiting the HIV protease enzyme from its function *late* in the HIV life cycle.
- Maraviroc (Selzentry), the first R5 coreceptor HIV entry inhibitor into CD4 cells, and raltegravir (Isentress), the first inhibitor of HIV's integrase enzyme, received FDA approval in August/ October 2007. Etravirine (Intelence) was FDA approved in January 2008.
- The role of the integrase enzyme in creating an HIV provirus.
- FDA approves rilpivirine (Edurant) as the 26th antiretroviral drug in 2011 and the second once-a-day combination drug, Complera. A third once-a-day combination drug, stribid a.k.a Quad FDA approved August 2012.
- Drug therapy for HIV raises life expectancy to nearly that of HIV-negative people!
- The Holy Grail for HIV therapy is to suppress HIV replication.
- Currently there are seven classes of antiretroviral drugs.
- Viral load is the number of HIV-RNA strands found at any one time in human plasma.
- Viral load is associated with HIV disease progression.
- Importance of viral load to CD4+ cell counts.
- Viral load is associated with HIV transmission.
- Anti-HIV drug combinations are extending lives.
- AIDS deaths are dropping in developed nations due in part to drug combination therapy.
- When to begin anti-HIV drug therapy is the big question.
- Strict adherence to drug regimens is essential but difficult to maintain.
- Drug resistance is easier to understand once you know how HIV replicates.
- Cost of antiretroviral drugs.
- Viatical (selling your life insurance) settlements.

- Salvage therapy, the kitchen sink approach—trying to save the patient.
- See Interactive HIV/AIDS map launched in mid-2011 by Emory University Rollins School of Public Health (AIDSVu.org).
- Dispensing current anti-HIV drug therapy requires an HIV/AIDS specialist.
- The *best* anti-HIV drug combinations are still unknown.
- Pre-exposure prophylaxis (PrEP) is presented as new method of prevention. The results of serodiscordant and PrEP studies showing the ability of antiretroviral drugs to prevent HIV transmission are presented.
- July 2012, FDA approves the use of Truvada as the first HIV prevention drug for use in HIV-negative people.
- Presentation against the push to test and treat infected individuals.
- Post-exposure prophylaxis (PEP) or morning-after drug therapy to prevent HIV infection looks promising.
- Scientists do not expect the production of an effective anti-HIV vaccine before 2015–2020.
- Ending 2013, globally, over 8 million people will be receiving antiretroviral therapy.
- Treatment as prevention—see pages 85–91, Sidebars 4.3 and 4.4 for discussion of the use of ART in a series of HIV prevention studies. For example, to prevent transmission between HIV serodiscordant heterosexual couples.
- HIV/AIDS therapy hotlines, and resources are listed.
- See disclaimer on page 103.

We are constantly humbled by the devastation that something so small, HIV, can launch upon something so large, a human. This chapter provides no final answers; there is no curative therapy, no truly outstanding therapies (drugs that benefit all HIV-infected without major side effects) against HIV, and, with the number of expensive anti-HIV drugs that are available, debate continues about the details on which drugs offer the best combination therapy and on the standard of care for HIV/AIDS patients. Because some 95% of HIV-infected people will eventually develop AIDS, and because 90% of all *new* HIV infections are occurring in developing nations, an inexpensive, easily taken, nontoxic, effective HIV-directed therapy is essential. Physicians need a drug that works against HIV as antibiotics once worked against a large variety of disease-causing bacteria.

BETTER DRUGS, BETTER TECHNOLOGIES, AND LINGERING PROBLEMS

Progress in the treatment of human immuno-deficiency virus (HIV) and AIDS has been just short of unbelievable! In the early 1980s, a diagnosis of AIDS was thought to be synonymous with death. Today, with available antiretroviral therapies, the life expectancy of HIV-infected persons nears that of age-matched uninfected persons. This chapter details some of the challenges and exciting breakthroughs in the development of antiretroviral drugs.

ANTIRETROVIRAL THERAPY OR ART

The ideal solution would be to prevent HIV from causing an infection. Then antiretroviral therapies would not be necessary. However, there are no means available to stop HIV from entering the body and infecting a limited number of cell types—primarily those cells displaying CD4 protein antigen receptor sites. Following HIV infection, there is a depletion of cells carrying the CD4 protein, especially the **T lymphocyte (T4) cells of the human immune system.** (See Chapter 5 for an explanation of cell types in the human immune system and their function.) With T4 or CD4+ cell loss (lymphocytes carrying the CD4 protein), over time immunological response is lost. Loss of immunological response leads to a variety of opportunistic infections (OIs). The suppression of the immune system and increasing susceptibility to OIs and cancers give HIV/AIDS a multidimensional pathology. (OIs are presented in Chapter 6.) Because HIV/AIDS is a multidimensional syndrome, it is unlikely that a single drug will provide adequate treatment or a cure.

An ideal goal for HIV drug investigators would be to find a drug that excises all HIV proviruses from the cell's DNA. It is very unlikely that this kind of drug will soon, if ever, be available. Alternatively, the elimination of all HIV-infected cells might be of comparable benefit, as long as irreplaceable cells are not totally lost through the process. In essence, this is the goal that the human immune system sets for itself, yet falls short of reaching, in the vast majority of HIV-infected individuals.

In the absence of a curative weapon, therapies must be designed to prevent the spread of the virus in the body. All of the FDA-approved antiretroviral therapies to date are presented in this chapter.

Most Americans have no direct contact with the U.S. Food and Drug Administration (FDA), but their lives literally depend on the effectiveness of the agency. Charged with assuring the safety of specific foods and all medicines, the FDA has oversight of 25% of the U.S. economy. One of the FDA's key functions is approving and monitoring prescription drugs—a job that is particularly crucial for people with HIV infection or other life-threatening diseases. The FDA is the American Gold Standard of endorsement! (See Point of Information 4.1.)

The Dark Age of Antiretroviral Therapy

Between the years 1981 and 1987, when hundreds of thousands in the United States and millions worldwide had already become HIV infected and many thousands had already died, there were no effective drug therapies against HIV. Physicians offered anything and everything they thought held promise. This was truly an **age of darkness across Planet Earth**. Even in March 1987 when researchers tried zidovudine (ZDU, aka AZT)—a long-abandoned cancer treatment drug, a nucleoside analog—the atmosphere that prevailed was still one of trying anything that might help. Luckily, this drug slowed the replication of HIV, and everyone immediately took notice. Continued drug research put them on the road to investigating nucleosides as antiretroviral medications—but it took another four years before a second antiretroviral drug, didanosine (DDI), reached the market and another four years to market the first protease inhibitor. This began the advent of highly active antiretroviral therapy (**HAART**).

[Pre HAART Era: No Effective HIV Treatment, 1981–1996 (15 years)]

[Post HAART Era: Effective HIV Treatment, 1996–2013 (17 years)]

POINT OF INFORMATION 4.1

THE FDA'S ROLE IN HIV/AIDS

The Food and Drug Administration (FDA) is a regulatory agency that enforces the Food, Drug, and Cosmetic Act and the Public Health Service Act, ensuring that drugs and biologics are safe and effective for their intended uses and properly labeled. The FDA's activities help protect all consumers in the United States, regulating some trillion dollars' worth of products that constitute approximately one-fourth of total consumer expenditures in the United States. The FDA sets standards for and monitors all prescription and nonprescription drugs; all blood products, vaccines, and tissues for transplantation; all medical devices and equipment, and all radiation emitting devices; all animal drugs and feed; nearly all domestic and imported foods except for meat and poultry; and all cosmetics.

FDA responsibilities include a variety of HIV/AIDS-related issues. The agency primarily serves a review and oversight function in areas related to drugs, biologics, and medical devices for the prevention and treatment of HIV/AIDS, and AIDS-related conditions.

WHERE IS THE CURE? IS IT TIME TO REVISIT THIS QUESTION? NO LEADING RESEARCHER HAS PUBLICLY UTTERED THE WORD "CURE" SINCE THE 1990s. HOWEVER, IN FEBRUARY 2011 THE PRESIDENT-ELECT OF THE INTERNATIONAL AIDS SOCIETY AND NOBEL PRIZE WINNER FRANÇOISE BARRÉ-SINOUSSI LAUNCHED A CALL FOR A CURE FOR HIV/AIDS. THERE IS A NEW OPTIMISM IN THE AIR!

WHY DO WE NEED A CURE? WON'T ANTIRETROVIRAL DRUGS BE ENOUGH?

HIV/AIDS treatment is a complex area and there are many different treatments available—some treat the virus itself, others treat the symptoms and illnesses caused by the virus. However, none is a cure for HIV or AIDS. It is important to be clear about the distinction between a treatment that may cure or prevent an illness related to HIV infection with a cure for HIV (or AIDS) itself. It also is important not to describe drugs used to slow the growth of the virus as cures. Again, there is no cure for HIV.

A cure for HIV is a necessity: 38 million people worldwide are living with HIV, and 25 million more will be infected in each of the coming decades (a total of 300 million by 2100). The lifelong treatment of these people would be logistically difficult, expensive, and could result in drug resistance, treatment failure, and onward transmission of drug-resistance HIV—in short, a public health nightmare without end.

To cure HIV infection three events must occur: (a) stopping HIV replication, (b) identifying all HIV reservoirs, (a major barrier because HIV persists in a latent stage), and (c) eliminating all such reservoirs. According to the AIDS policy project, the NIH spends about 3% of its research budget on finding a cure. In 2012, that came to $96,000,000.

Can We Be on the Way to a Cure?

So what kind of cure can there be? Why is "the cure word" re-emerging now? Should scientists and the layman be asking about a cure without the possibility of a vaccine in the near future? Currently there are two types of cure under discussion: a *sterilizing* cure and a *functional* cure.

A STERILIZING CURE VERSUS A FUNCTIONAL CURE AND THE PROBLEM OF HIV LATENT RESERVOIRS

Sterilizing Cure—A sterilizing cure against a virus, prevents a disease such as the vaccines made against viruses, that cause polio, measles, or smallpox. As a corollary, the cure stops any transmission of the virus. Such sterilizing cures are possible because the body's immune system produces virus-specific neutralizing antibodies when challenged with an inactive version of the virus—antibodies that inactivate that specific virus. In the near future—perhaps the next five to ten years—no such vaccine will be available to prevent the transmission of HIV. In fact, a sterilizing cure against HIV may not be possible! HIV may be the most extraordinarory disease-causing agent ever encountered by modern science. **HIV is a very unique virus, a unique pathogen!**

The Problem of HIV Latency As It Relates to an HIV Cure

Once HIV enters the body, it infects memory CD4+ cells and perhaps other cells in the brain, lymph nodes, and precursor blood cells, where it remains dormant, or rests quietly out of reach of antiretroviral drugs. These dormant (or latent) cells containing HIV act as reservoirs that become active and release the virus in the absence of ART. Douglas Richman and colleagues (2009) make the following four points with regard to eradicating HIV from the body:

1. Discontinuation of ART allows HIV to be released from latent reservoir cells.
2. Patients successfully treated with ART for longer than 10 years exhibit no appreciable decrease in the size of the latent reservoir.
3. The persistence of latently infected memory CD4+ cells precludes their elimination by ART alone for the lifetime of the patient.
4. No one has any idea of how many HIV reservoirs there are.

Although there is ample evidence that current ART will not cure HIV infections, investigators are reluctant to say that it can't be done someday. No one wants the infamy similar to that of past IBM president Thomas Watson, who said in 1943, "I think there is a world market for maybe five computers," or Pierre Pachet, professor of physiology in the late 1800s who said, "Louis Pasteur's theory of germs is ridiculous fiction."

For now it looks like HIV eradication will be, at best, very difficult, but not trying to achieve the goal of a cure is unacceptable.

UPDATE 2012—In July 2012, David Margolis published in *Nature* that a cancer drug called vorinostat can cause the release of HIV from its hidden cellular reservoirs. Stay tuned.

Renewed Hope: A Functional Cure—A functional cure is for HIV-infected persons. It would be the use of ART to reduce HIV to undetect-able levels and strengthen the immune system enough to hold the disease in check upon discontinuation of ART. In this case, the patient would live out his or her expected life span. Because the virus is undetectable, it would be unlikely to be transmitted. Both conditions are critical in regard to thinking "cure." Even so, "unlikely to be transmitted" means there is no sterile immunity; that is, some people would transmit HIV. It may, however, be possible to achieve a functional cure—a lifetime without symptoms, disease progression, or prolonged ART—if a short course of HIV therapy is started immediately and aggressively in people newly infected with the virus. And if this proves possible, there's hope of doing away with the need for expensive and potentially toxic treatment in others who have been living with HIV. Following Fauci's logic, the world may be able to treat its way out of this pandemic. However, besides the logistical and monetary demands it presents, a functional cure leaves two critical assumptions to be addressed: **one,** that early ART will provide personal health benefits that override long-term drug toxicities, and **two,** that ART will provide lasting prevention of HIV transmission.

A growing number of experts believe that a functional cure, whereby HIV is disabled and/or the immune system is strengthened sufficiently to hold off disease progression when ART is discontinued, is an achievable goal in the very foreseeable future. This ART-free remission may be a more realistic goal than the complete eradication of HIV.

However, the realization that the price of keeping tens of millions of people on ART for the rest of their lives is not a check that any nation is prepared to write.

There is no doubt that in the search for a cure, science often takes two steps forward and then one step back. However, scientists are heading in the right direction, and the pace is dramatically quickening. The take-home message: A CURE IS POSSIBLE; IT'S FINALLY IN SIGHT AND HOPEFULLY SOON WITHIN REACH. UNTIL THEN AIDS REMAIN FATAL.

In 2010, *POZ Magazine* polled its readers on three questions, each regarding their view on an HIV/AIDS cure. The three questions were:

1. Do you think a cure will be found in your lifetime?
2. Do you think a cure for HIV/AIDS will ever be found?
3. Do you think enough money is being spent on finding a cure?

CLASS QUESTION: The question remains: Is it time to think of a cure for HIV—sterilizing, functional, or otherwise? **Your response is?**

The readers' responses to the questions were:

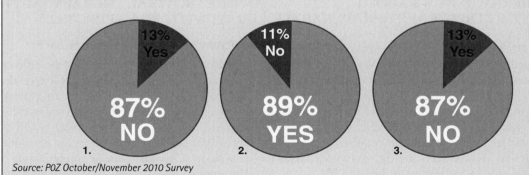

Source: POZ October/November 2010 Survey

A CURE—SIDELIGHTS INTO THE FUTURE?

In 2008, major worldwide media covered the story of an HIV-positive leukemia patient Timothy Ray Brown (Figure 4-1) in Berlin, Germany, who had possibly been "cured" of HIV after a bone marrow or stem cell transplant to treat his cancer. The man's transplant specialist used stem cells from a donor with a rare genetic mutation that prevented his CD4+ cells from producing CCR5 (R5) receptors, and thus rendered him virtually immune to HIV. Since the transplant in 2006, the leukemia patient has not received antiretroviral therapy, and scientists have been unable to locate HIV in his body. Some have called this a possible cure. Even if the patient turns out to have lost HIV permanently, it is unlikely that stem cell transplants are going to become a routine treatment for HIV patients. Not only do the transplants often cost at least a quarter of a million dollars, but patients also typically receive whole-body radiation or high-dose chemotherapy to get rid of leukemic stem cells and make space for the transplanted cells—a process called reconditioning—and both treatments come with a high risk of serious side effects and death.

Update 2013—Ending 2012, (69 months) Tim Brown continues to demonstrate an un-detectable viral load (HIV). It should also be mentioned that in mid-2009 two other patients similar to Timothy Brown received similar treatment. No HIV was found in either patient after four years of testing!

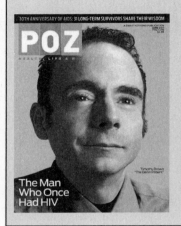

FIGURE 4-1 Timothy Brown, a.k.a. "The Berlin Patient." Brown, diagnosed with HIV in 1995, is an American who was in treatment for leukemia in Germany and required a stem cell transplant. His doctor, Gero Heutter, destroyed Brown's immune system using chemotherapy and radiation and rebuilt it with donated bone marrow. Heuter chose a donor who had a genetic mutation that made his CD4 cells immune to HIV. The transplant worked, and Brown no longer has HIV. When word of Brown's cure got out, it was big news. But the global media coverage created much confusion. He had friends e-mailing him saying, "Congratulations! We're happy for you." What few understand is that Brown's cure involved hundreds of thousands of dollars of experimental science, a rare and almost impossible-to-replicate set of conditions and the threat of death and a year in the hospital. In addition, there are strains of HIV that bind to other receptors to cause an infection. A widely applicable cure is still not here. *(From POZ Magazine, June 2011, cover photo. Copyright 2011 by POZ Magazine. Reprinted courtesy of Smart + Strong/POZ.)*

THE GOOD NEWS ABOUT ANTIRETROVIRAL THERAPY (ART)

In 2009 it was reported that ART worked well regardless of the subtype of HIV and individuals infected with it. They found little difference in the proportion of patients achieving and maintaining an undetectable viral load when analyzed according to their subtype. Immune restoration, measured by the increase in number of CD4+ cells, was also similar across the subtypes studied. These studies are important because the dominant HIV subtype in Western Europe and the United States is subtype B. Therefore, most clinical trials and observational studies have been performed in populations where subtype B predominates. This is despite the fact that this subtype represents only 12% of global HIV infections, with subtype C contributing approximately 48%. (Gevetti et al., 2009, see Chapter 3 pages 64 and 65.)

ANTIRETROVIRAL THERAPY (ART) DRUGS WITH FDA APPROVAL

Gold Standard = Holy Grail of ART

The **gold standard** for determining the efficacy (effectiveness) of a new treatment is that it alters the disease in a way that is beneficial to the patient. Therefore, the end points most often used in clinical trials of therapies for a disease such as HIV/AIDS include prolongation of life or the extension of time before a significant disease complication.

But studies using these end points require large numbers of patients and/or the passage of considerable amounts of time. **Surrogate markers** (that is, physiological measurements that serve as substitutes for these major clinical events) can eliminate this problem if their validity and correlation with clinical outcome in people can be confirmed. The use of surrogates has the potential to shorten the duration of clinical trials and expedite the development of new therapies.

The **Holy Grail** for HIV therapy is to suppress HIV replication to undetectable levels—less than 50 copies of HIV-RNA per milliliter of blood plasma.

Major Surrogate Markers Used to Evaluate Antiretroviral Therapy (ART)

The **T4 or CD4+ immune cell number** and **viral load** (the number of HIV-RNA strands in blood plasma) are the two most studied and commonly used surrogates (alternates) for clinical efficacy of antiretroviral therapies. They are imperfect measurements, however, because changes in T4 or CD4+ cell number per microliter of blood (a very, very small drop) and RNA strands per milliliter of blood (about 5 drops of blood) are only partially explained by the effects of therapy. T4 or CD4+ cell counts exhibit a high degree of day-to-day variation in individuals, and methods used to count these cells are difficult to standardize.

The Disconnect between CD4+ Cell Count and Viral Load with Regard to Their Clinical Benefits

Recent investigations have shown that there is a T4 cell level and viral load level **disconnect.** This means that viral suppression by itself does not always predict immunological and clinical benefit. T4 cell counts and viral load can be clearly dissociated during treatment: T4 cells can increase in the presence of a high viral load, remain stable, or drop. **Clinical benefit,** however, is more closely associated with the level of T4 cells than with viral load. Recent data support the hypothesis that T4 cell depletion during HIV infection occurs largely as a result of the immune system's inability to generate new mature cells, and that the main effect of antiretroviral therapy is to help restore the immune system's ability to produce new T4 cells (Perrin et al., 1998; Telenti et al., 1998; Deeks et al., 1999; Clark et al., 1999; Hellerstein et al., 1999; Rodriguez et al., 2006).

THE HIV MEDICINE CHEST: ART DRUGS RECEIVING FDA APPROVAL

The T4 or CD4+ cell count is the most immediate indicator of immune function. In the United States the average person who walks into an HIV clinic has a T4 or CD4+ cell count of about 180 cells per milliliter of blood plasma. This average person needed to start treatment years before they were diagnosed. The expected or "normal" T4 or CD4+ cell count is between 600 and 1200.

The evolution of treatment for HIV should be considered one of the most important accomplishments in the history of modern medicine. The introduction of protease inhibitors in the mid-1990s, along with insights into viral dynamics and the importance of using multiple active agents in combination, marked the beginning of the highly active antiretroviral therapy (HAART) era and substantially improved survival rates for individuals infected with HIV. In less than two decades, 26 unique antiretroviral therapies in over 30 different formulations have been developed—a feat virtually unparalleled in the history of medicine.

There have been no examples since the discovery of penicillin in 1929 that rivals the development of antiretroviral drugs in controlling a previously fatal disease. Of the 26 FDA-approved antiretroviral drugs to date, 17 are in common use against HIV.

A Delicate Balance

For most HIV medicines to work properly, their bloodstream levels must be precise. Too much, and they're toxic. Too little, and they fail to keep the virus in check.

The number and kinds of HIV drugs, their recommended mixtures, and their timing and dosage change almost continuously. This can be a source of tremendous confusion for patients and medical practitioners alike.

Processing Drugs

Our body recognizes drugs as foreign substances. It removes them, usually in urine or in bowel movements. Many drugs are removed unchanged by the kidneys in urine. Other drugs must be processed by the liver. Enzymes in the liver change drug molecules, and then they are eliminated in urine or in bowel movements. When you take a pill, the drug goes from the stomach into the intestines and then into the liver before circulating to the rest of the body. If the drug is easily broken down by the liver, then very little of the drug reaches the body. But if the drug interacts in the liver, its movement and amount available to the body can be altered. A number of ARVDs can slow or speed up the action of liver enzymes, causing an increase or decrease in the blood levels of said drugs. And the change in liver enzyme activity can also affect the levels of other drugs that are also processed by the same liver enzymes. For example, protease inhibitors and non-nucleoside reverse transcriptase inhibitors are processed by the liver and cause many drug interactions. A few of the ARVDs slow down the kidneys. This increases the blood levels of substances that are normally removed by the kidneys.

The Bottom Line

Many ARVDs can interact with other medications, drugs, or herbal products, and the list of interactions is always growing. These interactions can lead to serious or fatal overdoses of some drugs, or can drop drug levels too low to do any good. You and your physician should carefully review the information that comes with each medication (the package insert). Ask for this information for each drug that you are taking. Also, be sure that a doctor reviews all medications, drugs, supplements, or herbs you are taking.

Eating Or Not Can Alter ARVD Levels

Oral drugs pass through the stomach into the intestines. Most drugs are absorbed faster if the stomach is empty. For some drugs this is a good thing, but it can also cause side effects. Some drugs need to be taken with food so that they are broken down more slowly to reduce side effects. Others should be taken with fatty foods because they dissolve in fat and are absorbed better. Caution: stomach acid is needed for some

medications. They should not be taken at the same time as antacids.

FDA-Approved Antiretroviral Drugs

From March 1987 through 2012, 26 individual anti-HIV drugs and seven combination drugs have received FDA approval for use in persons infected with HIV. There are at least 33 FDA-approved drugs when combination pills and reformulations are included. Other drugs have been FDA-approved for **expanded access use** where standard regimens have failed (Table 4-1).

Seven Classes of Antiretroviral Drugs

Cellular targets of these drugs can be seen in Figure 4-2. All seven classes of antiretroviral drugs are classified by the stage of the HIV life cycle they affect. The bottom line is that they all do the same thing—prevent HIV from replicating—but they each do it in different ways.

Each of the eight nucleoside/nucleotide analogs, sometimes referred to as **nukes,** on entering an HIV-infected cell interferes with the virus's ability to replicate itself (Figure 4-3). That is, when any of the eight nucleoside/nucleotide analogs are incorporated into a strand of HIV DNA being newly synthesized, it stops further synthesis of that DNA strand. The nucleoside analog stops the HIV enzyme, reverse transcriptase, from joining the next nucleoside into position.

Focus on the Eight Single (non-combination) Nucleoside/ Nucleotide Analogs (NRTIs)

Each of the eight drugs has limited effectiveness as a **monotherapy.** The principal limitations are: (1) they are not 100% effective in stopping HIV reverse transcriptase from making HIV DNA; (2) positive clinical effects are short-term, they are not sustained; (3) each drug has its own set of toxic side effects; (4) individually they do not delay the onset of AIDS; and (5) HIV rapidly becomes resistant to each of them. Other nukes are in development.

Table 4-1 Choices: Antiretroviral Therapy (ART); Nucleoside Analogs, Non-Nucleosides, Protease Inhibitors, Entry Inhibitors, and Integrase Enzyme Inhibitors: The Average Pharmacy Charge per Month for a Typical HIV Drug Regimen Is about $2000

Name	FDA Approved	Cost/Year[a]
1. Nucleoside analog (reverse transcriptase inhibitor–NRTIs)		
Zidovudine, ZDU (Retrovir)/AZT	March 1987	$ 3,552
Didanosine, ddI (Videx)	October 1991	$ 5,112
Zalcitabine, ddC (Hivid)	June 1994	$ 3,013.89
Stavudine, d4T (Zerit)	June 1994	$ 6,012
Lamivudine, 3TC (Epivir)	November 1995	$ 6,084
Combivir (Zidovudine/lamivudine)	September 1997	$12,432
Abacavir (Ziagen)	December 1998	$ 7,992
Trizivir (Ziagen/Retrovir/Epivir)	November 2000	$20,808
Tenofovir (Viread)[b]	October 2001	$12,000
Emtricitabine (Emtriva)	July 2003	$ 6,492
Truvada (emtricitabine/tenofovir)	August 2004	$16,800
Epzicom[d] (Epivir/Ziagen); Kivexa outside USA	August 2004	$13,668
Atripla (Sustiva/Viread/Emtriva)	July 2006	$25,992
Complera (emtricitabine/ripivirine/tenofovir DF)[f]	August 2011	$25,380
Stribild (emtricitabine/tenofovir/elvitegravir/cobicistat)	August 2012	Est. $31,000

These are potent in combination with other drugs; used alone, they lead to HIV resistance. *ZDV (AZT), d4T, 3TC,* and *abacavir* penetrate the blood-brain barrier. Common side effects: lactic acidosis. *Seven* new nucleoside analogs are in some phase of testing in the United States.[c]

Non-nucleoside compounds (non-nucleoside analog reverse transcriptase inhibitors–NNRTIs)		
Nevirapine (Viramune)	June 1996	$ 7,428
Delavirdine (Rescriptor)	April 1997	$ 4,788
Efavirenz (Sustiva, Stocrin)	September 1998	$ 8,760
Etravirine (Intelence)	January 2008	$12,336
Rilpivirine (Edurant)	May 2011	$ 9,768

2. Non-nucleoside analog reverse transcriptase inhibitors (NNRTIs, or non-nukes) may interact with other *cytochrome p450-processed drugs:* protease inhibitors, oral contraceptives, etc. NNRTIs have a mixed ability to penetrate the blood-brain barrier. Common side effect: mild rash. Some doctors build up drug doses slowly to avoid rash; the other worry is that dose building increases risk of drug resistance.

3. Protease inhibitor drugs (PI)		
Saquinavir mesylate (Invirase)	December 1995	$ 3,384
Ritonavir (Norvir)	March 1996	$ 3,744
Indinavir (Crixivan)	March 1996	$ 6,912
Nelfinavir (Viracept)	March 1997	$10,944
Saquinavir (Fortovase)	November 1997	$ 3,396
Amprenavir (Agenerase)	April 1999	off the market
Kaletra (Lopinavir/Novir)	September 2000	$10,116
Atazanavir (Reyataz)	June 2003	$22,524
Fosamprenavir (Lexiva)	October 2003	$11,628
Tipranavir (Aptivus)[d]	June 2005	$ 4,020
Darunavir (Prezista)	June 2006	$17,796

PIs are very potent and may interact with other drugs using cytochrome p450 metabolic pathways. Potentially life-threatening if taken with Seldane, Hismanal, Propulsid, Halcion, or Versed. Avoid rifabutin, Nizoral, rifampin. Poor absorption may affect potency. Common side effects: liver toxicity, hypoglycemia, flatulence, bloating, lipodystrophy (fat distribution). Seven new protease inhibitors are now in some phase of testing in the United States. In addition, there are at least 28 other antiretroviral drugs being investigated.

OTHER DRUG CLASSES

4. Entry or Fusion Inhibitors—bar HIV from entering immune cells		
T-20 (Enfuvirtide, Fuzeon)	March 2003	$ 44,604[c]
Maraviroc[d] (Selzentry, the first CCR5 co-receptor antagonist)	August 2007	$ 14,436
FP21399		
PRO 542 and 140[e]		
TNX-355, a monoclonal antibody (ibalizumab)—CXCR4 receptor blockers AK6:02 Glaxo		
873180—CCR5 blocker		
TBR-652—CCR5 blocker		

(continued)

Table 4-1 (continued)

5. Integrase Strand Transfer Inhibitors—prevent HIV DNA from entering human DNA

Raltegravir (Isentress) (MK 0158)	October 2007	$16,092
Dolutegravir (S/GSK1349572)	—	—

6. NEW DRUG CLASSES (not yet approved)
Zinc Finger
 —disrupts polyprotein formation essential
  for HIV replication
Azodicarbonamide (ADA)
Antisense Drugs
 —prevent viral function
  HGTV43
Assembly Inhibitors[d]

7. Maturation Inhibitors: Bevirmat (PA-457); Vivecon (MPC = 9055)

[a] Cost is based on prescription prices as found in Jacksonville, FL, Walgreen pharmacies, 2012.

[b] Tenovir is the first nucleotide analog approved for HIV treatment. It blocks HIV replication similar to the nucleoside analogs.

[c] Prevent the viral proteins from assembling into the HIV capsid that houses viral RNA, enzymes, etc.
There are now drugs that interfere with at least nine different mechanisms in the process by which HIV attaches itself to specific cell types, enters them, enters the cells' DNA, makes copies of itself, and exits the cell.

[d] Maraviroc is the second FDA entry inhibitor drug. Raltegravir is the first FDA HIV integrase enzyme inhibitor drug. TNX-355 and HGS004 are monoclonal antibodies against CCR5.

[e] PRO 140 is a laboratory-made antibody that binds to CCR5.

[f] Complera contains one NNRTI and two NRTIs.

USE OF NON-NUCLEOSIDE ANALOG REVERSE TRANSCRIPTASE INHIBITORS

Non-nucleoside reverse transcriptase inhibitors (NNRTIs), sometimes referred to as **non-nukes,** are a structurally and chemically dissimilar group of antiretrovirals that can be used effectively in triple-therapy regimes. The mechanism of action of NNRTIs is distinct from that of nucleoside analogs, even though both *prevent* the conversion of HIV-RNA into HIV DNA. Nucleoside RT inhibitors stop HIV replication by their incorporation into the elongating strand of viral DNA, causing chain termination. In contrast, NNRTIs are not incorporated into viral DNA but inhibit HIV replication directly by binding noncompetitively to the RT enzyme. NNRTIs at first appeared to offer hope. All five tested did inhibit the RT-HIV enzyme. But this inhibition was short-lived because HIV-resistant mutants for each of the non-nucleoside RTIs were found within weeks of their use. The primary advantage of using NNRTIs in therapy is to delay the use of protease inhibitors. But they are associated with liver damage.

The key to future success in using the reverse transcriptase inhibitors (RTIs) is finding RTIs that work in cells that are not undergoing division. Most RTIs currently in use work only in cells that are dividing (dividing cells must replicate their DNA). Other non-nukes are in development.

FDA-APPROVED PROTEASE INHIBITORS

Recall from Chapter 3, pages 57, 58 and 62 that some HIV genes code for **reverse transcriptase** (RT), **integrase,** and **protease** enzymes. Later on in the reproductive cycle of HIV a specific **protease** is required to process the precursor GAG and POL proteins into mature HIV components, GAG proteins, and the enzymes integrase and protease (Erickson et al., 1990). If protease is missing or inactive, noninfectious HIV are produced. Therefore, inhibitors of protease enzyme function represent an **alternative** strategy to the inhibition of reverse transcriptase in the treatment of HIV infection (Figures 4-4 and 4-5).

The **protease inhibitors,** made up of a small number of amino acids (up to 15), bind to

Targets of Antiretroviral Drugs: Generalized Scheme

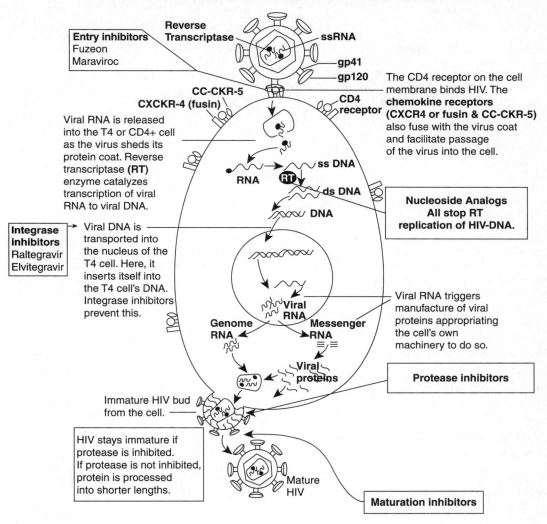

Entry inhibitors
Fuzeon
Maraviroc

Reverse Transcriptase

ssRNA

gp41
gp120

CC-CKR-5
CXCKR-4 (fusin)

CD4 receptor

The CD4 receptor on the cell membrane binds HIV. The **chemokine receptors (CXCR4 or fusin & CC-CKR-5)** also fuse with the virus coat and facilitate passage of the virus into the cell.

Viral RNA is released into the T4 or CD4+ cell as the virus sheds its protein coat. Reverse transcriptase **(RT)** enzyme catalyzes transcription of viral RNA to viral DNA.

RNA   RT   ss DNA

ds DNA

DNA

Nucleoside Analogs All stop RT replication of HIV-DNA.

Integrase inhibitors
Raltegravir
Elvitegravir

Viral DNA is transported into the nucleus of the T4 cell. Here, it inserts itself into the T4 cell's DNA. Integrase inhibitors prevent this.

Viral RNA

Genome RNA   Messenger RNA

Viral RNA triggers manufacture of viral proteins appropriating the cell's own machinery to do so.

Viral proteins

Protease inhibitors

Immature HIV bud from the cell.

HIV stays immature if protease is inhibited. If protease is not inhibited, protein is processed into shorter lengths.

Mature HIV

Maturation inhibitors

FIGURE 4–2 The diagram shows five classes of FDA-approved antiretroviral drugs used in therapy. These drugs attack five different targets. All 26 FDA-approved individual antiretroviral compounds are represented with respect to their anti-HIV activity. The nucleoside analogs act early after infection, while the protease inhibitors act later in the HIV life cycle, after viral proteins have been synthesized into long strands. Those strands of amino acids contain the individual HIV proteins that become functional after they are cut into their appropriate amino acid sequence lengths. NOTE: The enzyme integrase is required for HIV DNA to enter human DNA. Drugs called integrase and **maturation inhibitors** are in development. (See Table 4-1.)

the protease active site and inhibit the activity of the enzyme. This inhibition prevents cleavage of the long HIV proteins, resulting in the formation of immature *noninfectious* viral particles.

As research progressed, scientists found that HIV protease is distinctly different from human protease enzymes, so a drug that blocks HIV protease should not affect normal human cell

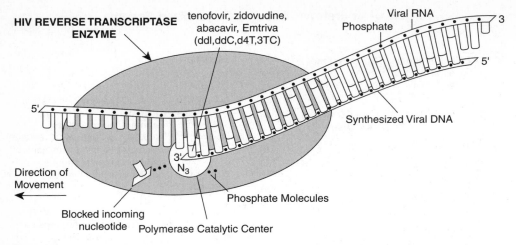

FIGURE 4-3 Incorporation of Nucleoside/Nucleotide Analogs Preventing HIV Replication. Zidovudine (ZDV) is a synthetic thymidine analog that is widely used in the treatment of HIV disease and AIDS. HIV-RT is 100 times more sensitive to ZDV inhibition than is the **human transcriptase.** The incorporation of zidovudine-triphosphate into HIV DNA by the action of HIV reverse transcriptase terminates DNA chain extension because polymerization, or the incorporation of the next nucleotide adjacent to the azide N_3 group, cannot occur. Similar blockage of DNA replication occurs when ddI, ddC, d4T, or 3TC are used. Abacavir is the first 2' deoxyguanosine analog to be used.

function. This means that HIV protease blockers are specific to HIV protease. Entering 2013, some 16 HIV protease-inhibiting drugs were under study, 6 were in clinical trials, and 10 had received FDA approval.

FDA-Approved Combination/Combined Therapy Drugs

What Is Combination Or Combined Antiretroviral Therapy (cART) Drug Medications?

Combination or combined medications used in ART are pills, tablets, or capsules that contain more than one drug to fight HIV. Pharmaceutical companies have been working hard to make their medications easier to take. Part of this effort has been to combine more than one medication in a single unit. These combinations are referred to as fixed-dose combinations, or FDCs.

Seven drug combinations have been FDA-approved. Combivir is a combination of nucleosides zidovudine and lamivudine. Kaletra is a protease inhibitor combination containing

lopinavir/Norvir. Trizivir is the first to contain three nucleoside analogs—Ziagen (abacavir), Retrovir (zidovudine or AZT), and Epivir (3TC). Truvada is a combination of the nucleo-sides emtricitabine and tenofovir. Epzicom combines Epivir and Ziagen. For costs of each combination therapy see Table 4–1.

What Are "PK Boosters" and Why Are They Used?

When some medications are taken by mouth, their levels in the blood are very low. For them to fight HIV, they have to be taken at high doses. Another possibility is to "boost" the low blood levels. This is done by slowing down the processing (metabolism) of these drugs. A drug that slows down the metabolism is called a "PK booster." PK stands for "pharmacokinetic." This refers to the way medications are processed by the body.

Seven drug combinations have been FDA-approved. Combivir, Kaletra, Trizivir, Truvada, Epzicom, Atripla, the first once-a-day pill and Complera, the second once-a-day pill was

A. Why HIV Protease is Essential for HIV Replication

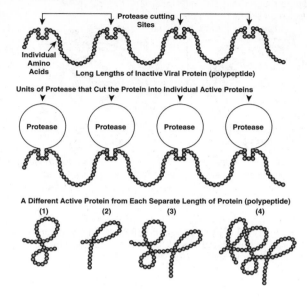

Protease cutting Sites

Individual Amino Acids

Long Lengths of Inactive Viral Protein (polypeptide)

Units of Protease that Cut the Protein into Individual Active Proteins

Protease   Protease   Protease   Protease

A Different Active Protein from Each Separate Length of Protein (polypeptide)

(1)   (2)   (3)   (4)

B. How HIV Protease Inhibitors Inhibit Viral Protease Function

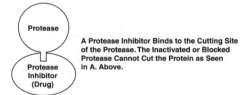

Protease

Protease Inhibitor (Drug)

A Protease Inhibitor Binds to the Cutting Site of the Protease. The Inactivated or Blocked Protease Cannot Cut the Protein as Seen in A. Above.

FIGURE 4-4 Function of Protease and Protease Inhibitors. **(A)** The function of HIV protease is to release the individual replication enzymes, core proteins, and envelope proteins so that HIV can develop into mature, infective HIV. **(B)** Blocking the production of these essential HIV proteins using protease inhibitors produces immature, non-infective HIV. The action (cutting of protein lengths into active HIV components) of HIV protease occurs during and just after HIV buds out of the cell. Also see Figure 4-5.

FDC approved in August 2011. For the cost of each combination therapy see Table 4–1.

ENTRY INHIBITORS AND PROBLEMS

Entry inhibitors make it possible for the first time to stop HIV from entering a cell. Thus, there are now drugs to target HIV before and after it enters a cell (Figure 4-2)! Fuzeon was FDA-approved in 2003 but has the drawback of being an injection drug. In August 2007, **Maraviroc/Selzentry** was FDA-approved. Maraviroc is the first attachment inhibitor drug. When HIV infects a cell, it attaches to the outside surface of cells displaying the CD4 protein. It uses the CD4 molecules to attach to the cell before fusing with it. Maraviroc blocks the receptor called an R5 molecule. When Maraviroc blocks this receptor, HIV cannot infect that cell. This is the first member of a new class of oral drugs in a decade. An inhibitor of the R5 receptor was long sought because it was shown **not** to be vital to health and survival. Fourteen entry inhibitors are in development.

Problem with Entry Inhibitors

Maravivoc/Selzentry will only be effective against CD4+ cells using the R5 receptor. It will not be effective against HIV that target the R4 receptor (and will have a limited effect against HIV with the ability to target both receptors). Because R4-targeting HIV is more common in people who have been infected with HIV for

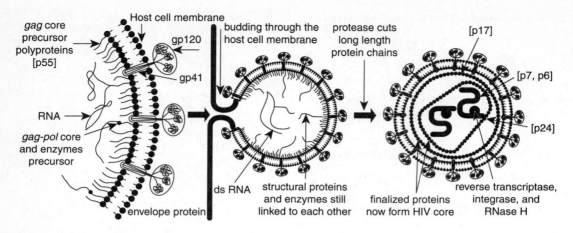

FIGURE 4-5 Representation of HIV Assembly. During the budding process, the viral GAG and GAG-POL polyproteins assemble at the cell membrane together with viral RNA to form immature HIV. These polyproteins are then cleaved by the HIV-coded protease enzyme to provide the structural and functional (enzyme) proteins essential to form the *mature*, infectious viral core. *(Adapted from Vella, 1995)*

SIDE ISSUE 4.1

YOUNG ADULTS IN SOUTH AFRICA SMOKING ANTIRETROVIRAL DRUG EFAVIRENZ: A NEW DRUG ADDICTION IN THE MAKING

Young adults in KwaZulu-Natal, South Africa, are becoming addicted to at least one antiretroviral drug as of mid-2009. They learned that if they smashed efavirenz tablets and rolled the powder into cigarette papers, they would get a quick high after smoking the drug. According to drug researchers, there is no medical benefit using the drug in this manner. And what is not known is whether using the drug in this manner will promote HIV resistance to the drug.

Thanks in part to America's help in making antiretrovirals available in underdeveloped nations, antiretroviral drugs like efavirenz are available and cheap. Now, the revelation that at least one antiretroviral drug can be used as a recreational drug has intensified the black market for antiretroviral drugs.

One 17-year-old male said, "Once you start there is no turning back. I want to stop using but I can't."

HIV-infected people are now being robbed of all their antiretroviral drugs, not just Efavirenz tablets. The various drugs are ground up and mixed in with marijuana and smoked. The mixture is called "Whoonga"—less a word than an exclamation. The cost is about $3 per hand-rolled cigarette. This mixture has become widespread in spite of no evidence to support that any of the antiretroviral drugs are hallucinogenic or addictive.

Could this addiction to antiretroviral drugs turn a success story in the use of antiretrovirals against HIV into a health crisis? Only time will tell.

How Did This Happen?

How efavirenz became a source of addiction is not known, but speculation abounds. One possibility is that people taking prescribed efavirenz said the drug can cause vivid dreams. An HIV patient may have increased his or her intake to heighten those dreams.

Today, efavirenz is being sold by people who should be taking it. Some of the drug is obtained by robbing patients and government-supplied pharmacy stocks. The use of efavirenz for drug-induced highs can be traced back to young adults in 2007.

several years, the people who are most likely going to be using Selzentry will be those whose CD4+ cells are displaying the R5 receptor or a mixture of R5 and R4 receptors.

INTEGRASE INHIBITORS

Each time HIV reproduces itself, it uses its integrase protein to insert a copy of its genome (HIV-DNA) into the DNA of a chromosome. That viral copy becomes a permanent archive of the virus's genes or its genetic program, like a tiny file burned onto a computer hard drive.

By interfering with integrase, the integrase inhibitors prevent HIV/DNA from integrating into the CD4 cell's DNA, thus stopping HIV replication.

Update for 2013: Coming a long lasting integrase inhibitor that could change Antiretroviral therapy!

Preliminary data presented at the 2012 interscience conference on antimicrobial agents and chemotherapy suggest that the integrase inhibitor–S/GSK744 could be taken once every three months. This will, if FDA approved, have enormous implications for therapy and prevention. What is causing the excitement is that the drug remains at inhibitory concentrations out to at least 12 weeks. In addition, the drug is active against a broad range of HIV-l subtypes and HIV-2 and HIV does not easily form mutations to lessen the effect of this drug.

Note: Studies on this drug were published as abstracts and presented at this conference. These data and conclusions about this drug should be considered preliminary until Published in a peer reviewed journal.

Maturation Inhibitors

Maturation inhibitors disrupt processing of the viral GAG protein by preventing the conversion of the capsid precursor (p25) into the mature capsid protein (p24). Although maturation inhibitors target the same enzymatic step as protease inhibitors, their methods of action differ. The lead candidate in the maturation inhibitor class is bevirimat (formerly PA-457) (Table 4-1, page 75). Vivecon, a new maturation inhibitor, is in Phase 2 trials.

DEVELOPMENT AND SELECTION OF HIV DRUG-RESISTANT MUTANTS

Drug resistance is easier to understand once you know a little bit about how HIV works. HIV, like all viruses, is a parasite; it needs a human cell in which to reproduce. The first thing HIV does when it enters your body is look for a place to make its home. Its target? Your immune system— in particular, cells known as CD4+ (or T4 or helper T) cells. The fact that HIV enters these particular cells is bad news because CD4+ cells control your immune system, which your body uses to fight off infections.

HIV is a virus elusive to drugs. Scientists have spent the last 26 years designing drugs to fight it. But HIV adapts (develops resistance) to each new drug (Figure 4-6).

Development of Drug-Resistant Nucleoside Analog Mutants

HIV reverse transcriptase, the enzyme that copies (transcribes) HIV-RNA into HIV DNA, is *unable* to correct transcription errors during nucleic acid replication. Because there is no repair or correction of mistakes (as occurs in human cells), there are about one to five mutations in each new replicated HIV DNA/HIV-RNA strand (Coffin, 1995). This means that each new virus is different from all other HIV that is being produced because new virus is being produced at a rate of 1 billion to 10 billion per day! There will be 1 billion to 10 billion new HIV mutants produced each day in one person. Thus, virtually all possible drug mutations, and perhaps many combinations of mutations to drugs, are generated in each patient daily (Ho et al., 1995; Wain-Hobson, 1995; Wei et al., 1995; Hu et al., 1996; Mayers, 1996; Clavel, 2004).

DEVELOPMENT OF HIV DRUG RESISTANCE TO PROTEASE INHIBITORS

HIV drug-resistant mutants have now been found for every FDA-approved antiretroviral drug! Given that a typical newly infected patient

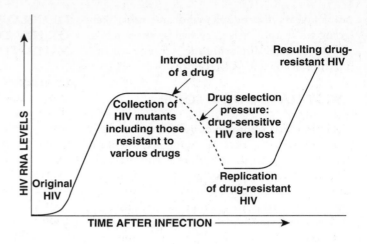

FIGURE 4-6 Enrichment of Drug-Resistant HIV. The development of drug-resistant HIV variants in an individual limits available treatment. This drug-resistant HIV is transmitted such that the recipient becomes infected with one or more drug-resistant HIV variants. Drug-resistant mutants occur by accident. The virus doesn't "figure out" the mutations to create in order to survive the drugs taken.

with HIV is in his or her 30s, delivering 40 years of medications to achieve the promise of a normal life span is a major challenge in the face of such high rates of resistance development. The problem of HIV resistance is a race between the virus and the pharmaceutical companies; will the pipeline provide drugs quickly enough to maintain options for patients with a multiple-drug resistant virus? In 2010, James Khan and Sally Blower reported that HIV mutants are almost as infectious as the wild-type strains of HIV (wild-type refers to the strain of HIV most found or in highest number in the study). The authors of the study state that 60% of drug-resistant HIV strains circulating in San Francisco are infectious enough to cause self-sustaining mini-epidemics. According to the researchers, one reason resistance is increasing stems from the protocols applied in developed countries, which call for early treatment to help keep patients healthy. But the longer a patient is using drug treatment, the greater the chance he or she will become resistant to it. Thus, there is an urgency to develop new drugs as the older ones are discarded because of HIV's resistance to them. In 2000, between 1% and 5% of HIV patients worldwide had drug-resistant strains. In 2011, between 10% and 30% of new patients were already resistant to the drugs. In Europe, it was 10%; in the United States, 15%.

Selection of Drug-Resistant Mutants

Based on the large number of mutant HIV produced in any one person, it is not surprising that HIV emerges with resistance to drugs used in antiretroviral therapy. Such strains are referred to as **drug-resistant mutants.** HIV drug-resistant mutants are selected to reproduce most effectively under conditions of selective pressure exerted by the presence of the drugs. Those HIV able to resist the drugs continue to multiply; those that are sensitive to the drugs are destroyed (Figure 4-6).

The Demise of Monotherapy and The Rise of HAART

It took seven years before David Cooper, an AIDS-drug therapy researcher, declared 1995 the year of the "demise of monotherapy for HIV and the rise of combination drug therapy" (Simberkoff, 1996; Stephenson, 1996). The **standard of therapy** became that *all* ART drugs must be used in combination and that each combination include two nucleoside reverse transcriptase inhibitors and a protease or a non-nucleoside inhibitor. Initially, the use of three or more drugs in combination was referred to as **HAART, or Highly Active Antiretroviral Therapy.** HAART now refers to all approved uses of ART. The HAART era really began in March 1996 after the FDA approved ritonavir and indinavir, two protease inhibitors, which dramatically shifted medication strategies: According to the latest U.S. treatment guidelines (March 2012), the recommended regimens are Combivir or Truvada or Atripla (see Table 4-1). The goal of using ART is to suppress HIV replication or viral load. As a result of a large reduction in HIV, fewer T4 or CD4+ cells become infected and die, so the end result is more CD4+ cells remain to divide. Thus, it appears that ART causes an increase in T4 or CD4+ cells over time, but the increase is not from an increase in new CD4+ cell production. Rather, the increase is due to cell division of existing CD4+ cells saved by ART drugs.

The reasoning is to keep the viral load low so that sexual transmission of HIV becomes less likely, and to prevent HIV mutation by reducing its ability to replicate. A number of clinical trials have demonstrated that only about half the patients placed on ART for the first time are able to achieve maximal suppression—undetectable or less than 50 copies of HIV-RNA per milliliter of blood plasma. Where ART works, most people reduce their viral load to 50 copies within 24 to 32 weeks. Less is known about the long-term durability of this suppression. Of those who achieve this undetectable viral load, the majority will experience a viral rebound during the first year of therapy, and most everyone will experience the rebound if they stop taking the drugs (Back, 2001). (See Sidebar 4.3.)

HOW COMBINATION OR COMBINED DRUG THERAPY CAN REDUCE THE CHANCE OF HIV DRUG RESISTANCE

Combination drug therapy works because a single strand of RNA, the genetic material of HIV, must be a multiple mutant, that is, it must carry a genetic change to become resistant to *each* new drug used. So, the greater the number of drugs used, each capable of stopping HIV replication, the greater the number of genetic changes that must occur in a single RNA strand of the virus. For reasons of explanation, say that the chance of change in one nucleotide of HIV for resistance to a single drug occurs in one RNA strand during the production of 10,000 (10 thousand) or 1×10^4 such strands. This is a reasonable figure. Then to have a second nucleotide mutation occur in that same single strand for resistance to a second drug, again at 1×10^4 means that only one RNA strand in 100 million or 1×10^8 would carry both genetic changes. For three separate nucleotide mutations occurring in one RNA strand then, it would be $(1 \times 10^4) \times (1 \times 10^4) \times (1 \times 10^4)$ or only one RNA strand out of 1,000,000,000,000 (1 trillion) would carry a resistance to all three drugs at the same time. But as small as this number is, recall that 1 billion to 10 billion genetically different RNA strands are produced each day in one individual. **In short, HIV can change or mutate at every nucleotide or base daily!** Also, individual RNA strands can exchange nucleotides in a process called recombination. This increases the chance of multiple resistant RNA strands. This is why it is so important to slow the replication of HIV—fewer rounds of replication mean fewer RNA strands, thus fewer possibilities of producing HIV that are resistant to HIV drug cocktails (Figure 4-7). Current HIV drug cocktails, especially those using one or more protease inhibitors, quickly and significantly reduce HIV replication—this is why people on these combination therapies must take them on schedule, in prescribed doses, and maybe for the rest of their lives.

BOX 4.1

PROTEASE INHIBITORS: EXTENDING LIFE; THE DOWNSIDE OF THIS GIFT—RECOVERY?

THE LAZARUS EFFECT: A RETURN TO FUNCTIONAL STATUS

In November 1995, one man in his late 40s wrote his obituary—he had been fighting off HIV disease, then AIDS, for over 13 years. In another case, the man's T cell count was zero. He was on oxygen and morphine. Funeral arrangements were made, and his friends and family were on a death vigil. They are but two examples of several thousand men, beginning in 1999, all under age 50, who had given up hope—they believed they were a short step away from death. Some ran up huge debts—maxed out all their credit cards and gave lavish gifts. Some regretted the way they had lived or not lived to this point, some became very angry, some made peace with themselves and others, but *all* felt death was imminent. *Then it happened*—the results of combination therapies using nucleoside and non-nucleoside reverse transcriptase inhibitors and protease inhibitors *dropped viral load counts* to unmeasurable or undetectable levels in people with HIV disease and AIDS patients. And, those with significantly lowered viral loads demonstrated surprising recovery—their T4 cells rebounded in some cases from below 200 back up to 500 or more. These **"AIDS cocktails,"** as the combination therapies were soon called, gave people with AIDS a new chance at a productive life for the first time since the beginning of the pandemic in the United States in 1981.

CAN THERE BE A DOWNSIDE TO SUCH A MIRACLE?

Of course the most tragic downside is the fact that not all who would benefit from the drug cocktail can tolerate the drugs or afford them—but that is not the issue that is relevant to the question per se. No, this question pertains to a downside, if any, for people who can tolerate the drugs and have access to these drugs.

WHAT KIND OF PROBLEMS EXIST?

Guilt

Many who now feel "new" again feel *guilty* because these drugs are not available to all who need them—the poor and the uninsured in the United States and those in underdeveloped nations.

Reestablishing Relationships

Depending on how long and how severe the illness, the affected became more or less isolated—even "best" friends stopped calling or dropping by. Some who also had AIDS died, while some were too sick to care or mourn them; but now that they have recovered? What now? **Ending year 2013, about 660,000 people in the United States will be on antiretroviral therapy, which includes protease inhibitors. These drugs are not yet deemed necessary to the other about 970,000 HIV-infected in the United States. To date they are mostly unavailable in developing nations.**

Ability to Work Again—Loss of Disability Pay

Disability insurance has been a cocoon of safety for many now experiencing "new" life. Traditionally, people with AIDS received disability checks until death. But suddenly it is not so certain that this will be the case. People who were expected to die are going to be coming back. Nobody is prepared for this. Now that drug cocktails have extended life expectancies, it is expected that these people will be reevaluated and lose their disability payments. They will have to go back to work.

Across the United States, AIDS groups are deluged with calls from patients who are excited, confused, or frightened about the prospect of ending disability status and returning to work. In Miami, a psychologist has begun weekly seminars on résumé writing and job interviews for AIDS patients who have not worked in years. At AIDS Project Los Angeles, counselors field 100 calls each week on return-to-work issues.

POLITICAL DOWNSIDE

As scientists dare ask whether HIV eradication may be possible in some people in the near future (two to five years), the press may be promising more than the scientists can deliver, but the press can and does influence political will. If the political will to fight this disease **weakens** due to the **premature declaration of victory,** this may be the greatest downside of all!

CAN AN HIV DRUG PREVENT HIV INFECTION AS IN "TREATMENT AS PREVENTION (T as P)"—PRE-EXPOSURE PROPHYLAXIS (PrEP)?

Will a Pill a Day Prevent HIV Infection?

PrEP is an experimental, unproven strategy that aims to reduce the risk of acquiring HIV through the use of once-daily antiretrovirals by HIV-negative people. As the new report (Anticipating the Results of PrEP Trials: A powerful new HIV prevention tool may be on the horizon. Are we prepared?) notes, by mid-2011 there were more people enrolled in PrEP trials than in vaccine and microbicide efficacy trials combined. Perhaps the closest precedent for pre-exposure prophylaxis is the use of the anti-retroviral drugs AZT, nevirapine, and/or other of these drugs to **prevent** mother-to-child transmission of HIV during pregnancy and delivery and during breast-feeding.

A number of HIV/AIDS physicians in New York, San Francisco, and Florida began giving Viread (tenofovir) to people who believed they might have been exposed to HIV. Although none of these people became HIV positive at the time, it is not hard evidence that tenofovir can prevent HIV infection or HIV transmission—still, the possibility is intriguing, and interesting enough for the National Institutes of Health, Centers for Disease Control and Prevention, and Bill and Melinda Gates Foundation to fund three separate human studies to determine whether a drug or combination of drugs can prevent HIV infection. Entering 2011 there were nine clinical trials worldwide to determine the effectiveness of PrEP.

UPDATE 2011/2012—Pre-Exposure Prophylaxis (PrEP) Studies Show That Certain Antiretroviral Drugs Can Prevent HIV Infection

[July 2012, FDA Approves The Use of TRUVADA As The First Prevention Drug-Healthy Uninfected People can Take TRUVADA To Prevent Their Infection!]

Recent clinical trials have dramatically confirmed some 10 years of observations on the early use of antiretroviral therapy (ART) to reduce the risk of transmitting HIV between sexual couples. Data reported from specific studies that show a reduction in HIV transmission between men having sex with men (MSM) in 2010 and between HIV serodiscordant (one sexual partner being HIV positive) heterosexual couples in 2011 clearly show that the use of two antiretroviral drugs, tenofovir (TDF) or a combination of tenofovir and emtricitabine called Truvada (TDF/FTC) prevented HIV transmission. A brief discussion of these studies is presented:

1. Pre-exposure Prophylaxis Initiative (iPrEx) Trials—November 2010

Data from this study was reported by Robert Grant and 33 co-authors (Grant et al., 2010). The clinical trials were conducted at 11 sites in six countries (Peru, Ecuador, Brazil, the United States, South Africa and Thailand). These locations were selected because of the high prevalence (between 10% and 28%) of HIV infection among men (MSM) and transgender women having sex with men. (The premise here is that safer sex methods will not succeed with gay men.) The study began in June of 2007 and ended in December 2009. Results from the iPrEx study revealed that, overall, those taking the drug Truvada were on average 44% less likely to become infected than those on placebo pills (a sugar or non-drug pill). Also reported from the study is that those who were adherent—took Truvada strictly according to schedule and did not miss a dose were 73% less likely to become infected. Updated data presented at the 2011 Conference on Retroviruses and Opportunistic Infections (CROI) supported the 2010 findings even suggesting that the risk reduction for those on ART was 92%.

WHY WAS THE STUDY CONDUCTED ON MSM AND TRANSGENDERED WOMEN WHO HAVE SEX WITH MEN?—Because of the disproportion of these people becoming HIV infected worldwide. For example, in the United States MSM account for 53% of new HIV infections and that numbers appear to be rising.

COST OF iPrEx STUDY—The trial cost about $43.6 million, of which National Institute of Allergy and Infectious Diseases (NIAID) contributed $27.8 million and the Bill and Melinda Gates Foundation paid $15.7 million. Gilead donated the drugs used in the trial and paid travel costs for some of the researchers.

In a latter study (Juusola et al., 2012), researchers at Stanford University found that using AIDS drugs to prevent infection among men who have sex with men (MSM) and are at high risk of HIV infection would be expensive, but could also reduce infection rates significantly. The authors estimate that if 20% of high-risk individuals—MSM who have five or more sexual partners a year—took the drug Truvada as a form of pre-exposure prophylaxis (PrEP), it could prevent 41,000 new infections over 20 years. The cost would be about $16.6 billion. In contrast, the team estimated that giving the drug daily to all MSM in the United States would cost $495 billion over the same 20-year period, including the cost of drugs and healthcare visits. In brief, use in high-risk MSM would provide substantial health benefits at a lower cost, although the budgetary effect would still be sizable.

Comment: Pre-exposure prophylaxis among MSM remains an exciting, and now potentially cost-effective, prevention, especially among high-risk MSM. However, the implementation challenges should not be overlooked. Who will prescribe PrEP, and who will pay for it? How will high-risk MSM be identified, and will they agree to use and adhere to PrEP? Finally, will other HIV preventions be equally (or more) effective while also being more affordable?

2. FEM-PrEP STUDY, April 2011

This was an NIAID trial to explore both PrEP and a vaginal microbicide gel as prevention for male-to-female HIV transmission. However, this trial was stopped in early 2011 because an equal number of women were infected among those taking Truvada and those taking a placebo. The conclusion was that "it is highly unlikely" that Truvada protects women against HIV infection. Why the gender difference in reaction to Truvada is unclear at this time. (See iPrEx study above.)

UPDATE 2012—Data from the FEM-PrEP study was re-evaluated. This was presented at the 2012 19th Conference on Retroviruses and Opportunistic Infections. Scientists who had analyzed trial participants' blood samples found that only a quarter who became infected had any tenofovir/emtricitabine in their blood. That suggests they had failed to take the drug. Researchers were uncertain why so few participants took the pill. Adherence, taking your drugs on time every time, as discussed on pages 97 and 102 is crucial to a successful treatment outcome! It would appear that the lack of adherence doomed these trials to failure.

COST OF FEM-PrEP STUDY—$26 million. Funded by United States Agency for International Developent (USAID) and Bill and Melinda Gates Foundation.

3. VOICE

In another trial called VOICE (Vaginal and Oral Interventions to Control the Epidemic) begun in September 2009, the VOICE study involved more than 5,000 HIV un-infected women in South Africa, Uganda, and Zimbabwe. The trial was designed to test the safety, effectiveness, and acceptability of two different HIV prevention strategies: an investigational microbicide gel containing tenofovir

and oral tablets containing tenofovir either along or co-formulated with the drug emtricitabine. The tablets, known by the brand names Viread (tenofovir) and Truvada (tenofovir plus emtricitabine), had been taken daily in an approach known as pre-exposure prophylaxis, or PrEP. After routine review of the study data in September 2011, the Data Safety Monitoring Board (DSMB) recommended that the investigators stop evaluating oral tenofovir because the study would be unable to show that tenofovir tablets have a different effect than placebo tablets at preventing HIV infection among the study participants. Further, the DSMB recommended that the VOICE study continue as designed to evaluate the oral Truvada tablet. These data should be available in 2013. FACTS 001, another major safety and effectiveness trial of tenofovir gel that uses a dosing strategy different from VOICE's, launched in 2011 with 2,200 women in South Africa; results are expected in 2014.

COST OF VOICE STUDY—$110 million funded by NIAID and the Eunice Kennedy Shriver National Institute of Child Health and Human Development.

4. HIV Prevention Trials Network (HPTN052) Trials—May 2011, Editors of *Science* cite the results of this study as "The 2011 Scientific Breakthrough of The Year." That TasP or T4P works gives new hope and optimism for the future.

This study was to determine if any of 11 different antiretroviral drugs would prevent HIV transmission between HIV *serodiscordant heterosexual* couples. The major drug used in these studies was TRUVADA. The studies took place in Africa, Asia and the Americas. The couples had CD4 counts between 350 and 500. Results of these studies revealed that if any of the 11 drugs were started immediately after an HIV positive test there was a 96% reduction in the risk of HIV infection of their uninfected partner (NIAID, 2011). This study showed for the first time that treatment of HIV infected people almost completely blocked their transmission of HIV. The obvious implication is that wide spread treatment of the infected will slow the rate of infection. (Condoms offer about an 85% reduction in HIV transmission. It is suggested that persons with HIV always practice safer sex regardless of when ART is started.)

Acknowledging the HPTN 052 study results led Secretary of State Hillary Rodham Clinton and President Barack Obama to call for the creation of "an AIDS-free generation." In short, the use of ART especially using Truvada for T as P or T4P genie is out of the bottle, so to speak, and as ART continues to improve in terms of tolerability, affordability, and convenience, its application for personal and public health is inevitable. Hopefully, the 2011 ART breakthrough will allow for significant reduction in new HIV infections. The CDC has been trying to achieve 25% reduction in new infections—perhaps now this goal is attainable! In July 2012 the World Health Organization endorsed the concept of using drugs to prevent infection in high-risk HIV negative people.

PROBLEM: Critics of the study say that the HPTN 052 data do not speak to transmission via men having sex with men—especially anal sex. Likewise, this was not a study of ART to reduce transmission by needle sharing. These are limitations and extrapolation to anything other than penile–vaginal sexual transmission of HIV would be just that, extrapolation. Perhaps the critics are saying that some or much of the greatness of this study is being assumed rather than assured? Finally, those taking ART as preventive will require repeated HIV testing to make certain they do not become HIV positive. Here one must consider their lifestyle and their level of risk taking.

And, no amount of money will be adequate to treat all of the uninfected. It is clear that even if you take the most efficient way of doing TasP—the number of people who will eventually need to be on treatment with the amount of money available is not enough to treat those people. And we must add in the cost to treat the infected. In short, the world will make a decision how much all of these lives matter. Currently, Truvada costs about $17,000 per person annually.

An Uncomfortable Finding at the 2012 19th International AIDS Conference, July 22–27.
In an uncomfortable finding for advocates of treatment as prevention, a study of heterosexual couples of differing HIV status in Uganda has found no difference in the rate of HIV infections in the negative partner when the positive partner was taking antiretroviral therapy (ART) and was virally suppressed, when compared to couples where the positive partner was not on treatment. The finding came from an "in the field" study of HIV patients attending the TASO clinic in Jinja, Uganda, and their spouses or partners. While researchers cannot explain why its results are so different from randomized controlled trials such as HPTN 052 (presented above), which found that putting the HIV-positive partner on ART (Truvada) reduced the HIV transmission rate by

96%, it does serve as a warning, as presenter Josephine Birungi said, that "It may be difficult to extrapolate the results of randomized controlled trials to real-life situations in low-income countries" (Abstract TUACO 103 Washington DC, 2012).

COST OF THE HPTN052 STUDY—$73 million funded by the National Institute of Allergy and Infectious Diseases (NIAID).

5. Partners PrEP—July 2011
These studies were conducted in Kenya and Uganda to determine if once a day Truvada or once a day Tenofovir would lower the risk of HIV transmission between serodiscordant heterosexual couples. The studies were conducted by researchers from the University of Washington. The results of these studies showed that using Truvada lowered the risk of HIV infection of their uninfected partner by 73%. Using Tenofovir lowers the risk by 62%. The Partners PrEP studies showed that where Tenofovir was used alone it was about as effective as using Truvada. The two drugs are available generically in many countries at about $0.25/pill.

COST OF PARTNERS PrEP STUDY—$63 MILLION. Funded by the Bill and Melinda Gates Foundation.

6. TDF2 Study—July 2011
These CDC studies were similar to those carried out at the University of Washington. To provide evidence that a once daily dose (pill) of an antiretroviral drug could or would reduce the risk of HIV infection to uninfected men or women who would then become exposed to HIV through heterosexual sex (this study is not quite the same as dealing with serodiscordant sexual couples as used in the Partners PrEP studies.) The CDC studies were conducted in partnership with the Botswana Ministry of Health. The studies using Truvada showed a 63% to 78% reduced risk of HIV infection in the uninfected partner. Both men and women were equally protected. These data mirrored the data that came from the Partners PrEP studies discussed above.

COST OF TDF2 STUDY—$27 million. Funded by the Centers for Disease Control and Prevention (CDC)
Because pregnant and breastfeeding women were excluded from participation in PrEP trials, further evaluation of available data will be needed before any recommendations can be made regarding the use of PrEP for women during conception, pregnancy, or breastfeeding.

SUMMARY

In reviewing the antiretroviral drug prevention studies presented in 2010, 2011 and 2012 it becomes clear that the use of these drugs for prevention in addition to treatment is a fundamental change in a global approach to lowering the incidence of HIV infection. Used alongside condoms, clean needles, syringes, and circumcisions add an enormous force in overcoming the transmission of HIV. The studies presented show that internationally individuals at high risk of HIV infection who took a daily tablet containing and HIV medication—either the anti-retroviral medication tenofovir or tenofovir in combination with embricitabine or by taking one or more of 9 other antiretroviral drugs—experienced significantly fewer HIV infections that those who received a placebo pill. These findings are clear evidence that this new HIV prevention strategy, called pre-exposure prophylaxis (or PrEP), sub-stantially reduces HIV infection risk. This is an extremely exciting finding for the field of HIV prevention. Now, more than ever, the priority for HIV prevention research must be on how to deliver successful prevention strategies, like PrEP, to populations in greatest need. But, the question now is **how** to best use this new knowledge given that there are not sufficient funds or resources to treat all those for whom ART is clinically required. **How** do you provide ART for 38 million people living with HIV hoping for a longer life and lower their chances of transmitting HIV or **how do you provide ART to say 100 million people to prevent their becoming infected?** OK, so the world can't, at the moment, afford the necessary drugs in addition to all the other challenges this disease demands of society. The question becomes **how** do we use the findings and available funding to make the best of all possibilities? In short, if treatment early, a 96% decrease in transmission is possible. And if you treat all HIV-negative people in the medium to high risk populations, theoretically, at least, the world could see the light at the end of the tunnel—HIV as just another successfully treatable human disease.

Treatment As Prevention (T as P or T4P): Are We Expecting Too Much?

To be sure, things are looking up when it comes to the use of antiretroviral drugs and preventing the transmission of HIV. But, are we assuming too many good things too quickly? The hype over the results of studies presented in this SIDEBAR has been extensive and has led to politicians and scientists alike declaring that the "End of AIDS is here," etc. **Questions: (a)** How will you get 38 million people to take their antiretroviral drugs on time, each time, every day? Providing they had access to them? And **(b)** what of the many millions of HIV negative people who want to prevent their infection? Does anyone think at the moment that these people will adhere to a drug regimen when most all of the drugs have moderate to serious side effects? The answers to both (a and b) are they won't! For example, over the last 17 years (1995 through 2012) and at least over the last five years, regardless of the available, well-tolerated, once-a-day drug therapy, only **19%** of those 1.63 million infected in the United States have undetectable levels of HIV (Gardner et al., 2011). This means the other 81% do not have their virus under control. The CDC claims that 28% have their virus under control but their data is less convincing (November 29, 2011). **Why? What do you think are some of the Reasons for this failure to keep viral loads undetectable?**

TENSION AMONG THE HIV/AIDS TREATMENT/PREVENTION SCIENTISTS

With all the good news, as discussed above, their remains a tension among scientists who (a) want to treat the infected to prevent the transmission of HIV and (b) those who believe available resources should be used to target the uninfected, at risk, population who can't control their exposure to HIV. Julio Montaner of the B.C. Center for Excellence in HIV/AIDS in Vancouver, a long-time advocate of using treatment as prevention, cites the HPIN052 trials as major evidence that treatment is prevention. However, other trials discussed above show that giving antiretroviral drugs to the uninfected also reduces the risk of becoming HIV infected—which is also treatment—prevention. Perhaps the two approaches need not be in competition. In fact, PrEP should enable the use of early treatment. In addition, PrEP should be a major incentive to get tested for HIV. If found positive, receive treatment. If found negative, receive treatment to help stay negative. Additional advantages are : with the acceptance of PrEP stigma related situation should drop! And PrEP should also reduce the number of persons who don't know their HIV status (specifically those who are infected and don't know it) as a test will be required before receiving treatment. One major disadvantage is that non-infected people taking the drugs may adopt riskier behaviors because they feel protected—a phenomenon known as risk disinhibition. Montaner however likes his "big picture" approach. Treatment will stop death, stop progression and stop transmission while PrEP only works in defined situations"

AUTHOR'S COMMENT—Perhaps it is time to recognize that now treatment is prevention in most if not all situations! The bottom line is that treatment as prevention isn't just about preventing illness, it is also about maintaining health. However, having effective ART is of no consequence if the drugs cannot reach those in need. In August 2012, the CDC issued updated interim guidance on the use of once-a-day Truvada to prevent HIV, saying providers should consider prescribing it for heterosexual women and men who are at high risk of infection. U.S. health officials previously advised doctors to give Truvada only to high-risk men who have sex with men (MSM).

CLASS DISCUSSION—(A) Is treatment as prevention or T4P leading to a cure, possible in your lifetime? Present real life scenarios as to how this might occur. Include politics, funding, care, drugs and social networking into your presentation as to whether this can or cannot occur. (B) When do you think its justifiable to treat someone in order to protect others? (C) In this time of tight resources, who should receive "breakthrough" antiretroviral drugs? Those already infected/sick or those who want to avoid becoming infected/sick? Defend your selection. (Keep in mind that the medical profession does not know how PrEP will work out in the world at large and PrEP does not prevent other sexually transmitted diseases.)

For more information on efforts to evaluate and plan for PrEP implementation in the United States, visit www.cdc.gov/hiv/prep (http://cdc.gov/hiv/prep).
For complete list of PrEP trials being conducted, see http://www.avac.org/ht/a/GetDocumentAction/i/3113.

QUICKTAKE 4.1

A SKEPTICAL LOOK AT "TEST AND TREAT" (TASP OR T4P)

In *Journal Watch HIV/AIDS Clinical Care* April 9, 2012, Abigail Zuger gave an interesting perspective on the recent fervor or zeal that is mounting for universal TasP or T4P with respect to reducing HIV infections. She offers a logical counterpoint to the recommendation to treat everyone. She does not share the enthusiasm of public health officials, politicians, or members of guideline committees and their recommendations. Specifically, Zuger feels the strategy, which calls for universal voluntary HIV testing and immediate ART for all who test positive, is a mistake! With regard to adherence, it turns out that in the aggregate, HIV-infected patients actually behave quite similarly to others (people taking medication for other diseases). For instance, in a large Swiss study in which HIV infected patients were followed for a median of almost five years, only about 50% had self-reported medication adherence that was consistently good, while 30% had adherence that was consistently poor or worsened over time. A British study found that even when adherence was measured with the best-case surrogate (an available supply of pills), about 50% of patients went through a period of missing 40% or more of their doses. Electronic monitoring techniques find rates of adherence

of 50% to 80% in various groups of HIV-infected patients. And although various intensive interventions can certainly improve adherence, their benefits are fleeting. A recent study showed that even the most intensive possible intervention—a period of directly observed therapy—did not change medication-taking habits appreciably over the long term. As for the anecdotal data, she said, "Well, where to begin? In our busy urban clinic, some patients are as precise with their medications over years and decades as anyone might wish. The rest offer up a true symphony of reasons for non-adherence. Some are too depressed, distracted, drug-addled, disengaged, blasé, or suspicious to take their medications consistently. Some sell the drugs on the black market, and some share them with friends and partners. Some work out their own schedule of treatment interruptions, contrary to all medical advice. One patient of mine, a nurse, actually took half a regimen for a solid calendar year. (The upshot: The pharmacokinetics of that regimen made him a very lucky guy, and he had an undetectable viral load at the end of that year.) Another patient was less fortunate: She couldn't get to her refills for a month—and her virus could never be controlled again." In theory, people interact with medications in only one way: They take them. But in the real world, people lose their medications, forget them, give them away (sell them), and forget to pick them up. Making treatment the default position means that we will just see more of all these behaviors with a rapid rise of resistance to all drug classes. She believes that a strategy of test and treat is really not that at all. It is actually a strategy of test and prescribe with no guarantees as far as the treatment part goes. Invested patients will be treated; the rest will not. In theory, physicians will wisely discriminate between the two, but there too the theory is problematic. We all know that when the default position is treat, most doctors will do just that because it is far easier to hand over a prescription than to consider all the ramifications of disease and treatment in a focused, ongoing dialogue that may run months or even years. Few of us have the mental strength to run counter to a prevailing slogan for so long. She asks, does it make any sense that we are calling loudly for nationwide antibiotic stewardship while at the same time considering unleashing a tide of antiretrovirals? Sometimes I look at the multidrug-resistant gram-negatives [bacteria] in our intensive care unit and think ahead a few decades to the day when fearsome multidrug-resistant HIV strains begin to land in our clinics. That's when we will bitterly rethink test and treat. Perhaps it will never happen this way, but microbiology and human psychology both suggest otherwise.

Finally, James Shelton (2012) presents information that supports the perspectives of Zuger (presented above). In his article he states that the use of anti-retroviral drugs (ARVs) as a magic bullet to eliminate HIV is not as simple as it sounds. He identifies a variety of obstacles to achieving impact with ARVs at the population level. For one thing, he says, identifying the infected but untreated population is daunting; globally [over 8] million of the estimated [38] million infected individuals are currently on treatment. He also cautions that very early infections, when HIV-positive individuals are more infectious, allow for rapid transmission, accounting for approximately one-third of transmission in generalized epidemics, while a test to detect acute or early infection remains unavailable. In sub-Saharan Africa about 40% of all new infections were transmitted during early HIV infection. Furthermore, the author asserts that adherence to a lifetime regimen of ARVs is still problematic, particularly for those whose experience side effects and warns that drug resistance may increase when ARVs are provided on a more massive and long-term scale. In contrast to the above information by Zuger and Shelton, Reuben Granich and colleagues (2009) suggest that universal voluntary testing and immediate ART could reduce the number of HIV/AIDS deaths by 55% by year 2050.

TESTING OF ANTI—HIV DRUGS FOR POST-EXPOSURE PREVENTION (PEP)

The Forum—A nurse pricks her finger on a needle. A woman has sex with her HIV-positive husband and the condom breaks. A woman is raped by a man who is HIV-positive. A child is sodomized by an HIV-positive male. A prison guard is bitten by an HIV-positive inmate. A couple has unprotected sex—a one-night stand. These were some of the cases brought up by experts as they debated whether doctors should be prescribing AIDS drugs as a morning-after or *post-exposure prophy-laxis* or *prevention* (PEP) treatment for those exposed to HIV. A PEP treatment consists of taking ART drugs as soon as possible after exposure to HIV.

In mid-October 1997, San Francisco became the first city in the United States to offer new PEP drugs to individuals trying to prevent HIV infection.

TIMING IS EVERYTHING

72-Hour Window—The standard of practice for about five years at most medical centers is to offer antiviral drugs promptly when healthcare workers of AIDS patients are stuck with needles or come into contact with body fluids from infected patients. New federal guidelines recommend ART drug treatment using three antiretroviral drugs each day for 28 days, starting no later than 72 hours after exposure. This costs $600 to $1000.

Resources—The following resource is available for consultation regarding HIV PEP: PEPline http://www.ucsf.edu/hivcntr/Hotlines/PEPline
Telephone: 1-888-448-4911

As of the beginning of 2013 about 1900 American healthcare workers have received PEP care—40 have become HIV positive, but they admitted to continuing to practice high-risk behavior. Regardless, over the past 17 years, PEP has become the standard of care for occupational exposure to HIV.

What Are Disadvantages of PEP?—In addition to expense, many of the drugs have serious side effects such that people do not complete PEP. However, one of the biggest fears about PEP is that people will return to unsafe sexual and drug-using practices if they believe that PEP will prevent them from becoming infected. There is some evidence that treatment advances, including PEP, may be leading to increasing incidence of unsafe sex in the United States. For example, rates of gonorrhea among men who have sex with men have recently increased for the first time since the early 1980s. There is a wide spectrum of situations to consider, but there are no absolutes when it comes to the right choices regarding PEP. PEP after HIV exposure is recommended because of the knowledge that in some cases it works. It is well recognized that the use of ZDV in pregnant women dramatically reduced vertical transmission of HIV to newborns. It is therefore conceivable that the use of antiretroviral medication following sexual exposure to HIV will also be effective. However, studies to date remain controversial (Pinkerton et al., 2004 updated).

In a study by Charlie Sayer and colleagues (2008), post-exposure prophylaxis is becoming increasingly available for individuals reporting sexual risk behavior. The number of gay men presenting for such treatments has increased following targeted advertising campaigns and the publication of professional guidelines. There is now robust evidence that post-exposure prophylaxis can prevent HIV infection. But there have still been reports of infection despite using treatment following possible sexual exposure to the virus. In many instances these infections can be attributed to ongoing sexual risk behavior.

Caution—Clearly this is not a morning-after pill. The treatment is not foolproof, but it offers an important safety net to prevent HIV infection in certain cases. It shouldn't be considered a substitute for more reliable ways to avoid getting infected with HIV, such as abstinence, monogamy, or condom use.

FINALLY THE QUESTION, DOES PEP WORK?

The CDC said that PEP is not recommended for habitual drug users who share needles or for people who frequently engage in risky sex. Those people would have to take antiretroviral drugs practically nonstop, which the health agency does not endorse.

DISCUSSION QUESTION: With your current knowledge about HIV/AIDS, if you knew that you had just been exposed to HIV would you ask for immediate therapy? Why?

PEPline (888) 448-4911: A Post Exposure Prophylaxis Hotline

Combined or Combination Drug Cocktails: Success Breeds Danger

Combination drug cocktails work well initially because they are attacking the strains of HIV that are least resistant to the drugs. But the result of that success is to encourage the rapid spread of HIV strains that are highly resistant to the drugs, which could give rise to a new and even more dangerous AIDS epidemic among people most at risk for the disease (Figure 4-7, page 92 and Figure 4-8, page 92).

Several separate research investigations, using two new types of sensitive diagnostic tests, found evidence suggesting that about 30% of individuals newly infected with HIV are carrying forms of the virus that are already resistant to one of the 26 drugs, and 14% are resistant to two of the drugs used in American combination therapy. In Great Britain, 13% of the HIV infected are resistant to three of the main classes of antiretroviral drugs.

Mutations that confer resistance to nucleoside analog reverse transcriptase inhibitors, nonnucleoside reverse transcriptase inhibitors, and protease inhibitors have all been identified in HIV-infected Americans who have never been treated with antiretroviral drugs.

In summary, the frequency of genetically variant HIV within an HIV population is influenced by the mutation rate, fitness of the mutant to survive, the size of the available HIV pool for genetic recombination, and the number of HIV replication cycles.

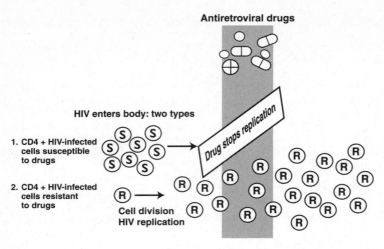

Drug-resistant variants
become predominant

FIGURE 4–7 Drug-Resistant Variants Become Predominant through the Selection Process.

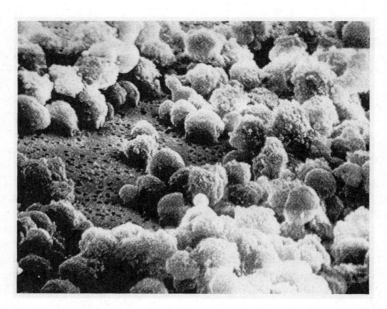

FIGURE 4–8 Production of HIV. Each dark hole in the T4 cell membrane represents the emergence of one new HIV that came off the membrane and is loose in the body. Each HIV-infected T4 cell is producing about 3000 to 4000 viruses at any time. Each HIV in this photograph is genetically different from any other HIV being released from this T4 cell and most likely genetically different from any other HIV in the body. T4 or CD4+ cells live for about 80 days in a non-HIV-infected person and about 25 days in an HIV-infected person. (*Source: Courtesy of the Centers for Disease Control and Prevention, Atlanta*)

HIV Coinfection and Superinfection

Coinfection—This is an infection with at least two genetically different strains of HIV from the **same** clade or group, for example clade B. (Not to be confused with coinfection meaning infected with two completely different viruses like HIV and HCV or hepatitis C). In February 2000, the first documented case of **HIV coinfection** was reported at the 7th Conference on Retroviruses and Opportunistic Infections. An HIV-infected male became infected, more or less simultaneously, with a second strain of HIV, one more aggressive than the other strain of HIV he carried.

Superinfection—This is an HIV-infected person at some point in time, becoming infected with a second strain of HIV. Superinfection may involve infections from **different** clades or subtypes, for example A and E or B and C.

Third-Line Regimens: Salvage, Mega, or GigaHAART Therapy

Under current definition, a treatment-experienced, or so-called salvage HIV-infected person, is one who has failed at least three HIV regimens that include at least one drug from each approved drug class. Salvage therapy is the use of substitute drugs that will continue to suppress viral replication when standard therapy fails. There is no "single recipe" for salvage therapy. Although the HIV salvage population is on the rise as the life expectancy of people with HIV increases, they are still underrepresented in new clinical trials because sponsors of new drugs do not expect the drugs to be effective in salvage patients. The reasons that HIV drug regimens lose their effectiveness are as varied as the people who are undergoing treatment with them. Treatment failures, which can occur in up to 60% of patients, can develop in those with a prolonged history of sequential HIV therapy because of built-up resistance. They also can occur in people who fail to comply with their prescribed therapy or who are given a poorly suited regimen at the outset.

How Many People Are on Salvage Therapy?

Throughout the developed world, about 1 in 10 AIDS patients now requires some form of salvage therapy because he or she carries HIV resistance to the drugs. About 1 in 50 of these patients is resistant to all 26 FDA-approved antiretroviral drugs. In 2002, French scientists began to use mega HAART or giga HAART therapy for those with limited treatment options. The theory behind using a larger number of drugs is that not all the virus in a person's body is going to be resistant to all the drugs. By using many drugs with different mechanisms of blocking HIV from reproducing, it may still be possible to achieve a potent anti-HIV effect. This salvage or rescue regime consists of the following drugs: three to four nucleoside reverse transcription inhibitors (NRTIs), hydroxyurea, one or two non-NRTIs, and three to four protease inhibitors. Continued studies will determine the safety and effectiveness of mega/giga HAART therapies.

Available Drug-Resistance Tests

Generally speaking, there are two types of drug-resistance tests available to HIV-positive patients: genotypic and phenotypic assays. Because genotypic testing provides results in one to two weeks—compared to the two- to five-week turn around associated with phenotypic testing—it is the preferred choice for patients who have yet to start treatment.

Genotypic Analysis/Testing

Genotypic testing examines the actual genetic structure—genotype—of HIV taken from an infected person (a standard blood sample is all that is required). The HIV is examined for the presence of specific genetic mutations that are known to cause resistance to certain drugs.

Establishing a list of genetic mutations or changes in HIV or RNA related to drug resistance is called a **genotypic analysis** or test and indicates a given HIV's genetic resistance to a given drug. Each HIV genetic change or mutation to a drug is listed by a license-plate-looking name such as "K103N" (the most common mutation found in those taking non–nucleoside transcriptase inhibitors (NNRTIs)). The first letter (K) is the code for the amino acid lysine in the wild-type HIV. The number (103) identifies the position of the three DNA bases (codon) coding for this amino acid. The second letter (N) is the code for the "changed" amino acid (asparagine) in the mutant sample. That is, because asparagine is now in the code instead of lysine, This copy of HIV is mutant! Lysine has been replaced with asparagine! Note that when HIV becomes resistant to one drug, it can, at the same time, become resistant to others that function in the same manner (cross-resistance). The suspected degree of drug resistance, as suggested from genotypic analysis, can be measured directly by adding the drug in question to an HIV-cell culture and determining the HIV's ability to reproduce.

Phenotypic Analysis/Testing

Phenotypic testing results are easier to interpret than genotypic testing results because they do not require the expert interpretation of complex mutation patterns. Put simply, a sample of a person's HIV is produced in the laboratory. A dose of one drug is added. The rate of reproduction (amount of HIV produced) is compared to the rate of the wild-type virus. If the test sample grows more than the wild type, it is considered resistant to the medication. The drug susceptibility data provide information for the clinician to select a treatment effective against the viral population circulating in the patient's blood. The main use of phenotypic assays at present is to identify those antiretroviral drugs that still retain activity against the infected person's virus. They are also useful to detect transmission of drug-resistant virus and to monitor HIV patients during early viral rebound. In essence, phenotypic testing provides information to target antiretroviral therapy against the predominant HIV variant in the patient.

Phenotype testing is very expensive at $800 to $1000 per test. Because of the time element (about two to five weeks) and cost, such testing is not readily available. Thus, patients rely on the cheaper (about $200 to $400) and faster (one to two week) genotypic testing. Most third-party payers do not cover these tests.

In general, resistance tests can't predict which drugs will work—only the ones that don't—which is why they're mostly recommended to help people whose regimens are failing.

VIRAL LOAD: ITS RELATIONSHIP TO HIV DISEASE AND AIDS

Viral load is a measurement of the quantity of HIV circulating in blood plasma. Throughout the 1980s and early 1990s, before antiretroviral drugs became available, it took, on average, 10 years for an HIV infection to progress to AIDS because the body controlled HIV. When containment was lost, HIV continued to multiply, and illness and death followed. In the mid-1990s, scientists began measuring the level or number of HIV-RNA strands in blood plasma. They found that HIV was rapidly replicating from the day of infection! A relationship was quickly established that the infectiousness of an HIV-positive person is directly linked to that person's viral load. Viral load then refers to the number of HIV-RNA strands in the blood plasma or **serum** of HIV-infected persons (a discussion of HIV-RNA production is provided in Chapter 3, pages 54–55). In general, two to six weeks after HIV exposure, infected individuals develop a high level of blood plasma HIV-RNA. Methods now exist to quantitate the amount of HIV-RNA in the blood plasma or serum of HIV-infected people.

Possible Side Effects of Viral Load

It is known that in the case of chronic untreated or, in some cases, treated infections, immune system reactions can lead to damaging episodes of inflammation. It is now clear that even in persons on ART, HIV patients more commonly express heart, kidney, bone, and liver disease and diabetes than HIV-uninfected people of similar ages. It is now believed the presence of HIV—any viral load, even if low—can trigger immune system-caused inflammation and associated bodily damage.

The reduction of viral load with the use of antiretroviral drugs can reduce inflammation and immune cell activation, and slow the destruction of the immune system and collateral organ and tissue damage. (See Point of Information 4.2, pages 97–98.) For measurement of viral load, see Chapter 13, page 397.

Viral Load Testing Is The Most Important Indicator of Response To Antiretroviral Therapy

If a person is not taking anti–HIV drugs, his or her viral load will be monitored during regular clinic visits to provide clues about the likely course of HIV disease if left untreated. Among people with the same T4 or CD4+ cell count, those with higher viral loads tend to have more rapid disease progression than those with lower viral loads.

Physicians recommend viral load testing for the following reasons:

♦ to help you make decisions about starting or changing drug treatment for HIV;

♦ to find out your risk for disease progression;

♦ to show how well your drug regimen is working: viral suppressions generally achieved in 12–24 weeks.

♦ to help determine your HIV disease stage.

Undetectable And Suppressed Viral Load

Undetectable There is no normal amount of HIV since it is not normally present in the body. A viral load lab report will list the lowest amount of virus that the particular test can detect. There is strong evidence that an undetectable viral load in a person with HIV is associated with a lower risk of transmission. For example, the risk of sexual transmission has been shown to be lowest in a person with HIV when their viral load is less than 1000 copies/ml. However, that risk is not zero. Similarly, a pregnant woman with an undetectable viral load is known to have a very low risk of transmitting the virus to her baby during labor and delivery. And similarly, the risk of transmission in that situation is not zero, but very low. **There is no completely safe level of viral load.**

An undetectable viral load has been proposed as the gold standard of HIV treatment by the guidelines used in the past few years. Suppressing viral load below the limits of detection results in the greatest reduction in the risk of death or illness. Undetectable viral load is one of the aims of antiretroviral therapy. However, the definition of "undetectable" viral load is constantly changing as the technology used to measure viral load improves. An undetectable viral load result indicates that a specific viral load test cannot find any HIV in a given blood sample. An undetectable result does not mean that the blood is free of HIV. In fact, most people with undetectable viral load have HIV in their blood, as well as in lymphoid tissue and bodily fluids. Samples with very low levels of HIV, for example below 50 copies/ml, are described as having a viral load that is undetectable, or below the level of detection. The higher an individual's viral load before starting treatment, the greater the reduction in viral load required to bring it down to undetectable levels. For this reason, some clinicians recommend more aggressive treatment to people with very high viral load compared to people with lower viral load (Palmer et al., 2008). (See Point of Information 4.2, pages 97–98.)

Suppressed—the virus is considered suppressed when there are 400 or fewer copies of HIV per milliliter of blood.

When Is Viral RNA Found in Blood Plasma?

Plasma is a transparent yellow fluid that makes up about 55% of blood volume. Removing fibrinogen and blood clotting factors from plasma results in **serum.**

HIV-RNA strands are present during *all stages* of the disease, and the viral load increases with more advanced disease (Piatak et al., 1993; Saksela et al., 1994). Following infection with HIV, there is usually a rapid increase of HIV proteins and RNA followed by a lengthy period of viral RNA replication at lower but measurable amounts (Figure 4-9). In well-characterized groups with known dates of HIV seroconversion (when an HIV-infected person's serum

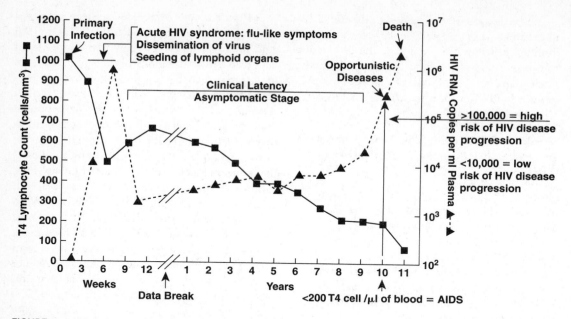

FIGURE 4-9 Clinical Course of HIV Disease as Related to T4 or CD4+ Cell Count and Level (number of HIV-RNA Copies (Viral Load) in Plasma. In an Average Patient without Antiretroviral Therapy: Primary Infection to Death. During primary infection (the time period between infection and development of HIV antibody), HIV-RNA levels spike *(triangles)* and HIV disseminates throughout the body. This is followed by an abrupt drop in measurable HIV-RNA in the blood (probably due to the production of HIV antibody), followed by a steady rise in HIV-RNA until death. Over these same time periods, there is a continuous loss of T4 cells *(squares)*. Note that the asymptomatic stage can be quite long—on average about 10 to 12 years, at which time T4 cell counts drop and HIV-RNA copies increase to levels where there is high risk of opportunistic infections.

changes from sero-negative to seropositive, HIV antibodies become measurable), a high viral load immediately after seroconversion (Mellors et al., 1995) and at three years after seroconversion (Jurriaans et al., 1994) appear to be strong predictors of HIV disease progression.

MEDICAL COMPLICATIONS ASSOCIATED WITH ANTI-RETROVIRAL THERAPIES (ART)

The term "medical complications" is used herein to describe clinical problems in the management of HIV infection. Most doctors now agree that not everyone infected with HIV needs to take antiretroviral drugs. But everyone with HIV does need medical monitoring and care and access to treatment when and if

appropriate. Because those taking antiretroviral treatment have had a fraction of the death rate of those without treatment does not necessarily mean that one's chance of survival will be correspondingly increased by antiretrovirals. The reduced death rates reflect the benefit of treatment for those who have needed and responded to it. (Bozzette et al., 2001; Freedberg et al., 2001).

For those who think HIV/AIDS is over—it is not.

For those who think the drugs are working well—they do for some people, for a number of years.

Management of HIV/AIDS: Treat Early, Treat Late?

Building the Ship as It Sails—There are at least three major decisions that have to be made early

POINT OF INFORMATION 4.2

CURRENT PROBLEMS USING ANTIRETROVIRAL THERAPY

First, Duration: Many patients ask how long they will have to continue therapy; how long will they have to be harnessed to pills and doctors?

Second, Adherence or Compliance—Taking Your Drugs On Time—Every Time: You don't have to like them, you just have to take them! Healthcare providers have been dealing with the issue of client **adherence** or **compliance** for centuries. The medical literature shows that it is difficult for patients to adhere to even the simplest treatment regimens. Factors associated with poor adherence include perceived need of medication, unstable housing, mental illness, and major life crises. Also adding to adherence problems are pill burden, pill size, frequency and timing of dose, dietary and/or water requirements or restrictions, liquid formulations, unpleasant drug taste, adverse events, storage requirements, number of prescriptions, and other factors such as the number of copayments, refills, and medication bottles.

Skipping only a few pills can trigger the emergence of **drug-resistant strains of HIV.** This could create a condition worse than the initial infection because the drug-resistant virus could overwhelm the individual taking the drugs and anyone else to whom the individual transmitted the virus.

In a recent analysis by Blaschke et al. (2012), researchers compiled data on more than 16,000 patients with various medical conditions who participated in 95 studies of medication adherence, as measured by electronic monitoring devices. By day 100 of treatment, about 20% of patients had stopped their medications permanently, and about 10% had begun to take their daily doses erratically. After a year, almost 40% had stopped treatment completely, and barely 50% were taking the medications correctly. One HIV-infected person said, "When you have been taking meds for as long as I have, you just get tired of taking them!"

Class Adherence Experiment: For an HIV class experience on adherence at the University of North Florida, 50 students aged 18–24 were asked to take either three or four different-colored M & M candies representing four different antiretroviral drugs, at three specified times per day between six in the morning and midnight for three days (Friday through Sunday). They were given the colored M & Ms and a dosing schedule sheet to record their compliance. After completion of the experiment, class compliance at 100%, 90%, 80%, and 70% was zero! Their overall comment—now we can better

relate to what it must be like for those who must be compliant to drug schedule.

DISCUSSION QUESTION: Do you think the results would be much different in your college or university HIV/AIDS class?

Clearly much more needs to be done to improve rates of adherence, or many patients will be embarking on a rapid route to resistance and treatment failure.

Third, Drug Costs in America: Larry Kramer, a cofounder of Gay Men's Health Crisis, states that the cost of his drugs to combat AIDS, which do not include a protease, amounts to about $19,000 a year; this does not include visits to his doctor or the batteries of blood tests he routinely requires. A *New York Times* article estimated that drugs for someone with symptomatic AIDS cost about $70,000 a year. In response, a New York University adjunct law professor and gay-rights advocate wrote a letter to the editor saying that his drugs cost $84,000 a year using protease inhibitors; the annual drug cost can exceed $150,000. At these prices, how many of the nation's HIV infected will be able to afford proper HIV therapy? **AT THESE PRICES PEOPLE HAVE TO CHOOSE WHETHER TO PAY RENT, BUY FOOD, OR PAY FOR THEIR MEDICINE—SOME CHOICE! MANY PEOPLE WITH HIV/AIDS TURN TO VIATICAL OR LIFE INSURANCE SETTLEMENTS.**

The viatical industry started in 1989 because people with AIDS were becoming bankrupt due to their medical expenses. Selling a life insurance policy is called viatification. If you want to sell a life insurance policy, you can sell it directly to a viatical investment company. A viatical investment company finds investors who want to buy life insurance policies, and it finds people who want to sell their policies. The company pays the person selling their policy a percentage of the policy's value, and when the person dies, the company receives the life insurance benefits and pays the investors.

Fourth, Effectiveness of Antiretroviral Therapy Causing Complacency among High-Risk Groups: Success using ART has led to complacency with regard to high-risk sexual behavior, which in turn has resulted in a rise in numbers of new HIV infections. Regardless of whether the ARTs are effective in blocking HIV replication, there is evidence that HIV-infected people are more susceptible to a number of cancers and other health conditions that are considered rare in the general population. This occurs

Chap. 4   Anti-HIV Therapy   **97**

because the virus causes nonrepairable damage to the immune system.

Fifth, Side Effects: The paradox of HIV treatment is that sometimes the cure feels worse than the disease, especially when treatment begins before symptoms arise. Sometimes the cure also looks worse than the disease. For example, abnormal fat redistribution or **lipodystrophy** can appear at a time when a person's HIV might otherwise be invisible—both to others and to him- or herself.

Lipodystrophy occurs particularly on the abdomen—central obesity, referred to as the **protease paunch** (Figure 4-10)—and on the back between the shoulder blades, called **"buffalo hump"** (Figure 4-11) and may include a loss of fatty tissue in the arms, legs, and face. Women may experience narrowing of the hips and breast enlargement. HIV-infected children placed on HAART therapy also experienced lipodystrophy (Vigan et al., 2003).

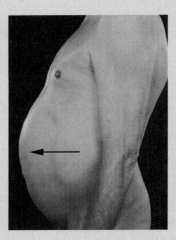

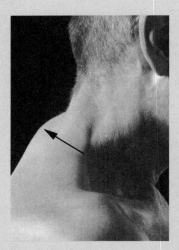

FIGURE 4-10 Protease Paunch—Also Referred to as Crix Belly. This lipid disorder (lipodystrophy) occurs in many patients using protease inhibitors for anti-HIV therapy. In addition to the visual effects of antiretroviral therapy, there are a number of dangerous side effects—see text for details. (*Photograph courtesy of Dr. David Cooper.*)

FIGURE 4-11 Buffalo Hump. The enlargement of a cervicodorsal fat pad. Buffalo hump develops after the use of protease inhibitors for anti-HIV therapy. In addition to the visual effects of antiretroviral therapy, there are a number of other dangerous side effects—see text for details. (*Photograph courtesy of Dr. David Cooper.*)

in the management of HIV/AIDS patients. The **first** is when to begin antiretroviral therapy, the **second** is which drugs to use to initiate treatment, and the **third** is how long to administer a given therapy.

During the last 17 years, clinicians have faced a dilemma of choice when advising asymptomatic people with established HIV infection on when to begin highly active antiretroviral therapy (HAART) and what drugs to use. Begin early, some researchers advise, because later there will be a higher virologic hurdle to overcome. Begin later, others recommend, and save potent drugs until the person's immune system begins to fail. If therapy is started too early, cumulative side effects of the drugs used and the development of multidrug resistance may outweigh the net benefits. If therapy is started too late, increases in disease progression and mortality outweigh the benefits.

In order to assess the very best time to initiate antiretroviral therapy, one needs to know the goal of antiviral therapy. Most HIV/AIDS physicians would agree that the goal is multidimensional: to prolong life while improving the quality of life; to suppress HIV replication to the limits of detection for as long as possible; to select the best possible therapy for the individual; and to minimize costs and side effects to drug therapy. With these goals in mind, and the drugs available to suppress HIV replication and extend life with quality, the first question remains "When should one begin antiretroviral therapy?"

Side Effects of ART

HIV/AIDS really is not yet manageable if it is not survivable. Rounding out what has been learned about antiretroviral drug toxicity is that HIV drugs are implicated in lipodystrophy, heart problems, bone loss (hip replacement), inter-cellular malfunctions called mitochondriosis (my-toe-con-dree-o-sis), lactic acidosis, and liver and kidney dysfunction and failure. Mitochondriosis is mitochondrial dysfunction—some side effects include fat redistribution syndrome, commonly referred to as lipodystrophy. "Lipo" (short for lipodystrophy) is an umbrella term for the gain or loss of fat where you weren't quite expecting it. (See Point of Information 4.2, pages 97–98.) Additional side effects associated with mitochondrial toxicity, which interrupts cellular energy production and leads to fatigue, are shortness of breath, weight loss, rapid heartbeat, hair loss, numbness and pain in the hands, arms, feet, and legs, muscle disease, heart disease, inflammation of the pancreas, increased blood acidity, and kidney irregularities. Add in various opportunistic infections and the drug toxicities required to treat them, and one finds many surviving HIV/AIDS patients have become multidrug resistant. These people require stronger and more toxic remedies month after month and year after year. Ultimately one eventually dies, either from infection or from complications from treatments.

The leading cause of HIV/AIDS-related death in the United States now that ART is available to most is HIV-caused inflammation which is known to be associated with liver failure, cardiovascular events, diabetes, and a variety of cancers and premature aging. Some researchers are suggesting that Acquired Immuno Deficiency Syndrome is becoming the new Acquired Inflammation Disease Syndrome.

U.S. Department of Health and Human Services (DHHS) Guidelines and International Antiviral Society-USA (IAS-USA) Recommendations for the Use of Antiretroviral Therapy in HIV-Infected Adults and Adolescents (July 2012)

There are no "one size fits all" treatment guidelines. Over the last 17 years it has been learned that antiretroviral therapy is becoming more individualized.

In general, the DHHS guidelines and IAS-USA recommendations are the most aggressive on when to start therapy, followed by French guidelines. The Brazilians are the least aggressive, recommending dual nucleoside therapy for those with earlier disease and lower viral loads. Overall, the various guidelines involve expensive strategies that can only be used in more developed countries, or in the wealthier sectors of less developed countries.

When to Start ART—San Francisco and New York City now recommend ART for everyone with HIV regardless of CD4 count and viral load. Current United States treatment guidelines agree with that aggressive standard. They also recommend ART for all HIV-infected individuals regardless of CD4 count. Treatment is also recommended at any CD4 count for people with additional conditions, including pregnancy, HIV associated nephropathy, hepatitis B or C, older age, high viral load, rapid CD4 decline, and high risk for heart disease. In the minds of many HIV experts, ART is now the default—recommended unless there's a good reason not to treat. Reasons why not to treat? People who aren't ready or willing to start should wait until they are. Some people have no way to pay for treatment, an increasingly common scenario

GLOBAL AVAILABILITY OF HIV DRUG THERAPY

Table 4-2 Estimated Antiretroviral Drug Coverage for People with HIV/AIDS in Highly Affected Countries, 2013

Estimated % of Antiretroviral Drug Coverage of Those Who Need Them

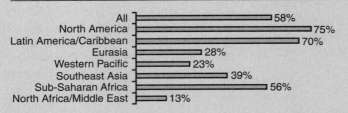

All	58%
North America	75%
Latin America/Caribbean	70%
Eurasia	28%
Western Pacific	23%
Southeast Asia	39%
Sub-Saharan Africa	56%
North Africa/Middle East	13%

Estimated number receiving ART, over 8 million people in low- and middle-income countries ending 2013. About 75% are being supported by U.S. dollars.

Estimated number who need ART, based on the new WHO Guidelines, is about 16 million.

Adapted from Kaiser Education Tutorials. *Current State of the Global HIV/AIDS Epidemic*, 2006 updated.

The goal of the World Health Organization was to have 10 million people on antiretrovirals by 2010. They were far short of their goal. The new goal is 15 million people on ART by 2015.

Of the estimated 54% worldwide receiving ART, about 70% live in sub-Saharan Africa. Ninety percent of those living with HIV/AIDS do *not* know they're infected!

In 2020, of the estimated 40 million people needing ART, about 22 million will be receiving ART. It is estimated that by 2050 some 70 million people in sub-Saharan Africa will be HIV positive, and about 30 million will be receiving ART. The falling mortality from HIV/AIDS due to ART is increasing HIV prevalence and the number of people living with HIV who need life-long therapy.

THINKING POSITIVE, BUT WHAT IF?

For the first 31 years (1981–2012) of this pandemic, people have been told that HIV/AIDS kills. But now various organizations, the WHO, NIH, UNAIDS, and others are saying to the globally HIV infected that you can now live with this disease. The attempt here is to repackage and remarket a still-lethal disease into one with which if people will just educate themselves and find a source of antiretroviral drugs globally, all will be well in the world of HIV/AIDS. The push in this message is to tell everyone their health is in their hands. With the latest estimates, that 16 million people who need antiretroviral drugs about half have access to them, the new message may be meaningless. **First,** for every five people newly infected, three die without access to ART in their lifetime. **Second,** although about one million people began ART for the first time in 2010, there were 2.5 million new HIV infections. For every

person going into treatment, two or three are going to the back of the line. **Third,** while new medicines and improved services help people infected with HIV/AIDS live longer and more productive lives for those in the developed nations that can access them, the economic burden is high. This means that HIV is not just a health issue, it's also an issue in economics. Antiretroviral regimens can cost from $25,000 to over $100,000 per year.

LATE TREATMENT, NO TREATMENT, AND ADHERENCE

Despite ever-widening access to ART, the Joint United Nations Program on HIV/AIDS (UNAIDS) estimates that through 2012 only 22 countries provided antiretrovirals to at least 50% of people who needed them. Yet in the world's developed countries, even those with universal free access, surprisingly large numbers of people start treatment late, never get started, or have a hard time sticking with their regimens (schedules/adherence).

GLOBAL ANGER: POLITICS AND PEOPLE

In many parts of the world, entire societies are composed of families surviving on less than $2 a day. And these societies are besieged by HIV/AIDS.

Widening gaps in access to antiretroviral drugs, creating glaring differences in life expectancies for America's HIV-infected population versus the vast majority of AIDS-affected people in the world, have become pivotal sources of global political anger. Resentment is building in both middle-income and poor nations; as the wealthiest nine nations thrive, the poorest nations witness the evaporation of previous development gains, rising foreign debts, and rising mortalities. Resentment can translate into support for anti-European and anti-Americanism in many forms. In 2004, the imams of northern Nigeria, for example, convinced mothers to shun polio vaccination for their children, on the premise that America put HIV in the vaccine—a successful propaganda campaign that has so far spawned a resurgence of crippling polio epidemics in Nigeria and at least 16 other predominately Muslim nations. Though many pharmaceutical companies have fought to protect high pricing schemes and patents at the expense of global access to affordable medicines, American firms have taken the brunt of the blame and are the target of a special anger bent on ignoring European and American medical patent rights in all their forms.

UNAIDS: TREATMENT AS PREVENTION

Everyone Wants to Do Things Smarter, Faster, and Better with Regard to Treatment of HIV/AIDS

The reality is that treatment today is complicated. From starting HIV therapy to maintenance, the treatment process works, but each step is cumbersome and expensive. Up to 80% of treatment costs are not for the drugs but for the system to get the drugs to a person and to keep them on them. Globally, about a half of the people who need antiretrovirals get them. HIV testing is underutilized, meaning that most people do not know they are HIV positive until they begin to show signs and symptoms of AIDS. Further, antiretrovirals vary with respect to costs, effectiveness, and tolerability. In addition, resistance to the drugs occurs, making it necessary to maintain costly laboratories to monitor individual treatments.

To offset some of these problems, the 2010 UNAIDS OUTLOOK report outlines a radically simplified HIV treatment platform called Treatment 2.0 that should reduce the number of new HIV infections, cut deaths, and reduce costs.

---

even in the United States. Also, we don't know what to do with long term non-progressors and elite controllers—people whose viral loads are already undetectable without therapy. Assuming normal and stable CD4 counts, it would be hard to show a benefit to starting ART in those individuals. How did we get to this point, where ART is recommended for virtually everyone else? First, we're recognizing that HIV isn't just a disease of immunosuppression due to CD4 decline. Untreated HIV has consequences even for people with high CD4 counts, because of the inflammation and immune activation caused by ongoing replication of the virus. Shutting off viral replication may help to reduce the long-term risk of conditions such as heart disease, cognitive decline, loss of bone density, and malignancies by reducing HIV-associated inflammation. Also treating people with HIV lowers their risk of infecting others. In fact, the HPTN052 study demonstrated that ART was 96% effective at preventing transmission to HIV-negative partners, a far greater efficacy than we've seen with any other form of prevention

so far, including condoms, circumcision, microbicides, vaccines—probably even abstinence. Put simply, if everyone with HIV were on treatment with an undetectable viral load, we would see virtually no new HIV cases. Evidence of the benefit of early ART is clear, but the decision to treat early must also consider the cost of therapy, in order to weigh the costs against the benefits. Once-daily regimens are now the norm; a growing number of single-tablet regimens (STRs) are becoming available; tolerability and safety are high. Weighing the financial cost against the benefits is more complicated, since it involves economics and politics rather than science. This is where the prevention benefits of ART become so important. Some people may be unwilling to pay for universal ART for individuals, but if universal treatment can slow or even stop the epidemic, perhaps they'll see it as money well spent.

Bottom line: Early treatment is a triple winner. The HIV infected fare better, their sexual partners are protected and it is cost effective, thus a "benefit trifecta."

Also, the results of recent studies by Michel Funk (2011) and Daniel Kuritzkes (2011) show that (a) starting HIV therapy when the person's immune system is still strong does not reduce the risk of AIDS or death and (b) there was little benefit when ART was started at CD4 counts between 500 and 800.

Serious Problems with Starting ART Early

Starting ART at around a 500 CD4+ cell count presents some difficult problems, such as:

1. **Enormous cost**—In the United States, many thousands of people would be put on ART years earlier than at CD4+ cell counts of 200 or 350. Think worldwide—many millions of people would require ART even earlier. Who would pay for it and for how long?

2. **Adherence**—The longer someone is on ART, the more difficult it is for them to adhere to their drug schedule.

3. **Drug resistance**—The longer someone is on ART, the greater the chance of developing drug resistance.

4. **Drug related toxicities**

5. **Unknown long term risks of ART**

Over the last 17 years, ART has transformed a life-ending disease into a life-changing one, wherein most of the HIV infected are living into their senior years! However, Laurie Garrett, a senior fellow for global health at the Council on Foreign Relations, urges caution when it comes to believing the world can treat its way out of this pandemic. Garrett stated in 2008 that "It is troubling that formerly militant activists, United Nations agency leaders, government health officials, the American foreign policy establishment, religious leaders, scientists, and physicians fail to see AIDS treatment for what it is: a stop-gap measure to tide humanity over until we can collectively reach what ought to be our real goal—stopping HIV's spread, entirely [finding a vaccine?]. On an individual basis living with AIDS is a proper goal; on a population basis it is catastrophic."

Summary

The development of antiretroviral therapy for HIV infection represents one of the most remarkable accomplishments in medical history. Beginning with the introduction of zidovudine in 1987, progress in this area has transformed a uniformly fatal disease into a chronic condition that can be largely controlled in patients with appropriate combinations from among 26 antiretroviral agents licensed for this purpose. However, despite the tremendous success of antiretroviral therapy, major uncertainties remain. Many of the current recommendations for treatment are based on the outcomes of large clinical trials rather than on an understanding of the fundamental science underlying successful therapy.

The goal of an antiretroviral therapy is to reduce viral replication to below the limit of detection of standard clinical assays (HIV-RNA < 50 copies/mL). In patients achieving this treatment goal, clinically significant viral evolution stops, and CD4+ cell counts increase. However, the infection cannot be cured with antiretroviral therapy alone because of the virus's ability to persist in a stable latent reservoir. Nevertheless, patients generally experience positive clinical outcomes as long as suppression of HIV is maintained.

Resistance

Looking at the problem of resistance, it's now known that unless the virus is virtually eliminated from the blood—again, an unlikely prospect—it's only a matter of time before a viral mutant emerges that is resistant to therapy. Current estimates are that the virus mutates once each time it copies itself—over 1 billion times a day. It's like going to Las Vegas. HIV just keeps spinning its bases (its genetic building blocks), looking for a jackpot.

Side Effects

Concerns about serious drug side effects and drug resistance linked to long-term use of HIV combination therapies have replaced optimism, causing a growing number of people on therapy to reconsider the benefits versus the risk of potent antiviral therapies and to seek alternative approaches. In response, pharmaceutical manufacturers have worked to simplify drug regimens and create more potent, less toxic products.

Adequacy: The Dance of a Lifetime

At the moment, current treatments are inadequate. And, once they begin, for now, one must take them for his or her lifetime! Improved ART has given people more time, but it has not provided a cure. At best, antiretroviral drugs have slowed disease progression and extended life. The drugs are complicated to administer, require close medical monitoring, and can cause significant side effects. They are also very costly and, as a result, are inaccessible to the majority of people living with HIV/AIDS in underdeveloped nations.

Although dramatic progress has been made with the increase in access to ART in the developing world, several challenges remain. **First,** as with prevention services, most of the increase in the initiation of ART occurred in Africa. Injection drug users, the primary driver of the epidemic in many countries in Eastern Europe, have limited access to ART, primarily because their behavior is punishable by law. Similar issues exist with men who have sex with men in many parts of the developing world. **Second,** most of the patients initiating ART do so at advanced stages of HIV disease with low CD4+ cell counts, which has been associated with poorer treatment outcomes compared with initiation at higher CD4+ cell counts.

Ending 2013 over eight million people will be on ART. Worldwide, about 38 million people will have been infected. In addition, 2011 studies show that MSM and heterosexual HIV-discordant couples can take preventive ART so as not to transmit HIV to others. In addition, the provision of antiretroviral drugs to HIV-negative people will create an enormous cost for drug supplies, delivery systems, monitoring, and medical care. Who is going to pay? Where will the money come from?

CAUTION:

Consumers should be aware that there are no over-the-counter or online drugs or dietary supplements available to treat or prevent STDs/HIV/AIDS. Appropriate treatment of STDs and/or HIV/AIDS can only occur under the supervision of a healthcare professional. There are many FDS-approved medications available for treating these conditions, but all do require a prescription.

DISCLAIMER

Knowledge about HIV/AIDS changes rapidly. This textbook is designed for educational purpose only and is not engaged in rendering medical advice or professional services. The author does not accept any responsibility for the accuracy of the information or the consequences arising from the application, use, or misuse of any of the information contained herein, including any injury and/or damage to any person or property as a matter of product liability, negligence, or otherwise. No warranty, expressed or implied, is made in regard to the contents of this material. Verify all information independently. This material is not intended as a guide to self-medication. The reader is advised to discuss the information provided here with a doctor, pharmacist, nurse, or other authorized healthcare practitioner and to check product information (including package inserts) regarding dosage, precautions, warnings, interactions, and contraindications before administering any drug, herb, or supplement discussed herein.

Some HIV/AIDS Therapy Information Hotlines

For HIV/AIDS treatment information, call:

The American Foundation for AIDS Research: 1-800-39AMFAR (392-6237)

AIDS Treatment Data Network: 1-800-734-7104

AIDS Treatment News: 1-800-TREAT 1-2 (873-2812)

National HIV Treatment: 1-800-822-7422

For information about AIDS/HIV clinical trials conducted by National Institutes of Health and Food and Drug Administration-approved efficacy trials, call:

National AIDS Clinical Trials Information Service (ACTIS): 1-800-TRIALS-A (874-2572)

For more information about HIV infection, call:

Drug Abuse Hotline: 1-800-662-HELP (4357)

Pediatric and Pregnancy AIDS Hotline: 1-212-430-3333

National Hemophilia Foundation: 1-212-219-8180

Hemophilia and AIDS/HIV Network for Dissemination of Information (HANDI): 1-800-424-HANDI (424-2634)

National Pediatric HIV Resource Center: 1-800-362-0071

National Association of People with AIDS: 1-202-898-0414

Teens Teaching AIDS Prevention Program (TTAPP) National Hotline: 1-800-234-TEEN (8336)

General information:

English: 1–800–332–2636

Spanish: 1–800–344–7432

TDD Service for the Deaf: 1–800–243–7889

General information for healthcare providers:

National Clinician's Post-Exposure Treatment: 1–888–448–4911

HIV Telephone Consultation Service: 1–800–933–3413

Review Questions

(Answers to the Review Questions are on page 463.)

1. Can HIV infection be cured?

2. What is a surrogate marker?

3. From _____ 1987 through 2007 _____ individual and combination anti-HIV drugs were FDA-approved.

4. How many FDA-approved anti-HIV drugs are nucleoside or nucleotide analogs?

5. How do nucleoside analogs inhibit HIV replication?

6. What are the two major problems in the use of nucleoside and non-nucleoside analogs in HIV therapy?

7. What is HIV viral load? What can its quantitative measurement reveal?

8. How do non-nucleoside drugs inhibit HIV replication?

9. Briefly describe the goal of HIV combination drug therapy.

10. After starting antiretroviral therapy, what is an acceptable target for viral load that indicates the therapy is effective?
    A. 50 copies/mL
    B. 5000–10,000 copies/mL
    C. 10,000–15,000 copies/mL
    D. No acceptable target level has been set.

11. HIV escapes the effects of HIV antiretroviral drugs by
    A. inactivating the drugs.
    B. disguising itself as an immune cell.
    C. pretending to be a harmless virus.
    D. changing its genetic makeup.

12. When HIV mutates to a drug, it can cause
    A. the virus to become less "fit."
    B. the drug to become less effective.
    C. other drugs to become less effective.
    D. all of the above.

13. When your virus becomes resistant to a drug in your drug combination, your _____ may go up.

A. temperature
B. CD4 cells
C. doctor bills
D. viral load

14. True or False: Resistance is all-or-nothing—the drugs work perfectly or not at all.

15. True or False: Mutations take years to develop, so missing one day's dose of meds will not contribute to resistance.

16. Cross-resistance is a problem for which class of drugs?
    A. Protease inhibitors
    B. Nukes
    C. Non-nukes
    D. All three classes

17. Which of the following is not an important issue when choosing a drug regimen?
    A. Potential side effects
    B. Easy dosing schedule
    C. High genetic barrier
    D. All three are important.

18. True or False: ART has lowered the number of deaths in the United States.

19. Antiretroviral therapy (ART) is less than ideal because
    A. it does not eliminate latent HIV infection.
    B. its cost is too great for 90% of AIDS sufferers.
    C. it often has severe side effects.
    D. some HIV strains are resistant to it.
    E. All of the above.

20. Prior to 1994, which group was usually omitted in FDA clinical trials?
    A. African Americans
    B. Asians
    C. women
    D. minorities

21. An HIV viral load test can
    A. assess your risk for disease progression.
    B. assess how well your drug regimen is working.
    C. determine your HIV disease stage.
    D. all of the above.

22. The surge in HIV-RNA copies in the plasma three to six weeks after infection
    A. is known as Acute HIV Syndrome.
    B. is a period of HIV dissemination in the body.
    C. is when the lymphoid organs are seeded.
    D. all of the above.

23. True or False: The 2010 report on the iPrEX study showed that **antiretroviral** drugs are very effective in HIV prevention.

The Immunology
of HIV Disease/AIDS

For most, immunity is simply there when it's needed, like the umbrella sitting by the door. But the immune system's elegance—honed by millions of years of warfare with invaders of every kind—shouldn't be confused with simplicity. The immune system is a thing of beauty—subtle enough to distinguish dangerous invaders like viruses from benign interlopers such as food; clever enough to recognize when the body's supposedly friendly cells turn cancerous and should be eliminated. But the immune system can also go seriously awry. When it begins attacking healthy tissues, the result can be any one of 80 autoimmune diseases such as lupus or rheumatoid arthritis. It's the price we pay for having such a dynamic, finely balanced system.

THE IMMUNE SYSTEM

All living organisms are continually exposed to substances that are capable of causing harm. Most organisms protect themselves against such substances in more than one way—with physical barriers, the skin for example, or with chemicals that repel or kill invaders. Animals with backbones, **vertebrates,** have these types of general protective mechanisms, but they also have a more advanced protective system called an **immune system.** The immune system is a mind-numbing, incredibly complex network of organs containing cells that recognize foreign substances in the body and destroy them. Like a security force, it protects vertebrates against pathogens, or infectious agents, such as viruses, bacteria, fungi, and other parasites. Within the body of a healthy adult, such microbial cells are estimated to outnumber human cells by a ratio of ten to one!

Although there are many potentially harmful pathogens (agents that cause diseases), no pathogen can invade or attack all organisms because a pathogen's ability to cause harm requires a susceptible victim, and not all organisms are susceptible to the same pathogens. For instance, the virus, HIV, that causes AIDS is strictly a human pathogen; it does not cause a disease in any other animal. Similarly, humans are not susceptible to the viruses that cause canine (dog) distemper or feline (cat) leukemia. This is because the cells in different animals carry their own specific receptors or protein fragments wherein each **receptor** on a given cell only allows a specific cellular product or environmental agent to attach. The receptor is like a doorknob that a given pathogen can attach to.

An Explanation of the Importance of Cell Receptors: They are Biological Conduits for Information Transfer

In the study of cells, the term **receptor** is used to describe any molecule that interacts with and subsequently holds on to some other molecule. The receptor is like the hand, and the object held by the hand is commonly called the **ligand.** The interaction between the receptor and ligand implies **specificity;** a receptor known to bind with substance X would not normally bind with a different substance. For example, a two-slotted electrical wall outlet is a receptacle (receptor) for a two-pronged plug (ligand). A three-pronged plug will not fit into this receptacle. Depending on the type of two-slotted receptacle, even some two-pronged plugs may not fit.

All Cells Have Receptors: Where Are Cell Receptors Located?

Receptors are classified into five families and can be found inside or on the outside of a cell, and especially embedded within all the membranes that a given cell may have. In humans, there are organ systems present, and a given receptor may be found associated only with a particular type of cell that composes a particular type of tissue that makes up a particular organ.

What Do Receptors Do?

Receptors allow cells to recognize specific ligands and to receive extracellular messages. And, they are critical to the life of all cells, whether the cells represent an animal, a plant, a fungus, or a bacterium. Every function, response, interaction, pathway, process, and other term you might think of that concerns the moment-to-moment existence of a cell is controlled by various receptor/ligand-induced systems. Essentially, you are what your genetically coded receptors allow you to become. In Chapter 3, pages 50–51, there is an explanation of receptors that restrict the types of virus that can attach to certain cell types. In particular the ligand, in this case HIV, attaches almost exclusively to the CD4 (protein) receptor of a specific population of T lymphocytes (100% of T4 or CD4+ lymphocytes, 50% of macrophages and monocytes, 5% of B cells, and a smaller percentage of glial cells, chromaffin cells in the lower gut and vaginal lining, and retinal cells in the eye). Several human diseases are associated with alterations in cell-surface receptors, e.g., HIV/AIDS.

Function of the Immune System

A man dies because his body rejected a heart transplant; a woman is crippled by rheumatoid arthritis; a child goes into a coma that is brought on by cerebral malaria; another child dies of an infection because of an immunodeficiency; an elderly man has advanced hepatic cirrhosis caused by iron overload. These five clinical situations are diverse, yet all have one thing in common: a malfunction of the human immune system.

The immune system filters out foreign substances, removes damaged and dead cells, and acts as a security system to destroy mutant and cancer cells. It is composed of a number of specialized cells, several organs, and a group of biologically active chemicals. The human immune system is like a jigsaw puzzle—many parts come together to form an overall defense against disease-causing agents. If parts of the immune system are missing or damaged, illness may occur due to an immune deficiency.

Separating Friend from Foe: How the Immune System Decides

Skin prevents disease-causing agents from entering the body. But they can enter through body openings, cuts, or wounds. Whether the invader is a life-threatening bacterium or a relatively harmless cold virus, your immune system must control it—if it does not, the harmless may become the harmful! A single infectious microorganism or virus that survives and multiplies may cause a severe illness. Some infectious agents resemble the body's own cells. How do immune cells know which to attack and which to ignore? The answer is, once something foreign (an agent) enters the body, it triggers an **immune response** if the body does not recognize the substance or agent as a part of itself or **"self."** All body cells have special molecules, called **class I proteins,** on their membranes that are like flags or bar codes with the word "self" on them. (See Figure 5-1 and Point of Information 5.1, page 116.) The cells of the immune system try to destroy anything present in the body that is not carrying the self molecules— anything that is **"nonself."** Nonself is any substance or agent that triggers the creation of antibodies (very specific body proteins that react against [anti] anything foreign that gets into the [body]). Such nonself substances are called **antigens.** Antigens may be whole viruses or organisms or parts of viruses, organisms, or their products.

In general, most cellular organisms that damage cells do so from the outside by producing toxic chemicals or in some way externally interfering

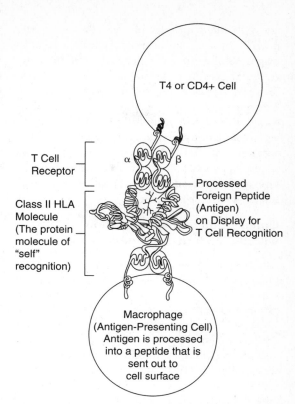

FIGURE 5-1 Interaction Between a Human Leukocyte Antigen "Self" Protein (HLA), a Foreign Peptide (Antigen), and a T Cell Receptor. The diagram represents the trimolecular interaction of a processed antigen into a peptide that is being presented on the surface of the antigen-presenting cell to a T4 cell. The presence of the class II HLA self-identity marker and the presence of the foreign peptide stimulate the T4 cell into action. *(Adapted from Sinha, 1990.)*

with the cell's metabolism. But viruses invade or enter different cell types, forcing them to produce viral replicas at the expense of the cells' own essential metabolic functions. Gradually, like a machine wearing out, host cells start to malfunction and die. The best thing a virus can do is find a host cell that does not die and that can produce replicas indefinitely. In a biological time frame, new disease-causing viruses are often very deadly to new hosts. If a new virus strain is too deadly, it kills its host before other hosts are infected, and the ensuing epidemic dies out. For example, the **Ebola virus** makes its victims very weak shortly after infection and kills them in 7 to 14 days. This virus kills quickly, vanishes, and turns up somewhere else. Its origin is still unknown. Over biological time, successful viruses like the human herpes virus and their new hosts learn to accommodate each other. This will most likely happen with human-HIV associations, but how many people over how many years will have to die before human cells learn to accommodate HIV is unknown. Perhaps it will never happen. Smallpox virus has been infecting humans for thousands of years and has never been accommodated by humans.

Cooperation and Coordination within the Human Immune System

The basic premise of the immune system is simple: to coordinate the activities of various cell types in order to provide extended, if not lifelong, protection against disease-causing pathogens. Usually, this cooperating system works flawlessly, quashing diseases before they can kill their host and sparking an immunity to provide protection against future attacks. Sometimes, however, the system fails and infection and disease prevail—and there is no greater example of this than HIV, a pathogen that almost always succeeds in circumventing and manipulating the body's immune defense to facilitate its own survival.

HUMAN LYMPHOCYTES: T CELLS AND B CELLS

The hallmark of the human immune system is its ability to mount a highly specific response against virtually any foreign entity, even those never seen before in the course of evolution. It is able to do this because of the number of different kinds of cells called lymphocytes. Lymphocytes are a type of white blood cell. About 15% to 40% of white blood cells are lymphocytes. Within the family of lymphocytes are some of the most important cells within the human immune system. The human immune system contains about 2 trillion (2×10^{12}) lymphocytes, but this is a relatively small number when compared to the 100 trillion cells in the body (see Box 5.1, Figure 5-4, page 110). Most mature lymphocytes recirculate continuously, going from blood to tissue and back to blood again as often as one to two times per day. They travel among most other cells and are present in large numbers in the thymus, bone marrow, lymph nodes, spleen, and appendix (Figure 5-2).

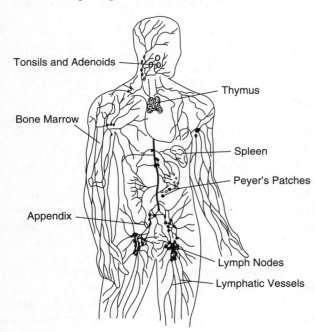

Tonsils and Adenoids

Thymus

Bone Marrow

Spleen

Peyer's Patches

Appendix

Lymph Nodes

Lymphatic Vessels

FIGURE 5-2 Organs of the Human Immune System. The organs of the immune system are positioned throughout the body. They are generally referred to as lymphoid organs because they are concerned with the development, growth, and dissemination of lymphocytes, or white cells, that populate the immune system. Lymphoid organs include the bone marrow, thymus, lymph nodes, spleen, tonsils, adenoids, appendix, and the clumps of lymphoid tissue in the small intestine called Peyer's patches. The blood and lymphatic fluids transport lymphocytes to and from all the immune system organs. Gut-associated lymphoid tissue contains 50% to 60% of the body's lymphocytes, and those lymphocytes, according to Peter Anton at UCLA, contain six times more CD4 receptors than do CD4+ or T4 cells circulating in the blood. Other lymphoid tissue contains about 98% of lymphocytes, and blood contains about 2%. These data may mean that the gut is the preferred site of HIV replication in untreated patients.

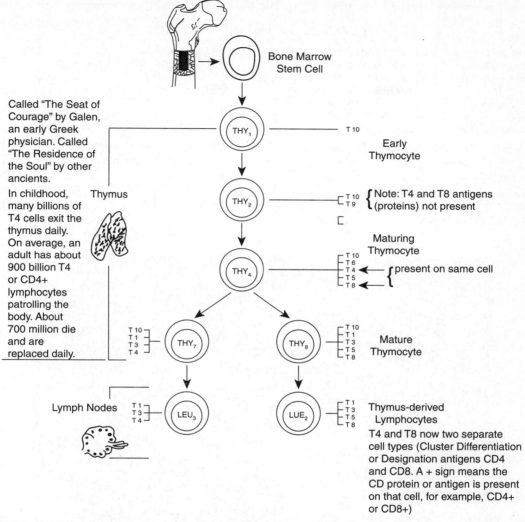

Called "The Seat of Courage" by Galen, an early Greek physician. Called "The Residence of the Soul" by other ancients.

In childhood, many billions of T4 cells exit the thymus daily. On average, an adult has about 900 billion T4 or CD4+ lymphocytes patrolling the body. About 700 million die and are replaced daily.

Thymus

Lymph Nodes

Bone Marrow Stem Cell

THY₁ — T 10 — Early Thymocyte

THY₂ — T 10, T 9 — Note: T4 and T8 antigens (proteins) not present

THY₄ — T 10, T 6, T 4, T 5, T 8 — Maturing Thymocyte — present on same cell

THY₇ — T 10, T 1, T 3, T 4 — Mature Thymocyte

THY₈ — T 10, T 1, T 3, T 5, T 8

LEU₃ — T 1, T 3, T 4

LUE₂ — T 1, T 3, T 5, T 8 — Thymus-derived Lymphocytes

T4 and T8 now two separate cell types (Cluster Differentiation or Designation antigens CD4 and CD8. A + sign means the CD protein or antigen is present on that cell, for example, CD4+ or CD8+)

FIGURE 5-3 T Lymphocyte **Cluster Differentiation (CD)** Antigen in Humans. The CD marker or antigen on a T cell tells something about what the cell does. For example, the CD4 and CD8 T cells have different jobs to do. Stages of thymic differentiation (that is, the presence of the different antigens or proteins on their membrane surfaces) are defined on the basis of reactivity to monoclonal antibodies. Schematic pictures of cells represent thymocytes within specific stages of a defined phenotype: T1–T10.

By 1968, lymphocytes had been divided into two classes: **lymphocytes called B cells** that are derived from and mature in bone marrow, and **lymphocytes called T cells** that are derived from bone marrow but travel to and mature in the thymus gland (Figure 5-3). T cells make up 70% to 80% of the lymphocytes circulating in the body. Circulating T cells are a heterogeneous group of cells with a wide range of different functions. When a T cell encounters another cell, it uses various probes or detecting devices on its surface—known as receptors—to examine the fragments displayed on an antigen-presenting cell's surface (Figure 5-1). The fragments displayed on the antigen-presenting cell (APC) disclose to the scanning T cell whether the APC being scanned is

BOX 5.1

HOW LARGE IS A TRILLION? A BILLION?

The human body is made up of many trillions of cells. For example, the human immune system contains at least a trillion lymphocytes dedicated to destroying foreign substances that endanger health. But, a trillion of anything is a very large number. Can we really appreciate just how large a trillion of something is? Perhaps the following will help.

1. One trillion seconds equals 31,700 years.

2. One trillion minutes equals 1,901,000 years.

3. A stack of 1 trillion one-dollar bills would reach a height of 69,000 miles.

4. It would take a person 11.5 days to count to 1 million and 31,688 years to count to 1 trillion—1, 2, 3, 4, 5 . . . !

5. A stack of 1 trillion HIV would be over 62 miles high (diameter of HIV = 1000 angstroms:
$(1 \times 10^{12})(1000)$
$(1 \times 10^{-10}) = 1 \times 10^5$ meters = 62.15 miles).

In billions:

1. One billion seconds ago it was 1960.

2. One billion minutes ago, Jesus was alive.

3. One billion hours ago, our ancestors were living in the Stone Age.

4. One billion days ago no one walked on the Earth on two feet.

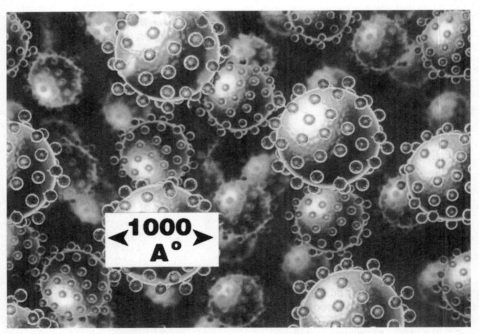

FIGURE 5-4 Dimensions of HIV in Angstroms. HIV has a diameter of 1000 angstroms (Å). It would take 254,000 HIV laid side by side to equal 1 inch in length. *(Illustration courtesy of the author)*

normal and to be left unharmed, or infected and to be destroyed. The protein fragments are cupped inside tiny holders called class II major histocompatibility complexes (class II MHCs). To be more specific, each individual T cell expresses a receptor **(T cell antigen receptor, TCR),** which recognizes a ligand (a com-pound that fits a particular receptor) composed of an antigenic peptide, 8–15 amino acids long, bound to a **self-major-histocompatibility-complex (MHC) molecule** (also referred to as **HLA-human leukocyte antigen system**). Thus, a T cell does not directly recognize a soluble antigen, but rather recognizes an antigen displayed on the surface of an **antigen-presenting cell (APC)** like a B cell or macrophage. There are about 10 billion APCs located in the lymphoid organs. The receptors of T cells are different from those of B cells because they are "trained" to recognize fragments of antigens that have been combined or complexed with HLA class II molecules. As T cells circulate through the body, they scan the surfaces of body cells for the presence of foreign antigens that have become associated with the HLA molecules. The antigen present on the APC signals to the T cell whether the APC should be left unharmed or whether the APC is infected and should be destroyed. This function is sometimes called **immune surveillance.**

The Cytotoxic and Helper (T4 or CD4+) Lymphocytes

Two of the important kinds of T cells are **cytotoxic** or **killer T** lymphocytes (CTL) and **helper T** lymphocytes. Killer T cells carry the **CD8 protein antigen** on their surface and are called T8 or CD8+ cells. CD8 or T8 cells are suppressor cells that bring an end to an immune response that is no longer needed. Helper T cells carry the **CD4 protein antigen** on their surface and are called **T4** or **CD4+ cells.** The CD4 and CD8 proteins or antigens located on their respective T lymphocytes act similar to a bar code or a number on a football jersey; the proteins or antigens identify the cell type. Killer or CTL T cells bind to cells carrying a foreign antigen and destroy them. But CD4+ or T4 cells do not kill cells directly; they interact with B cells and CTL cells and help them respond to foreign antigens. The CD4+ or T4 cell has the role of a quarterback in football; it calls the plays for the rest of the lymphocyte team.

Normal CD4+ cell counts vary between 500 and 1200 per microliter (μL) of blood while CD8+ cell counts range between 375 and 1100. This balance between CD4+ and CD8+ cells must be maintained. It is the CD4+ count that drops dramatically in HIV-infected people.

WHY CD4+ CELLS ARE IMPORTANT IN HIV INFECTION—WHAT IT MEANS

CD4 cells are distributed throughout the body in the blood, lungs, heart, intestines, brain, etc. The vast majority of all CD4 cells are out in the tissues, not floating in the blood. They can find and attack infection best at the source in the tissues of the body. However, CD4 counts are measured in the liquid part of the blood, so in essence one is looking only at the top of a very large iceberg. As that iceberg bobs in and out of the water, the amount we see goes up and down. That is, as the CD4 cells move in and out of the blood to the tissues, the number can fluctuate. The CD4 percentage can be more stable since the proportion of T cells that are CD4 is consistent between what is in the blood and tissues (just like the content and makeup of the part of the iceberg above and below the water line).

When HIV infects humans, the cells it infects most often are CD4+ cells. The virus becomes part of the cells, and when they multiply to fight an infection, they also make more copies of HIV. When someone is infected with HIV for a long time, the number of CD4+ cells they have (their CD4+ cell count) goes down. This is a sign that the immune system is being weakened. The lower the CD4+ cell count, the more likely the person will get sick. There are millions of different families of CD4+ cells. Each family is designed to fight a specific type of agent. When HIV reduces the number of CD4+ cells, some of these families can be totally wiped out. You can lose the ability to fight off the particular agents those families were designed for. If this happens, you might develop an opportunistic infection (see Chapter 6, page 134, on Opportunistic Infections).

THE CD4+ CELL COUNT— WHY IT MATTERS

The CD4+ cell value bounces around a lot. Time of day, fatigue, and stress can affect CD4+ test results. It's best to have blood drawn at the same time of day for each CD4+ cell test, and to use the same laboratory. Infections can have a large impact on CD4+ cell counts. When your body fights an infection, the number of white blood cells (lymphocytes) goes up. CD4+ and CD8+ counts go up, too. Vaccinations can cause the same effects. CD4+ cell counts should not be checked until a couple of weeks after recovery from an infection or a vaccination.

The Loss of T4 or CD4+ Lymphocytes When Compared to T8 or CD8+ Lymphocytes and Its Biological Impact

The ratio of CD4 cells to CD8 cells is often reported. This is calculated by dividing the CD4 value by the CD8 value. In healthy people, this ratio is between 0.9 and 1.9, meaning that there are about 1 to 2 CD4 cells for every CD8 cell. In people with HIV infection, this ratio drops dramatically, meaning that there are many times more CD8 cells than CD4 cells.

Ashley Haase, director of the University of Minnesota Microbiology Department, estimated that healthy young adults harbor approximately 200 billion mature CD4+ cells in the body at any given time. In HIV-positive patients, this total number is halved by the time the CD4+ cell count falls to 200 cells/μL of blood. In the more advanced stage of HIV disease, the destruction of parenchymal lymphoid spaces is so extensive that a total body CD4+ cell count has not even been attempted (Haase, 1999).

It is believed that T4 cells recognize only those antigens of viruses, fungi, and other parasites; and trigger only those parts of the immune system necessary to act against these agents. Indeed, the viruses, fungi, and other parasites produce the majority of opportunistic infections when the T4 cells have been depleted by HIV.

It was unknown if B cells begin to malfunction soon after HIV infection. In late 2001, investigators at the National Institute of Allergy and Infectious Diseases (NIAID) reported that the presence of HIV in infected patients causes B cells (a) to produce excessive amounts of nonessential antibodies, (b) to fail to respond to physiological signals, and (c) to be at risk of becoming cancerous. Some of these changes can be reversed with the use of antiretroviral drugs (Moir et al., 2001).

In Summary

The two types of lymphocytes, B cells and T cells, play different roles in the immune response, though they may act together and influence each other's functions. The part of the immune response that involves B cells is often called **humoral immunity** because it takes place in the body fluids. The part involving T cells is called cellular immunity because it takes place directly between the T cells, other cells, and their antigens. This distinction is misleading, however, because strictly speaking, all adaptive immune responses are cellular—that is, they are all initiated by cells (the lymphocytes) reacting to antigens. **B cells** may initiate an immune response, but the triggering antigens are actually eliminated by soluble products that the B cells release into the blood and other body fluids. These products are called **antibodies** and belong to a special group of blood proteins called **immunoglobins.** When a B cell is stimulated by an antigen that it encounters in the body fluids, it transforms, with the aid of T4 cells, into a larger cell, a blast cell. The blast cell begins to divide rapidly, forming a clone of identical cells. Some of these transform further into plasma cells—in essence, antibody-producing factories. These plasma cells produce a single type of antigen-specific antibody at a rate of about 2000 antibodies per second. The antibodies then circulate through the body fluids, binding to the triggering antigen.

What Happens to the Immune System after HIV Infection

HIV enters the body via infected body fluids: blood, semen, and vaginal secretions. Once inside, HIV specifically infects active T4 or CD4+ cells. However, while HIV devastates CD4 or T4 cells, most of the time they cannot be infected because 95% of these cells are in a resting state when HIV cannot infect them. It is only when these cells become activated—rapidly multiplying to kill invading microorganisms—that HIV infects the cells, uses their genetic machinery to replicate, and eventually kills the cells. The resting CD4 cells' antiviral protection derives from the protein APOBEC3G (a-po-beck), an enzyme that could have evolved in mammals as a natural antiviral defense. HIV has a protein, called VIF (viral infective protein), that appears to disarm these cells by neutralizing APOBEC (see explanation in Chapter 3, pages 60–61). APOBEC exists in lightweight and heavyweight versions. In resting cells, the lightweight APOBEC is lethal to HIV. But when T cells are activated, the free-floating, lightweight APOBEC proteins are gathered into the heavyweight complexes that are vulnerable to HIV.

In 2008, Mario Santiago and colleagues reported that the APOBEC gene in mice contains a second gene, Rfv3, that is responsible for producing the **neutralizing antibody** necessary for surviving the **Friend virus.** It possesses the ability to make the HIV-neutralizing antibody that is missing in humans. Scientists are now searching for a way to apply the mouse APOBEC/Rfv3 findings to humans.

Use of Absolute vs. Percentage T4 or CD4+ Cell Count

Doctors use a test that counts the number of T4 or CD4+ cells in a cubic millimeter or μL (microliter) of blood. About 2% of the body's T4 cells are in the blood; the rest are in tissues such as lymph nodes. Changes in your T4 cell count (observed as results of a test that only measures levels in blood) may reflect the movement of cells into and out of the blood, rather than changes in the total number of T4 cells in your body. The *absolute* CD4 count is obtained by multiplying the estimated percentage of CD4 cells in a blood sample by the total number of white blood cells in the body. It is the absolute CD4 count of about 350 that is used as the criterion to start antiretroviral therapy (ART).

A metaphor that can be used to describe the differences between percent and absolute CD4 counts is that the absolute count is like measuring the total number of red cars on the highway at any one time—if measured at rush hour, there would be more than at midnight. The real question, however, is how many red cars are there in the city (or CD4s in your body); presumably, the percentage of red cars remains the same at rush hour and at midnight. Percentage is a way to smooth over variations in the traffic or CD4 cells in multiple samples.

In some cases, in order to help understand changes in your absolute T4 count, a physician may determine what proportion of a blood sample's lymphocytes are T4+ cells. This is called the T4 or CD4+ **percentage.** This percentage is more stable than a CD4 count over time. In HIV-negative people a normal result is between 30% and 50%. This means that 30% to 50% of your lymphocytes are CD4+ cells. This means that the immune system is still functioning properly regardless of the CD4+ count. A T4 percentage that falls below about 15% is understood to reflect damage to the immune system and a risk of serious infections. Most people with HIV find that their T4 count falls over time.

Monitoring CD4+ Counts

It is useful to have a T4 or CD4+ count measured regularly for two reasons: (1) to monitor one's immune system and help one decide whether and when to take antiretroviral drugs (ARD) and treatments to prevent opportunistic infections (OI); and (2) to help monitor the effectiveness of any anti-HIV drugs being taken. If your T4 or CD4+ count is persistently below 350, your immune system is weakened and you are at a gradually increasing risk of OI the further it falls. If it drops below 200–250 you are at increased risk for serious OI (Figure 5-5). At 350 both European and U.S. treatment guidelines now recommend beginning ART. One effect of ARD is to improve the state of the immune system. This is crudely reflected in an increase in the T4 or CD4+ count. Evidence suggests that the cells' ability to fight OI is also improved. For example, people taking ARD who find their T4 count rises and stays above 250 cells may no longer need to take drugs that may have been prescribed to prevent *Pneumocystis* pneumonia (PCP) or other opportunistic infections. Monitoring the changes in your T4 count while you

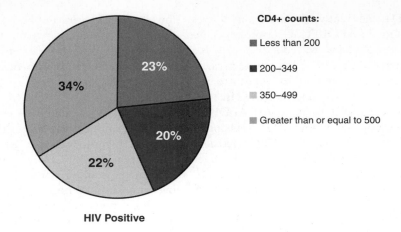

CD4+ counts:

■ Less than 200

■ 200–349

■ 350–499

■ Greater than or equal to 500

HIV Positive

Nationally representative sample of the civilian, noninstitutionalized household population aged 18–49 years. Source: CDC/NCHS, National Health and Nutrition Examination Surveys, 1999–2006 (Updated).

FIGURE 5-5 Estimated CD4+ Count, by HIV Status: United States, 1999–2011. The CD4 cell value bounces around a lot. Time of day, fatigue, and stress can affect the test results. Infections can also have a large impact on CD4 cell counts. When your body fights an infection, the number of white blood cells (lymphocytes) goes up. CD4 and CD8 counts go up, too. Vaccinations can cause the same effect.

are taking ARD can help the doctor decide whether the treatment is working or whether it is time to try different options. A fall in T4 count would be a sign the treatment is not working and may need to be switched to a new regimen. However, the T4 count isn't the only consideration when making these decisions; viral load results, how well you feel, and which treatments have been used before are also considered.

Understanding the Results

Factors other than HIV can affect your T4 or CD4+ count including infections, time of day, smoking, stress, and which lab tests the blood sample. So it is very important to watch the trend in your CD4+ count over time, rather than to place too much emphasis on a single test that may be misleading. Doctors will normally suggest measuring the T4 or CD4+ count every three to six months if one has a relatively high count and no symptoms and is not taking ARD. They may suggest more frequent counts if decisions have to be made (such as whether to start treatments),

HIV-related symptoms develop, or if the decline in CD4+ cells appears to be increasing.

The Antibody (See Sidebar 5.1, page 115 and Point of Information 5.1, page 116)

Antibodies are Y-shaped molecules that bind to specific foreign proteins, or pieces of protein, called antigens.

When antibodies on the surface of a B cell snag an undesirable or foreign protein, *both disappear inside the cell.* Eventually, as previously discussed, a bit of the foreign protein may reemerge, attached to a self-recognizable protein molecule called a **class II protein** (Figure 5-1, page 107). The pair, the small piece of foreign protein attached to a self class II protein, acts as a red flag to T4 cells, which set off an aggressive immune response.

(For an excellent review of the concept of antigen processing and presentation, see Unanue, 1995; for class I and class II proteins, Strominger et al., 1995; for the concept of self, Zinkernagel, 1995; for cell-mediated immunity, Doherty, 1995).

B Cells Make Antibodies and Release Them into the Bloodstream

After an antibody and virus join, they are digested by macrophages or cleared from the blood by the liver and spleen. Some B cells and T cells become memory cells, which are stored by the immune system. Memory cells appear to recall their history and remember the antigen they have previously encountered. However, if the antigen, say a virus, has mutated (changed), as the flu virus does yearly, previous antibodies will not affect it. New antibodies must be created to neutralize or cancel out the new mutant virus. While this antibody production is taking place, the viral invader has time to multiply and infect new cells, and the infected person suffers the symptoms of the flu.

Can the Immune System Remember HIV Exposure?

The immune system works because it produces antibody against an antigen and in addition creates immune memory cells. But this does not appear to occur when the immune system is exposed to HIV. Yes, antibody is made, but when HIV disappears (is reduced to below measurable levels using

---

SIDEBAR 5.1

MEASURES AND COUNTERMEASURES: THE HUMAN IMMUNE SYSTEM VS. VIRUSES

A war has existed between humans and viruses that invade human cells and cause disease. Probably from the first encounter, prehuman to first humans, viruses became able to *hide* inside human cells. The immune system in turn adapted by developing a means of surveying and identifying cells containing a hidden virus. Viruses then adapted by deceiving the immune surveillance system; the immune system then evolved a better means to *mark* cells carrying the virus. This game of hide-and-seek between the virus and the immune system continues. Learning the means by which the virus attempts to trick the immune system carries over into the study of tumor cells. They must also escape the immune system's surveillance system and do so by using several of the same ploys used by the virus. From what microbiologists have learned so far, different viruses have evolved different ways of getting rid of expression of class I proteins, the flagpole of self-proteins. But the mechanisms are amazingly different in different viruses. Examples are:

Cytomegalovirus (CMV)—A virus that may cause birth defects in the fetus and the rapid onset of blindness in people with AIDS. On entering a cell, CMV stops self-identity proteins from reaching the cell membrane. If the class I proteins can't reach the membrane neither will pieces of CMV. The immune system is blinded to the fact the CMV is inside the cells. The immune system counters with a natural killer cell that destroys all cells that do not contain a self protein on their surface! But CMV over time evolved a means to produce a fake self protein that passes for the real one. The natural killer cells are successfully fooled.

Adenovirus—The virus causing common colds. This virus can also stop self proteins from reaching the membrane carrying identifying pieces of virus. Further, this virus is able to make the cell divide so it can replicate itself. The cell then becomes cancerous (replication out of control), and begins to destroy itself—but the virus has evolved a way to stop the cell's self-destruction, so the cell continues to divide. The process is similar to what happens in tumor cells.

HIV—This virus has the most deadly scheme of all. This virus infects cells of the immune system—most often the T4 cells that are essential to the initiation of the immune response. Similar to other viruses, HIV has to disable the self-alerting system. One of HIV's genes, called **nef** (negative effector), makes a protein that attaches to the self-proteins, just inside the cell's membrane. The other end of the nef protein carries an address label, readable by the cell's internal sorting system that directs proteins to their proper place. The message carried by the nef protein says, in the cell's sorting code, "Haul to garbage dump and recycle," tricking the infected cell into pulling down its self-proteins and destroying them. The nef protein also tags the CD4 proteins for destruction in the same way. Like the self-proteins, the CD4s stick up through the cell membrane. What does HIV gain from having the cell destroy CD4 proteins? That's the million-dollar question investigators are working on. The reason may be to prevent other viruses from entering the cell or because in latching onto the CD4 proteins, the nef protein dislodges and energizes another protein that is known to activate the T cells. The cell's activation to make more HIV may be the answer.

antiretroviral therapy or HAART), so does the immune defense against it. There are few if any memory cells to protect the body should HIV rebound or break through drug suppression replication. In the mid–1990s, Francis Plummer and colleagues at the University of Nairobi stunned scientists when they announced the discovery of a group of Kenyan female prostitutes who appeared resistant to HIV infection, surviving infection for years despite more than six customers a week without condom protection in a society where upward of 20% of their customers were likely to be HIV positive. Vaccine researchers were ecstatic because the discovery offered evidence that people could successfully become immune to HIV—something some scientists had argued might be impossible. But at the Seventh Conference on Retroviral and Opportunistic Infections (2000) Plummer's group had distressing news: 10% of the apparently resistant prostitutes became HIV positive from 1996 to 1999. Their infections coincided with the women's decisions to *decrease their exposure* to HIV by having fewer customers or insisting that the men wear condoms. Kevin De Crock, an

HIV investigator, said, "It suggests that HIV antigen stimulation is required for the maintenance of resistance." De Crock said it may be that the immune system is not capable of remembering without a constant presence of HIV (too few memory cells made?). This would appear to be an HIV catch 22—to control HIV it must be present, but the control will over the long run be insufficient to stop the progression to AIDS.

ANTIBODIES AND HIV DISEASE

Resistance to HIV does not seem to be the same as the more common examples of immunity. The body's protective countermeasures against measles and mumps are absolute. Years after exposure, there is no hint within the body of the foreign agents that cause those diseases. After children become immune to mumps, they can no longer infect other people. Immunity to these diseases occurs because the immune system makes neutralizing antibody, antibody that binds to and directly inhibits or neutralizes the function of infectious agents. Memory immune cells are able to produce neutralizing or cancelling antibody whenever these infecting agents enter the body. In contrast, it has been shown that although the immune systems of most people initially produce neutralizing HIV antibodies, the continued evolution of HIV in their bodies results in a series of mutant HIV that are not efficiently neutralized or cancelled via antibody response. Thus over time, the ratio of effective neutralizing antibody production to new virus production becomes disproportionate, that is, more virus exists than effective neutralizing antibody. At this time the level of T4 or CD4+ cells begins to drop (See Point of Information 5.2, page 117). T4 cells drop because antibodies to HIV reduce circulating HIV in the plasma (viral load) without affecting HIV replication or cell-to-cell spread of HIV. This means that the production of mutant HIV to existing antibody never ceases, resulting in continued T4 cell infection and loss. Eventually there are too few T4 cells to ward off opportunistic infections (see Chapter 7, specifically page 165, for additional

PATHOLOGISTS BELIEVE THEY HAVE FOUND A CONSTANT ANTIGENIC SITE THAT MAY ALLOW FOR THE PRODUCTION OF NEUTRALIZING ANTIBODIES

HIV researchers at the University of Texas Medical School at Houston believe they have uncovered the Achilles heel in HIV. The weak spot is hidden in the HIV envelope protein gp120. This protein is essential for HIV attachment to host cells. Normally the body's immune defenses can ward off viruses by making antibodies that bind and neutralize the virus. However, HIV is constantly changing so that the antibodies produced after infection do not control disease progression to AIDS. For the same reason, there is no HIV vaccine that stimulates production of protective antibodies. The constant site, a small stretch of amino acids numbered 421–433 on gp120, is under study as a target for drug inhibition. Sudhir Paul, pathology professor at the University of Texas Medical School at Houston, said, "Unlike the changeable regions of its envelope, HIV needs at least one region that must remain constant to attach to cells. If this region changes, HIV cannot infect cells. HIV would lose if this constant region provoked the body's defense system. For now, B cells are fooled into making abundant antibodies to the changeable regions of HIV but not to its constant region cellular attachment site." **Immunologists call such regions superantigens.** HIV's antibody evasive action is unmatched. No other known virus evades the body's defenses in this manner.

How Do Scientists Attack HIV's Constant Region?

To attack HIV's constant region, Paul's group has engineered antibodies with enzymatic activity, also known as **abzymes,** which can attack the constant region of the HIV in a precise way. Paul said, "The abzymes recognize essentially all of the diverse HIV forms found across the world. This solves the problem of HIV changeability. The next step is to confirm this theory in human clinical trials. Unlike regular antibodies, abzymes will inactivate HIV permanently. A single abzyme molecule can inactivate thousands of virus particles while regular antibodies inactivate only one virus particle. The abzymes, instead of passively binding to the target molecule, are able to fragment it and destroy its function. This work indicates that naturally occurring catalytic antibodies, particularly those of the Immunoglobin A (IgA) subtype, may be useful in the treatment and prevention of HIV infection."

Where Did the Abzymes Come From?

The abzymes are derived from HIV-negative people with the autoimmune disease lupus and a small number of HIV-positive people who do not require treatment and do not progress to AIDS. Immunological events in lupus patients can generate abzymes to the constant region of HIV. A minority of HIV-positive people also start producing the abzymes after decades of the infection. Paul said, "This is an entirely new finding. It is a novel antibody that appears to be very effective in killing HIV. The main question now is if this can be applied to developing a vaccine and possibly used as a microbicide to prevent sexual transmission" (Planque et al., 2008).

information on T4 cell replacement and HIV production).

The rapid production of HIV mutants without the same rapid production of a neutralizing or cancelling antibody against each mutant means that sometime after infection, much if not most of the antibody in some people may be nothing more than useless antibody copy (antibody to the initial strain or strains of HIV). In these people, HIV disease would most likely progress more swiftly than in persons whose immune system can keep up with the production of somewhat useful antibody to match the formation of HIV mutants. This may be one important reason why some people progress to AIDS and death so rapidly when compared to other HIV-infected people.

Immune Activation: A Clue to AIDS Progression?

Recently, researchers have suggested that a natural process called **immune activation** may determine why infection with HIV progresses differently in different people.

Immune activation occurs whenever immune system cells detect foreign invaders and send out chemical signals to draw other cells into the fight. It occurs at the beginning of any infection and, in the case of HIV, seems to remain engaged throughout. Researchers speculate that HIV turns this normally beneficial response into a cellular malfunction.

Since the early days of HIV/AIDS, scientists have realized that a higher-than-normal proportion of immune cells become and stay activated in a person with HIV than in someone responding to another infection. Ironically, activation makes immune cells more vulnerable to the infection. That's because, when activated, immune cells begin allowing HIV to hijack their cellular machinery in order to copy its viral genes.

Infection-Enhancing Antibodies

Ramu Subbramanian and colleagues at the University of Montreal (2002) reported that infection-enhancing antibodies (IEAs) make up most of the antibody humoral response to HIV infection. Their results show that the anti-HIV humoral immune response consists of a mixture of antibodies that may inhibit or enhance HIV infection and whose ratios may vary in different stages of the infection. Seventy percent of blood serums from HIV-infected persons contained IEAs. Such antibodies enhance HIV's ability to infect cells!

HIV Protected from Human Antibodies

Humans create antibodies against a number of HIV proteins, namely the envelope proteins (gp120), the transmembrane protein (gp41), and the proteins of HIV's core (gp24). But, *antibodies cannot enter cells*. The antibody can only attack HIV in the plasma. Plasma is the fluid part of the blood and does not include the blood cells. Once inside a host cell, *HIV is protected from antibodies.* Such cells, monocytes, and macrophage and dendritic cells carry HIV internally. All these cell types serve as **HIV reservoirs** in the body. In addition, these cells travel to all distant points within the body and deliver HIV. The self antiretroviral chemicals that these cells generate appear to be ineffective against their hidden traveling companion, HIV (Moir et al., 2000; Olinger et al., 2000).

HIV ERADICATION CURRENTLY NOT POSSIBLE BECAUSE OF INFECTION OF LATENT RESTING CD4+ CELLS AND IMMUNOLOGIC MEMORY CELLS

HIV latency or dormancy is a consequence of the normal physiology of CD4+ T lymphocytes. At any given time, most CD4+ T lymphocytes are in a resting state. Resting lymphocytes are profoundly quiescent or quiet cells with a low metabolic rate and a unique morphology characterized by a small cytoplasmic volume. In adults, about half of the resting cells are **naïve,** meaning they have yet to encounter an appropriate antigen. The remaining cells are memory cells that have previously responded to an antigen. Antigen-driven responses involve a burst of cellular division and differentiation, giving rise to **memory cells.** These cells have an altered pattern of gene expression enabling long-term survival and rapid responses to the same antigen, should they meet again in the future. With regard to HIV, the virus infects immunologic memory cells, creating a reservoir of HIV within the body. That is, within these memory cells HIV gene expression is largely or completely silenced. In the absence of HIV gene expression, latent cells differ from their uninfected memory cells only by the presence of HIV DNA integrated into the memory cells' DNA. It is difficult to envision any targeting mechanism that will allow specific elimination of this reservoir of HIV-infected dormant or silent memory cells because they cannot be distinguished from the uninfected memory cells.

HIV Reservoirs

Perhaps the most disturbing discovery concerning HIV reservoirs in 2001 is the work of Robert Siliciano at Johns Hopkins University. This discovery is disturbing because little is known about memory cells' life span and whether they can be eradicated. Memory cells are programmed to sit and wait for viruses to attack; their job is to keep a record of the germs that the body has previously encountered so that the immune system will be ready the next time it is confronted with those antigens. What HIV has done is tap into the most fundamental aspect of the immune system—a person's immunological memory. It's the perfect mechanism for the virus to ensure its survival. Because the cells are the immune system's memory, they must survive for a long time, creating a latent or dormantly infected reservoir of HIV in the body. This reservoir is the single biggest obstacle to getting rid of HIV. In 2010, Kathleen Collins and colleagues reported that HIV, after infection, remains dormant in long-living bone marrow cells, a reservoir of infection very resistant to ART (HAART) and the body's immune responses. When these progenitor cells, ancestors to our blood cells, begin converting into red blood cells, HIV can reactivate and continue to multiply and move out to infect other cells. In brief, three major HIV reservoirs are now known: memory cells, macrophage, and bone marrow cells. Anthony Fauci, director of the National Institute of Allergy and Infectious Diseases, said, "We are not going to be eliminating these reservoirs. Whether you can measure it or not doesn't seem to have a significant impact on the clinically relevant phenomenon of what happens when you stop taking the drug."

Once HIV gets inside these cell reservoirs as a **provirus,** it is likely to remain there for the rest of the cell's life (person's life) unless some other antiviral mechanism within the body or some chemical agent is able to destroy the provirus. To date, no such drug has been found to be effective against the HIV provirus.

Deleting HIV (Provirus) from Cellular Reservoirs

In 2008, Pauline Chugh and colleagues (2008) reported on the steps HIV takes to hide out in macrophage cells (one of two major cell types that act as HIV reservoirs; the other is the memory T cells). The research team found that HIV produces a protein that turns on a particular cell survival pathway. After a multistep process, it activates an enzyme called **Akt** that in turn prevents cell suicide. They placed macrophage in laboratory dishes and added drugs known to block the **Akt** pathway. The drug miltefosine blocked the formation of the **Akt** protein, and those treated cells died. This drug is already known to be safe to humans as it is used to treat Leishmaniasis patients (an intestinal disease of humans and other animals caused by the protozoan Leishmania). The real problem is how many macrophages are infected. If too many are infected, how will their loss affect the body's immune system? Miltefosine may be a first and very meaningful step in eliminating one of the two main HIV reservoirs in the body.

In September 2009, Robert Siliciano and colleagues reported on their screening of 2400 chemicals, 17 of which stimulated HIV to replicate in HIV-infected latent cells. The best of the 17 chemicals, one they called "5HN" is found in the leaves, bark, and roots of the black walnut tree. Their research also revealed the presence of at least one additional, unidentified latent reservoir in the body. It should be mentioned that there is no test to determine if a person is a carrier of latent HIV-infected cells. The best means, at the moment, to determine if one has such cells, is to drug treat to undetectable levels of HIV and then stop therapy and see if HIV levels rebound (increase).

IMMUNE SYSTEM DYSFUNCTION

When HIV first arrives in the body, there are no immune memory T cells that know how to deal with it. The body has never experienced HIV. As with any other first exposure to an infection, it is the job of **naïve** or **unexposed T cells** to respond (Figure 5-6, page 120). Returning to the scene in the lymph nodes, naïve T4 or CD4+ cells get recruited to fight HIV and in turn they become infected. As these infected T cells begin to divide, HIV is able to replicate and release new viruses from each infected cell. Viral load counts in the blood will usually rise rapidly during this period, which is called **primary** or **acute infection.** During the acute phase HIV also creates latent HIV reservoirs in lymphoid tissue. During this period, a small fraction of the T cells that are activated to fight HIV revert

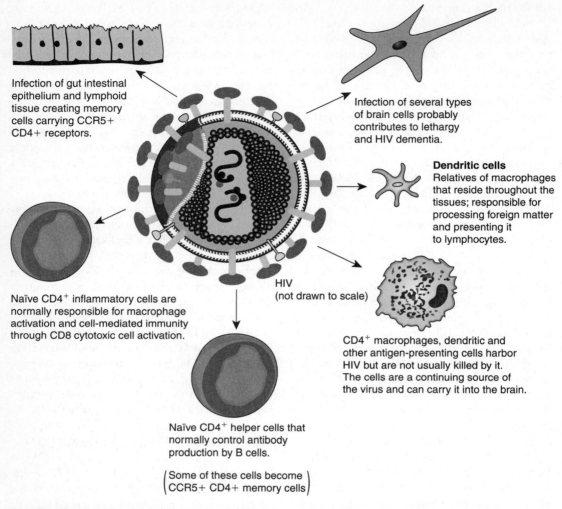

Infection of gut intestinal epithelium and lymphoid tissue creating memory cells carrying CCR5+ CD4+ receptors.

Infection of several types of brain cells probably contributes to lethargy and HIV dementia.

Dendritic cells
Relatives of macrophages that reside throughout the tissues; responsible for processing foreign matter and presenting it to lymphocytes.

Naïve CD4$^+$ inflammatory cells are normally responsible for macrophage activation and cell-mediated immunity through CD8 cytotoxic cell activation.

HIV (not drawn to scale)

CD4$^+$ macrophages, dendritic and other antigen-presenting cells harbor HIV but are not usually killed by it. The cells are a continuing source of the virus and can carry it into the brain.

Naïve CD4$^+$ helper cells that normally control antibody production by B cells.

(Some of these cells become CCR5+ CD4+ memory cells)

FIGURE 5-6 HIV's Favorite Cellular Targets. On entering the body, HIV attaches to those naïve T lymphocyte cells carrying CD4+ CCR5+ receptors. Certain of the infected T cells revert back to a resting stage, becoming memory cells infected with HIV or silent reservoirs of HIV in the body. *(Adapted from Eugene Nester, Microbiology, McGraw-Hill Publishing Company.)*

back to a resting, or memory, state. As the cells rest or become dormant, so do the viruses they harbor. In effect, HIV causes two infections: an active infection that spreads via infected T4 cells to other parts of the body, including the brain, and a dormant, or latent infection that persists in lymphoid tissue to become HIV cell reservoirs.

If this process is allowed to continue unchecked, the large pool of naïve T cells becomes slowly drained. To understand why, think of the lake metaphor. The water flows out of the lake at a rate greater than the amount of water coming in, so if the siphoning isn't stopped, the lake eventually empties. Studies have shown that the naïve T cell pool does indeed dwindle in HIV infection. In fact, a recent study shows that the loss of newly produced naïve T4 cells is strongly linked to disease progression.

ORIGINAL ANTIGENIC SIN

Although there are many facets to immune system dysfunction that investigators have yet to understand, there is one phenomenon that may help us to understand why some diseases leave people with immunity against future attacks while other diseases, like dengue (ding-ee) fever, make people sicker the second time around. Or why some HIV-infected people fare better immunologically and live longer without antiretroviral drugs than others. The explanation for this phenomenon may have to do with **"original antigenic sin"** (OAS). OAS is defined or recognized by the manner in which the immune system responds to vaccination against a disease. In OAS, vaccination creates memory cell DNA sequences that *increase* susceptibility to future exposure to the same disease. For example, if the vaccine were to use "virus A" (HIV), the immune system would learn to recognize it and attack. Later, if a very similar but not identical form of the type A virus (or mutant HIV) were to show up, the body would mobilize against the original type A (HIV) and produce immune cells that might not be fully effective against the new invader, a changed or mutant type A or HIV. In second infections, the immune system does not make new antibodies that exactly fit the antigen but instead looks in its memory cells to see if any antibody messages already exist to do the job. Because the memory cells already know something about the attacking virus, in effect they are halfway round the track when the gun goes off. So the immune system goes on the attack (makes antibodies) directed at the "original" cause of the disease, type A virus or HIV. This is "Original Antigenic Sin." The advantage is that a response can be quickly mobilized. The disadvantage is that the response is shaped by previous antigen, and it may not be the best fit to the current form of that antigen (the sin). This idea was originally developed in studies of influenza, which is caused by a virus that changes or mutates so often that new vaccines have to be developed annually. OAS would mean that no new batch of flu vaccine will be 100% effective. How effective the vaccine will be depends on the effects of the OAS—how close the antibodies, now produced, fit the new mutant flu virus or how structurally close these antibodies are to the originally formed antibodies. The more similar the antibodies, the less effective they will be against new mutant flu viruses or perhaps HIV.

For clarification, if a person's white blood cells or B cells are making four antibodies against four antigen sites that worked against one variety of the flu virus, and he or she contracts another variety of the flu virus that shares only two of those antigenic sites, then his or her immune system will be predisposed to make antibodies against only the two sites the different flu viruses have in common. That is, the immune system mounts an attack *directed at the original form of the virus.* Moreover, the immune system will never learn to recognize the two new antigenic sites that are present on the new flu strain, choosing instead to go with what worked in a prior case of infection. Over time, as the flu virus continues to mutate and has progressively less in common with the original "remembered" antigenic sites, the immune system becomes less prepared to recognize newer flu strains. In effect, the immune system forgoes whole classes of random combinations that might actually work against the new mutant flu virus in favor of tried-and-true varieties, carried in the memory bank, that will not.

How Invading HIV Gets to the T4 or CD4+ Cell: Dendritic Cells Just Doing Their Job!

Based on the recent investigations of American and Dutch scientists, it appears that HIV hijacks immune cells to enter the body's immune system.

Dendritic cells are the watchdogs of the immune system. They are located just below the skin surface and under moist mucosal tissue on surfaces like those of the mouth, gut, genital, and urinary tracts. When dendritic cells see a foreign invader such as a microorganism or virus, they capture it, shred it, and display pieces of proteins from the invading pathogen on their surfaces.

These displayed proteins serve to alert other immune system cells such as T4 cells that the body is under attack. What recent investigations now show is that HIV attaches to dendritic cells and hitches a ride into the lymphoid tissues where it then infects T4 cells. The dendritic cell has finger-like projections that carry a protein receptor called **DC-SIGN** (dendritic cell-specific protein). HIV adheres to DC-SIGN and is carried from the mucosal lining of the cervix or rectum to the lymph nodes where it transfers HIV to the T4 cells through their coreceptors CXCR4 (R-4) and CCR5 (R-5) (Steinman, 2000; Geijtenbeek et al., 2000). Thus, another puzzle piece is in place toward the complete understanding of how HIV successfully attacks the human immune system.

Dendritic Trojan Horses

According to Melissa Pope (2002), as capable as dendritic cells are of kicking off a multipronged immune response to any invading pathogen that crosses their paths, something goes wrong when they are confronted with HIV. Herein lies the paradox. The very cells that should be activating the immune system against this pathogen end up facilitating the virus infection. It is now known that some dendritic cells can actually become infected with HIV and replicate the virus. It also appears that the R-5 receptor on immature dendritic cells permits infection and replication to occur.

Understanding the Mechanism of HIV Entry and Tropism

To understand CD4+ cell entry inhibitors, presented in Chapter 4, pages 79 and 81, some basic knowledge of the mechanism of viral entry is necessary. HIV needs to make at least two attachments to the CD4+ cell before it finds itself within the cell. First, the virus must bind to the CD4 component on the CD4+ cell surface—specifically, to one of the envelope proteins of the virus, gp120. This gp120 to CD4+ binding induces a conformational change, or a change in the shape of the outer portion of the cell, which then allows for the next step, the HIV coreceptor binding. In this step, the virus uses one of two additional receptors on the CD4 cell, the CCR5 (R-5) and/or CXCR4 (R-4) receptors (coreceptors).

Tropism

Tropism means "an innate turning." In the case of HIV, it is the virus's preference for using one coreceptor versus another that is referred to as viral tropism. The HIV strain in most individuals uses the CCR5 coreceptor (and is called a CCR5 or R-5 tropic virus). Some HIV use the CXCR4 or R-4 receptor. Some individuals harbor HIV that uses both types of coreceptors (dual/mixed). Receptor binding eventually allows for the fusion of HIV to the CD4+ cell to take place with subsequent HIV penetration into the cell. The fusion step is the site of activity for the drugs Fuzeon and Maraviroc. Inside the cell, other drug-targeted sites block HIV replication. (See Table 4–1, pages 75–76, and supportive information within Chapter 4.)

How HIV Enters T4 or CD4+ Cells and Macrophages

HIV researchers have known since 1984 that human CD4 cell membrane receptors alone (or chemokine coreceptors) are sufficient for binding HIV to the T4 lymphocyte membrane, but CD4 receptors are not sufficient for HIV envelope fusion with the T4 cell membrane or for HIV penetration or entry into the cell's interior. This knowledge has enticed many groups of AIDS researchers to search for additional receptors, coreceptors to CD4, that HIV uses to enter a cell after binding to it.

THE SEARCH FOR ADDITIONAL RECEPTORS (CORECEPTORS) TO CD4: FUSIN OR CXCKR-4 (R-4)

In May 1996, Ed Berger (Figure 5-7, page 123) and colleagues reported finding a receptor that allowed syncytium-inducing (SI) strains of HIV (HIV that causes T4 cells to form clusters—they attach to each other) to enter T4 cells. Strains of

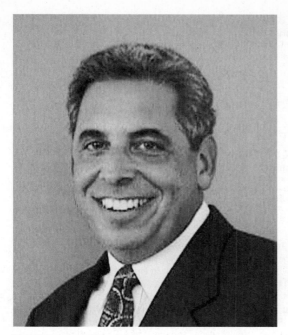

FIGURE 5-7 Edward A. Berger, Chief of the Molecular Structure Section, Laboratory of Viral Diseases at the National Institute of Allergy and Infectious Diseases. In spring 1996 he and colleagues discovered the first coreceptor, **R-4** or **FUSIN**, that HIV needs to complete its attachment and entry into T4 lymphocytes. In 2007 he received the Bernard Fields Memorial Lecture Award. *(Photograph courtesy of National Institutes of Health.)*

HIV that do not induce T4 cell syncytium formation (NSI) could not enter T4 cells. Berger and colleagues named this T4 cell receptor **FUSIN**. In August 1996 Conrad Bleul and colleagues identified a chemokine, **CXC stromal cell-derived factor-1 (SDF-1)** that binds to the FUSIN receptor and blocks HIV entry. They named this chemokine **R-4.** This coreceptor functions preferentially for T cell line-tropic HIV strains.

CCKR-5 (R-5) RECEPTOR

Within two months after the FUSIN receptor data were reported an additional coreceptor called CCKR-5 (R-5) was found. This coreceptor

functions mainly in macrophage cells. Members of the research teams who have contributed to the discovery of the R-5 receptor believe that macrophage-tropic or M-tropic (or non-syncytium inducing [NSI]) HIV strains occur in greatest number early on after HIV infection and then, sometime later during HIV disease, the predominant HIV strain shifts to HIV strains that use the FUSIN receptor (R-4) on T4 cells. HIV, by shifting receptors, may be avoiding the suppressive activity of the chemokines that block the R-5 receptor. Figure 5-8, page 124 shows a diagram of this suggested **receptor swap** that occurs sometime during HIV disease progression. One of the great unsolved puzzles of HIV disease is *why,* during disease progression, does HIV lose its ability to infect macrophage and become T cell tropic? *Why* does HIV switch to other cell receptors?

Figure 5-9, page 125 represents the use of R-5 and/or R-4 as necessary HIV attachment sites in conjunction with CD4 to enter a T lymphocyte or macrophage. HIV coreceptor switching R-5 to R-4 occurs in about half of those in treatment.

EMERGENCE OF HIV STRAINS THAT VARY IN THEIR LETHAL ABILITIES

During the course of HIV disease, viral strains emerge in an infected person that differ widely in their ability to infect and kill different cell types, as well as in their rate of replication. Scientists are investigating why strains of HIV from people with advanced disease appear to be more virulent and infect more cell types than strains obtained earlier from the same person. Part of the explanation may be the expanded ability of the virus to use other coreceptors, such as R-4.

HIV is truly the Houdini virus of all viruses to date. This virus has the ability to change in response to the human immune system. And not in any predictable pattern. HIV mutates into new forms and escapes—like Houdini, but from the immune system.

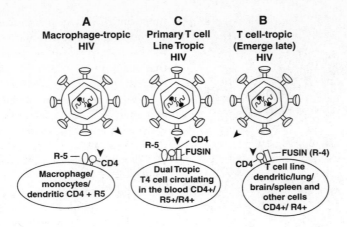

A
Macrophage-tropic HIV

C
Primary T cell Line Tropic HIV

B
T cell-tropic (Emerge late) HIV

R-5 — CD4
Macrophage/ monocytes/ dendritic CD4 + R5

R-5   CD4
FUSIN
Dual Tropic T4 cell circulating in the blood CD4+/ R5+/R4+

FUSIN (R-4)
CD4   T cell line dendritic/lung/ brain/spleen and other cells CD4+/ R4+

FIGURE 5–8 Viral Tropism: Coreceptors Required for HIV to Enter Human Cells. HIV can be broadly divided into two classes: those more suitable (tropic) to infecting macrophage, a major reservoir of HIV, and those that infect T4 cells in the lymph nodes or other tissues. HIV usually uses one of two coreceptors, R-5 or R-4, to enter the CD4+ lymphocyte. (A) Macrophage-tropic HIV isolates infect macrophages but fail to infect HIV T cell lines, (B) while T4 HIV strains fail to infect macrophage. But HIV of both classes efficiently infect T4 cells (C) isolated from peripheral blood mononuclear cells (PBMC). Macrophage-tropic HIV appear to be preferentially transmitted by sexual contact and constitute the vast majority of HIV present in newly infected individuals (Zhu, 1993). The T-tropic viruses generally appear late in the course of infection during the so-called "phenotypic switch" that often precedes the onset of AIDS symptoms (Conner et al., 1994). The molecular basis of HIV-1 tropism appears to lie in the ability of envelopes of macrophage-tropic and T-tropic viruses to interact with different coreceptors located on macrophage or T4 cells. Macrophage-tropic viruses primarily use R-5 (80%), R-4 (20%), and less often R-3 and R-2, newly described chemokine receptors, while T-tropic HIV tend to use FUSIN (R-4) (Hill et al., 1996; Moore, 1997; McNicholl et al., 2008).

IN SEARCH OF GENETIC RESISTANCE TO HIV INFECTION

At this point in the HIV/AIDS pandemic it is believed that about 95% of HIV-exposed people are susceptible to HIV infection and HIV disease progression. This statement is made because it has long been known that some persons who have deliberately avoided safer sex practice and who have had unprotected sex with HIV-infected persons failed to become HIV-infected! The question that has continued to puzzle HIV investigators is, how can multiple HIV-exposed persons remain uninfected? Pieces of that puzzle began to fall into place when two gay males came forward who, despite repeated unprotected sex with companions who died from the disease, remained HIV negative. Neither quite understood why he was spared, but they pressed scientists to come up with the answer. HIV investigators Rong Liu and coworkers (1996) and Michel Samson and

coworkers (1996) reported that repeated HIV-exposed but uninfected people have a 32-nucleotide deletion in the gene that produces the R-5 receptors on macrophage. The protein produced by this gene is severely damaged and does *not* reach the cell surface to act as an R-5 chemokine receptor. Without R-5 receptors, the envelope of HIV cannot fuse with the envelope of macrophage to gain entrance into the cell. Thus, most people who carry both defective R-5 genes, **homozygotes** (they received one defective gene from each parent) are resistant to HIV infection. This resistance is not absolute because some people carrying the 32-nucleotide deletion have become infected! If one is **heterozygous** (that is, one carries one defective gene and one normal gene), one will produce the R-5 receptor that HIV needs to penetrate macrophage, but they are fewer in number. Thus, there are fewer R-5 receptors, so there are fewer R-5 receptors available for HIV attachment. As a result, heterozygous

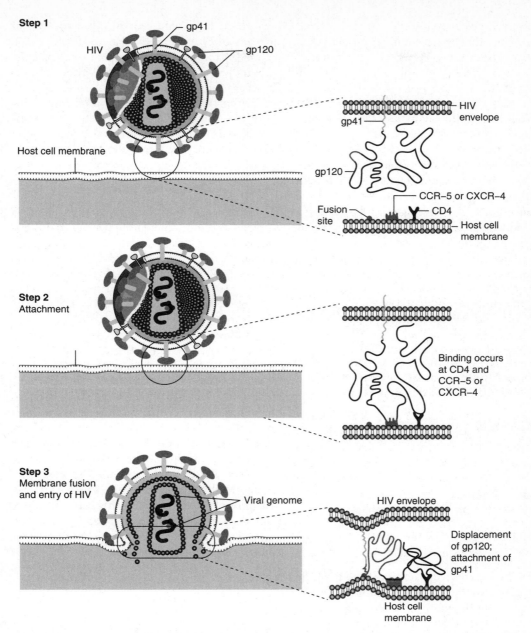

FIGURE 5-9   Attachment and Entry of HIV into a Host Cell, Schematic Representation of CD4 Receptor Binding Step 1: Virion in close proximity to the cell membrane; blow-up showing gp120 protein and sites of reaction with host cell receptors. **Step 2:** Initial contact of gp120 is with CD4. Attachment to a chemokine receptor such as R-5 or R-4 must occur before membrane fusion and entry of the viral genome can take place. **Step 3:** Membrane fusion probably is mediated by gp41.

* In their publication on how HIV enters a cell, Kosuke Miyauchi and colleagues (2009) report that HIV can also enter cells through the process of endocytosis after HIV anchors itself to the host cell receptors. The cell's membrane engulfs HIV, forming a vesicle around HIV which then releases its contents into the cell's cytoplasm. This finding may suggest new therapeutic avenues for targeting HIV.

people are *less* resistant to HIV infection than the homozygous mutant (receptorless) people, but are *more* resistant than people who have two normal genes (homozygous normal) who are the most susceptible to HIV infection (O'Brien, 1998).

Michael Marmor and colleagues (2001) reported that white gay males who are heterogeneous were 70% less likely to become HIV-infected than those without the mutation. Survival analysis also shows that disease progression is slower in R-5 deletion heterozygotes than in individuals with the normal R-5 gene. Jesper Eugene-Olsen and colleagues (1997) reported that individuals who are heterozygous for the 32-base-pair deletion in the R-5 gene have a slower decrease in their T4 cell count and longer AIDS-free survival than individuals with the wild-type gene for up to 11 years of follow-up.

Sean Philpott and colleagues reported in 1999 that children who inherit the R-5 mutation are protected from vertical HIV infection (mother to newborn via breast milk).

Will the Mutant R-5 Gene Protect People from All Subtypes of HIV?

This genetic defect, the 32-nucleotide deletion, prevents infection only with the strain of HIV (Subtype B) that is transmitted sexually and is prevalent in the United States and Europe. It does not necessarily protect against other strains of HIV transmitted through intravenous drug use or blood transfusions, or strains prevalent in Africa.

Should Everyone Be Tested for the Presence of the R-5 Gene?

Researchers agree that getting tested for the gene would not be difficult, but it would not be of great value because the tested person could still be infected by other strains of HIV. It must be assumed that most people do not carry a pair of defective R-5 genes because 95% or more of HIV-exposed people become HIV-infected.

Who Carries the Defective R-5 Gene?

Perhaps most surprising, HIV investigators found that the homozygous genetic defect is common: **It is present in about 10% of whites of Northern European descent.** But it appears to be absent in people from Japan and Central Africa; about 20% of whites are heterozygous for this gene.

Recent studies conducted at Stellenbosch University show that the R-5 gene deletion is virtually absent in the South African black population. Most likely there are other genes involved in the complexity of susceptibility to infection.

Why Does This Gene Exist?

Scientists speculate that the mutant form of R-5 protected against some disease that afflicted Europeans but not Africans. The obvious candidates would be the Black Death of 1346, the plague, and/or smallpox. Both lethal diseases are at least 700 years old, enough time for genetic selection to take place. Those without the mutant R-5 gene died, the survivors reproduced, and the gene became dispersed within the surviving population. Stephen O'Brien said that the chance of this gene *randomly* reaching its current frequency in the white population is about zero. Raymond Weinstein (2011) states that the CCR5 (R5) mutation first appeared in Northern Europe about 3500 years ago in a single person. This mutation provided resistance to smallpox. This same mutation confers resistance to HIV. Therefore, it is speculated that the explosive spread of HIV may be related to the eradication of smallpox. Thus, the presence of variola, the virus that causes smallpox and its vaccine, may have inhibited the spread of HIV. The idea that a mutant gene can confer protection against a specific infection is not new. The mutation that causes sickle cell anemia provides people carrying one copy of it with resistance (but not immunity) to malaria. There is some evidence that the cystic fibrosis mutation may protect against typhoid fever.

These ideas for why the R-5 gene exists remind us that we carry a genetic record of the diseases of the past and that, at least for some, those genes have once again come to the rescue. In contrast to mutant forms of genes being beneficial is the report by He Weijing and colleagues (2008) that the mutant form of the

Duffy Antigen Receptor for chemokines, which helps protect people living in sub-Saharan Africa from malaria common to the region, could make them more susceptible to HIV infection. The researchers estimated that this gene mutation could account for about 11 percent or 2.7 million HIV infections in Sub-Saharan Africa. This study does have its skeptics who say that the prevalence of HIV infection among those who carry the mutation versus those who do not is barely statistically significant.

T4 CELL DEPLETION AND IMMUNE SUPPRESSION

Means by Which T4 Cells May Be Lost

1. *Filling CD4 Receptor Sites*—There is evidence from in vitro studies that HIV can attack CD4 receptor sites in at least two ways. First, HIV can attach, via its gp160 "spikes," to CD4 receptor sites. Second, HIV is capable of releasing or freeing its exterior gp120 envelope glycoprotein, thereby generating a molecule that can actively bind to CD4–bearing cells (Gelderblom et al., 1985). As a result of filling the receptor sites on the T4 cells, the T4 cells lose their immune functions; that is, the T4 cell does not have to be infected with HIV to lose immune function.

2. *Syncytia Formation*—The formation of syncytia involves fusion of the cell membrane of an infected cell with the cell membranes of uninfected CD4 cells, which results in giant multinucleated cells.

3. *Apoptosis*—Programmed cell death, or **apoptosis** (a-po-toe-sis), is a normal mechanism of cell death that was originally described in the context of the response of immature thymocytes to cellular activation.

In a typical day, 60 billion to 70 billion cells die. Much of this normal cellular turnover involves apoptosis. When apoptotic pathways are defective, insufficient cell death can lead to cancers and autoimmune diseases, and excessive cell death can result in neurodegeneration or stroke.

4. *Cofactors May Help Deplete T4 Cells*—HIV-infected people who are asymptomatic show a wide variation in HIV disease time and progression to AIDS. It is believed that cofactors may be responsible for some of the time variation with regard to disease progression.

Many agents may act as cofactors to activate or increase HIV production. Although, in general, it is not believed that any cofactor is necessary for HIV infection, cofactors such as nutrition, stress, and infectious organisms have been considered as agents that might accelerate HIV expression after infection. Three new human herpes viruses (HHV-6, 7, and 8) may be cofactors and play a role in causing immune deficiency. They have been shown to infect HIV-infected T4 cells and activate the HIV provirus to increase HIV replication. Cytomegalovirus, Epstein-Barr virus, hepatitis B and C viruses, and tuberculosis have also been associated with increased HIV expression. Over time, investigators expect to find other sexually transmitted diseases that behave as cofactors associated with HIV infection and expression.

Drugs may also be cofactors in infection. Used by injection–drug users (IDUs), heroin and other morphine-based derivatives are known to reduce human resistance to infection and produce immunological suppression.

Blood and blood products may also act as cofactors in infection because they are immunosuppressive. Because blood transfusions save lives, their long-range effects are generally overlooked. Transfusions in hemophiliacs, for example, result in lowered resistance to viruses such as cytomegalovirus (CMV), Epstein-Barr, and perhaps HIV.

IMPACT OF T4 CELL DEPLETION

The overall impact of T4 cell depletion is multifaceted. HIV-induced T4 cell abnormalities alter the T4 cells' ability to produce a variety of inducer chemical stimulants such as the **interleukins** that are necessary for the proper maturation of B cells into plasma cells and the maturation of a subset of T cells into cytotoxic cells (Figure 5-10). Thus the critical basis for the

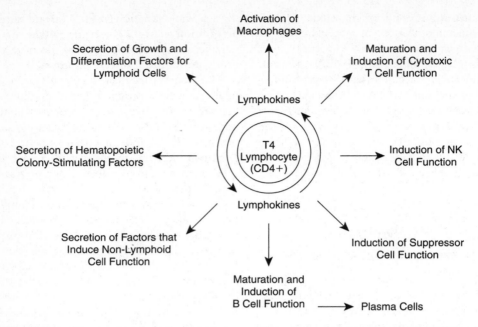

FIGURE 5-10 The T4 or CD4+ Cell Role in the Immune Response. T4 lymphocytes are responsible directly or indirectly for inducing a wide array of functions in cells that produce the immune response. *(Adapted from Fauci, 1995.)*

immunopathogenesis of HIV infection is the depletion of the **T4 lymphocytes,** which results in profound immunosuppression.

Presumably, with time, the number of HIV-infected T4 cells decreases to a point where, in terminal AIDS patients, *few normal T4 cells exist.*

ROLE OF MONOCYTES AND MACROPHAGES IN HIV INFECTION

Some scientists now believe that T4 cell infection alone does not cause AIDS. They believe that equally important to T4 cell infection are **dendritic, monocyte,** and **macrophage** infection (Bakker et al., 1992). Monocytes change into various types of macrophages (given different names) in order to search and destroy foreign agents within tissues of the lungs, brain, and interstitial tissues, tissues that connect organs. Despite the name changes, all forms of macrophages basically work the same way: They ingest things. Some macrophages travel around

within the body; others become attached to one spot, ingesting.

Macrophages, like dendritic cells, are often the first cells of the immune system to encounter invaders, particularly in the area of a cut or wound. After engulfing the invader, the macrophage makes copies of the invader's antigens and displays them on its own cell membrane. These copies of the invader antigens sit next to the self molecules. In effect, the macrophage makes a "wanted poster" of this new invader. The macrophage then travels about showing the wanted poster to T4 or CD4+ cells, which triggers the T4 cells into action. Macrophages also release chemicals that stimulate both T4 cell and macrophage production and draw macrophages and lymphocytes to the site of infection.

Macrophage: Trojan Horses

Macrophages may play an important role in spreading HIV infection in the body, both to other cells and to HIV's target organs. First, HIV enters a macrophage and spreads from macrophage to macrophage before the immune system is alerted. Second, macrophages, in their different forms, travel to the brain, the lungs, the bone marrow, and to various immune organs, carrying HIV to these organs.

HIV's ability to infect brain tissue is particularly important. The brain and cerebrospinal fluid (CSF) are specially protected sites. CSF cushions the brain and the spinal cord from sudden and jarring movements. The blood-brain barrier, a chemical phenomenon, normally stops foreign substances from entering the brain and the CSF. But HIV-infected monocytes can pass through this barrier. For HIV, monocyte-macrophages are Trojan horses, enabling HIV to enter the immune-protected domain of the central nervous system—the brain, the spine, and the rest of the nervous system.

HIV-infected macrophages have proven to be a major problem in efforts to control and stop HIV infection. Some become reservoir cells protecting HIV from immune destruction.

The investigators suggest that in order to eradicate HIV, a way must be found to target and eliminate HIV-infected macrophage.

WHERE DO T4 OR CD4+ CELLS BECOME HIV INFECTED?

The Human Gut-Associated Lymphatic Tissue (GALT)—Gut-associated lymphoid tissue is the largest component of the human lymphoid system and contains the highest number of CD4+ T cells. Persistent depletion of CD4+ T cells in the gut is due to ongoing HIV replication even though ART achieves undetectable plasma viral loads.

Despite 29 years (1983–2012) of research on HIV, debates continue about the path from infection to immunological mayhem and failure. There is abundant evidence that HIV preferentially infects and decimates T4 or CD4+ lymphocytes, and some researchers have long argued that direct killing alone causes the profound CD4+ loss that is the hallmark of AIDS. That prompted David Ho

to once wear a button saying, "It's the virus, stupid." Another camp contends that HIV infects a relatively small number of CD4+ cells and indirectly causes the massive death of uninfected CD4+ cells by activating them, a process that leads to their premature death.

The studies of Daniel Douek and colleagues (2004–2005) indicated there was both a direct and indirect killing of CD4+ cells beginning with the primary infection of CD4+ cells in **gut-associated lymphatic tissue (GALT).** Douek and colleagues present fascinating and galvanizing evidence on how HIV blazes through CD4+ cells starting in the lymphatic tissue of the gut (Figure 5-11), then moving into lymph nodes and the blood. Regardless of how HIV enters the body at infection, HIV attaches to CD4+ cells that have surface receptors known as CCR5 (R-5). The vast majority of CD4+/R-5+ cells reside in the gut. The investigators provide a startling photograph taken during colonoscopies. Whereas the uninfected person's ileum had mounds of lymphoid tissue that contained CD4+/R-5+ (Figure 5-11a), the landscape of the ileum of a person recently infected by HIV was scraped clean (Figure 5-11b). The investigators noted, "You have absolutely no GALT at all—it's completely wiped out." This is absolute evidence that direct killing caused this loss. These investigators provide compelling evidence for a rapid and profound depletion of R-5+ and CD4+ cells in the GALT of patients in the first several weeks of HIV infection. GALT is the major reservoir for activated CD4+ cells in the body. Thus, about 50% of the body's memory CD4+ cells are lost within about two weeks after infection by the direct effects of HIV. Interestingly, while there is a significant increase in peripheral blood CD4 cell counts after six months on antiretroviral therapy, there is no increase in GALT CD4 cell counts. Thus CD4 depletion in GALT may not be reversible. This may explain treatment failure in some patients. As the disease progresses to a chronic infection, indirect killing—which takes place, to a large degree, in the lymph nodes—creates additional CD4+ cell loss. The investigators propose that

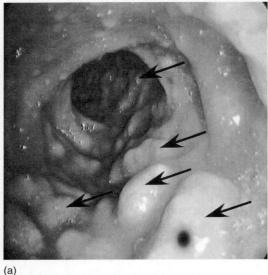 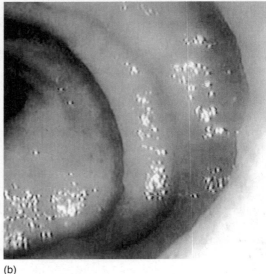

(a)   (b)

FIGURE 5-11   Gastrointestinal Tract Endoscopy: Before and After. (a) The interior lining of the gut of an uninfected person showing numerous lymph node patches. (b) The gut lining stripped of lymph node patches in an HIV-infected person. *(Photographs from Brenchley et al.,* Journal of Experimental Medicine, 2004, Vol. 200, pp. 749–759. *Copyright © The Rockefeller University Press. Reprinted by permission.)*

when HIV destroys GALT immunity, other pathogens flourish, which in turn overactivates the lymph production of CD4+ cells, many of which will soon die even though they are uninfected. "Just as the inflammation caused by hepatitis destroys the liver, chronic inflammation of the lymph nodes or immunitis destroys their architecture, leading to massive buildup of collagen, causing fibrosis."

The investigators showed that the greater the amount of collagen in lymph nodes, the less able infected people were to respond to antiretroviral drugs. This may mean that the differences in individual collagen levels may determine their response to drug therapy. The most important ramifications of this improved understanding of how HIV causes disease could be in vaccine research. A vaccine that triggers immune responses in the GALT may best prevent the initial HIV infection.

A separate study on GALT, by Moraima Guadalupe and colleagues (2006) and Liliana Belmonte and colleagues (2007), showed that even when blood tests show that viral load is undetectable and CD4+ or T4 cell counts are responding well to HIV treatment, there is likely ongoing viral replication and immune system damage occurring in the gut. In other words, HIV replication in the gut is not influenced by HIV drugs. These investigators explained that GALT accounts for 70% of the body's immune system, and restoring GALT function is crucial to ridding the body of HIV. They concluded that blood measurements of viral load and CD4+ cell counts do not provide an accurate analysis of what is happening in GALT.

The Human Lymph Nodes And Follicular Dentritic Cells—The **lymph nodes,** which are pea-sized capsules that trap foreign invaders and store immune cells, are all over the body and are connected by vessels much like those that transport blood (Figure 5-2, page 108). Deep within the lymph nodes researchers have found millions of viruses. Based on those data, Fox suggested that HIV uses the lymph nodes as places to meet up with immune cells. Infected T4 cells leave the lymph nodes and new

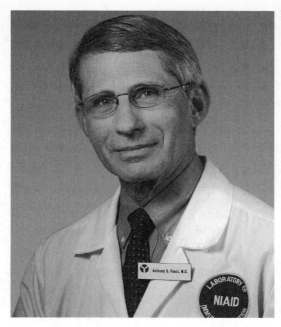

FIGURE 5-12 Anthony S. Fauci, M.D., Director, National Institute of Allergy and Infectious Diseases, National Institutes of Health, Associate Director of NIH for AIDS Research. He received the 2001 Annunzio Humanitarian Award for his impact on the understanding and treatment of infectious diseases/AIDS. In 2007 he received the Mary Woodard Lasker Public Service Award, The Kober Medal—the highest honor of the Association of American Physicians—and the National Medal of Science, bestowed by the president of the United States. *(Photograph courtesy of National Institute of Allergy and Infectious Diseases.)*

uninfected cells arrive to become infected. Years later, when enough GALT and lymph node immune cells have been killed, the patient's defenses become so impaired that he or she is vulnerable to any one of a wide array of opportunistic infections—AIDS has arrived.

Anthony Fauci (Figure 5-12), the head of the National Institute of Allergy and Infectious Diseases (NIAID), and Sonya Heath and colleagues (1995) agree that there are many more HIVs in the lymph nodes than in the blood. Studies in Fauci's laboratory have shown that there are many millions of HIV particles stuck to what are known as **follicular dendritic cells (FDCs),** located in hotspots of immune activity in the

lymph tissue called germinal centers of an infected individual.

The follicular dendritic cells, which have thousands of long, feathery, squid-like tentacles emanating from them and whose normal function is to filter and, acting like flypaper, trap antigens for presentation to antibody-producing B lymphocytes, serve as highly effective collection centers for extracellular HIV particles. Virtually every lymphocyte in a lymph node is enmeshed in the processes of these cells. Follicular dendritic cells themselves are susceptible to HIV infection, and they appear to place huge numbers of virus particles into intimate contact with other cells that are susceptible to HIV infection (Haase et al., 1996; Knight, 1996). FDCs also serve as latent reservoirs for HIV.

During the clinically latent phase, the lymph nodes of an infected individual are slowly destroyed.

In the final phase of an infection, the follicular dendritic network completely dissolves and the architecture of the lymph node collapses to produce what Fauci called a "burnt-out lymph node," or Douek's equivalent of collagen-caused lymph node fibrosis. With regard to HIV-caused CD4+ cell death, Douek states that with the initial infection of CD4+ cells, rapid renewal of lost CD4+ cells essentially means there will be more cells for HIV to infect! "Unlike any other viruses that we know of, unlike any other diseases, HIV is a virus that generates its own targets." With this collapse, large amounts of HIV are released into the circulatory system, and an ever-increasing number of peripheral cells are infected with HIV (Edgington, 1993).

Implications of a High HIV Replication Rate

Based on Ho and colleagues' kinetic studies of viral replication, it can be estimated that the population of HIV undergoes between 3000 and 5000 replication cycles (**generations**) over the course of 10 years, producing a minimum of 10^{12} (1 trillion) HIV in an HIV-infected person. This creates a lot of opportunity for HIV RNA evolution because genetic mutations occur most commonly during replication. Some mutations will weaken HIV in such a way as to expose it to attack by the immune system. But other mutations will aid the virus, speeding its replication and increasing the chances it can evade the immune system. Because HIV gets so many chances to replicate, it evolves and mutates, and those strains with the greatest replication efficiency gradually win out. This is Darwinian evolution going on in one patient.

In 1996 the hope was that Highly Active Antiretroviral Therapy (HAART) could wipe out HIV. This hope was based on two ideas, both later proved to be wrong: that the drugs would completely stop the virus from reproducing, and that there were no reservoirs where the HIV could hide. But HIV has the uncanny ability to reestablish itself in a variety of cell types. Even the most rigorous attempts to reduce or eliminate HIV from these reservoirs have failed. Scientists had vastly underestimated the extent of virus activity in an HIV-infected person, particularly during the asymptomatic or clinically latent phase. These and other recent studies should satisfy the major unanswered question concerning HIV disease/AIDS, which was, "Where is the virus?" During the 1980s, it was difficult to find medium to high levels of HIV in persons with HIV disease or even in those persons in the later stages of AIDS. We now know that there are large amounts of HIV present early on in the gut and lymph nodes of HIV-diseased people and in viral reservoirs. Perhaps the most troubled group of researchers now may be those currently developing AIDS vaccines. (See Chapter 9, pages 275–278, for a discussion about possible HIV vaccines.)

Summary

After a healthy person is HIV-infected, he or she makes antibodies against those viruses that are in the bloodstream, but not against those that have become integrated as HIV proviruses in the host immune cell DNA. Over time the immune system cells that are involved in antibody production are destroyed. Evidence is accumulating that cofactors such as nutrition, stress, and previous exposure to other sexually transmitted diseases that increase HIV expression are associated with HIV infection and HIV disease. Agents that suppress the immune system may also play a significant role in establishing HIV infection. In short, HIV infection is permanent. HIV attaches to CD4-bearing cells and enters those cells using one or more of at least four chemokine receptors, **R-2, R-3, R-4 (FUSIN),** and **R-5.** These coreceptors allow HIV to fuse with the cell membrane and enter the cell after HIV attachment to the CD4 receptor. As seen in Chapter 3, pages 49–66, HIV undergoes rapid genetic change, and, as far as is known, attacks only human cells—mostly of the human immune system. It is also known that the body's natural immune response against HIV is inadequate in containing or controlling the virus. Indeed, since the discovery of HIV, there is only one documented case in which an individual's immune system has ever completely eradicated the virus following established infection. (see Sidebar 4.2, pages 71–72, on the Berlin Patient). It has recently become quite clear that large amounts of the virus are produced within weeks after HIV infection. The virus remains, for the most part, in the gut and lymph nodes until very late in the disease process.

Review Questions

(Answers to the Review Questions are on page 463.)

1. Which cell type is believed to be the main target for HIV infection? Explain the biological impact of this particular infection.

2. What is CD4, where is it found, and what is its role in the HIV infection process?

3. Is there a period of latency after HIV infection— a time when few or no new HIV are being produced?

4. True or False: HIV is the cause of AIDS.

5. True or False: HIV primarily affects red blood cells.

6. True or False: Lymphocytes have a major role in the immune response to antigens.

7. True or False: All T and B lymphocytes inhibit or destroy foreign antigens.

8. True or False: CD4 and CD8 molecules are antibodies.

9. True or False: HIV belongs to the family of retroviruses.

10. True or False: Cytotoxic and suppressor T lymphocytes are the main targets of HIV.

11. True or False: The latent period is that time between initial infection with HIV and the onset of AIDS.

12. True or False: HIV can spread to infect new cells after it buds out of infected cells.

13. True or False: HIV causes the gradual destruction of cells bearing the CD4 molecule.

14. The most effective use of T4 cell counts in the clinical management of patients with HIV infection is for:

A. determining when to initiate therapy.
B. assessing risk of disease progression.
C. deciding on prophylaxis for opportunistic infections.
D. measuring the antiretroviral effect of initial therapy.

15. What cells of the immune system are the prime targets of HIV?

16. Which cells destroy body cells infected by viruses?

A. B cells
B. memory cells
C. CTL or killer T cells
D. helper T cells

Opportunistic Infections and Cancers Associated with HIV Disease/AIDS

CHAPTER HIGHLIGHTS

- Suppression of the immune system allows harmless agents to establish harmful opportunistic infections (OIs).
- OIs respond well to Highly Active Antiretroviral Therapy (HAART).
- OIs in AIDS patients are caused by viruses, bacteria, fungi, and protozoa.
- In the United States, about 95% of the HIV infected are coinfected with herpes 1 and/or 2. About 40% are coinfected with hepatitis C, and 36% are coinfected with tuberculosis.
- Annually, March 24 is recognized as World Tuberculosis (TB) Day.
- Nearly one-third of the world's population is infected with *Mycobacterium tuberculosis.*
- About 1.5 million people with tuberculosis are coinfected with HIV.
- About 13 million people in America have a latent TB infection.
- Human Herpes Virus-8 is believed to be the cause of Kaposi's sarcoma.
- The cost of treating OIs can be very high.
- There are two types of Kaposi's sarcoma (KS): classic and AIDS-associated.
- Cancers associated with HIV/AIDS are presented.
- Human papilloma virus and HIV infections
- KS is rarely found in hemophiliacs, injection drug users, and women with AIDS.
- The clinical presentation of OIs has been impacted by the use of antiretroviral therapy.

WHAT IS AN OPPORTUNISTIC DISEASE?

Humans evolved in the presence of a wide range of parasites—viruses, bacteria, fungi, and protozoa that do not cause disease in people with an intact immune system. But these organisms can cause a disease in someone with a weakened immune system, such as an individual with HIV disease. The infections they cause are known as **opportunistic infections** (OIs), meaning, OIs occur after a disease-causing virus or microorganism, normally held in check by a functioning immune system, gets the **opportunity** to multiply and invade host tissue after the immune system has been compromised. For most of medical history, OIs were rare and almost always appeared in patients whose immunity was impaired by either cancer or genetic disease.

With improved medical technology, a steadily growing number of people become severely immunosuppressed because of medications and ra-diation used in bone marrow or organ transplantation and cancer chemotherapy. HIV disease also suppresses the immune system. Perhaps as a corollary to their increased prevalence, or because of heightened physician awareness, OIs seem to be occurring more frequently in the elderly, who may be rendered vulnerable by age-related declines in immunity. New OIs are now being diagnosed because the pool of people who can get them is so much larger, and, in addition, new techniques for identifying the causative organisms have been developed. However, most of the infections considered opportunistic are not reportable to state or federal governments, which interferes with a clear-cut count of their growing numbers.

Although OIs are still not commonplace, they are no longer considered rare—they occur in tens of thousands of HIV/AIDS patients. But despite this increase, physicians and their patients have reasons to be optimistic about their ability to contain these infections. The reasons are: (1) In a massive federal effort, driven by the HIV/AIDS epidemic, researchers are finding drugs that can prevent or treat many of the OIs; and (2) various antiretroviral drug therapies have shown promise for warding off OIs by boosting patients' immune systems (Figure 6-1).

THE PREVALENCE OF OPPORTUNISTIC DISEASES

The prevalence of OIs in the United States is very high. There are about 500,000 HIV-seropositive individuals with T4 or CD4+ cell counts below 200/μL of blood. Worldwide, there are between 12 and 18 million HIV infected with a T4 or CD4+ cell count of 200 or less. More than 100 microorganisms—bacteria, viruses, fungi, and protozoa—can cause disease in such individuals, even though only a fraction of these (17) are included in the current surveillance definition for clinical AIDS. In a large survey from the Centers for Disease Control and Prevention (CDC), such

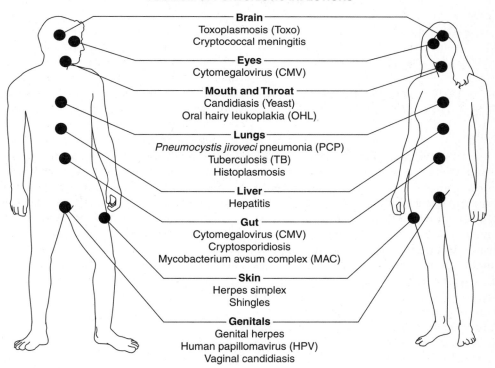

COMMON OPPORTUNISTIC INFECTIONS

Brain
Toxoplasmosis (Toxo)
Cryptococcal meningitis

Eyes
Cytomegalovirus (CMV)

Mouth and Throat
Candidiasis (Yeast)
Oral hairy leukoplakia (OHL)

Lungs
Pneumocystis jiroveci pneumonia (PCP)
Tuberculosis (TB)
Histoplasmosis

Liver
Hepatitis

Gut
Cytomegalovirus (CMV)
Cryptosporidiosis
Mycobacterium avsum complex (MAC)

Skin
Herpes simplex
Shingles

Genitals
Genital herpes
Human papillomavirus (HPV)
Vaginal candidiasis

FIGURE 6-1 HIV and Opportunistic Infections.[1,2] HIV doesn't kill anybody directly. Instead, it weakens the body's ability to fight disease. Infections that are rarely seen in those with normal immune systems can be deadly to those with HIV. People with HIV can get many infections (called *opportunistic infections,* or OIs). Some of these illnesses can be prevented; others can only be combated after their onset.

[1]For Kaposi's Sarcoma, see Figure 6-7, page 149.
[2]See Table 6-1, page 140.

OIs were diagnosed in 33% of individuals at one year and in 58% at two years after documentation of a T4 cell count below 200/μL. In late 2009 the CDC presented its latest guidelines for prevention and treatment of OIs in HIV-infected persons. The new treatments for OIs have extended the survival of AIDS patients, but they have also opened new issues. With the growing proportion of longer-term HIV/AIDS survivors, new OIs have become prominent, together with concerns about cost, compliance, drug interactions, and quality of life (Laurence, 1995; *MMWR*, 1995b). The six most common AIDS-related OIs are bacterial pneumonia, candidal esophagitis, pulmonary/disseminated TB, mycobacterium avium complex disease, herpes simplex reinfection, and *Pneumocystis* pneumonia or PCP (Figure 6-2, page 137). The year 1997 marked the first time, since the HIV/AIDS pandemic began in the United States, that the incidence of AIDS-defining OIs among HIV-infected persons fell in number from the previous year's total. The reason: the use of antiretroviral drugs.

OPPORTUNISTIC INFECTIONS IN HIV-INFECTED PEOPLE

HIV/AIDS is a devastating human tragedy. It appears to be killing about 95% of those who demonstrate the symptoms. One well-known American surgeon said, "I would rather die of any form of cancer rather than die of AIDS." This statement was not made because of the social stigma attached to HIV/AIDS or because it is lethal. It was made in recognition of the slow, demoralizing, debilitating, painful, disfiguring, helpless, and unending struggle to stay alive.

Because of a suppressed and weakened immune system, viruses, bacteria, fungi, and protozoa that commonly and harmlessly inhabit the body become pathogenic (Figure 6-2, page 137). Prior to 1998, about 90% of deaths related to HIV infection and AIDS were caused by OIs, compared with 7% due to cancer and 3% due to other causes. Now, with the use of antiretroviral drugs, OIs cause less than 50% of deaths. Liver and kidney organ failure, heart disease, and various cancers are on the increase as the cause

of death in HIV/AIDS patients. (See Point of Information 6.1, page 138.)

HIV-Related Opportunistic Infections Vary Worldwide

The course of HIV infection tends to be similar for most people: Infection with the virus is followed by seroconversion (HIV test changes from negative to positive) and progressive destruction of T4 or CD4+ cells. Yet the opportunistic infections and malignancies that largely define the symptomatic or clinical history of HIV disease vary geographically. People with HIV and their physicians in different regions confront distinct problems, mainly because of differences in exposure, in access to diagnosis and care, and in general health.

Comparisons between the data about opportunistic infections in different countries must be made with care. But most developing nations lack the facilities and trained personnel to identify opportunistic infections correctly; consequently, their prevalence may be underreported. Clinicians in developed countries can order sophisticated laboratory analyses to identify pathogens. Those in developing countries must rely on signs and symptoms to make their diagnoses. Oral candidiasis and herpes zoster are easy to diagnose without laboratory backup because the lesions are visible. While some pneumonias and types of diarrhea can be specified, others, such as extrapulmonary tuberculosis, cytomegalovirus infections, cryptococcal meningitis, and systemic infections such as histoplasmosis, toxoplasmosis, microsporidiosis, and nocardiosis, go underreported due to the lack of laboratory facilities.

Socioeconomic Factors

Geography explains much about the varying patterns of opportunistic infections, but a decisive factor is often financial capacity. On the most fundamental level, money is needed to create an infrastructure that limits exposure to pathogens. Thus, while few people with HIV in wealthy countries develop certain bacterial or protozoal infections, they are a major cause of

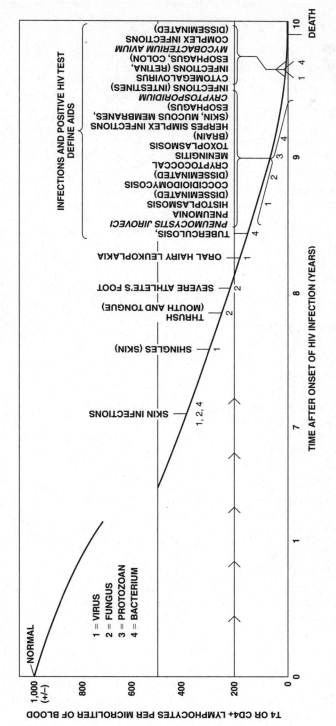

FIGURE 6–2 General Progression of Opportunistic Infections in Untreated Adolescents/Adults After HIV Infection. Normal T4 or CD4+ cell count in adolescents/adults is, on average, about 1000/μL of blood. There is a relationship between the drop in T4 lymphocytes and the onset of opportunistic infections (OIs). The first sign of an OI begins under 500 T4 cells/μL. As the T4 or CD4+ cell count continues to drop, the chance of OI infection increases. Note the variety of OIs found in AIDS patients with 200 or less T4 cells/μL.

THE CHANGING SPECTRUM OF OPPORTUNISTIC INFECTIONS

Prior to 1995 there was hardly any standardized use of protective agents to block the infectious complications or opportunistic infections (OIs) associated with HIV-induced immunodeficiency. Now there is an array of drugs that can be used in strategies to prevent or delay nearly all the major OIs. With this advancement has come the need to weigh the pros and cons of the various strategies. Cost, antimicrobial resistance, drug interactions, and pill overload are all important considerations.

EFFECT OF ANTI-HIV THERAPY ON OPPORTUNISTIC INFECTIONS

As presented in Chapter 4, the use of anti-HIV combination drug therapy has produced a number of unexpected results in patient response to those drugs. Soon after combination therapy began, physicians witnessed a rather confusing or unusual presentation of OIs. In some cases certain OIs improved, in others the situation deteriorated. Such changes in OI expression are occurring now, at a time when hundreds of thousands of HIV-infected Americans are on **Highly Active Antiretroviral Therapy (HAART)** or simply ART.

TREATMENT IN THE HAART (ART) ERA

HAART or in short, ART therapy appears to help the human immune system. When HIV patients take antiretroviral medicines that control HIV replication, their immune systems begin to recuperate in ways that are puzzling and controversial. For example, patients recover immunity to some deadly opportunistic infections but appear unable to fight diseases for which they were vaccinated as children, for example, tetanus, or to target HIV itself. Collectively, such observations indicate ART patients can only raise successful immune responses against pathogens they see regularly. For example, cytomegalovirus is an organism found in almost everybody's blood, so the immune systems of ART patients see the pathogen constantly and generate cells and antibodies that attack it. But tetanus is something people rarely encounter, so ART patients, unlike their HIV-negative counterparts, fail to raise immune responses against it. The ultimate irony is that ART, when successful, destroys all but a few million HIVs that are forced into hiding.

Recent studies suggest that the incidence of esophageal candidiasis and, by inference, other forms of *Candida* infection has fallen by 60% to 70% in patients treated with ART. The use of ART dramatically changed the epidemiology of opportunistic infections and is clearly associated with gradual recovery of the immune system (Powderly et al., 1998; Ledergerber et al., 1999).

This information aside, when HIV is controlled with the antiretroviral drugs, immunity to infections—other than HIV—usually starts to return. As a result, some opportunistic infections go away without specific treatment; and sometimes patients can stop prophylactic treatment for certain opportunistic diseases. However, entering year 2013, it is still unclear who can stop prophylaxis safely, and who cannot.

Studies from 1998 through 2012 using protease inhibitor drugs in ART have shown that few patients whose T4 level rose to and stayed over 200 to 300 per microliter of blood (μL) developed an OI. This is the strongest evidence to date that immune reconstruction is occurring with antiretroviral drug therapy, and suggests that it occurs early and with quite modest improvements in T4 cell levels. The implication is that the search for immunorestorative therapy other than with the current antiretroviral is somewhat less urgent than previously believed, though still a clear priority.

VIRAL LOAD RELATED TO OPPORTUNISTIC INFECTIONS

HIV clinicians have recently looked at the predictive value of plasma HIV RNA for the development of three OIs: PCP, CMV, and MAC. Using a database of patients participating in AIDS Clinical Trial Groups (ACTG), for every 1-log increase in plasma HIV RNA level, the risk of developing one of these OIs was increased two- to threefold. Plasma HIV RNA level was predictive of an increased risk of an OI independent of T4 cell count, which also predicted OI risk. This information confirms that maintaining control of viral replication may be a critical component of preventing OIs in HIV-infected people.

death in poor areas that cannot provide clean water and adequate food storage facilities.

Financial resources also affect clinicians' abilities to diagnose HIV/AIDS and, when appropriate, to provide the proper medicine. People with HIV/AIDS in Africa often die of severe bacterial infections because they don't have the antibiotics or the clinical care they need. They don't survive long enough to develop diseases such as PCP.

United States, Europe, and Africa—The United States and Europe on one end, and Africa on the other, represent the global extremes of financial resources for health care. The most common opportunistic infections each region faces reflect the overall quality of health care, sanitation, and diet. For example, Thailand and Mexico belong to the large group of nations that have intermediate incomes and correspondingly intermediate patterns of HIV complications (Harvard AIDS Institute, 1994).

HIV/AIDS patients rarely have just one infection (Table 6-1). The mix of OIs may depend on lifestyle and where the HIV/AIDS patient lives or has lived. Thus, a knowledge of the person's origins and travels may be diagnostically helpful. (Note: a number of the symptoms listed in the CDC definition of HIV/AIDS can be found associated with certain OIs presented.)

Sporozoan Disease—Malaria

Although the disease occurs in many parts of the world, including Asia, Latin America, the Middle East, and parts of Europe, it poses the greatest problem in sub-Saharan Africa, where 81% of malaria cases and 91% of deaths occurred mostly in children under five years of age. This region of the world is particularly hard-hit by malaria due to several factors: sub-Saharan is home to a species of mosquito, Anopheles, that can transmit malaria parasite very efficiently; most of the region's cases are caused by the Plasmodium falciparum parasite, which causes the most severe and life-threatening form of malaria; poverty and limited health infrastructure make the mounting of effective prevention and treatment efforts difficult; and drug-resistant strains of the parasite have also emerged in the region, acting as another barrier to malaria control. In sub-Saharan Africa, the situation is also worsened by the presence of other diseases, especially HIV/AIDS. Both HIV/AIDS and malaria affect similar geographic areas and risk groups, causing dual public health crises. Increasing knowledge regarding the interactions between HIV/AIDS and malaria suggests that HIV positive individuals may be more susceptible to malaria illness because of their weakened immune systems and may be less likely to respond to standard treatments for malaria. There is also evidence to suggest that severe malarial episodes can temporarily lead to an upsurge in HIV viral load, thereby leading to increased morbidity in individuals co-infected with HIV and malaria.

Fungal Diseases

In general, healthy people have a high degree of innate resistance to fungi. But a different situation prevails with opportunistic fungal infections, which often present themselves as acute, life-threatening diseases in a compromised host (Medoff et al., 1991).

Because treatment seldom results in the eradication of fungal infections in HIV/AIDS patients, there is a high probability of recurrence after treatment (DeWit et al., 1991).

Fungal diseases are among the more devastating of the OIs and are most often regional in association. AIDS patients from the Ohio River Basin, the Midwest, or Puerto Rico have a higher-than-normal risk of histoplasmosis (histo-plaz-mo-sis) infection. In the Southwest, there is increased risk for coccidioidomycosis (kok-sid-e-oi-do-mi-ko-sis).

In the southern Gulf states, the risk is for blastomycosis (blast-toe-my-co-sis). Other important OI fungi such as *Pneumocystis jiroveci* (nu-mo-sis-tis yer-row-vet-see), *Candida albicans* (kan-di-dah al-be-cans), and *Cryptococcus neoformans* (krip-to-kok-us knee-o-for-mans) are found everywhere in equal numbers. Because of their importance as OIs in AIDS patients, brief descriptions of histoplasmosis, candidiasis, *Pneumocystis* pneumonia, and cryptococcosis are presented.

Histoplasmosis (Histoplasmacapsulatum)— Spores are inhaled and germinate in or on the body (Figure 6-3, page 141). This fungal pathogen is endemic in the Mississippi and Ohio River Valleys. Signs of histoplasmosis include prolonged influenza-like symptoms, shortness of breath, and possible complaints of night sweats and shaking chills. Histoplasmosis in an HIV-positive person

Table 6-1 Some Common Opportunistic Diseases Associated with HIV Infection

Organism/Virus	Clinical Manifestation
Protozoa	
Cryptosporidium muris	Gastroenteritis (inflammation of stomach-intestine membranes)
Isospora belli	Gastroenteritis
Taxoplasma gondii	Encephalitis (brain abscess), retinitis, disseminated
Fungi	
Candida sp.	Stomatitis (thrush), proctitis, vaginitis, esophagitis
Coccidioides immitis	Meningitis, dissemination
Cryptococcus neoformans	Meningitis (membrane inflammation of spinal cord and brain), pneumonia, encephalitis, dissemination (widespread)
Histoplasma capsulatum	Pneumonia, dissemination
Pneumocystis jiroveci	Pneumocystic pneumonia (PCP)
Bacteria	
Mycobacterium avium complex (MAC)	Dissemination, pneumonia, diarrhea, weight loss, lymphadenopathy, severe gastrointestinal disease
Mycobacterium tuberculosis (TB)	Pneumonia (tuberculosis), meningitis, dissemination
Viruses	
Cytomegalovirus (CMV)	Fever, hepatitis, encephalitis, retinitis, pneumonia, colitis, esophagitis
Epstein-Barr	Oral hairy leukoplakia, B cell lymphoma
Hepatitis C (HCV)	Liver cirrhosis or cancer (major reason for liver transplants)
Herpes simplex	Mucocutaneous (mouth, genital, rectal) blisters and/or ulcers, pneumonia, esophagitis, encephalitis
Papovavirus J-C	Progressive multifocal leukoencephalopathy
Varicella-zoster	Dermatomal skin lesions (shingles), encephalitis
Cancers	
Kaposi's sarcoma	Disseminated mucocutaneous lesions often involving skin, lymph nodes, visceral organs (especially lungs and GI tract)
Primary lymphoma of the brain	Headache, palsies, seizures, hemiparesis, mental status or personality changes
Systemic lymphomas	Fever, night sweats, weight loss, enlarged lymph nodes

Patients with compromised immune systems are at increased risk for all known cancers and infections (including bacterial, viral, and protozoal). Most infectious diseases in HIV-infected patients are the result of proliferation of organisms already present in the patient's body. Most of these opportunistic infections are not contagious to others. The notable exception to this is tuberculosis.

Disclaimer: This table was developed to provide general information only. It is not meant to be diagnostic nor to direct treatment.

(Adapted from Mountain-Plains Regional Education and Training Center HIV/AIDS Curriculum, 4th ed., 1992 updated, 1997; and from MMWR 2002.)

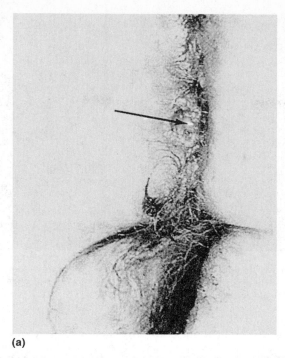

(a)

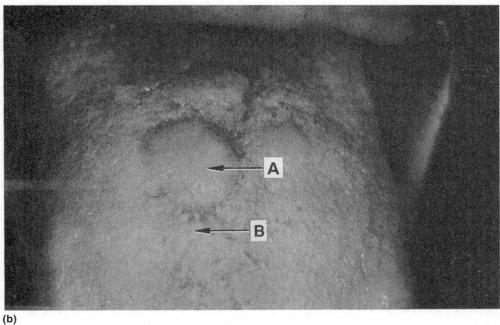

(b)

FIGURE 6–3 **(a)** Anal Histoplasmosis. Histoplasmosis is caused by *Histoplasma capsulatum* and causes infection in immunocompromised patients. **(b)** AIDS patient's tongue showing multiple shiny, firm *Histoplasma* erythematous nodules (see arrow A) and thrush (see arrow B). *(A, Courtesy of the Centers for Disease Control and Prevention, Atlanta; B, Courtesy of Marc E. Grossman, New York.)*

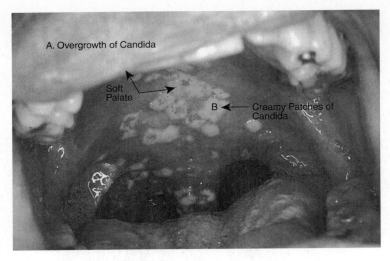

A. Overgrowth of Candida

Soft Palate

B ← Creamy Patches of Candida

FIGURE 6-4 Thrush **(a)** An overgrowth of *Candida albicans* on the soft palate in the oral cavity of an AIDS patient. **(b)** Creamy patches of candida that can be scraped off, leaving a red and sometimes bleeding mucosa. *(Centers for Disease Control/Dr. Sol Silverman, Jr., DDS)*

is considered diagnostic of AIDS. In about two-thirds of AIDS patients with histoplasmosis, it is the initial OI. Over 90% of cases have occurred in patients with T4 cell counts below 100/μL (Wheat, 1992).

***Candidiasis or Thrush* (Candida albicans)**— This fungus is usually associated with vaginal yeast infections. It is a fungus quite common to the body and in particular inhabits the alimentary tract. It is normally kept in check by the presence of bacteria that live on the linings of the alimentary tract. However, in immunocompromised patients, especially those who have received broad spectrum antibiotics, candida multiplies rapidly. Because of its location in the upper reaches of the alimentary tract, if unchecked, it may cause mucocutaneous candidiasis or **thrush,** an overgrowth of candida in the esophagus and in the oral cavity (Figure 6-4, page 142). Mucosal candidiasis has been associated with AIDS patients from the very beginning of the AIDS pandemic (Powderly et al., 1992). In women, overgrowth of candidiasis also occurs in the vaginal area.

Oral or esophageal candidiasis causes thick white patches on the mucosal surface and may be the first manifestation of AIDS. Because other diseases can cause similar symptoms, candidiasis by itself is not sufficient for a diagnosis of AIDS.

***A New Name for* Pneumocystis Carinii *Is* Pneumocystis Jiroveci *(yee-row-vet-see)*—**In September 2002, James Stringer and colleagues, based on DNA evidence, reported that *Pneumocystis carinii* is the species that infects rats and that *Pneumocystis jiroveci* infects humans. Given the compelling evidence that the human form of *Pneumocystis* is a separate species, the most important objection to designating it as such has been the problem that this name change could create in the medical literature, where the disease caused by *P. jiroveci* is widely known as *Pneumocystis carinii* pneumonia. This problem can be avoided by taking the species name out of the disease name. Under this system, PCP refers to *Pneumocystis* pneumonia. This simple modification accommodates the name change pertaining to the *Pneumocystis* species that infects humans. Furthermore, adopting this change makes the acronym appropriate for describing the disease in every host species, none of which, except rats, is infected by *P. carinii.* In summary, the acronym PCP will be retained in the literature. But the causative agent will be referred to as *Pneumocystis jiroveci* or Pj pneumonia where necessary.

In this book, PCP will be used with the understanding that it is caused in humans by *Pneumocystis jiroveci*.

Virtually everyone in the United States by age 30 to 40 has been exposed to *P. jiroveci*. It lies dormant in the lungs, held in check by the immune system. Prior to the HIV/AIDS epidemic, PCP was seen in children and adults who had a suppressed immune system, as in leukemia or Hodgkin's disease, and were receiving chemotherapy. In the HIV/AIDS patient, the onset of PCP is insidious—patients may notice some shortness of breath and they cannot run as far. It causes extensive damage within the alveoli of the lungs.

Prior to 1981, fewer than 100 cases of PCP infection were reported annually in the United States; yet 80% of AIDS patients develop PCP at some time during their illness. This is one of the few AIDS-related conditions for which there is a choice of relatively effective drugs. The first of these to be made available was the intravenous and aerosolized versions of pentamidine. There are frequent recurrences of this infection. PCP accounted for a diagnosis of AIDS in over 65% of AIDS cases in 1990. In 1994 it had fallen to 20% due to available therapy (Ernst, 1990; Murphy, 1994). The triad of symptoms that almost always indicates the onset of PCP during HIV disease is fever, dry cough, and shortness of breath (Grossman et al., 1989). PCP is unlikely to develop in people with HIV disease unless their T4 cell count drops below 200 (Phair et al., 1990). Regardless, PCP remains the most common, serious OI among those HIV infected in the United States.

Viral Diseases

Hepatitis—Viral-caused hepatitis which can lead to liver cirrhosis (fibrosis of the liver) and cancer. Although there are five primary hepatitis viruses, A, B, C, D, and E, hepatitis C is the most damaging and at this time there is no vaccine against it. (The first ever World Hepatitis Day was held on July 28, 2011.)

Hepatitis C—Hepatitis means an inflammation or swelling of the liver. Viruses can cause hepatitis. Alcohol, drugs (including prescription medications), or poisons can also cause hepatitis. In late 1999, **hepatitis C** caused by the hepatitis C virus **(HCV)** was classified as an OI because the relative risk for liver-associated death is increased sevenfold in HIV-positive people compared to non–HIV-infected individuals. It is estimated that 200 million people worldwide are infected with the hepatitis C virus. About 5 million of the infected live in America.

HIV/HCV Means Double Trouble

The hepatitis C virus (HCV) is now at least four times as widespread in America as HIV. It kills between 10,000 and 15,000 each year and is predicted to kill 30,000 a year by 2012. Its transmission is similar to that of HIV. About 30% of people living with HIV infection in America, about 250,000 people, are believed to be co-infected with the HCV. Among some groups, primarily HIV-positive current and former intravenous-drug users, the coinfection rate is thought to be about 90%. According to the National Hemophilia Foundation, the coinfection rate among HIV-positive hemophiliacs is equally high. For those who become infected with HCV, the virus produces no symptoms for 10–30 years. Then symptoms like fatigue, joint and abdominal pain, nausea, and lapses in concentration begin to set in. Because doctors have not traditionally screened patients for the virus, many people do not even know they are infected until their livers show signs of serious damage. Studies now indicate that HIV can greatly speed the progression of hepatitis C. That means that many with HIV may suffer advanced liver disease (cirrhosis of the liver) after just 5 or 10 years, even as the antiretroviral drugs boost their life expectancies. Studies on HCV's effects on HIV/AIDS patients have been contradictory, but the coinfection has been associated with a higher risk of progression to HIV disease and AIDS. The antiretroviral drugs used to fight HIV, particularly the protease inhibitors, place a great strain on the liver, the organ whose function is to metabolize them. Over the last 13 years (2000–2012), hepatitis C coinfections have been and will most likely continue to be the second leading cause of liver failure and death in HIV/AIDS patients. Some people infected with both viruses find that their bodies have great difficulty tolerating many HIV/AIDS and HCV drugs. At present, there is no national policy for dealing with this virus.

Herpesviruses

Because of a depleted T4 or CD4+ cellular component of the immune system, AIDS patients are at particularly high risk for the herpes family of viral infections: cytomegalovirus, herpes simplex virus types 1 and 2, varicella-zoster virus, and Epstein-Barr virus. (See Figure 8–9a, b, page 224.)

Cytomegalovirus (CMV)—This virus is a member of the human herpes virus group of viruses. CMV is the perfect parasite. It infects most people asymptomatically. When illness does occur, it is mild and nonspecific. There have been no epidemics to call attention to the virus. Yet CMV is now considered the most common infectious cause of mental retardation and congenital deafness in the United States. It is also the most common viral pathogen found in immunocompromised people (Balfour, 1995).

The virus is very unstable and survives only a few hours outside a human host. It can be found in saliva, tears, blood, stool, and cervical secretions, and in especially high levels in urine and semen. Transmission occurs primarily by intimate or close contact with infected secretions. The incidence of CMV infection prior to the beginning of HAART therapy in 1996 varied from between 30% and 80% depending on the geographical community tested. In the 1980s, over 90% of homosexual males tested positive for CMV (Jacobson et al., 1988).

CMV infection of people with HIV usually results in prolonged fever, anemia (too few red blood cells), leukopenia (too few white blood cells), and abnormal liver function. *CMV also causes severe diarrhea and HIV-associated retinitis resulting in eventual blindness* (*Emergency Medicine*, 1989; Lynch, 1989).

Prior to HAART therapy, 75% of HIV/AIDS patients had an eye disease, with the retina the most common site (Russell, 1990). The retina, which is a light-sensitive membrane lining the inside of the back of the eye, is also part of the brain and is nourished by blood vessels. HIV-related damage to these vessels produces tiny retinal hemorrhages and small cotton wool spots—early indicators of disease that are often detected during a routine eye examination (Figure 6-5). Since the beginning of HAART therapy, CMV retinitis has fallen to about 5% in HIV/AIDS patients.

In unusual circumstances, the virus can produce dramatic symptoms, such as loss of vision

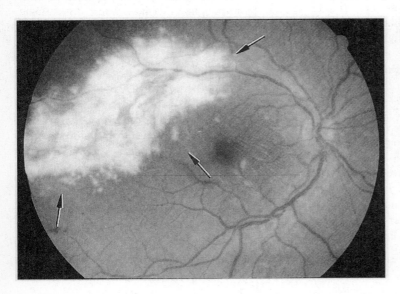

FIGURE 6-5 Cytomegalovirus Retinitis. The disease, as seen in this photograph, involves the posterior pole of the right eye. Fluffy white infiltrate (**cotton wool spots**) with a small amount of retinal hemorrhage can be seen in the distribution of the superior vascular arcade. *(Courtesy of Scott M. Whitcup, M.D., National Eye Institute, National Institutes of Health, Bethesda, Md.)*

within 72 hours. Without treatment, CMV can destroy the entire retina in three to six months after infection.

Herpesviruses Types 1 and 2 (HSV-1 and -2)— The name *herpes* comes from the Greek *herpein*—"to creep." Members of the *Herpesviridae* family have been identified in a variety of animals, and they all share certain features, including an ability to establish latency following primary infection, as well as a potential to reactivate and cause further disease. Herpes infections are among the most commonly diagnosed infections among the HIV/AIDS population. Almost all HIV-infected individuals (95%) are coinfected with HSV-1 and/or HSV-2. Both viruses cause *severe* and progressive eruptions of the mucous membranes. HSV-1 affects the membranes of the nose and mouth. Also, when herpetic lesions involve the lips or throat, 80% to 90% of the time they either precede or occur simultaneously with **herpes caused pneumonia** (Gottlieb et al., 1987). Bacterial or fungal super-infections occur in more than 50% of herpes-caused pneumonia cases and are a major contributory cause of death in HIV/AIDS patients.

Mortality from HSV pneumonia exceeds 80% (Lynch, 1989). Herpes may also cause blindness in HIV/AIDS patients. The following is from Paul Monette's *Borrowed Time:*

> I woke up shortly thereafter, and Roger told me— without a sense of panic, almost puzzled—that his vision seemed to be losing light and detail. I called Dell Steadman and made an emergency appointment, and I remember driving down the freeway, grilling Roger about what he could see. It seemed to be less and less by the minute. He could barely see the cars going by in the adjacent lanes. Twenty minutes later we were in Dell's office, and with all the urgent haste to get there we didn't really reconnoiter till we were sitting in the examining room. I asked the same question—what could he see?—and now Roger was getting more and more upset the more his vision darkened. I picked up the phone to call Jamiee, and by the time she answered the phone in Chicago he was blind. ***Total blackness, in just two hours!***
>
> The retina had detached. (An operation on retinal attachment was successful and sight was restored. The cause of the retinal detachment was a herpes infection of the eyes.)

HSV-2 affects the membranes of the vagina, penis, and anus, causing severe ulcers in and on these organs.

Herpes Zoster Virus (HZV)—Like herpes simplex, this virus has the potential to cause a rapid onset of pneumonia in HIV/AIDS patients. Untreated HZV pneumonia has a mortality rate of 15% to 35%. HZV is now monitored as an early indicator that HIV-positive people are progressing toward AIDS.

Protozoal Diseases

An increasing number of infections that have not been observed in immunocompromised patients are being found in AIDS patients. Two such infections are caused by the protozoans *Toxoplasma gondii* and *Cryptosporidium muris*.

Toxoplasma gondii—*T. gondii* is a small intracellular protozoan parasite that lives in vacuoles inside host macrophages and other nucleated cells. It appears that during and after entry, *T. gondii* produces secretory products that modify vacuole membranes so that the normal *fusion* of cell vacuoles with lysosomes containing digestive enzymes is blocked. Having blocked vacuole-lysosome fusion, *T. gondii* can successfully reproduce and cause a disease called **toxoplasmosis** (Joiner et al., 1990). It can infect any warm-blooded animal, invading and multiplying within the cytoplasm of host cells. As host immunity develops, multiplication slows and tissue cysts are formed. Sexual multiplication occurs in the intestinal cells of cats (and apparently only cats); oocysts form and are shed in the stool (Sibley, 1992). Transmission may occur transplacentally, by ingestion of raw or undercooked meat and eggs containing tissue cysts or by exposure to oocysts in cat feces (Wallace et al., 1993).

In the United States, 10% to 40% of adults are chronically infected, but most are asymptomatic. *T. gondii* can enter and infect the human brain, causing **encephalitis** (inflammation of the brain). Toxoplasmic encephalitis develops in over 30% of AIDS patients at some point in their illness (Figure 6-6). The signs and symptoms of cerebral toxoplasmosis in AIDS patients may include

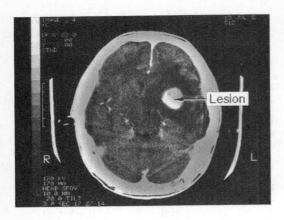

FIGURE 6-6 *Toxoplasma gondii* Lesions in the Brain. Radiographic imaging shows a deep ring-enhancing lesion located in the basal ganglia. *(Courtesy of Carmelita U. Tuazon, George Washington University.)*

fever, headache, confusion, sleepiness, weakness or numbness in one part of the body, seizure activity, and changes in vision. These symptoms can get worse and progress to coma and death unless toxoplasmosis is promptly diagnosed and treated. Thus, for most AIDS patients, it is believed that *T. gondii* is latent within their bodies and is reactivated by the loss of immune competence.

Cryptosporidium—*Cryptosporidium* is the cause of cryptosporidiosis and is a member of the family of organisms that includes *Toxoplasma gondii* and *Isospora.* Its life cycle is similar to that of other organisms in the class Sporozoa. Oocysts are shed in the feces of infected animals and are immediately infectious to others. In humans, the organisms can be found throughout the GI tract. *Cryptosporidium* causes **profuse watery diarrhea** of 6 to 26 bowel movements per day with a loss of 1 to 17 liters of fluid (a liter is about 1 quart). It is an infrequent infection in AIDS patients, usually occurring late in the course of disease as immunological deterioration progresses.

Studies of transmission patterns have shown infection within families, in nursery schools, and from person to person, probably by the fecal-oral route. The infection is particularly common in homosexual men, perhaps as a consequence of

anilingus (oral-anal sex). About 15% of people with HIV/AIDS are infected with this parasite.

Bacterial Diseases

There is a long list of bacteria that cause infections in HIV/AIDS patients. These are the bacteria that normally cause infection or illness after the ingestion of contaminated food, such as species of *Salmonella.* Others, such as *Strep-tococci, Haemophilus,* and *Staphylococci,* are common in advanced HIV disease. A number of other bacteria-caused sexually transmitted diseases such as syphilis, chancroid, gonorrhea, and chlamydial diseases are also associated with HIV disease.

One difference between AIDS and non–AIDS individuals is that bacterial diseases in AIDS patients are of greater severity and more difficult to treat. Two bacterial species, *Mycobacterium avium intracellulare* and *Mycobacterium tuberculosis,* are of particular importance as agents of infection in AIDS patients.

Mycobacterium avium intracellulare (MAI)—Over the past 40 years, MAI has gone from a rare, reportable infection to something that is common in most large American communities. Unlike tuberculosis, which is almost exclusively spread person to person, MAI is, in most instances, environmentally acquired. MAI exists in food, animals, water supplies, and soil and enters people's lungs as an aerosol when they take showers.

MAI occurs in about 25% of people with HIV disease and has been implicated as the cause of a nonspecific **wasting syndrome.** AIDS patients demonstrate **anorexia** (inability to eat), weight loss, weakness, night sweats, diarrhea, and fever. Some patients also experience abdominal pain, enlarged liver or spleen, and malabsorption. In contrast to viral infections, this bacterium rarely causes pulmonary or lung problems in AIDS patients. Among persons with AIDS, the risk of developing disseminated MAI increases progressively with time. AIDS patients surviving for 30 months had a 50% risk of developing disseminated MAI. It appears most HIV-infected persons will develop disseminated MAI if they do not first die from other OIs (Chin, 1992).

World Tuberculosis (TB) Day

World TB Day is observed on March 24 each year and commemorates the date in 1882 when Dr. Robert Koch announced the discovery of *Mycobacterium tuberculosis,* the bacterium that causes tuberculosis (TB). Worldwide, TB remains one of the leading causes of death from infectious disease. An estimated two billion plus persons (i.e., one-third of the world's population) are infected with *M. tuberculosis.* Each year, approximately nine million persons become ill from TB; of these, nearly two million die from the disease. World TB Day provides an opportunity for TB programs, nongovernmental organizations, and other partners to describe problems and solutions related to the TB pandemic and to support worldwide TB control activities.

Tuberculosis dates back to at least 4000 B.C. and was present in ancient Egypt, Greece, Rome, and India. Known as consumption, it was responsible for one in five deaths in 17th-century London.

Tuberculosis (TB) is now the leading cause of illness and death in people infected with HIV. TB is spread almost exclusively by airborne transmission. TB has been observed in elephants, cattle, mice, and other animal species.

The disease can affect any site in the body, but most often affects the lungs. When persons with pulmonary TB cough, they produce tiny droplet nuclei that contain TB bacteria, which can remain suspended in the air for prolonged periods of time. (With respect to transmission, the cough to TB is like sex to HIV.) Anyone who breathes air that contains these droplet nuclei can become infected with TB. It has been suggested that there is a minimal chance of inhaling HIV in blood-tinged TB sputum (Harris, 1993).

In 1989, the goal was set to eliminate TB in the United States by 2010. In 2010, there were 11,281 cases of TB. Most of these cases were among foreign-born persons in the United States.

An estimated 10 to 15 million Americans are infected with TB bacteria. About 10% of these otherwise healthy persons who have latent tuberculosis infection (TB lives in the body without causing illness) will become ill with active TB at some time during their lives. With HIV disease, the risk is 10% per year. It has been estimated that through year 2012, over 16 million HIV-infected people worldwide will be coinfected with TB. No two diseases are more inextricably linked. HIV infection severely weakens the immune system, allowing TB to become active. A person with an HIV infection is 20 times more likely to express the symptoms of TB than a non-HIV-infected person. HIV accelerates the disease! Were it not for HIV, global TB infections would be declining. Without effective drug therapy for TB, millions of coinfected (HIV/TB) Africans will die of TB over the coming years. HIV/AIDS researchers believe that to end HIV/AIDS the international community must first end TB.

Tuberculosis is not generally considered to be an OI because people with healthy immune systems contract TB. After infection with *M. tuberculosis* about 5% of immunocompetent individuals will develop TB (Daley, 1992).

TB: THE LEADING CAUSE OF DEATH AMONG HIV-POSITIVE PEOPLE WORLDWIDE

According to the World Health Organization, TB worldwide is the leading cause of death in HIV-infected people. About 1.5 million HIV-infected individuals develop TB each year and about 470,000 of those die from TB. Globally, TB was estimated to account for 20% of AIDS-related deaths each year from 2000 through 2012. In the United States, 14% of the HIV infected are also coinfected with TB.

Other Opportunistic Infections

Other opportunistic infectious organisms and viruses and the diseases they cause and possible therapies are listed in Table 6-1, page 140.

From diagnosis until death, the AIDS battle is *not* just against its cause, HIV, but against those organisms and viruses that cause OIs. Opportunistic infections are severe, tend to be disseminated (spread throughout the body), and are characterized by multiplicity. Fungal, viral, protozoal, and bacterial infections may be controlled for some time but are rarely curable.

CANCER OR MALIGNANCY IN HIV/AIDS PATIENTS

Common sense tells us that viruses should be cleared from our bodies just like any other invading pathogen. However, many are not cleared entirely and are able to persist by establishing latent or dormant infection. In many cases, virus-host interactions have evolved over the millennia such that viruses reproduce, remain viable, and are transmitted. During this time, host immune systems contain these viral infections and prevent severe illness or death. Examples of such viruses include herpesviruses and papillomaviruses. Herpesviruses that can establish latent and long-term infection in host humans include cytomegalovirus (CMV) or human herpesvirus 5 (HHV-5), Kaposi's sacoma–associated herpesvirus (KSHV) or human herpesvirus 8 (HHV-8), and Epstein-Barr virus (EBV). Many of the viruses that become latent in the body—for example, HPV, CMV, and EBV—are quite common in the human population but do not always lead to the development of a cancer. It is now known that infection with HIV changes the playing field, and the environment of immunosuppression may eventually tip the scale in favor of these viruses, leading to an increased risk of cancer.

Malignancy (ma-lig-nan-cy)

The word "malignancy" means a cancer. Specifically, cancer is an abnormal growth of cells that divide uncontrollably and may spread to other parts of the body. There are many kinds of cancer, which can involve just about any part of the body.

HIV infection carries with it a high susceptibility to certain cancers. Because of the severe and progressive impairment of the immune system, host defense mechanisms that normally protect against certain types of cancer are lost.

Cancer is a significant cause of mortality and morbidity in people infected with HIV; in fact, 30% to 40% will develop a malignancy or cancer during their lifetime. The majority of cancers affecting HIV-positive people are those established as *AIDS-defining* Kaposi's sarcoma (KS),

non-Hodgkin's lymphoma, invasive cervical cancer, and progressive multifocal leukoencephalopathy (oral and anal). However, other types of cancer, *non-AIDS defining* but AIDS associated or opportunistic, also appear to be more common among those infected with HIV. While not classified as AIDS-defining, these malignancies are rising in the HIV/AIDS community (Table 6-2).

Of the four types of HIV/AIDS-associated cancers, KS occurs with the greatest frequency and is discussed in some detail. The other three cancer conditions are briefly described. (For a review of HIV/AIDS-related cancers, read Hessol, 1998; Grulich, 2000; Newcomb–Fernandez, 2003.)

Kaposi's Sarcoma (cap-o-seas sar-co-ma)

No other HIV/AIDS-related opportunistic disease attacks and singles out one segment of the population as KS does with HIV-positive gay men. Men with KS outnumber women approximately 19 to 1; HIV-positive homosexual men with KS outnumber heterosexual men almost as significantly. KS is extremely rare in hemophiliacs with HIV.

Table 6-2 Some Non-AIDS-Defining Cancers with Increased Incidence in the HIV-Infected Population

Leukemia	Esophagus	Kidney
Multiple myeloma	Lip	Colorectal
Skin cancer	Tongue	Brain and CNS
Penile	Stomach	Heart
Vulva/Vagina	Larynx	Angiosarcoma
Leiomyosarcoma	Hodgkin's disease	Squamous cell
Burkitt's lymphoma	Pancreas	carcinoma
Pharynx	Liver	

Note: The four most frequent non-AIDS cancer-related deaths are lung cancer; cancer of the gastrointestinal tract, including liver cancer; blood-related cancers such as leukemia and Hodgkin's disease; and anal cancer. Considering that HIV-positive patients are living longer due to the use of antiretroviral therapy, researchers believe that death rates due to non–AIDS-related cancers will likely continue to overshadow death rates associated with classic AIDS-related cancers. *(Adapted from Jennifer Newcomb-Fernandez in RITA 9:5–10, 2003; Hessol et al., 2007 and Patel et al., 2008.)*

HIV infection represents an overwhelming risk factor for the development of KS, which was rare in the United States (incidence less than 1/100,000/year) before the HIV epidemic. It is an aggressive disease, with involvement of the gut, lung, pleura, lymph nodes, and hard and soft palates.

In the United States, Kaposi's sarcoma is at least 300 times more common in people with HIV/AIDS than in the general population.

KS was first described by Moritz Kaposi in 1877 as a cancer of the muscle and skin. Characteristic signs of early KS were bruises and birthmark-like lesions on the skin, especially on the lower extremities. KS was described as a slow-growing tumor found primarily in elderly Mediterranean men, Ashkenazi Jews, and equatorial Africans.

Kaposi's sarcoma as described by Moritz Kaposi is called classic KS, and it differs markedly from the KS that occurs in AIDS patients (Figure 6-7). Classic KS has a variable prognosis (forecast), is usually slow to develop, and causes little pain **(indolent).** Symptoms of classic KS are ulcerative skin lesions, swelling **(edema)** of the legs, and secondary infection of the skin lesions.

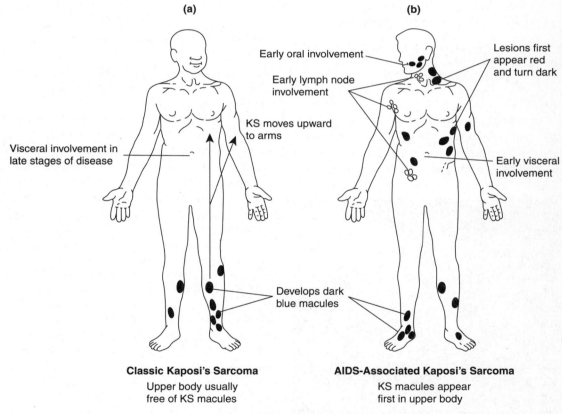

(a)

Early oral involvement

Early lymph node involvement

KS moves upward to arms

Visceral involvement in late stages of disease

Develops dark blue macules

Classic Kaposi's Sarcoma
Upper body usually free of KS macules

(b)

Lesions first appear red and turn dark

Early visceral involvement

AIDS-Associated Kaposi's Sarcoma
KS macules appear first in upper body

FIGURE 6-7 Classic and AIDS-Associated Kaposi's Sarcoma. **(a)** Patients with classic KS (non-AIDS-related) demonstrate violet to dark blue bruises, spots, or macules on their lower legs. Gradually, the lesions enlarge into tumors and begin to form ulcers. KS lesions may, with time, spread upward to the trunk and arms. The movement of KS appears to follow the veins and involves the lymph system. In the late stages of the disease, visceral organs may become involved. **(b)** For AIDS patients, initial lesions appear in greater number and are smaller than in classic KS. They first appear on the upper body (head and neck) and arms. The lesions first appear as pink or red oval bruises or macules that, with time, become dark blue and spread to the oral cavity and lower body, legs, and feet. Visceral organs may be involved early on and the disease is aggressive. However, death is not caused by KS.

Kaposi's Sarcoma and HIV/AIDS

The HIV/AIDS epidemic has brought a more virulent and progressive form of KS marked by painless, flat to raised, pink to purplish plaques on the skin and mucosal surfaces that may spread to the lungs, liver, spleen, lymph nodes, digestive tract, and other internal organs. In its advanced stages it may affect any area from the skull to the feet (Figure 6-8, page 150). In the mouth, the hard palate is the most common site of KS (Figure 6-9, page 150) but it may also occur on the gum line, tongue, or tonsils.

The prevalence of KS among gay men in 1981 was 77%; by 1987, it had fallen to 26% and by 2004 to less than 5% in gay men on HAART.

Human Herpesvirus Is the Kaposi's Virus— Most HIV/AIDS researchers now believe that HIV is not the primary pathological agent for Kaposi's sarcoma; rather, they believe a herpesvirus is the primary cause.

In December 1994, Yuan Chang and colleagues reported that they found DNA sequences that appear to represent a *new human herpesvirus (HHV-8)* in KS tissue. Evidence continues to

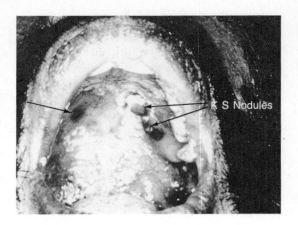

FIGURE 6-9 Oral Kaposi's Sarcoma. KS can be seen on the hard palate and down the sides of the oral cavity. *(Courtesy of Nicholas J. Fiumara, M.D., Boston.)*

accumulate indicating that HHV-8 is the infectious agent responsible for KS (Kledal et al., 1997; Said et al., 1997).

Many research papers on whether herpesvirus 8 causes KS have been published in recognized scientific/medical journals. It appears there is a cause-and-effect relationship; HHV-8/KS.

The work of Charles Rinaldo and colleagues (2001) reveals that healthy non–HIV-infected people who carry HHV-8 have a healthy immune response and control the virus. HIV-infected persons who carry HHV-8 have a poor immune response to the virus, which then becomes a precursor for the expression of KS.

The Kaposi's virus may have entered the same population in which HIV is endemic, which would explain why the two are often transmitted together. HIV may produce the right conditions for Kaposi's development by causing growth factor production, and possibly by suppressing the body's immune defenses against cancer.

Lymphoma (lim-fo-mah): Cancer of the Lymph Glands

Lymphomas are the second most common cancer in HIV and are now the seventh most common cause of death for people with AIDS. A lymphoma is a neoplastic disorder (cancer) of the

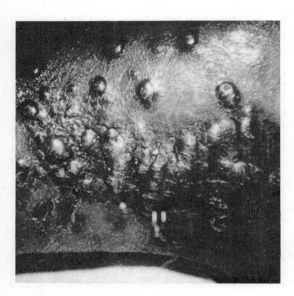

FIGURE 6-8 Kaposi's Sarcoma on Lower Leg of an AIDS Patient. *(Courtesy of Nicholas J. Fiumara, M.D., Boston.)*

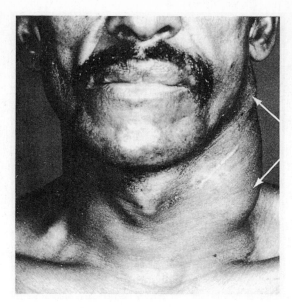

FIGURE 6-10 HIV/AIDS Patient Demonstrating a Lymphoma of the Neck. *(Courtesy of the Centers for Disease Control and Prevention, Atlanta.)*

lymphoid tissue (Figure 6-10). B cell lymphoma occurs in about 1% of HIV-infected people, but makes up about 90% to 95% of all lymphomas found in people with HIV disease (Herndier et al., 1994; Scadden, 2002). Although it occurs most often in those demonstrating persistent generalized lymphadenopathy (swollen lymph glands), the usual site of lymphoma growth is in the brain, the heart, or the anorectal area. The most common signs and symptoms are confusion, lethargy, and memory loss. Lymphomas are increasing in incidence primarily due to the extension of the life span of AIDS patients because of medical therapy (Tables 6-1 and 6-2).

AIDS-Related Lymphomas (ARL)

AIDS-related lymphomas (ARL) are a heterogeneous group of aggressive non-Hodgkin's lymphomas occurring 60-fold more frequently in HIV-infected individuals than in the non–HIV-infected population. ARL shortens life more than any other commonly occurring cancer in HIV infection. Some changes in the distribution and outcome of ARL have been documented since the advent of HAART. These changes vary among the various forms of ARL. While the incidence of ARL in HIV infection has decreased overall since the beginning of HAART in 1995, there has been no change within any patient grouping defined by CD4+ T cell counts.

Non-Hodgkin's Lymphoma

The risk of non-Hodgkin's lymphoma (NHL, also referred to as AIDS-related lymphoma) is substantially increased in the HIV-infected population, with risks ranging from about 100 to 200 times that of the general population. Many agree that the risk of developing NHL increases with lower CD4+ T cell counts and further progression of HIV infection. Moreover, NHL is more prevalent in HIV-positive women than in high-risk HIV-negative women, indicating that immunosuppression, rather than other risk factors, is associated with the increased incidence of NHL in the HIV-positive community. No definitive conclusions can be drawn regarding the effect of HAART on the incidence of NHL, although it continues to be one of the most common malignancies afflicting those with HIV infection.

Progressive Multifocal Leucoencephalopathy (*leuco* means white; *encephalo* means brain; *pathy* means disease)

Progressive multifocal leucoencephalopathy (PML) is an opportunistic infection caused by a papovavirus (Jamestown Canyon virus [JCV]) affecting about 5% of AIDS patients. It is usually fatal within an average of 3.5 months, and there is no treatment. In a few patients spontaneous improvement and prolonged survival have been reported. Some observations have indicated that cytosine arabinoside, a potent antiviral, may reverse the symptoms of PML. Symptoms of PML include altered mental status, speech and visual disturbances, gait difficulty, and limb incoordination (Guarino et al., 1995).

Invasive Cervical Cancer

Though invasive cervical cancer (ICC) is considered an AIDS-defining condition, the association between HIV and cervical cancer is somewhat inconsistent. Some analyses report no increase in incidence that is coincident with the AIDS epidemic and no correlation between immunosuppression and increased risk of developing the cancer. Indeed, HIV-positive women with ICC tend to have higher CD4 T cell counts than HIV-positive patients with other malignancies. Still, other studies report that HIV-positive women are approximately five to nine times more likely to have ICC than are seronegative women, and this cancer accounts for 55% of AIDS-related malignancies in some settings. Moreover, the clinical course becomes even more aggressive when CD4 T cell count is low. Decreased CD4+ cell counts are associated with an increased risk of becoming infected with the human papillomavirus (HPV). HPV is associated with almost all cases of cervical cancer, and women who are HIV infected are even more likely to be coinfected with HPV. The use of HAART does not appear to affect the incidence of ICC.

Human Papillomavirus (HPV)

HPV infects about 6 million people in the United States annually and is spread mainly through sexual contact. There are over 100 viruses known as human papillomavirus (HPV). They are common. One study found HPV in 77% of HIV-positive women. HPV is transmitted easily during sexual activity. It is estimated that 75% of all sexually active people between ages 15 and 49 get at least one type of HPV infection. Some types of HPV cause common warts of the hands or feet. Several types of HPV cause genital warts on the penis, vagina, and rectum. (See Figure 8-10a, b, page 225.) Those with HIV can get worse sores in the rectum and cervical areas. HPV can also cause problems in the mouth or on the tongue or lips. Other types of HPV can cause abnormal cell growth known as dysplasia. Dysplasia can develop into anal cancer in men and women, or cervical cancer, or cancer of the penis.

Summary for HIV and Cancers

The cancer prognosis for people infected with HIV tends to be worse compared to seronegative cancer patients regardless of the type of cancer (Table 6-2). Perhaps because of a suppressed immune system and impaired immune surveillance, cancers take a more aggressive clinical course in those infected with HIV. HIV-positive patients typically present with more advanced cancer at the time of diagnosis, and the average age of diagnosis is usually younger in HIV-positive patients compared to seronegative patients; this is particularly true with lung and testicular cancers.

The Impact of ART

Preliminary data suggest that with the exception of KS, ART has not had a significant impact on cancer incidence in the HIV-positive population, although it may be premature to draw any definitive conclusions at this time. Widespread availability of ART has only occurred within the last 17 years, and many of the cancers discussed require many years to develop.

While the goal of antiretroviral therapy is the suppression of HIV replication, failure to accomplish this objective is common in clinical practice. Also, data suggest that the continuing efficacy of present antiretroviral therapy may allow more HIV-infected patients to survive with long-term mild to moderate immunosuppression, thereby placing such patients at risk for the development of lymphoproliferative disorders such as Hodgkin's and non-Hodgkin's lymphomas. Indeed, recent data suggest that 23% to 50% of patients receiving ART developed Hodgkin's and non-Hodgkin's lymphomas despite effective HIV suppression and high CD4 T cell counts. These results substantiate the idea that the development of lymphomas in HIV-infected individuals is a complex process.

HIV Provirus: A Cancer Connection

In early 1994 AIDS investigators reported that HIV, on entering lymph cell DNA, activated nearby cancer-causing genes (oncogenes). The evidence suggests that HIV itself may trigger cancer in an otherwise normal cell.

These findings may mean that a variety of retroviruses that infect humans may also cause cancer (McGrath et al., 1994). Such findings raise concerns for developing an HIV vaccine. Using a weakened strain of HIV to make the vaccine may, when used, increase the incidence of lymphoma and other cancers.

DISCLAIMER

This chapter is designed to present information on opportunistic infections in HIV/AIDS patients. The author does not accept any responsibility for the accuracy of the information or the consequences arising from the application, use, or misuse of any of the information contained herein, including any injury and/or damage to any person or property as a matter of product liability, negligence, or otherwise. No warranty, expressed or implied, is made in regard to the contents of this material. This material is not intended as a guide to self-medication. The reader is advised to discuss the information provided here with a doctor, pharmacist, nurse, or other authorized healthcare practitioner and to check product information (including package inserts) regarding dosage, precautions, warnings, interactions, and contraindications before administering any drug, herb, or supplement discussed herein.

Summary

There was a time when living with HIV meant having to dodge one opportunistic infection (OI) after another. In the absence of potent and durable HIV therapy, it was not a question of when, but rather, which OI would put you down.

One of the gravest consequences of HIV infection is the immunosuppression caused by the depletion of the T4 or CD4+ helper cell population; suppressed immune systems allow for the expression of opportunistic diseases and cancers. The OI, end organ failures, and cancers kill AIDS patients, not HIV per se. It is the cumulative effect of several OIs that creates the chills, night sweats, fever, weight loss, anorexia, pain, and neurological problems.

KS is characterized as a cancer that can spread to all parts of an AIDS patient's body. About 20% of AIDS patients, mostly gay men, have KS. It is not usually found in hemophiliacs, injection-drug users, or female AIDS patients.

OIs are no longer the plague on top of the plague that they once were, at least in the United States and other places where ART is widely available. That means that the people most at risk for serious OIs are those unaware of their HIV infection, those without access to or not ready to start antiretroviral therapy, and those who are not able to adhere to HIV treatment. In addition, there are the people who are veterans of the HIV battle and have exhausted all treatment options or whose CD4 cell counts remain stuck below 200 even though their HV is controlled.

Despite the dramatic declines in the incidence of opportunistic infections (OIs) in the United States, they remain an important cause of morbidity and mortality for HIV-infected persons. Previously separate guidelines on the prevention and treatment of OIs have recently been combined into an updated single document (Brooks et al., 2009).

Review Questions

(Answers to the Review Questions are on page 463.)

1. Define opportunistic infection (OI).

2. Which OI organism expresses itself in 80% of AIDS patients? Where is it located and what does it cause?

3. Which of the protozoal OI organisms causes weight loss, watery diarrhea, and severe abdominal pain?

4. Which of the bacterial OIs causes "wasting syndrome," night sweats, anorexia, and fever?

5. True or False: Kaposi's sarcoma (KS) is caused by HIV. Explain.

6. Name the two kinds of KS.

7. True or False: KS affects all AIDS patients equally. Explain.

8. True or False: Candidiasis and ulceration may be present in patients with HIV infection.

9. True or False: Oral candidiasis occurs frequently with HIV infection.

10. True or False: The use of combination anti-HIV drug therapy, especially those combinations containing a protease inhibitor, have substantially decreased the severity and number of OIs in AIDS patients.

A Profile of Biological Indicators for HIV Disease, Progression to AIDS, and Hope

CHAPTER HIGHLIGHTS

- What is known and what is missing from our understanding of HIV/AIDS.
- Why all the fuss about HIV/AIDS?
- Clinical signs and symptoms of HIV infection and AIDS are presented.
- Stages of HIV disease vary substantially.
- HIV fitness, its ability to replicate.
- HIV replication is rapid and continuous in HIV-infected lymphoid cells.
- The relationship of HIV to inflammation, heart attacks, strokes, etc.
- AIDS Dementia Complex and other neurological impairments.
- Viral load indicates current viral activity.
- T4 or CD4+ cell counts indicate degree of immunologic destruction.
- Information on long-term survival is presented.
- Serological changes after HIV infection are presented.
- The rate of clinical HIV disease progression is variable among individuals infected with HIV.
- The development of AIDS over time is discussed.
- Elite controllers and long-term survivors, with and without drug therapy. **Updated 2012.**
- Classification of HIV/AIDS progression is presented.
- Clinical indicators to track HIV disease progression are listed.
- Diarrhea is the most common gastrointestinal sign and symptom of HIV/AIDS infection.
- Humanized mice may become a model animal system in which to study the pathology of HIV/AIDS.
- Clues to pediatric AIDS diagnosis are presented.
- See the Interactive HIV/AIDS Map produced by Emory University, Rollins School of Public Health (AIDSVu.org).

I WILL SHARE WITH YOU MY DESIRES
BUT NOT MY DISEASE
I WILL SHARE WITH YOU MY DREAMS
BUT NOT MY ISOLATION.

–Author Unknown

THE PREDICTION

In 2010, the United States Office of National AIDS Policy said, "The United States will become a place where new HIV infections are rare, and when they do occur, every person, regardless of age, gender, race/ethnicity, sexual orientation, gender identity, or socio-economic circumstance will have unfettered access to high-quality, life-saving care, free from stigma and discrimination."

HIV has the vexing capacity to do the right thing for itself and the wrong thing for those it infects.

WHAT IS KNOWN AND WHAT IS MISSING FROM OUR UNDERSTANDING OF HIV/AIDS: THE NEW CRISIS

Scientists know more about HIV than any other virus known to humans—yet one of the most important unanswered questions about HIV remains: How does HIV actually cause immune damage? What is the exact mechanism that makes HIV harmful to humans? To date, scientists say that HIV infects susceptible CD4+ cells, and

POINT OF VIEW 7.1

HIV/AIDS: A NEW FIRST IMPRESSION APPEARED ON HUFFINGTONPOST.COM. IT IS BEING CROSS POSTED HERE WITH MINOR EDITS.

IF ONLY HIV/AIDS HAD MADE A DIFFERENT IMPRESSION!

I wonder where we'd be right now if those first few cases of AIDS had been found in straight white guys. If the disease hadn't been initially referred to as "gay cancer" or GRID (gay-related immunodeficiency disease). If HIV/AIDS hadn't been associated from the start with lifestyle, rather than biology. Here we are, entering the fourth decade of HIV in our lives. And much of our country, the world still thinks HIV/AIDS is not so much a viral disease as it is the inevitable result of a bad decision. Never mind that about half of all people in the United States who become infected with HIV are heterosexual and that most people who get it are not injection drug users. Or that it whittles away the immune system in the same manner regardless of a person's sex, gender, race, age, education level, wealth, geographic location or the manner in which the person was infected. It's always the first impression that matters. And that first impression was that HIV/AIDS was something sinners got for doing things they shouldn't: having sex with men, using drugs, acts of which God does not approve. That first impression persists to this day. It's a twisted, tightened, pulsing knot of assumption, judgment, fear and moral superiority, and it lies at the core of our society's willful ignorance of HIV ("surely, I'm too pure for HIV/AIDS to affect me") and intolerance of those who have it. Well, except for HIV/AIDS children. They win our pity, since they're innocent, powerless victims. HIV/AIDS prevention specialists talk, talk, and talk, within the HIV/AIDS field about how to stem the tide of new infections. A tide, incidentally, that has flooded the United States steadily for years, so that now more than 1.5 million Americans are living with HIV and about

60,000 more join the ranks each year. Among the hardest hit groups? African American women and people living in the rural South. Some talk about the need for universal, routine HIV testing; some talk about the need for worldwide access to HIV treatment; some talk about the need for wealthy countries, such as the United States, to pump more money into the fight against HIV/AIDS. All of these are valiant ideas. And all of them are futile if we can't find a way to reteach our communities about what HIV is, who gets it, and why having it doesn't make you a bad person. Because you're not going to get tested if you're afraid of how your family, your friends, your boss, your religion, or your community will treat you if the test is positive. And you're not going to get treatment if you haven't been tested. And all the HIV funding in the world won't help you if you die in silence. In our culture today, if you have syphilis, gonorrhea, or chlamydia, you're a regular person with an infection. If you have HIV, you're a deviant. To beat this pandemic, each of us needs to sweep away that mistaken first impression and create a new one. We need to understand that living with HIV/AIDS is something to respect—not fear, or loathe, not revile, not discriminate against. HIV is a virus. People get it. It usually happens through sex, via needles, or during childbirth, just like a lot of other diseases. (And decidedly not, by the way, through spitting, sharing sandwiches, or shaking hands.) HIV can't be cured, and it's dangerous. But it can be prevented, it can be treated, and the pandemic can be stopped. Provided we each stop instinctively judging those who live with it, and instead start learning more about it. You can find this article online by typing this address into your web browser: http://www.thebody.com/content/art58529.html.

when those cells die off to where there is an insufficient number of CD4 cells remaining, the infected person becomes ill. The person then progresses to having AIDS and dies (unless put on ART). However, this is not the whole story. Bits and pieces of information, while themselves insufficient to complete the complex picture of HIV, do suggest that inflammation caused by HIV-induced inflammatory substances somehow causes other uninfected cells to die.

HIV-Induced Body-wide Inflammation

Inflammation is a process by which the body's white blood cells and chemicals protect us from infection and foreign substances such as bacteria and viruses. In some diseases, however, the body's defense system (immune system) inappropriately triggers an inflammatory response when there are no foreign substances to fight off. In these diseases, called autoimmune diseases, the body's normally protective immune system causes damage to its own tissues. The body responds as if normal tissues are affected or somehow abnormal.

Previously, it was assumed that the higher the CD4 count, the greater the level of protection. When CD4 counts were high, the risk for AIDS-defining opportunistic infections and other diseases was thought to be lowered, perhaps even nonexistent. However, serious conditions like heart, liver, and kidney disease in people with higher CD4 counts are occurring. Also occurring are more deaths in people whose CD4 counts are near 300. It appears that during the period of latency HIV is not silent, that CD4 levels may not indicate what is happening inside the body, and that inflammation may be affecting many organ systems. So the question is, how is this happening? To answer this, one can look at the SMART study, one of the first to reveal this effect. In this study, people who stopped their antiretroviral drugs when their CD4 count rose to about 350 had higher rates of AIDS-defining opportunistic infections and non-AIDS conditions, as compared with those who stayed on HIV drug therapy. They had higher amounts of virus in their blood, and those higher levels were associated with inflammation. In short, ongoing inflammation is associated with many chronic diseases. These include heart failure, kidney problems, diabetes, dementia, and frailty. HIV is a chronic infection. Even patients with an undetectable viral load make new virus. This may contribute to continuing inflammation. Antiretroviral medications reduce inflammation, but not to normal levels. Over time, HIV weakens the immune system. Old infections may come back. Almost everyone with HIV is also infected with cytomegalovirus (CMV). Latent CMV infection can become active in people with HIV, causing inflammation. Other infections or illnesses, like hepatitis, herpes, or many of the other infections that occur in the HIV infected may also be causing chronic inflammation.

It is known that untreated HIV increases inflammation in the body, and inflammation can result in heart attacks and stroke. HIV can increase the blood's ability to clot. HIV also causes premature aging and affects bone loss, type 2 diabetes, arthritis, and other metabolic events. For example, untreated HIV can affect lipid levels, distorting the body's fatty deposits, causing associated lipid disorders (see Figures 4-10 and 4-11, page 98). These HIV-associated attacks show that CD4+ counts and viral loads are not the only things that must be considered with regard to HIV. Something else is going on that scientists are not measuring. There are just too many unknowns remaining to believe we can readily conquer HIV/AIDS any time soon without a vaccine. Perhaps scientists need to understand more about how currently used antiretrovirals actually decrease some of that inflammation, how some of them may actually increase some of that inflammation, and how we can use our present drugs to better treat HIV infection, based on a true understanding of how the virus does its damage to the human body. (See Point of View 7.2, page 158.)

This chapter reveals some of what is known about the biological and medical signs and symptoms of this disease.

HIV DISEASE DEFINED

The diagnosis of AIDS in the 1980s was most often associated with a quick death. Mortality came quickly and was inevitable within a few months of the diagnosis. It was at the time, and still is, one of the few terminal diseases that elicits the question, *"How did you get it?"*

By the mid-1980s the CDC had learned enough about HIV infection to call it a disease. That made sense, as the vast majority of those who became infected became ill. HIV infection leads to the loss of T4 or CD4+ cells, which in turn produces a variety of signs and symptoms of a **nonspecific disease** with initial acute fever-associated illness or mononucleosis-like symptoms that may last up to four weeks or longer. After the initial symptoms, most individuals enter a clinically asymptomatic phase. (See Case in Point 7.1, below.) This means the infected person feels well while his or her immune system is slowly compromised. It has been shown that long-lasting symptomatic *primary* HIV infection predicts an increased risk of rapid development of HIV-related symptoms and AIDS, but it is not known whether the different responses to HIV infection are caused by viral factors, host factors, or both. Virulent (extremely infectious) strains of HIV have been characterized by their rapid replication,

syncytium (sin-sish-e-um) **inducing (SI)**— that is cell-fusing—capacity, and tropism (attraction) for various types of T cells. It is known that the biological properties of HIV strains in asymptomatic HIV-infected individuals with normal T4 or CD4+ cell counts may predict the subsequent development of HIV-related disease, and that patients who harbor SI isolates develop immune deficiency more rapidly. It is not clear whether the appearance of more virulent strains during the symptomatic phase of the infection is a cause or an effect of progressive imune deficiency (Nielson et al., 1993). Several studies have demonstrated that a long period of fever around the time of **sero-conversion** (the presence of detectable HIV antibody in the serum) is associated with more rapid development of immune deficiency (Pedersen et al., 1989).

Spectrum of HIV Disease

Because the immune system slowly falters, HIV disease is really a spectrum of disease (Figure 7-1, page 159). At one end of the spectrum are those infected with HIV who look, feel, and are perfectly healthy. At the opposite end are those with advanced HIV disease **(symptomatic AIDS)** who are visibly sick and require significant medical and psychosocial support. Between these two extremes, HIV-infected people may develop

---

CASE IN POINT 7.1

VARIATION OF INITIAL SYMPTOMS AFTER HIV INFECTION

Case I: Male, Age 35, Los Angeles, California

One evening, for no apparent reason, John began sweating profusely. Soon after, a red rash began on his arms, face, and legs and then covered his body. Simultaneously, breathing became difficult and he was rushed to an emergency room. By then he was shaking violently. After medication and a battery of tests his problem could not be defined. This brief illness passed, but some years later, during a blood screen for insurance purposes he came up HIV positive. He immediately reflected back on his earlier illness and its cause.

Case II: Male, Age 29, Los Angeles, California

This case is in marked contrast to Case I. Feeling the pinch of a sore throat, this male went to his physician for an antibiotic. On examination, he had a yeast infection that appeared far back in his throat. This raised suspicion and he agreed to an HIV test. It came back positive. He had no other illness. He was treated, the sore throat vanished, and he is thriving in a long asymptomatic period.

WHY ALL THE FUSS ABOUT HIV/AIDS?

Why has the U.S. federal government will have spent over $400 billion over the past 26 years (1987–2013) on just this one disease? More money has been spent on HIV/AIDS in its relatively short history than on any other human disease in our history. In addition, the public/private sector has spent a sum equal to or greater than the government over the same time period. (See Chapter 14, pages 439–455 for a breakdown of the billions of dollars spent on this disease.)

First, over the past years, HIV/AIDS has been killing about 2.5 million people each year worldwide. Through 2013, an estimated 30 million people will have died of AIDS worldwide. Malaria, TB, heart disease, cancer—no other disease is spreading or growing at this rate. Finally, HIV/AIDS campaigns in most countries are showing evidence of a slowdown in the spread of the epidemic. However, by the end of 2013, about 68 million people are expected to have been infected by HIV.

Second, this virus is mainly transmitted during sexual intercourse. Since few human societies talk openly and honestly about sex, this makes this disease difficult to discuss; and since sex is a very private activity, it makes the transmission of HIV very difficult to control.

Third, HIV has an extraordinary capacity for change and rapid global spread.

Fourth, there is a long asymptomatic period between infection and illness. On average, without ART, it takes about 10 to 12 years for someone infected with HIV to develop AIDS. During this time, HIV-infected people will show few if any recognizable symptoms, but they will be able to infect other people. This long asymptomatic period is rare in human infectious disease. People dying today represent those infected 10 to 20 years ago; the results of anything we do now to reduce transmission may not be apparent for years.

Fifth, HIV/AIDS has greater social repercussions than many of the more common diseases because of the age groups it attacks. Some diseases—measles and diarrhea, for example—affect mainly infants and children; others, such as heart disease and cancer, affect mainly the old. But because HIV is predominantly transmitted sexually, HIV/AIDS mainly kills people in their twenties through forties. A major increase in deaths among these age groups, society's most productive groups, has a much greater impact socially and economically than deaths that occur among children or old people would have.

Sixth, in the past, plagues were often marked by their lack of discrimination, by the way in which they killed large numbers of people with little regard for race, wealth, sex, or religion. But AIDS was different from the beginning. It immediately presented a political as much as a public health problem. Homosexuals, who until the pandemic had been mostly closeted in the United States, were suddenly at the heart of a health crisis as profound as any in modern American history.

Seventh, with respect to therapy, HIV disease/AIDS requires the use of some of the most expensive and toxic drugs in medical history.

Eighth, it is a disease that has severely stigmatized those who have it.

Ninth, it is a disease that has parents burying their children.

Tenth, this virus means there are other viruses in waiting. This has awakened our most primal fear; dying a horrible death by an unknown agent. Examples include the West Nile encephalitis virus that struck the New York City metropolitan area in the summer and fall of 1999, the SARS virus that struck in 2003, the avian flu virus that began its global spread in 2005, and a strain of the flu virus, H1N1, that began in the United States in 2009.

So why all the fuss about HIV/AIDS? It is caused by a unique virus that changes itself faster than a rumor making the gossip column of a tabloid. It is lethal, it is transmitted most often sexually, it affects people in their reproductive and most productive years, it is exceptionally expensive to treat, it defies our best scientists who are working to create a vaccine for preventing infection and transmission, and it is a disease that has severely stigmatized those who have it.

HIV has one requirement to continue its presence on earth: a human host!

illnesses, for example, opportunistic infections, that range from mild to serious. Symptoms can include persistent fevers, chronic fatigue, diarrhea, swollen lymph nodes, night sweats, skin rashes, significant weight loss, visual problems, chest pain, and fungal infections of the mouth, throat, and vagina. Illness from these conditions can be severe and disabling, and some people may die without ever being diagnosed with AIDS. Also, people with HIV disease may develop neurologic

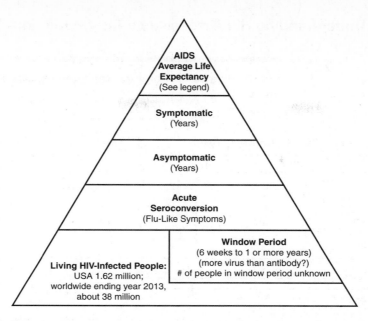

FIGURE 7-1 The HIV/AIDS Pyramid. This figure demonstrates that current AIDS cases are coming from an existing pool of HIV-infected persons. In the United States, of those infected, about 21% do not yet know they are HIV positive. Although both the asymptomatic and symptomatic periods may last for years, once a person is diagnosed with AIDS, the average life expectancy without AIDS drug cocktails is two to three years. Life expectancy for those now on combination drug cocktails depends on the state of the individual's immune system and response to antiretroviral therapy.

disorders, which can cause forgetfulness, memory loss, loss of coordination and balance, partial paralysis, leg weakness, mood changes, and dementia. These symptoms may occur in the absence of any other symptoms. The interval between initial HIV infection and the presence of signs and symptoms that characterize AIDS is variable and may range, in those who have not used antiretroviral drugs, from several months to a median duration of about 11 years (Figure 7-2, page 160).

Defining Eclipse, Incubation, and Latency

Eclipse Phase—Following transmission of HIV there is a period of about 10 days, known as the **eclipse phase,** before HV RNA becomes detectable in the plasma. Single-genome amplification and sequencing of the first detectable virus has shown that about 80% of mucosally transmitted HIV clades B and C infections are initiated by a single virus. Infectious molecular clones derived from these primary founder viruses could infect CD4 T cells with greater efficiency than they could infect monocytes and macrophages, which differs from the virus quasispecies (pools of genetically distinct HIV that evolved from the initial HIV that caused the infection) that arise later in the infection and can infect lymphoid and myeloid cell types with equal efficiency. Studies in rhesus macaques inoculated intrarectally with a complex SIV quasispecies also showed that productive infection arises from a single infecting virus, which supports the use of SIV infection of rhesus macaques as a model for HIV transmission and vaccine studies. In other studies in which macaques were infected experimentally, the first cells to be infected in the vaginal mucosa were found in a place of resident memory T cells that expressed the virus receptors CD4 and

Understanding HIV Disease as a Continuum to AIDS

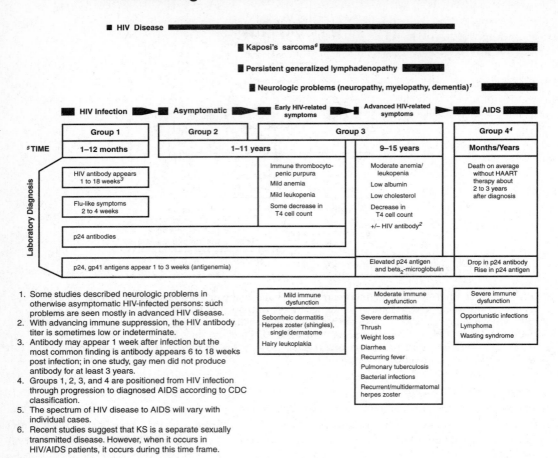

1. Some studies described neurologic problems in otherwise asymptomatic HIV-infected persons: such problems are seen mostly in advanced HIV disease.
2. With advancing immune suppression, the HIV antibody titer is sometimes low or indeterminate.
3. Antibody may appear 1 week after infection but the most common finding is antibody appears 6 to 18 weeks post infection; in one study, gay men did not produce antibody for at least 3 years.
4. Groups 1, 2, 3, and 4 are positioned from HIV infection through progression to diagnosed AIDS according to CDC classification.
5. The spectrum of HIV disease to AIDS will vary with individual cases.
6. Recent studies suggest that KS is a separate sexually transmitted disease. However, when it occurs in HIV/AIDS patients, it occurs during this time frame.

FIGURE 7–2 Adult/Adolescent Spectrum of HIV Infection, Disease, and the Expression of AIDS, no therapy involved. Seroconversion means that HIV antibodies are measurably present in the person's serum. With continued depletion of T4 or CD4+ cells, signs and symptoms appear, announcing the progression of HIV disease to AIDS. Although HIV antibodies have been found as early as 1 week after exposure, **most often seroconversion occurs between weeks 6 and 18; 95% within 3 months, 99% within 6 months** (see Figure 7–4). The level of an individual's infectiousness is believed to be greatest within the first months after infection and again when the T4 cell count drops below 200. **However, people who are HIV-infected can transmit HIV at any time.**

CC-chemokine receptor 5 (CCR5), which is consistent with the cell tropism of the cloned HIV founder virus. Homogeneity of the founder virus indicates that the established infection probably arises in a single location of infected mucosal CD4 T cells. Virus replication at this location might be supported by early innate immune responses that lead to the recruitment of additional susceptible T cells to the site (McMichael, et al., 2010).

Incubation and Latency—Because of the long delay in determining what happened after HIV infection and progression to AIDS, the terms **incubation** and **latency** are used, in many cases interchangeably, causing some confusion. In this chapter, the two terms are used with respect to *clinical* observations as follows: **Clinical incubation** is that period after infection through the window period or when anti-HIV antibody production is measurable. **Clinical latency** is the time period from detectable anti-HIV antibody production (seroconversion—the person now tests HIV-antibody positive) through the asymptomatic period—a time prior to the expression of opportunistic diseases. This time period, being asymptomatic and not on ART, may last from 1 to 22 years—the average being about 11 years. The beginning and end of these periods will vary from person to person and their susceptibility and expression of HIV disease and whether they begin drug therapy.

STAGES OF HIV DISEASE (WITHOUT DRUG THERAPY)

The course of the disease in the infected individual varies substantially. At the extremes are individuals who show either little evidence of progression (loss in T4 cells) 10 to 30 years following infection (about .3%) or extremely rapid progression and death within less than two to three years. In general, HIV-infected adults experience a variety of conditions, categorized into four stages: *acute infection, asymptomatic, chronic symptomatic,* and *AIDS.* (See Side Issue 7.1, page 163.)

Primary HIV Infection (PHI) or the Acute Infection Stage

The clinical syndrome of primary HIV infection was recognized and documented in 1985, about two years after the initial identification of the causative agent of AIDS. By 1991 it was known that this symptomatic period is associated with an explosive replication of the virus, which is then partially controlled as the external illness resolves spontaneously. Reports in 1993 further showed the population of HIV during this early period of infection to be quite homogeneous, in distinct contrast to the diverse quasispecies (mixture of HIV RNA strands) that are typically found in chronically

infected persons. The course and time frame of the infection are illustrated graphically in Figure 7-2, page 160. The course of primary HIV infection (PHI) is limited to a few weeks or months, whereas the entire course of HIV infection can span many years. Specifically, PHI is the period after infection with HIV but before the development of detectable antibodies or seroconversion (see Figure 7-3, page 164).

The acute stage usually develops in two to eight weeks during PHI. Up to 70% of infected individuals develop a self-limited (brief) illness similar to influenza or mononucleosis: high spiking fever, sore throat, headaches, and swollen lymph nodes. Some may develop a rash, vomiting, diarrhea, and thrush (yeast infection in the mouth). This is referred to as the **acute retroviral syndrome.** The symptoms generally last about one to four weeks and resolve spontaneously. The acute stage can be over quickly and easily missed. The acute phase is marked by high levels of HIV production, of 1 to 10 million copies per milliliter of blood. (Recall that only about 2% of all HIV is found in the blood.) During this phase, large numbers of HIV spread throughout the body, seeding themselves in various organs, particularly the gut and lymphoid tissues such as the lymph nodes, spleen, tonsils, and adenoids (Figure 7-3). During this time frame, HIV infects monocytes, macro-phage, T4 or CD4+ cells, and follicular dendritic cells. Within these safe havens, or reservoirs, HIV can persist for years despite Highly Active Antiretroviral Therapy (HAART). This pool of latently infected cells (cells that are not replicating their DNA) is established very early after HIV enters the body—even if the person takes drug therapy immediately after exposure to HIV.

Window of Infectivity

During acute primary infection, patients have extremely high levels of viral replication but a variable antibody immune response. The level of cytotoxic T lymphocytes (CTLs) targeted against HIV appears to increase significantly, an attempt by the cellular part of the immune system to contain the high rate of HIV replication.

SIDEBAR 7.1

DISGRUNTLED HIV PATIENT COMMENTS ON HIS HEALTHCARE PROVIDER

Patient: What kind of virus do I have? Doctor: Who knows? Is it already drug resistant and to which drugs? Don't know but your insurance will only pay for this kind of information once in a blue moon. Does my immune system have a natural ability to fight my virus? Who knows? One cannot readily have tests run to answer that unless they are being studied by the National Institutes of Health. Are my drugs working? Maybe, but we can't always tell for sure, until you lose a big chunk of your immune system. Are my drugs trying to kill me? That depends; how are you feeling today? Can you tell me if my pain is from my liver, gas, or mitochondriosis? We need more information but it is not available. Sorry your 10 minutes are up. And so it goes. Eventually you learn the best emergency rooms to visit in your area and start shopping for a viatical company to buy your life insurance. (Viaticals are discussed in Chapter 4, Point of Information 4.2, pages 97–98.)

Ignorance Prevails—In 2009, a gay male went to a local doctor and asked if he had experience with HIV/AIDS patients. He thought this to be a reasonable question. The doctor looked him and said, "Not if I can help it." Entering 2012, one study revealed that about 5 percent of Los Angeles County dentists refused to treat people who are HIV positive.

Clearly, there are numerous issues reflected in the preceding scenarios. One is that HIV/AIDS is not solely a physiological disease. While it undoubtedly comes with numerous medical challenges, it is also accompanied by a significant number of social and emotional obstacles. These obstacles can be, and often are, both frustrating and psychologically draining for many HIV-infected individuals, especially the recently diagnosed. Dealing with these issues necessitates the support and guidance of a caring and skilled healthcare team. Unfortunately, not all HIV-treating clinicians have the resources—or even the knowledge of their patients' social and emotional troubles—to effectively deal with them.

It is now believed that the increase in the presence of CTLs and chemical factors they produce brings about a milder illness and a reduction in HIV to a *lower set point*—a steady state of viral load. The higher this set point, the more rapidly HIV disease progresses to AIDS. At this time in HIV infection and in some cases for weeks or months, neutralizing antibodies to HIV are not measurable—thus antibody testing, whether at clinical labs or using a home testing kit, is negative. This period of high viral replication in the absence of detectable antibody is called the *window of infectivity before seroconversion, or window period*. During this period, patients may be highly infectious, about 10 times more infectious than in the asymptomatic stage. The viral burden in genital secretion is particularly high during this time. Mathematical models suggest that 56% to 92% of all HIV infections may be transmitted during this period of acute infection (Quinn, 1997; Wainberg, 2007).

A true state of **biological latency,** according to the work of Xiping Wei and coworkers (1995) and David Ho and coworkers (1995), does not exist in the lymph nodes at any time during the course of HIV infection. The Wei and Ho investigations show that from the time of infection HIV replication is rapid and continuous, and within two to four weeks the infecting HIV strain is replaced by drug-resistant mutants. Each day over 1 billion HIV are produced and mostly destroyed and millions of T4 cells are infected, dying, and replaced. Over time the immune system fails to destroy HIV and replace its T4 cell losses and HIV disease progresses. Also, over time, many T4 cells in the lymphoid organs probably are activated by the increased secretion of certain cytokines such as tumor necrosis factor-alpha and interleukin-6. T4 or CD4+ cell activation allows uninfected cells to be more easily infected and causes increased replication of HIV in infected cells. Other components of the immune system are also chronically activated, with negative consequences that may include the suicide of cells by a process known as programmed cell death or apoptosis and an inability of the immune system to respond to other invaders.

The National Institute on Drug Abuse (NIDA), part of the National Institutes of Health, selected David Ho as the 2011 recipient of the NIDA Avant-Garde Award for HIV/AIDS Research. Ho's proposal aims to develop a novel HIV therapy that could be administered monthly for the prevention and treatment of HIV/AIDS in drug abusers. Awardees receive $500,000 per year for five years to support their research. Ho was *Time*

HLABISA, AN AIDS-RAVAGED TOWN IN KWAZULU NATAL PROVINCE

In 1994, 10% of adults in Hlabisa (Sha-BEE-sa) were HIV infected. By 2004, over 30% or 75,000 people were HIV positive.

In the desperately crowded clinics and hospital wards, the scale of the epidemic is clear enough. This district of 250,000 people sits amid the hills of KwaZulu Natal, which has the highest adult rate of HIV infection of any province in South Africa. It is one of the few communities in South Africa in which government researchers have kept statistics on HIV infection rates for over a decade. Its story offers a rare and intimate look at one community ravaged by the plague. It marks the faces of young widows who trudge the road in somber capes and skirts, traditional mourning garb. It inspires the medicine makers who brew slivers of tree bark and bundles of dried leaves into elixirs sold in used Coca-Cola bottles. "Two spoons in the morning, two spoons in the afternoon," advises an herbalist who charges $1.25 a bottle. Chilled bodies that are often stacked one on top of another swamp the morgue.

FEAR, DENIAL, AND GUILT

Professional men in Hlabisa boast over beers about extramarital affairs and the pleasures of unprotected sex. Some church leaders burn condoms and assail people with the virus as sinners. Prominent community members die in silence because the disease is considered so shameful. The disease is so deadly and so frightening that many hospital employees are reluctant to call it by name. They say a patient is immune compromised, or that he suffers from "that disease." Others simply say, "You know what he's got." It is as if uttering the word might infect the tongue.

HEALTHCARE CHOICE: HOSPITAL OR HEALER?
Hospitals

On any given day there are more patients than available beds. In the male ward, 80% of men are HIV positive and about half the nursing positions are vacant. The first event in morning rounds is to count those who died of AIDS or a combination of HIV infection and tuberculosis. Of those who die, about half are under age 30! In the first six months of 2001, of 500 people who took HIV tests, 63% tested positive. One of the staff nurses has six children, four daughters and two sons. She leaves boxes of condoms on their bedroom dressers. The two things that give her the greatest sense of peace are taking her pills and watching those boxes empty. The children do not comment—she watches and replenishes the condom supply as needed.

Healers or Sangomas

In Southern Africa, a sangoma undergoes a long apprenticeship studying plant lore and making diagnoses that can include playing a guessing game with the patient, dancing into a trance, reading cast bones or waiting for the answer to come in a dream. In Hlabisa, physicians believe that virtually all their patients first visit a sangoma—a traditional healer.

Traditional Therapy

Because traditional Zulu medicine focuses chiefly on digestion, bile, and mucus, sangomas often give emetics or enemas. Some are simply dishwashing liquid or toothpaste. But others contain powerful herbs that can cause serious drug interactions. Enemas are used for anything from constipation to hysterical crying. However, enemas can rapidly dehydrate patients and send them into kidney or liver failure. For those who receive herbs causing them to throw up (emetics), it defeats the use of antiretroviral drugs.

magazine's 1996 Man of the Year for his work on HIV replication.

Asymptomatic HIV Disease Stage

Following acute illness, an untreated infected adult can remain free of symptoms from 6 months to a median time of about 11 years. During the asymptomatic period, measurable HIV in the blood drops to a lower level, but it continues to replicate and to destroy T4 cells within the lymph nodes while the body continues to produce new T4 cells and antibodies to fight the virus (Figure 7-4, page 165). An asymptomatic individual appears to be healthy and performs normal activities of daily living. During this period, if untreated, the infected lose about 60 CD4+cells/mm^3 per year.

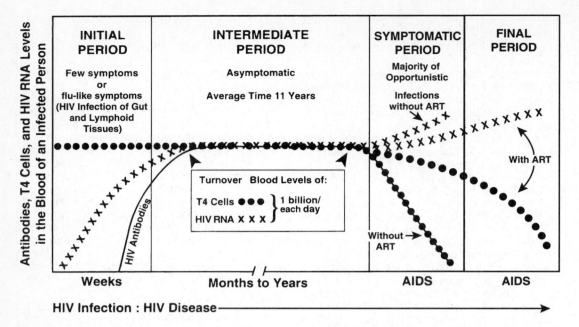

FIGURE 7-3 Relationship of T4 or CD4+ cells, HIV Antibodies, and HIV RNA Levels (Viral Load) Beginning with HIV Infection through AIDS. Within a week to weeks after HIV infection, HIV becomes seeded throughout the body's blood, gut, and lymph system. HIV reproduction (infection of T4 cells) begins almost immediately in the gut and lymph system. The T4 cell population also begins rapid reproduction to replace T4 cell loss. This is why the T4 graph line stays at the same level through the **asymptomatic** period. The immune system begins to turn out HIV antibodies, in general 6 to 18 weeks later (window period, see Figure 7–4). Note that during the asymptomatic period T4 cell and HIV replication and antibody production keep pace. With time, however, T4 cells fail to replace losses, HIV continues to replicate, antibody levels drop due to loss of T4 signals to B cells to produce antibodies, and opportunistic infections begin—the **symptomatic** period. Without therapy this period lasts on average about two to three years. For people using ART, the average number of years one can survive in the symptomatic period, when on drug therapy, is now between 15 and 30 years.

Chronic Symptomatic HIV Disease Stage

The symptomatic phase can last for months or years before a diagnosis of AIDS occurs. During this phase, as viral replication continues, T4 or CD4+ cells drop significantly. As the number of immune system cells declines, the individual develops a variety of symptoms such as fever, weight loss, malaise, pain, fatigue, loss of appetite, abdominal discomfort, diarrhea, night sweats, headaches, and swollen lymph glands. Ultimately, HIV overwhelms the lymphoid organs. The follicular dendritic cell networks break down in late–chronic–stage disease, and virus trapping is impaired, allowing spillover of large quantities of virus into the bloodstream. The destruction of

the lymph node structure seen late in HIV disease may stop a successful immune response against HIV and other pathogens as well. Individuals at this stage, with a T4 cell count of 500 or less/μL of blood, often develop thrush, oral lesions, and other fungal, bacterial, and/or viral infections. The duration of these symptoms varies, but it is common for HIV-infected individuals to have them for months at a time. Of those persons in the symptomatic stage and not using HIV drug therapy, about 30% developed AIDS-associated infections within five years. In most U.S. cities, 30% of people are diagnosed with HIV when their CD4+ count is already below 200. In Washington, D.C., 65% of people are below 200!

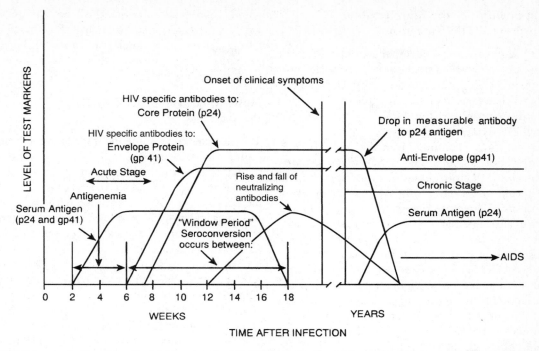

FIGURE 7-4 Profile of Serological Changes after HIV Infection for People Not on ART. The dynamics of antibody response to HIV infection were determined by enzyme immunoassays (EIA). Note that during antigenemia, specific HIV proteins (antigens) can be detected before seroconversion occurs. Perhaps other HIV proteins will allow even earlier detection of HIV infection. Once antibodies appear, some antigens like p24 and gp41 disappear only to show up again later on. Note also that although antibody production is a sign that the immune system is working, in HIV-infected people it is not working well enough. Although envelope and core protein antibodies are being produced as clinical illness begins, as the p24 antibody drops, the illness becomes more serious. *(Adapted from Coulis et al., 1987.)*

Response to ART

The CD4+ count typically begins to increase at four to eight weeks after viral suppression with ART and then increases an additional 50–100 cells/mm³/year in some patients. Normal CD4+ cell counts range between 600 and 1200 cell/mm³.

AIDS: Advanced HIV Disease Stage

The diagnosis of AIDS is a marker, not an end in itself. Currently, most people on ART recover from their first, second, and third AIDS-defining illnesses. People with AIDS are a very heterogeneous group—some feel well and continue working for several years, others are chronically ill, and some die rather quickly.

Patients with AIDS became an even more diverse group after the 1993 expansion of the Centers for Disease Control and Prevention's definition of AIDS. People in excellent health are diagnosed with AIDS if they test HIV positive and their T4 or CD4+ cell count is less than 200/μL of blood.

The final stage of HIV infection is called AIDS. During this time there is continued rapid viral replication that finally upsets the delicate balance of HIV production/T4 cell infection to T4 cell replacement. The virus largely depletes the cells of the immune system. It has been suggested that during the AIDS stage, serious immunodeficiency occurs when HIV diversity exceeds some threshold beyond which the immune system is unable to control HIV replication (Nowak et al., 1990; Wei et al., 1995; Cohen, 1995).

Opportunities for Interventions to Prevent HIV Infection

During the first week of infection, HIV must not only establish a small founder population of infected cells at the portal of entry but also expand that local infection in order to continue to disseminate cell free HIV and HIV-infected cells via lymphatic draining to establish a self-propagating infection. Given the small founder populations documented in SIV mucosal transmission (SIV from rhesus macaque animals) and inferred in HIV transmission, the first week of infection is a time of greatest vulnerability of virus and maximal opportunity for interventions that decrease viral reproductive rate, thereby eliminating infection at the portal of entry. Microbicides, or pre-exposure prophylaxis with antiretroviral drugs such as tenofovir, are in clinical trials to see if preventing viral reproduction at the portal of entry can prevent infection. Mucosal antibodies, ideally broadly neutralizing antibodies, could prevent establishment of the small founder population, as has been shown in rhesus macaques protected with a microbicide containing high concentrations of neutralizing monoclonal antibody. Perhaps even just binding antibodies to HIV could prevent establishment of the small founder population of infected cells and/or its expansion.

Finally the Question—How Long Will I Live; How Long Can an HIV-Infected Person Live?

How Long Will I Live?

This is one of the most pressing, frightening questions people with HIV face, whether they've been newly diagnosed or have been infected for some time. And like so many other questions related to HIV, the answer is frustratingly complex, confusing and ever-changing. How long will you live with HIV? It depends on who you are and where you live. Research suggests that one with HIV dies sooner if, for instance, he or she uses injection drugs, is coinfected with hepatitis, is depressed, or is pretty much any race and sex other than a white male. HIV-positive people in developed countries are likely to live longer than HIV-positive people in resource-poor countries, like those in sub-Saharan Africa or much of Latin America. Regardless, life will be longer if one has consistent access to quality health care.

How Long Can an HIV-Infected Person Live?

The average time someone survives from the moment of HIV infection until death continues to increase. At the beginning of the epidemic, the average time was about 10 years. Many people confuse the date of diagnosis with the date of actual infection. The latter date is most often not known. Many years may separate the dates of infection and diagnosis. For the United States, it currently is estimated at least 25% of persons infected with HIV today, utilizing drugs and treatments available, will survive on average for about 49 years. According to the Antiretroviral Therapy Cohort Collaboration 2008 report, if one lives in a high-income country, is currently age 20, and is on effective drug therapy, one can expect to live, on average, in their early 70s. In contrast, an HIV-negative 20-year-old can expect to live, on average, to about age 80. But averages are exactly that—averages. More precise estimates for individuals depend on current and past HIV RNA levels, current and past T4 or CD4+ cell counts, number of antiretroviral regimens used, adherence to therapy, response to therapy, and current health status. About 5% of HIV-infected persons are estimated to be long-term nonprogressors. That is, in the absence of therapy, these individuals maintain a T4 or CD4+ cell count of about 450 cells per microliter of blood and typically have HIV RNA levels of less than 5000 copies/mL of blood. It is not clear what immunologic features distinguish these individuals from the other 95% of HIV-infected persons. (See Box 7.2, pages 173–174.)

Regardless, thanks to years of HIV health advocacy, better understanding of HIV disease and its complications, and improved antiretroviral treatment regimens, people with HIV now are better able to maintain their health and live longer, even decades longer than they ever expected. For many, living longer with HIV brings new health challenges that positive people, clinicians, and researchers are only just beginning to understand.

Symptoms and Impairment

In the symptomatic stages of HIV disease, an individual's ability to carry on the activities of daily living is impaired. The degree of impairment varies considerably from day to day and week to week. Many individuals are debilitated to the point that it becomes difficult to hold steady employment, shop for food, or do household chores. It is also quite common for people with AIDS to experience phases of intense life-threatening illness and pain, followed by phases of seemingly normal functioning, all in a matter of weeks. For a good review on the mechanisms of HIV disease, read *The Immunopathogenesis of HIV Infection* by Giuseppe Pantaleo et al. (1993), Bucy (1999), and Yu (2000).

HIV Can Be Transmitted During All Four Stages

A person who is HIV-infected, even while feeling healthy, may unknowingly infect others. *The greatest risk of HIV transmission occurs within the acute period, the first several months after infection, and again when the T4 cell count drops below 200.*

HIV DISEASE WITHOUT SYMPTOMS, WITH SYMPTOMS, AND AIDS

Michael is a 31-year-old Hispanic male who complains of fatigue, headache, muscle aches, sore throat, and nausea. Physical assessment demonstrates a skin rash on his trunk and swollen lymph glands. His temperature is 98°F (37°C); other vital signs are within normal limits. Laboratory findings including white blood cell count, platelet count, and blood chemistry are normal. Michael states that his symptoms began one week ago. Subsequent laboratory testing will confirm that Michael has acute retroviral syndrome that accompanies primary HIV infection (PHI). But the odds are high that in almost every emergency room or physician's office in the country, Michael will be misdiagnosed. He is likely to be told that he has a viral infection, probably the flu, and sent home with instructions for supportive care.

A person may have no symptoms (be **asymptomatic**) but test HIV positive. This means that the virus is present in the body. Although he or she has not developed any of the illnesses associated with HIV disease, it is possible to transmit the virus.

In time, most people with HIV disease progress to AIDS. A person has AIDS when the defect in his or her immune system caused by HIV disease has progressed to such a degree that an unusual infection or tumor is present or when the T4 or CD4+ cell count has fallen below 200/μL of blood. In AIDS patients, a number of diseases are known to take advantage of the damaged immune system. These include opportunistic infections and tumors such as Kaposi's sarcoma or lymphoma, a malignancy of the lymph glands. The presence of one of the opportunistic diseases or a T4 cell count of less than 200/μL of blood, along with a positive HIV test, establishes the medical diagnosis of AIDS (see Chapter 1, page 28, Table 1-1). Thus the disease we call AIDS is actually the end stage of HIV disease. It is important to remember that AIDS itself is not transmitted—the virus is. AIDS is the most severe clinical form of HIV disease.

The term "full-blown AIDS" is often used on TV and in the press but not in this textbook. Terms such as advanced HIV disease or advanced AIDS are not only more accurate but also more meaningful.

PRODUCTION OF HIV-SPECIFIC ANTIBODIES

During the 29 years (1983–2012) since the discovery of HIV, scientists have constructed a serological or antibody graph of HIV infection and HIV disease. The graph reveals how soon the body produces HIV-specific antibodies after infection and about when the virus begins its reproduction. Different parts of the graph (Figure 7-4, page 165) have been filled in by Paul Coulis and colleagues (1987), Dani Bolognesi (1989), and Susan Stramer and colleagues (1989). The history of the HIV antibody is not yet complete, but the order of appearance and disappearance of antibodies specific for the serologically important antigens over the course of HIV disease has been described.

Note that Figure 7-4 shows that HIV plasma viremia (the presence of virus in blood plasma) and antigenemia (an-ti-je-ne-mi-ah—the persistence of antigen in the blood) can be detected as early as two weeks after infection. This demonstrates that viremia and antigenemia occur prior to seroconversion. Using HIV proteins produced by recombinant DNA methods (making synthetic copies of the viral proteins), antibodies specific for gp41 (a subunit of glycoprotein 160) are detectable prior to those specific for p24 (a core protein) and persist throughout the course of infection. Levels of antibody specific for p24 rise to detectable levels between six and eight weeks after HIV infection but may disappear abruptly. The drop in p24 antibody has been shown to occur at the same time as a rise in p24 antigen in the serum. This strange phenomenon is thought to be due to the loss of available p24 antibody in immune complexes—too little p24 antibody is being made to handle the new virus being produced. A sudden decrease in anti-p24 is considered by many scientists to be a prognostic indicator that people with HIV disease are moving toward AIDS.

Some AIDS researchers and healthcare professionals believe that 90% to 95% of those persons infected with HIV will eventually develop AIDS. Without antiretroviral drugs, approximately 50% of people with HIV disease will progress to AIDS within 8 years after infection. At 10 years 70% will have developed AIDS. After that, an additional 25% to 45% of the remainder will develop AIDS. (See Point of Information 7.1, page 169.)

Classification of HIV/AIDS Progression

There are several classifications that spell out the progression of signs and symptoms from HIV infection to the diagnosis of AIDS. The classifications were developed to provide a framework for the medical management of patients from the time of infection through the expression of AIDS. All classification systems are fundamentally the same—they group patients according to their stage of infection, based on signs that indicate a failing immune system (Royce et al., 1991).

The most widely accepted classification—because of its greater clinical applicability—comes from the CDC. The CDC classification uses four mutually exclusive groupings (Figure 7-5, page 169). The groupings are based on the presence or absence of signs and symptoms of disease, and clinical and/or laboratory findings and the chronology of their occurrence. (See Box 7.1, page 170 and Snapshot 7.2, page 171.)

PROGNOSTIC BIOLOGICAL MARKERS (BIOMARKERS) RELATED TO AIDS PROGRESSION

Biomarkers are described as anything that can be used as an indicator of a particular disease state.

The ideal marker would be able to predict HIV disease progression, be responsive to antiretroviral therapy, and explain the variance in clinical outcome due to therapy. It is, however, unlikely that any one marker will be able to fulfill all these criteria in HIV infection. Therefore, individual markers used to track HIV infection to AIDS are presented.

p24 Antigen Levels

p24 is a specific protein located in the core or inner layer of HIV. Because the immune system produces antibody against foreign protein, antibody is made against p24. A positive test for p24 antigen in the blood means that HIV production is so rapid that it overcomes the available

IS THE DIAGNOSIS OF AIDS IRREVERSIBLE? THAT IS, NOW YOU HAVE AIDS (THEN TREATMENT), NOW YOU DON'T?

Beginning with the use of combination therapy in 1995/1996, people have questioned the use of the term *AIDS* for people who, through the use of highly active antiretroviral therapy (HAART) returned to non-detectable HIV levels, good health, and CD4+ cell counts above 500 to 1000. The preferred or "normal" range of CD4+ cell counts is between 600 and 1200 per microliter of blood plasma.

The History of AIDS Definitions

The term *AIDS* was coined in 1982 as an epidemiological tool to help us quantify and track the epidemic. HIV had not yet been discovered, so there was no way to know whether someone was sick until they became ill with opportunistic diseases. A person was diagnosed with AIDS if he or she developed one of a number of specific opportunistic infections. These particular illnesses do not occur in people with normal and healthy immune systems. After HIV was discovered in 1983, and a test for HIV became available in 1985, being HIV-antibody positive became part of the new definition of AIDS. In 1993 the CDC changed the AIDS definition again to include people who demonstrated opportunistic infections and had a CD4+ cell count of 200/µL of blood or below.

The Irreversible Diagnosis of AIDS

Once diagnosed with AIDS, a person's carrier status is irreversible (but going from poor health to good health, and vice versa, is reversible!). AIDS is like herpes in this respect: the virus level drops, and the body appears to have gotten rid of the virus, but then it reappears in numbers sufficient to cause symptoms. In addition, even when it appears that the person recovered from the virus in the time between outbreaks, a low level of herpesvirus continues circulating in the body and is only kept in check by the person's immune system. Herpes is for life regardless of treatment. Scientists are searching for a preventive and therapeutic vaccine—a cure for the herpesvirus infection. Now substitute the words *AIDS* and *HIV* for herpes. The scenario is the same. AIDS is for life because HIV remains in the system, and without drug therapy the amount of HIV rises to levels that bring back the symptoms of AIDS.

The Cure Changes the Scenario

If a cure is found for herpes or AIDS, the disease will then be categorized as any other preventable and treatable disease.

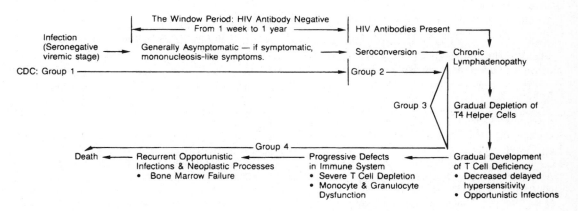

FIGURE 7–5 Clinical History of HIV Infection According to Centers for Disease Control and Prevention Groupings. Seroconversion means that HIV antibodies are measurably present in the person's serum. With continued depletion of T4 cells, various signs and symptoms appear announcing the progression of HIV disease into AIDS. Although HIV antibodies have been found as early as 1 week after exposure, most often seroconversion occurs between weeks 6 and 18 but may not occur for up to 1 year or more.

BOX 7.1

EVOLUTION OF HIV DURING HIV DISEASE PROGRESSION

HIV is a unique retrovirus. For example, mitosis, a form of cell division, is a requirement for the nuclear entry of most retroviral nucleic acids. In contrast, mitosis does not appear to be required for nuclear entry of HIV nucleic acids, particularly in terminally differentiated cells (for example, macrophages and dendritic cells) (Freed et al., 1994). In addition, HIV lacks any mechanism to correct errors that occur as its genetic material is being duplicated, so a few days or weeks after initial infection, there may be a large population of closely related, but not identical, viruses replicating in an infected individual. In the quasi-steady-state condition, there are successive generations of viral progeny, with each generation following the next by about 2.6 days. Approximately 140 generations of virus are produced over the course of a year and 1400 generations over the course of 10 years, allowing production of an extraordinary number of genetic variants or mutants. Some variants can provide preexisting drug-resistant forms or enable rapid development of resistance under drug pressure, and some enable the viral population to escape immune activity.

VIRAL POOL

The viral pool in an HIV-infected person is estimated to be about 10 billion viruses and each is genetically different from all other HIV in the pool. It is known from experimental data that about 1 in 1000 particles is infectious, so the infectious viral pool may be on the order of 10 million viruses. With a genome of approximately 10^4 nucleotides, and from 1 to 10 billion HIV variants made daily, mutations most likely occur at every nucleotide position on a daily basis (Ho, 1996). This creates an enormous potential for viral evolution. On average, the HIV that is transmitted to another individual will be over 1000 generations removed from the initial HIV infection. This extent of replication per transmitted infection (transmission cycle) is probably without equal among viral and perhaps bacterial infections (Coffin, 1995). Regardless of the underlying mechanism of immunodeficiency, it is becoming apparent that the force that is driving the disease is the constant repeated cycles of HIV replication.

LIFE SPAN OF HIV

Alan Perelson and colleagues (1996) reported data collected from five HIV-infected people after administering ritonavir through seven days. Each person responded with a similar pattern of decline in plasma HIV RNA. Their results: Infected T4 cells had an average life span of 2.2 days. Plasma HIV RNA had an average life span of 0.3 days. The results also suggest that the minimum duration of the HIV life cycle in human T4 cells is

1.2 days on average and that the average HIV generation time—defined as the time from release of a virus until it infects another cell and causes the release of a new generation of HIV—is 2.6 days. The lifetime of HIV in resting or latent T4 cells may range from 6 months to perhaps an infinite amount of time. Such cells can produce HIV when activated.

TREATMENT FAILURE

Virologic Failure

Failure to reduce the viral load to an undetectable level *or*
Failure to reduce the viral load by at least 2 to 2.5 $\log_{10}$ *or*
A persistent increase in viral load following a period of adequate suppression

Immunologic Failure

Failure to restore the T4 or CD4+ cell count to more than 200 cells/mm^3 *or*
Failure to significantly increase T4 cell count *or*
A persistent decline in T4 cell count after a period of immune reconstitution

Clinical Failure

Development of new opportunistic infections (OIs) *or*
Failure to resolve pretreatment OI, wasting, or dementia

(Adopted from Soloway et al., 2000.)

With new techniques for quantitating plasma HIV RNA, infected individuals can be evaluated for response to antiretroviral therapy.

THE BATTLE BETWEEN HUMANS AND HIV: MUTANT HIV EVOLVES TO OVERWHELM THE IMMUNE SYSTEM

As HIV multiplies and mutant forms are produced, the immune system responds to these new forms. But ultimately the sheer number of *different* viruses to which the immune system must respond becomes overwhelming. It's a bit like the juggler who tries to keep too many balls in the air: The result is disastrous. Once the immune system is overwhelmed, the latest escape mutant—which may not necessarily be the most pathogenic one to come along—will predominate and immune deficiency will progress. It appears as though HIV is outrunning the human body's potential to defend itself.

Perhaps the battle can best be seen in a statement by Sherri Lewis, an advocate for those with HIV/AIDS. "AIDS is a holocaust. It is a constant tsunami. It is the plane that flies through the World Trade Center every goddamned day."

A UNIVERSITY STUDENT'S MESSAGE TO HER CLASSMATES

"People want to know that you care before they care what you know. . . ."

James F. Hind

Worried about how she could make a difference in her generation's reaching out to help the HIV infected, this student felt that she could help her classmates become involved by raising a sensitive issue and asking them to think deeply about what she had to say. She said, "I asked myself how can I get your attention in a meaningful way? For example, if I were given an assignment to write a message so that all of you would feel differently about this pandemic once I shared it with you, what would I say?" She then went on to tell her classmates that "In writing this message, I would tell people our age to imagine their best friend coming to them and telling them they are HIV positive. Imagine your best friend has just told you that he or she is infected with HIV, that he or she will ultimately progress to AIDS and die. Suddenly, the person who you have grown up with, and whom you confide in for everything will over time become terminally ill with a condition that will cause him or her to visibly suffer. You will watch your best friend wither away, in pain, and there will be nothing you can do to help. Eventually, you will be at the funeral, and the cause of death will be AIDS. If your friend had only been cautious that ONE time, he or she would still be here today. Will you be careful? Will you help stop the spread of HIV?" (See Figure 7-6 a, b and Snapshot 7.3.)

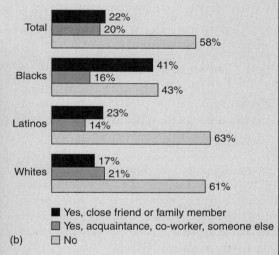

Total
22%
20%
58%

Blacks
41%
16%
43%

Latinos
23%
14%
63%

Whites
17%
21%
61%

■ Yes, close friend or family member
▨ Yes, acquaintance, co-worker, someone else
□ No

(b)

FIGURE 7-6 (b) Percentage of ethnic groups, by age, who say they personally know someone who now has AIDS, has died from AIDS, or has tested positive for HIV. "Kaiser Family Foundation *Survey of Americans on HIV/AIDS,* Part Three—Experiences and Opinions by Race/Ethnicity and Age" (#7140), The Henry J. Kaiser Family Foundation, August 2004. The 2009 and 2012 survey data were not significantly different. The information was reprinted with permission from the Henry J. Kaiser Family Foundation. The Kaiser Family Foundation, a leader in health policy analysis, health journalism and communication, is dedicated to filling the need for trusted, independent information on the biggest health issues facing our nation and its people. The Foundation is a non-profit private operating foundation based in Menlo Park, California.

What Do You Do When Your Best Friend Has AIDS?

(a)

FIGURE 7-6 (a) The Photograph Presents Its Own Message. *(Courtesy of the Centers for Disease Control and Prevention, Atlanta.)*

antibody (Figure 7-4). This raised p24 antigen level condition occurs at least twice: once shortly after infection and again during the AIDS period when the immune system is rapidly deteriorating and unable to produce sufficient antibody to deal with newly produced HIV.

Those who, during the early stage of HIV infection, test p24 antigen positive are likely to progress to AIDS earlier than those who test p24 negative. Thus, a positive p24 test is an early and serious warning sign for HIV-infected people (Escaich et al., 1991; Phillips et al., 1991a).

T4 and T8 Lymphocyte Levels

The most extensive use of data for AIDS progression risk identification involves the number of T4 or CD4+ and T8 or CD8+ cells circulating in the blood (Anderson et al., 1991; Burcham et al., 1991; Phillips et al., 1991b).

T4 cells and the ratio of T4 cells to T8 cells found in the blood have, since 1997, been widely used as prognostic indicators for AIDS progression. T4 cell counts, however, are not ironclad predictors of HIV disease progression. In some cases persons with HIV disease and very low (less than 50 or 100) T4 counts remain healthy; conversely, some HIV-diseased persons have relatively high counts (over 400) and are quite ill. *T4 counts are notoriously fickle*—their counts can vary widely between labs or because of a person's age, the time of day a measurement is taken, and even whether the person smokes (Sax et al., 1995).

Lymph Nodes, the T Cell Zones, T4 or CD4+ Cell Production, and HIV Infection

The T cell zone in the lymph nodes is involved with 98% of the body's T4 or CD4+ cells. It is also where 99% of HIV production occurs. As HIV replication continues it causes inflammation, scarring, and eventual destruction of the T cell zone. Newly produced T4 cells have little room in the scarred T cell zone to divide. If they divide there is a high probability they will become infected. With this new knowledge reported in 2003, researchers now believe they understand why some people respond well to antiretroviral drug therapy and have their T4 cell counts increase while others on drug therapy do not experience T4 cell increase. They believe the increase of T4 cells or lack of it is associated with the amount of T cell zone destruction.

Performing T4 or CD4+ Cell Counts in HIV-Infected People Continues to Be Essential

A major player in the body's immune system is the T4 or CD4+ cell. By binding with CD4+ cells, HIV can kill them and stop the associated production of antibodies, leaving the immune system weakened and vulnerable to opportunistic disease. Doctors gauge the health of the immune system by counting T4 or CD4+ cells. A healthy, HIV-negative adult has between 600 and 1200 CD4+ cells per cubic millimeter of blood. If the count falls below 350, the immune system has become significantly weakened.

BOX 7.2

DEVELOPMENT OF AIDS OVER TIME: RAPID, SLOW, NONPROGRESSORS, AND ELITE CONTROLLERS

HIV INFECTED AND THEIR PROGRESSION TO AIDS WITHOUT ANTIRETROVIRAL THERAPY

A spectrum of clinical expression of disease can occur after HIV infection. Approximately 10% of HIV-infected subjects progress to AIDS within the first two to three years of HIV infection **(rapid progressors).** People with greater than 50,000 HIV RNA copies/mL at six months after infection are the most likely to be rapid progressors. About 60% of adults/adolescents will progress to AIDS within 12 to 13 years after HIV infection **(slow progressors). Long-term nonprogressors (LTNPs)** are a subset of people who remain symptom-free with a CD4+ cell count at or above 500 for at least eight years after their HIV infection. Nonprogressors represent about 1% of HIV-positive individuals worldwide. (There are no internationally agreed upon and standardized definitions of LTNPs.)

To date, the only difference between progressors and LTNPs is that LTNPs have about 20 times more CD8+ cells than progressors. In LTNPs, researchers found that these CD8+ cells increase the production of two HIV-infected-cell-destroying proteins: perforin, which creates pores on the infected cell's surface, causing cell death, and granzyme B, a cytotoxin, a chemical that initiates an infected cell's death. Persons who progress rapidly to AIDS do not contain those CD8+ cells (Migueles et al., 2008). People with AIDS having low T4 cell counts who have survived for five years or more without therapy are usually described as long-term survivors (LTS). Some 6% of persons diagnosed with clinical AIDS are long-term survivors.

THE ELITE AND VIREMIC CONTROLLERS

A subset of HIV positive people do not need ART. They are considered elite.

Elite controllers, as defined by Steve Deeks, University of California at San Francisco, are HIV-positive people who have their viral load at undetectable levels or less than 50 copies of HIV RNA per mL for at least two years without using antiretroviral drugs. Is it possible that some of the elite controllers have eradicated HIV? Studies on this question by Hiroyu Hatano and colleagues (2009) reported that of elite controllers tested for HIV, 98% had plasma measurable HIV-RNA, often at levels higher than those found in people on antiretroviral therapy. But, it's hard to prove a negative. **Viremic controllers** are HIV-positive people whose immune systems have kept the virus under 2000 for at least one year without antiretrovirals. Neither group progresses to AIDS. Researchers believe it is unlikely that elite or viremic controllers can transmit the virus. Bruce Walker,

director of Partners AIDS Research Center at Massachusetts General Hospital, and colleagues initially enrolled 200 elite controllers to find out. The researchers have expanded the initial controller study to a five-year study involving 1000 elite and 1000 viremic controllers, in order to better understand the biological factors involved in controlling HIV in these people.

HIV/AIDS researchers estimate that one in 300 people (0.3%) living with HIV/AIDS worldwide are elite controllers. Clusters of elite controllers, or HIV-exposed seronegatives, have been found. They generally fall into one of three groups: (a) discordant couples (one infected), (b) those with high-risk sexual behaviors, e.g., commercial sex workers and men who have sex with men, and (c) non-sexually exposed individuals (exposed via injection drug use, newborns to infected mothers, and hemophiliacs (bleeding disorder)). The incidence of elite controllers found within these groups varies widely (Horton et al., 2010). The rarity of elite controllers became apparent in a recently published analysis of HIV-positive soldiers serving in the U.S. military. Elite controllers were just 0.55% of the 4586 persons in the military cohort-group of soldiers (viremic controllers made up 3.34%). This population offers perhaps the best natural history that scientists are likely to obtain, because all soldiers are regularly screened for HIV and all infections are identified fairly soon after they occur.

POSSIBLE EXPLANATION FOR ELITE CONTROLLERS?

One possibility is that these "HIV resistant" people have been infected with a heavily compromised, mutated strain of HIV. For example, they may carry HIV with a mutant or nonfunctional **nef** gene. In this case, **nef** minus HIV would not be able to activate CD4 lymphocytes. A few cases of **nef**-depleted HIV were discovered in blood-transfused people in the early 1980s. These people, some 30 years later, are still without the symptoms of HIV/AIDS. However, the R5 nucleotide mutation (discussed in Chapter 5, pages 124–126), which confers some resistance to HIV infection, is found in only a few elite controllers. For example, neither Robert Massie (infected in 1978 and currently thriving at age 57 following a liver transplant necessitated by a hepatitis C infection contracted from a blood transfusion) nor Kai Brothers (infected in 1981 via blood transfusion and currently thriving) nor Rob Rosenthal (infected in 1986 and currently thriving) carry the R5 mutation. It is possible that elite controllers inherited a unique set of HLA (human leukocyte antigen) molecules that sit on the surface of the T cells and identify the virus to the

— BOX 7.2 (continued) —

immune system, which then can kill the virus and the cell. Current research (2010, 2011) suggests that the presence of specific HLA genes may be the primary factor in the elite control people.

These **elite and viremic controllers** all have one thing in common, a functional squad of **memory T4 or CD4+ cells** that respond to HIV infection. Such people have an immune system that remembers HIV and controls it over time, or else they are infected with defective HIV that cannot promote their pathological condition.

The elite and viremic controllers are a very important group to study as they control infection without antiretroviral drug intervention and thus should provide valuable information on disease progression and how it is influenced by immunological, virological, and genetic factors.

HIV-INFECTED CHILDREN FOUND TO BE ELITE CONTROLLERS

At the 2009 16th Conference on Retroviruses and Opportunistic Infections, several investigators reported that about 5% of HIV-infected children ages 7 to 16 who were not on ART had reasonable CD4+ cell counts and were not progressing to AIDS. These findings are very important not only to finding a vaccine but regarding whether all infected children should be placed on ART, which is currently being done. The question is how to determine if a child is an elite controller at an early age.

Controllers are likely to be disproportionately represented among those who do not know their HIV status. Other controllers have been put on therapy early, perhaps before they needed to be. Doctors and patients simply do not know enough about this type of response and where to refer these patients to participate in a study. And finally, privacy laws hamper communications between controllers who might otherwise help to push the research forward. All of these factors contribute to making it difficult to identify and study HIV controllers.

UPDATE 2012—ARE HIV LONG-TERM NON-PROGRESSORS (LTNP) AND ELITE CONTROLLERS (EC) REALLY SLOW PROGRESSORS?

To learn more about these unusual group, Sundhiya Mandalia and colleagues (2012) analyzed medical records from all patients with HIV seen at Chelsea and Westminster Hospital in London between 1988 and 2010. LTNP were defined as individuals who were HIV positive for more than seven years, were ART-naïve, had no history of opportunistic illness (defined as any symptomatic manifestation of HIV disease), and had a stable normal CD4 cell count. They found that out of 5,417 people who belonged, by definition, to either of the two groups, few HIV positive people in this and other studies are LTNPs or Elite HIV controllers. Out of all current HIV patients seen at their hospital, 13 (0.2%) met the LTNP criteria, including three controllers (0.05%). The investigators suggest that even the few who appear to be LTNPs or EC will, over time, progress to HIV disease.

AIDS: LONG-TERM SURVIVORS WITH DRUG THERAPY

Current and continued use of AIDS drug cocktails containing at least one protease inhibitor has increased the number of long-term survivors. Survival after the onset of AIDS, without ART, has been increasing in industrialized countries from an average of less than one year to over five years at present. With therapy, on average, survival time has been increased by 8 to 30 years, depending on the case and therapy.

LONG-TERM UNDETECTABLE

The goal for antiretroviral drug therapy is to get the viral load or number of HIV to undetectable levels in the blood—that is, maintaining a viral load of less than 50 copies of HIV RNA per milliliter of blood. Using the new antiretroviral combination once- and twice-a-day drugs like Kaletra, Combivir, Truvada, and Trizivir has kept HIV at undetectable levels in some patients for seven years and counting (see Table 4-1, pages 75–76).

Further loss leads to immune suppression and the onset of opportunistic diseases.

Thus, accurate and reliable measures of T4 or CD4+ lymphocytes are essential to the assessment of the immune system of HIV-infected persons. The progression to AIDS is largely attributable to the decrease in T4 lymphocytes. Using

ART has allowed for an increase in CD4+ cell counts. Consequently, the Public Health Service (PHS) now recommends that T4 or CD4+ lymphocyte levels be monitored every six months to one year in all HIV-infected persons. The measurement of T4 cell levels has been used to establish decision points for initiating prophylaxis for a variety of opportunistic infections. Moreover, T4 lymphocyte levels are a *criterion* for categorizing HIV-related clinical conditions by CDC's classification system for HIV infection and surveillance case definition for AIDS among adults and adolescents (*MMWR*, 1997).

Levels of HIV RNA in the Blood: Viral Load

David Baltimore (Figure 7-7), the Nobel Prize–winning retrovirologist, and coworkers have found a useful clinical predictor of HIV disease progressors, *levels of HIV RNA in the blood. More RNA means more HIV,* and that makes patients get sicker sooner. HIV RNA is a more sensitive measure of HIV than other antibody type assays and may detect the virus earlier than it would be seen otherwise.

Since the reported work of Baltimore and others on the levels of HIV RNA in the blood, Denis Henrard and coworkers (1995) have concluded that the stability of HIV RNA levels suggests that an equilibrium between HIV replication rate and efficacy of immunologic response, *a set point,* is established shortly after infection and persists throughout the asymptomatic period of the disease (Figure 7-3, page 164). Thus, a defect in immunologic control of HIV

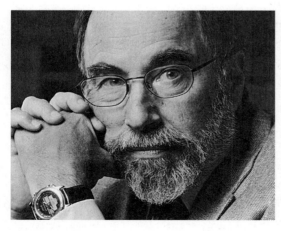

FIGURE 7-7 David Baltimore, 1975, Nobel Prize Molecular Biologist and President of the California Institutes of Technology. *(Photograph © David Baltimore.)*

infection may be as important as the viral replication rate for determining AIDS-free survival. Because individual steady-state levels of HIV RNA are established soon after infection, HIV RNA levels can, as Baltimore suggests, be useful markers for predicting clinical outcome. **Viral load measurements indicate the amount of current HIV activity (HIV replication). T4 cell counts indicate the degree of immunologic destruction.** Thus, the best monitor of disease progression is the use of both the T4 cell count and viral load (Voelker, 1995; Merigan et al., 1996; Katzenstein et al., 1996; Goldschmidt et al., 1997).

No current viral or immunological markers adequately reflect drug toxicities caused by therapy.

HIV INFECTION OF THE CENTRAL NERVOUS SYSTEM (CNS)

The nervous system has two parts. The brain and the spinal cord are the central nervous system (CNS). A wide variety of CNS abnormalities occur during the course of HIV infection. They result not only from the opportunistic infections and malignancies in the immunodeficient individual, but also from direct HIV infection of the CNS and through the toxic effects of ART. It was believed that because some brain cells contain CD4-like receptors they were receptive to HIV infection. In addition, other brain cells contain a glycolipid that allows for HIV infection (Ranki et al., 1995). However, more recent research shows that after HIV-infected monocytes migrate to the brain, become tissue macrophage, and release HIV, the virus *does not* infect brain cells; rather HIV resides in brain spaces, in the cerebrospinal fluid and it may cause an inflammation of the brain. In 2004, Yan Xu and colleagues reported that it is the molecular products of HIV and not the virus itself that cause nerve cell death, which leads to neurodegeneration and associated cognitive and motor dysfunctions. HIV investigators believe that HIV may invade the brain within a few weeks to months after HIV infection.

The CNS and Antiretroviral Therapy

HIV infection of the CNS has to be treated with antiviral drugs. Yet, the blood-brain barrier keeps many drugs out of the central nervous system. The barrier is a tight network of blood vessels that protects the brain and spinal cord from most infectious agents or poisons in the bloodstream. Several antiretroviral drugs do get through the blood-brain barrier. A special concern is that people with CNS problems may need extra help remembering to take their medications.

Genetic analysis and clinical studies have revealed that HIV in the cerebrospinal fluid (CSF) of some people with HIV/AIDS-related dementia evolves *independently* of the HIV in their blood, leading to at least two genetically distinct forms of the virus. This finding poses a new challenge for treatment of these patients, suggesting that drugs effective against HIV in their blood may not do the job in the central nervous system, and vice versa.

AIDS Dementia Complex

HIV/AIDS-associated dementia or AIDS Dementia Complex (ADC) is a progressive brain disorder that causes confusion, memory loss, difficulty with thinking and speaking, and balance problems.

ADC is characterized by severe changes in four areas: a person's ability to understand, process, and remember information (cognition); behavior; ability to coordinate muscles and movement (motor coordination); and/or emotions (mood). These changes are called ADC when they're believed to be related to HIV itself rather than to other factors that might cause them, such as other brain infections or drug side effects (Figure 7-8).

UPDATE 2012

Italo Mocchetti and colleagues at Georgetown University Medical Center found that even though HIV does not infect neurons, it tries to stop the brain from producing a protein growth factor called mature brain derived neurotrophic factor (mature BDNF). Mochetti says mature BDNF acts like food for brain neurons and a reduced amount results in the shortening of the axons and their branches that neurons use to connect to each other. When they lose this connection, the neurons dies. Mochetti believes that HIV stops production of mature BDNF because that protein interferes with the abilily of the virus to attack other brain cells. It does this through the potent gpl20 envelope protein that sticks out

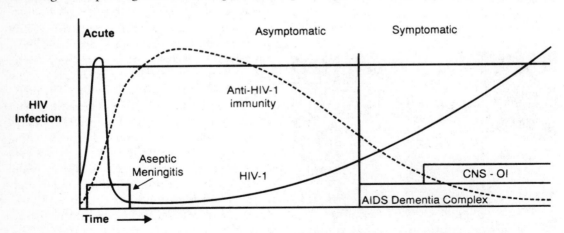

FIGURE 7-8 Central Nervous System Events after HIV Infection in Patients Not on ART. Note that aseptic meningitis (an inflammation of the membrane of the brain and spinal cord in the absence of viral or bacterial infection), when it occurs, occurs early after HIV infection. Although usually apparent later, AIDS dementia complex may begin during the early-late phase. The late phase represents the period during which major AIDS-defining opportunistic infections occur. The headings acute, latent, early-late, and late refer to periods after HIV infection. It appears that opportunistic infection of the brain occurs after the onset of ADC. *(Adapted from Price, 1988.)*

from the viral shell—the same protein that hooks on to brain macrophages and microglial cells to infect them. "In earlier experiments, when we dumped gpl20 into neuronal tissue culture, there was 30–40% loss of neurons overnight. That makes gpl20 a remarkable neurotoxin. The HIV infected patients who develop this syndrome are usually quite young, but their brains act old."

NEUROPATHIES (NERVE TISSUE DAMAGE) IN HIV DISEASE/AIDS PATIENTS

Soon after it enters the body, HIV colonizes in the brain and other nerve tissues. Within the compartment of the nervous system, the virus remains, often at high concentrations, and with time can lead to a spectrum of problems spanning from localized disease of the brain to distal peripheral neuropathy.

Neuropathies are functional changes in the peripheral nervous system; therefore, any part of the body may be affected. Although neuropathies are not OIs, they may result from the presence of certain OIs. **Peripheral neuropathy** is caused by nerve damage and is usually characterized by a sensation of pins and needles, burning, stiffness, or numbness in the hands, feet, legs, and toes. It is a common, sometimes painful, condition in HIV-positive patients, affecting up to 30% of people with AIDS. At autopsy, two-thirds of HIV/AIDS patients have neuropathies. Neuropathy has been a continuous problem for patients throughout the HIV/AIDS pandemic. It is most common in people with a history of multiple opportunistic infections and low T4 or CD4+ cell counts. There is a wide range of expression among patients with neuropathy, from a minor nuisance to a disabling weakness.

FINALLY, HOPE, A RENEWED HOPE FOR THE FUTURE OF THOSE WHO ARE HIV INFECTED

The word "Hope" is the last word in the title of this chapter. Hope and renewed hope is the here and now! This chapter reveals so much of what

has been learned about HIV, the virus, and HIV/AIDS, the progressively debilitating disease. Along with Chapter 4, this chapter presents how the infected can and do survive with an increased quality of life and life span. This chapter, like the material found on the inside cover, helps put a face on HIV/AIDS! Many thousands of HIV-infected people are back to bringing home paychecks, not hospital bills. At first HIV/AIDS was like a car wreck with you (the HIV infected) in it. You are standing in the middle of the street, you see the car coming (AIDS), you know what the impact means, but you can't get out of the way. Today, from Chapters 4 and 7 you learned that you can get out of the way—there is hope, and a lot of it, entering 2013. For example, just in 2010, several excitingly important advances were made: (a) a first vaginal microbicide gel was produced that offers women a level of protection against HIV infection, (b) two new neutralizing antibodies were discovered that are effective against 90% of known strains of HIV, (c) data from the first of nine 2011 Pre-Exposure Drug Prevention Studies (iPrEX—see Chapter 4, page 85, for more on the importance of this and other very important 2011 antiretroviral drug studies.) showed that Truvada, a combination antiretroviral drug, did offer protection from HIV infection if taken before exposure to HIV, (d) the pope of the Catholic Church opened the way for Catholics globally to use condoms to prevent HIV infection, and (e) United Nations officials announced that new HIV infections dropped about 20% over the past few years. We are on the verge of a significant breakthrough in the AIDS response. The vision of a world with zero new HIV infections, zero discrimination, and zero AIDS-related deaths has captured the imagination of diverse partners, stakeholders, and people living with and affected by HIV. New HIV infections continue to fall, and more people than ever are starting treatment. With research giving us solid evidence that antiretroviral therapy can prevent new HIV infections, it is encouraging that some 6.6 million people are now receiving treatment in low- and middle-income countries: about one-third of those in need. Just a few years ago, talking about ending the AIDS epidemic in the near term seemed impossible, but science, political support, and community responses are starting to deliver clear and tangible results. The critical question is no longer *"Can We End AIDS?"* but *"Will We End AIDS?"* Can the world garner the political and financial capital to do what science now says is possible?

Will 2013 truly by "the beginning of the end of AIDS?" Truly, pieces of the puzzle on how to cope with this pandemic are coming together, and **THAT IS HOPE.**

Summary

The clinical signs and symptoms of HIV infection and AIDS have been addressed in the previous chapters. The most often used classification systems to diagnose patients as they progress from HIV infection to AIDS come from the CDC. The CDC uses four groupings to identify the stage of illness from infection to AIDS. Both systems revolve around the recognition of a failing immune system, persistent swollen lymph nodes, and opportunistic infections. Mysteries still to be resolved are exactly why and how HIV kills cells, and why some people stabilize after the initial symptoms of HIV infection while others move directly on to AIDS.

One disorder that was not immediately recognized in AIDS patients is AIDS Dementia Complex (ADC), a progressive mental deterioration due to HIV infection of the central nervous system. ADC develops in over 50% of adult AIDS patients prior to death. Research has shown that some of the symptoms of this dementia can be reversed with the use of the drug zidovudine.

Review Questions

(Answers to the Review Questions are on page 463.)

1. Name the two major AIDS classification systems used in the United States.

2. What percentage of HIV-infected individuals will progress to AIDS in 5 years; in 15 years?

3. What is the neurological set of behavioral changes in AIDS patients called?

4. Name three body organs and their associated AIDS-related diseases.

5. True or False: Currently the single most important laboratory parameter that is followed to monitor the progress of HIV infection is the T4 cell count.

6. True or False: The average time from infection to seroconversion is two weeks. Explain.

7. True or False: Being infected with HIV and being diagnosed with AIDS are the same thing. Explain.

8. True or False: The average length of time from infection with HIV to an AIDS diagnosis is approximately two years.

9. Write a brief essay on: (a) In general, about how long HIV can reside in the body before one shows signs of HIV infection. (b) In general, about how long it takes the body to generate antibodies to HIV after infection.

10. The general signs and symptoms associated with HIV/AIDS include

    A. recurrent fever.

    B. weight loss for no apparent reason.

    C. white spots in the mouth.

    D. night sweats.

    E. all of the above.

11. If you were infected with HIV, you might show symptoms

    A. within a few weeks.

    B. within a year.

    C. in 10 or more years.

    D. any of the above.

12. All of the following symptoms are characteristic of AIDS, except

    A. fever.

    B. fatigue.

    C. diarrhea.

    D. blindness.

    E. weight loss.

13. Which of the following is a cause of T4 cell death in HIV disease?

    A. Replication of HIV lyses the cell.

    B. Infected cells are destroyed by cytotoxic T cells (T_C).

    C. Infected cells are attacked by natural killer cells.

    D. Cells are killed by fusion and syncytium formation.

    E. All of the above.

14. True or False. Because of the success in retroviral drug therapy, in 2011 the Public Health Service stated that CD4+ counts need only be monitored between six months and one year.

Epidemiology and Transmission of the Human Immunodeficiency Virus

---

CHAPTER HIGHLIGHTS

- First evidence of HIV-1, 1959, Central Africa.
- In 1985, HIV-2 was isolated in West Africa.
- Transmission of HIV into the United States may have been via Haiti.
- Behavior is associated with HIV transmission.
- HIV is not casually transmitted.
- HIV is not transmitted to humans by insects. Only people transmit HIV!
- HIV transmission is being reported from 194 countries and among all ages and ethnic groups.
- The transmission of HIV is like a biological chain letter from human to human.
- The four basic mechanisms of HIV transmission are sexual contact, needles and syringes, mother to child, and blood transfusions. All involve an exchange of body fluids.
- HIV enters the body through the mucosal lining of the vagina, vulva, penis, rectum, or mouth during sex.
- Globally, most acts of anal intercourse involve unprotected sex.
- A single copy of HIV can cause an HIV infection.
- One new route of HIV transmission has been discovered in the last 31 years: (1981–2012) prechewed food!
- First documented case of HIV transmission via deep kissing is presented.
- Highest frequency of HIV transmission in the United States is among homosexual and bisexual males and among injection-drug users.
- High-risk activities of gay males presented.
- Serosorting is preferentially picking sexual partners of the same HIV status.
- It has been found that most HIV-infected people do not infect others.
- Male circumcision prevents HIV transmission into males but does not affect women's HIV risk.
- Sperm washing: an effective means of providing HIV-free fertilizations.
- Swiss experts say HIV positive people with undetectable viral load and no sexually transmittable diseases **do not** transmit HIV.
- Other countries, HIV infection, by injection-drug use.
- There are about 16 million injection-drug users globally.
- The biological factor
- Knowing your sexual partner
- History's 10 most- known HIV-positive celebrities
- HIV/AIDS in the Caribbean.
- Worldwide, highest frequency of HIV transmission is among heterosexuals.
- Blood banks in several countries knowingly allowed the distribution of HIV-contaminated blood.

- HIV-infected athletes want to compete.
- Death due to HIV infection is placed in perspective.
- Interactions between HIV and sexually transmitted diseases are discussed.
- Criminalization of HIV transmission.
- Sexual assault with HIV.
- Prenatal HIV transmission generally occurs after the 12th to 16th week of gestation, most often during childbirth and breast-feeding.
- Zidovudine (ZDU or AZT) and nevirapine decrease perinatal HIV transmission.
- HIV and senior citizens.
- National HIV/AIDS resources phone numbers are listed.
- Play the game—see if you can tell who is HIV positive or not.

HIV INFECTION HAS NO LIMITS, FROM THE FETUS TO SENIORS IN THEIR NINETIES

EPIDEMIC/EPIDEMIOLOGY

When a population becomes infected with a contagious disease, an epidemic results. **Epidemic** is derived from Greek and means "in one place among the people." To understand how an infectious disease can spread or remain established in a population, investigators must consider the relationship between an infectious disease agent and its host population. The study of diseases in populations is an area of medicine known as **epidemiology** (ep-i-de-mi-ol-o-gy).

Complacency and HIV Infection

The spread of complacency among people who are at risk for HIV in the United States is demonstrated by the shocking increase in some groups of people at risk for HIV exposure. Their attitude, often expressed, is that HIV infection is "No big deal. It's like diabetes." But it is not, The complex balance of drugs that controls HIV is not like insulin. The virus can and does outsmart the medicines and the drug regimens can have terrible side effects. Complacency can lead to a false sense of security among people at risk for HIV infection.

The danger of complacency has been learned from earlier epidemics. Complacency about HIV infection is especially dangerous because the infection can remain hidden for years. Because many infected people remain symptom-free for up to 10 or more years, it is hard to be sure just who is infected with the virus. The more sexual partners, the greater the chances of encountering one who is infected and subsequently becoming infected.

With regard to HIV infection, it is your behavior that counts. The transmission of HIV can be prevented. HIV is relatively hard to contract and with exceptions, can be avoided.

The presence of HIV/AIDS is not isolated—the transmissibility of HIV between individuals and across borders and populations is what drives this global pandemic and makes it imperative that nations work together to prevent the continued transmission of HIV. On an individual level, IT IS NOT IMPORTANT HOW YOU GOT HIV, WHAT IS IMPORTANT IS HOW YOU LIVE YOUR LIFE WITH THE VIRUS.

How HIV Enters the Body

In order to enter the body, HIV is entirely dependent on the transfer of body fluid—through either HIV-contaminated drug injection equipment, semen, vaginal fluid, or breast milk. Using this knowledge makes HIV potentially avoidable.

In all cases, HIV is transmitted in one of two ways: first, as the virus itself, or second, within an HIV-infected cell. Both are carried in bodily fluids.

HIV and Sexual Transmission

The transmission of HIV is like a biological chain letter, with the number of human carriers or links (senders and recipients) increasing yearly.

Epidemiological data suggest that sexual transmission, in general, is relatively inefficient, in that exposure to HIV often does not produce infection. Regardless, sexual transmission of HIV now accounts for about 90% of infections worldwide. HIV is transmitted more efficiently intravenously than through sexual routes. However, worldwide the predominant mode of transmission of HIV is through exposure of mucosal surfaces of the vagina, vulva, penis, rectum, or mouth to infected sexual fluids (semen, cervical/vaginal, rectal) and during birth.

Factors Driving Sexual Transmission

There is evidence from around the world that many factors play a role in initiating a sexually transmitted HIV epidemic. Among the *behavioral*

and *social factors* are (a) condom use, (b) proportion of the adult population with multiple partners, (c) overlapping (as opposed to serial) sexual partnerships—individuals are highly infectious when they first acquire HIV and thus are more likely to infect any concurrent partners, (d) sexual networks (often seen in individuals who move back and forth between home and a far-off workplace [for example, migrant workers] and houses of prostitution), (e) age mixing, typically between older men and young women and children, and (f) poverty and in particular women's economic dependence on marriage or prostitution, robbing them of control over the circumstances or safety of sex.

Biological factors include (a) high rates of sexually transmitted infections, especially those causing genital ulcers, (b) low rates of male circumcision, and (c) high viral load—HIV levels in the bloodstream that are typically highest when a person is first infected and again in the late stages of illness.

While all these factors help spread the virus, it is not known exactly how much each of them contributes and to what extent they need to be combined in order to spread the epidemic. The issue of male circumcision is a good example. Many countries in which all boys are circumcised before puberty have very limited epidemics, and even in some countries with wider epidemics, circumcised men have lower HIV rates than uncircumcised men (see discussion on the benefits of male circumcision later in this chapter).

HIV: Other Routes of Transmission?

People do not "catch" HIV in the same way that they "catch" the cold or a flu virus. Unlike colds and flu viruses, HIV *is not,* according to the CDC, spread by tears, sweat, coughing, or sneezing. The virus *is* **not** transmitted via an infected person's clothes, phone, or toilet seat. HIV *is not* passed on by eating utensils, drinking glasses, or other objects that HIV-infected people have used that are free of their blood.

HIV *is not* transmitted through daily contact with infected people, whether at work, home, or

BOX 8.1

A NEIGHBOR'S STORY: PUBLIC IMAGE, PUBLIC FEAR

We have over the last 31 years witnessed educated people offering misrepresentation and fantasy about HIV infection and AIDS. We have listened to them distort the truth by presenting false perceptions rather than facts. If education is to become a major player in prevention of the spread of HIV, the mix of myth and fantasy must be replaced by reality—and this can be done by giving the proper respect to a new disease in our lifetime.

THE NEIGHBOR

Some neighbors were having a garage sale. Their friend came over and asked them a question about AIDS. They mentioned that he should talk to the professor next door and he came over to the house. He said, "I'm looking for the truth about who is and who isn't HIV infected and how I can tell people who are HIV infected from those who are not." I asked if he cared to share the reason for the questions and he immediately told me that he divorced three years ago and has been so frightened by the information he has seen on TV, heard on the radio, and read in the paper that he has remained celibate for three years and that it has truly affected his quality of life. He said, "I'm afraid to have sex with any woman I date because I believe almost every woman in Jacksonville and elsewhere carries HIV. It's driving me insane. My male friends are still having sex. Are they crazy or am I the fool?" I took the second question first. I assured him that his worst fears were correct. You can't tell the HIV positive from the HIV negative just by their appearance. Infected and noninfected all look alike—at

least in the early and middle stages of the disease. For the second question of who is and who is not HIV infected, I gave him some details relating to people's behavior, the particular behavioral risk groups and I said that if he did not belong to such groups or did not have a blood transfusion before 1985–1986, and that if he had some information about his sexual partner and did not change sexual partners too frequently and always used a condom, he could feel as safe as one can. The expression on his face went from concern to relief. He shook my hand repeatedly. He thanked me profusely and he said, "I feel like the media, the government, the gays, and everyone else has cheated me out of three years of my life. I can never get that back." I said, "Yes, to some degree that is true, but here you stand after three years still HIV negative. Would you like to exchange three years of free-wheeling sexual encounters for an HIV infection?" He agreed that he would not, but we both understood his point. We all need to understand his point. Misinformation—data skewed by ignorance or lack of education—causes fear. And failure to give an accurate representation of a disease, from both the medical and social vantage points, can cause a great deal of harm—in ways that most of us would not begin to contemplate. Did I give him the right advice? No, because I did not give him advice at all. I simply attempted to put things in their proper perspective. He did not leave me less afraid of dying of AIDS. He left me with the idea that he could have his sex life restored without dying from AIDS, provided he maintains his low-risk behavior.

—The Author

---

school. Insects *do not* transmit the virus. Kissing is also considered very low risk: There is only one documented case to prove that HIV is transmitted by kissing. Paul Holmstrom and colleagues (1992) report that salivary HIV antibodies are detected regularly in HIV seropositive subjects. The route of HIV into saliva is not fully understood. Both salivary glands and salivary leukocytes have been shown to harbor HIV. Gingival fluid (fluid seeping out of the gums) has been regarded as the main source of salivary HIV antibodies and infectious HIV.

In its 1990 supplemental guidelines for cardiopulmonary resuscitation (CPR) training and rescue, the Emergency Cardiac Care Committee of the American Heart Association (AHA)

noted that there is an extremely small theoretical risk of HIV or hepatitis B virus (HBV) transmission via CPR. To date no known case of seroconversion for HIV or HBV has occurred in these circumstances. (See Box 8.1, above)

WE MUST STOP HIV TRANSMISSION NOW!

Education and advocacy for risk reduction remain important tools for preventing HIV infection. Used alone however, they will never accomplish the objective of slowing the speed and extent of the virus's spread. This can only be achieved by combining educational and early intervention efforts with specific measures guiding those resources to the people who need them most: those who are already infected and to their sex and drug partners.

Ending year 2013, there will be about 1.37 million AIDS cases in the United States. Figure 8-1, page 183 breaks this number down according to means of HIV infection—sexual behavior, drug use, medical exigencies, and undetermined causes. Figure 8-2, page 183 gives a breakdown by transmission category for the 35,000 to 40,000 AIDS estimated cases for 2013.

EPIDEMIOLOGY OF HIV INFECTION

The first scientific evidence of human HIV infection came from the detection of HIV antibodies in preserved serum samples collected in Central Africa in 1959. The first AIDS cases appeared there in the 1960s. By the mid-1970s HIV was being spread throughout the rest of the world. The earliest places to experience the arrival of HIV were Central Europe and Haiti.

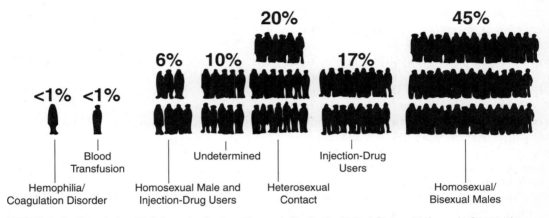

FIGURE 8-1 Cumulative AIDS Cases by Route of Transmission in the United States. At the end of 2013, there will be about 1.37 million AIDS cases in the United States. This diagram gives the percentage of adults and adolescents in each group. Groupings are according to the identification of risk factors—sexual preference, drug use, medical conditions, and others not associated with any of these. *(Courtesy of CDC, Atlanta—updated.)*

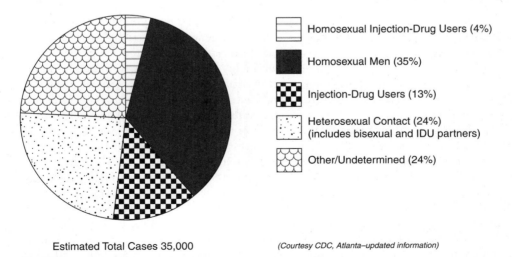

Estimated Total Cases 35,000   *(Courtesy CDC, Atlanta—updated information)*

FIGURE 8-2 Adult/Adolescent AIDS Cases by Transmission Category Estimated for 2013, United States.

Transmission into the United States may have been by tourists who had vacationed in the area of Port-au-Prince, Haiti (Swenson, 1988).

On entry into the United States the virus first spread among the homosexual populations of large cities such as New York and San Francisco. The first *recorded* AIDS cases in the United States occurred in retrospect, in 1979 in New York. The first *CDC-reported* AIDS cases were in New York, Los Angeles, and San Francisco in 1981. In all cases, the diagnosis of AIDS was based on clinical descriptions.

According to the CDC's first clinical AIDS definition, at least one case of AIDS occurred, in retrospect, in New York City in 1952 and another in 1959. Both males demonstrated opportunistic infections and *Pneumocystis jiroveci* pneumonia, a hallmark of HIV infection. This early evidence of AIDS suggests that the virus might have been in the United States, Europe, and Africa at about the same time (Katner et al., 1987). If HIV has been present for decades as suggested, its failure to spread may reflect a recent HIV mutation, a major change in social behaviors conducive to HIV transmission, or both. For example, the sexual revolution and the widespread use of birth control pills, which began in the 1960s, and the subsequent decrease in the use of condoms may have contributed to the transmission of HIV. (See Snapshot 8.1, page 185.)

TRANSMISSION OF TWO STRAINS OF HIV (HIV-1/HIV-2)

The spread of HIV-1 is global. The clinical presentation of AIDS caused by HIV-1 is similar regardless of geographical area.

HIV-2 is a genetically distinct strain. HIV-2 was first discovered in 1985 in West Africa. It is believed to have been present in West Africa as early as the 1960s. Clinical data demonstrate that HIV-2 has a reduced virulence compared to HIV-1 (Marlink et al., 1994).

It appears that HIV-2, like HIV-1, may spread worldwide. HIV-2 has already spread from West Africa to other parts of Africa, Europe, and the Americas. Both HIV-1 and HIV-2 are transmitted or acquired through the same kinds of exposure.

Because over 99% of global AIDS cases are caused by the transmission of HIV-1, only data that pertain to HIV-1 (HIV) will be presented unless otherwise stated.

THE TEN MOST COMMON FEARS IN THE U.S.A. ASSOCIATED WITH HIV TRANSMISSION—#10 BEING THE LEAST AND #1 BEING THE MOST FEARED

10. Swimming pool
 9. Coughing/sneezing
 8. Touching a piece of chewed gum
 7. Mosquito bites
 6. Public restrooms
 5. Eating at a restaurant
 4. Receiving a lap dance
 3. Sharing a drinking glass
 2. Shaking hands
 1. Kissing

IS HIV TRANSMITTED BY INSECTS?

In spite of convincing evidence of the ways in which HIV can be transmitted, it remains difficult for the general public to believe that a virus that appears to spread as rapidly as HIV is not either highly contagious or transmitted by an environmental agent. After all, there are many viral and bacterial diseases that are highly contagious and transmitted by insects. The question was asked: Is this virus being transmitted by insects?

Necessary data to resolve the question is available. Epidemiological data from Africa and the United States suggest that HIV is not transmitted by insect bites. If it were, many more cases would be expected among school-age children and elderly people, groups that are proportionally underrepresented among AIDS patients. In one study of the household contacts of AIDS patients in Kinshasa, Zaire, where insect

TOP 20 MYTHS ABOUT HIV/AIDS

Beginning with the least believable at number 20. If you do not recognize these statements as myth, you will by the time you complete this chapter/book.

20. HIV survives outside the body for very long periods of time.
19. Gambian President Yahya Jammeh can cure AIDS in three days.
18. Teenagers aren't really at risk.
17. Mostly gay men and drug users get it.
16. There is a cure, but only rich people like Magic Johnson can afford it.
15. You only need to get tested if you don't know your sex partner that well.
14. You can tell someone has AIDS just by looking at them.
13. Heterosexual women and their children are not at risk.
12. You shouldn't kiss, hug, or share a meal or drink with someone who is HIV positive or has AIDS.
11. Wearing the Red Ribbon is the only way to help fight the AIDS pandemic.
10. It's really only bad in developing, third-world countries.
 9. You don't hear so much about it anymore, so it must not be that bad.
 8. The U.S. government has the secret to cure HIV/AIDS locked away and only the rich and powerful receive this cure.
 7. You can get HIV by being around those who are HIV positive.
 6. You don't need to worry about HIV infection—the new drugs will keep you well.
 5. You are receiving treatment so you can't spread HIV.
 4. My partner and I are both HIV positive—there's no reason for us to practice safe sex.
 3. You can't get HIV from oral sex.
 2. In 2011, Stefanie Russell and colleagues reported that 28% of blacks, 24% of Hispanics, and 8% of whites thought it was "very or somewhat likely" that HIV/AIDS is "the result of a government plan to intentionally reduce the black population by genocide".
 1. In 2003, Jeremiah Wright, former long-time pastor to Barack Obama, said that the U.S. government had "lied" about not inventing HIV as a means of perpetrating black genocide. In April 2008 he said that he believes the U.S. government is "capable" of having invented HIV as a means of committing genocide against people of color (CNS News.com 4/28/08).

Other Rumors and Hoaxes Going Around

1. I received an e-mail warning that a man who was believed to be HIV positive was recently caught placing blood in the ketchup dispenser at a fast food restaurant. Because of the risk of HIV transmission, the e-mail recommended that only individually wrapped packets of ketchup be used.
2. A child in Florida tested HIV positive after being stuck by a used needle found on a playground.
3. HIV can easily be transmitted through contact with unused feminine (sanitary) pads.
4. The CDC has discovered a mutated version of HIV that is transmitted through the air.
5. Many people are getting stuck by HIV blood-containing needles in phone booth coin returns, movie theater seats, gas pump handles, and other places.
6. In 2010, a woman who posted online a video claiming to have infected 500 Detroit men with HIV said her action was a hoax designed to encourage testing for HIV. "If it scared people, my apologies for scaring them. I wanted them to know—one night of pleasure could lead to a life full of pain. Hopefully, the video will serve as a public service." In the video, she reads from a list of people she said she had infected with HIV and herpes. "You're all going to die." The video was viewed by hundreds of thousands of people. Health authorities report that walk-in traffic at the city's HIV testing clinics was up by 45% within one week. Police identified the woman and picked her up at a college where she said she is studying health administration. She agreed to take an HIV test; the results were negative. Law enforcement officials and legal experts said they are unsure whether she can or will be charged with a crime.

NOTATION: HIV IS ONLY CARRIED BY PEOPLE—ONLY PEOPLE CAN TRANSMIT HIV!

bites are common, not a single child over the age of 1 year had been infected with HIV, while more than 60% of spouses had become infected.

In 1987, the Office of Technology Assessment (OTA) published a detailed paper on the question of whether blood-sucking insects such as biting flies, mosquitoes, and bedbugs transmit HIV (Miike, 1987). The conclusion was that the conditions necessary for successful transmission of HIV through insect bites and the probability of their occurring rule out the possibility of insect transmission as a significant factor in the spread of AIDS. Jerome Goddard reported (1997) that blood-sucking arthropods (for example, mosquitoes and bedbugs), for good biological reasons, *cannot* transmit HIV. The virus has to overcome many obstacles. It must avoid digestion in the gut of the insect, recognize receptors on the external surface of the gut, penetrate the gut, replicate in insect tissue, recognize and penetrate the insect salivary glands, and subsequently escape into the lumen of the salivary duct. Webb and colleagues (1989) inoculated bedbugs intraabdominally (belly) and mosquitoes intrathoracically (chest) with HIV to enable the virus to bypass gut barriers. HIV failed to replicate in either. Some myths about HIV/AIDS in circulation can be found in Snapshot 8.1, page 185.

HIV TRANSMISSION

If most HIV-exposed people can become HIV infected, can *most* infected people *transmit* HIV to others? Most likely yes, but this is a difficult question as infection with HIV appears to depend on a large number of variables that involve the donor, recipient, and portal of entry. The most important variables are route of transmission, viral load, which subtype and variant of HIV is present, and the recipient's genetic resistance.

Global Patterns of HIV Transmission by Identification of Risk

Worldwide there are now three types or patterns of HIV epidemics unfolding. The first pattern is occurring in wealthy countries, such as the United States, where the epidemics are heterogeneous but predominantly involve *male-to-male* or men having sex with men (MSM) sexual transmission. After a long period of decline, those epidemics are now showing troubling signs of resurgence, largely due to unsafe sexual practices among gay men.

The second pattern is seen in sub-Saharan Africa and Latin America, driven by *heterosexual* transmission. Africa continues to have the largest numbers of people living with HIV and dying of AIDS.

The third pattern, labeled just as explosive by UNAIDS, has almost nothing to do with sex. It is driven by *needles shared among people who inject narcotics.* All over the world the narcotics-driven HIV pandemic seems to begin, unnoticed by government officials, in isolated communities of injection-drug users, spreads like wildfire, and then suddenly takes on national significance. The most disturbing examples of this phenomenon are the epidemics of Eastern Europe and Asia, which regionally are in the midst of an HIV explosion that was predicted some years ago. Injection-drug use–associated HIV infections are out of control in Russia, China, and Indonesia.

HIV TRANSMISSION IN FAMILY/HOUSEHOLD SETTINGS

Several studies of the family members of AIDS patients have failed to demonstrate the spread of HIV through household contact. The only cases in which family members have become infected involved the sexual partners of AIDS patients or children born to mothers who were already infected with the virus. Even individuals who bathed, diapered, or slept in the same bed with AIDS patients have not become infected. In one study, family members shared toothbrushes with the infected person and no one became infected.

Perhaps the best evidence *against* casual HIV transmission comes from studies of household members living with blood-transfused AIDS patients (Peterman et al., 1988). Transfusion infection cases are unique because their dates of infection are known retrospectively. Prior to the onset of AIDS symptoms, the families were unaware that they were living with HIV-infected individuals. Family life was not altered in any way, yet family members remained uninfected. In some cases, the transfusion patients were hemophiliacs who received weekly or monthly injections of blood products and became HIV infected. From the combined studies of these households, only the sexual partners of infected hemophiliacs became infected.

NONCASUAL TRANSMISSION

The routes of HIV transmission were established *before* the virus was identified. The appearance of AIDS in the United States occurred first in specific groups of people: homosexual men and injection-drug users. The transmission of the disease within the two groups appeared to be closely associated with sexual behavior and the sharing of IV needles. By 1982, hemophiliacs receiving blood products, as well as the newborns of injection-drug users and heterosexual female partners of AIDS patients demonstrated AIDS. Thirty one years of continued surveillance of the general population has failed to reveal other categories of people contracting HIV/AIDS (Table 8-1). It became apparent that the infectious agent was being transmitted within specific groups of people, who by their behavior were at increased risk for acquiring and transmitting it (Table 8-2, page 188). Clearly, an exchange of body fluids was involved in the transmission of HIV, even in the three cases of HIV being transmitted via prechewed food reported on by the CDC in 2008.

Bodily Fluids

With the announcement that a new virus had been discovered, further research showed that this virus was present in a number of body fluids. Thus, even before there was a test to detect this virus, the public was told that it was transmitted through body fluids exchanged during inti-mate sexual contact, contaminated hypodermic needles or contaminated blood or blood

Table 8-1 HIV Transmission and Infection[1]

CHAIN OF HIV INFECTION	
Agent causing the disease	HIV
Major reservoirs (source of HIV in the body)	Lymph nodes, intestines, blood, genitals
Replication site of HIV	Mostly inside T4+ or CD4-bearing lymphocytes
Portal of exit (how does HIV leave the body)	Mucosal openings, skin breaks, bleeding, or expulsion of body fluids
Transfer or transmission of HIV (from one human to another)	Via body fluids
Portal of entry (how does HIV enter the body)	Mucosal openings, skin breaks, areas of bleeding, injection, prechewed food

TRANSMISSION ROUTES

Blood Inoculation

Transfusion of HIV-infected blood and blood products
Needle sharing among injection-drug users
Needle sticks, open cuts, and mucous membrane exposure in healthcare workers
Use of HIV-contaminated skin-piercing instruments (ears, acupuncture, tattoos)
Injection with unsterilized syringe and needle (mostly in undeveloped countries)

Sexual Contact: Exchange of semen, vaginal fluids, or blood

Homosexual, between men
Lesbian, between women
Heterosexual, from men to women and women to men
Bisexual men and women

Perinatal

Intrauterine
Peripartum (during birth)
Breastfeeding

[1]To reduce the risk of spreading HIV, use condoms during sexual activity. Do not share drug injection equipment. If you are HIV infected and pregnant, talk with your doctor about taking anti-HIV drugs. If you are an HIV-infected woman, talk with your doctor about breast-feeding. Protect cuts, open sores, and your eyes and mouth from contact with blood and other bodily fluids. If you think you've been exposed to HIV, get tested and ask your doctor about taking anti-HIV medications.

products, and from mother to fetus. In addition, it was concluded that the widespread dissemination of the virus was most likely the result of multiple or repeated viral exposure because the

Table 8-2 Adult/Adolescent AIDS Cases by Sex and Exposure Categories, Estimated through 2013, United States

Male Exposure Category (75%)	Total No.
1. Men who have sex with men	426,234
2. Injection-drug use	263,859
3. Men who have sex with men and inject drugs	65,965
4. Hemophilia/coagulation disorder	10,148
5. Heterosexual contact:	142,078
a. Sex with injection-drug user	52,569
b. Sex with person with hemophilia	284
c. Sex with transfusion recipient with HIV infection	1,137
d. Sex with HIV-infected person, risk not specified	88,088
6. Receipt of blood transfusion, blood components, or tissue	5,074
7. Other/undetermined	100,000
Total male AIDS cases	1,014,842

Female Exposure Category (25%)	
1. Injection-drug use	155,609
2. Hemophilia/coagulation disorder	—
3. Heterosexual contact:	165,758
a. Sex with injection-drug user	66,303
b. Sex with bisexual male	8,951
c. Sex with person with hemophilia	1,160
d. Sex with transfusion recipient with HIV infection	1,492
e. Sex with HIV-infected person, risk not specified	87,852
4. Receipt of blood transfusion, blood components, or tissue	3,383
5. Other/undetermined	13,531
Total female AIDS cases	338,281
Total male/female cases	1,353,123
Total pediatric cases	16,877
Total AIDS cases	1,370,000

These calculations only give a general idea of risk. They can tell you which activities carry a higher or lower risk. They cannot tell you if you have been infected. If, for example, the risk is 1 in 100, it doesn't mean that you can engage in that activity 99 times without any risk of becoming infected. You might become infected with HIV after a single exposure. That can happen the first time you engage in a risky activity.

data from transfusion-infected individuals indicated that they did not necessarily infect their sexual partners. In other words, it was concluded

Table 8-3 How HIV Is Transmitted Worldwide, 2012

Exposure	Efficiency, %	% of Total
Blood transfusion/ blood products	>90	3
Perinatal	20–40	9
Sexual intercourse[a]	0.1–1.0	80
Injection-drug use	0.5–1.0	8

[a]Heterosexual intercourse over 70%
(Source: WHO/Global Programme on AIDS and UNAIDS, 2008, updated.)

Table 8-4 An Approximation of How an Estimated 2,263,000 Americans Became Infected with HIV, through 2012

226	—healthcare workers got infected from the blood or body fluids of patients;
30,324	—children infected through their mothers;
48,665	—people got HIV from infected blood or blood products;
158,410	—people did not know how they were infected, did not report their risk, or died before anyone could find out;
147,095	—people were infected who had both unprotected sex and shared needles;
565,750	—people were infected who shared needles;
1,312,540	—people were infected through unprotected sex.

(Based on data from HIV/AIDS Surveillance Report, CDC, Year-End Edition, 2006, updated.)

early on and later confirmed that this virus was not transmitted as easily as other blood-borne viral diseases such as hepatitis B, or viral and bacterial sexually transmitted diseases. Table 8-3 lists the means of HIV transmission worldwide. Table 8-4 lists the means of HIV transmission in the United States.

Mobility and the Spread of HIV/AIDS

Mobility is an important epidemiological factor in the spread of communicable diseases. This becomes particularly obvious when a new disease enters the scene. In the early stage of the HIV/AIDS epidemic, for example, the route of the virus could be associated with mobility.

The first HIV-infected people in some Latin American and European countries reported a history of foreign travel. In some African countries, spread of the virus could be traced along international roads. Today, increasing numbers of HIV infections have been observed to be associated with the relaxation of travel restrictions in Central and Eastern Europe.

Few countries are unaffected by HIV/AIDS. This has made it clear that restrictive measures such as refusal of entry to people living with HIV/AIDS and compulsory testing of mobile populations are *ineffective* measures to stop the spread of the virus. In times of increasing international interdependency, it is an illusion to think that this disease can be stopped at any border.

Number of HIVs Required for Infection

An article by Brandon Keele of the University of Alabama at Birmingham and colleagues (2008) revealed that most HIV infections can be traced back to the transmission of a *single* HIV that penetrates the body's defenses.

For the study, Keele and colleagues analyzed blood samples from 102 people who had recently become HIV infected. The investigators genetically analyzed the samples and were able to count generations of HIV. They found that the HIV in 76% of the infected people could be traced back to a single copy of the virus! The remaining 24% of infections were traced back to between two and five viruses. In the majority of cases, the single virus crossed the sexual mucosa and infected a single cell. Keele said, "That cell makes a lot of viruses; you have a firestorm of HIV replication over the next couple of weeks. Very quickly the person is populated by millions of viruses." The investigators believe the findings are significant because they indicate that if researchers are trying to develop a vaccine or microbicide to prevent HIV infection, the only thing it has to prevent, in most cases, is the transmission of a single virus. In addition, the investigators believe these findings help to clarify our understanding of the acute and early stages

of HIV transmission (discussed in Chapter 7, pages 161–167).

In striking contrast to a single copy of HIV crossing the sexual mucosa, it is known that for other sexually transmitted infectious agents like bacteria and spirochetes, many copies of these agents cross the mucosa to cause infection.

Keele said, "The findings are crystal clear; they will stand up to scientific study." So far they have!

Levels of HIV Found in Body Fluids

High levels of HIV have been isolated from blood, genital fluids (semen and vaginal), serum, and breast milk. Lower levels of HIV are found in saliva, tears, urine, lung fluid, and cerebrospinal fluid.

Cases of low levels of HIV in cell-free body fluids and within the cells of these fluids does not mean that HIV cannot be transmitted via these fluids or cells—it can, but the dose (number of viruses) is so small that the risk of infection is minimal. Also, no one has been identified as becoming infected with HIV due to contact with a body fluid on an environmental surface. CDC studies show that high concentrations of HIV in a drying fluid became 90% to 99% less infectious over several hours; thus the reason for the low number of healthcare workers contracting HIV infection after touching, being splashed by, or needle sticking themselves with blood containing HIV.

Highest Concentration of HIV in the Body

HIV is found in greatest numbers within T4 or CD4+ cells, macrophages, monocytes, dendritic cells, blood, vaginal fluids, and semen. Laboratory findings, along with overwhelming empirical observations, support the scientific conclusion that the major route of HIV transmission is through human blood and sexual activities involving exchange of semen and vaginal fluids. Semen carries significantly larger numbers of HIV than vaginal fluid. It appears that of all body fluids, these three contain the largest number

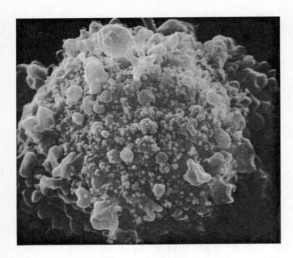

FIGURE 8-3 Electron Micrograph of an HIV-Infected T4 Lymphocyte. The T4 or CD4+ cell has produced a large number of HIVs that are located over the entire lymphocyte. Each HIV leaves a hole in the cell membrane. The photograph shows part of the convoluted surface of the lymphocyte magnified 20,000 times. *(Courtesy of The National Biological Standards Board, South Mimms, UK.)*

of infected lymphocytes (Figure 8-3), which provide the largest HIV concentration in a given area at a given time.

Presence of HIV-Infected Cells in Body Fluids

Blood—Red blood cells do not contain nuclei; therefore, they have no DNA for HIV to use to replicate itself. Recent observations indicate that both latent and HIV-producing cells are present throughout the course of infection in the blood. Thus it is probable that HIV-infected people harbor substantial numbers of HIV-infected CD4+, macrophage, and monocyte cells in their blood from soon after the initial infection through the terminal stage of the disease.

Semen—A single specimen of ejaculate (discharged semen) contains between 1 million and 10 million nonspermatozoal cells, and many leukocytes including T4 cells, macrophage, and monocyte cells.

Christopher Pilcher and colleagues (2007) reported that HIV in semen reached its peak at four weeks after infection, and HIV shedding was almost completely contained by week 10, reflecting perhaps the host immune response. Lee Harrison and colleagues (2000) reported on 93 HIV-positive men on antiretroviral drugs. Before drug treatment, 74% had detectable levels of HIV in their semen. After six months on therapy 33% had detectable HIV in their semen.

Starting at the Source—Human Semen/ Sperm—It has been shown that the majority of HIV infections worldwide result from the sexual transmission of HIV, yet the cellular and molecular mechanisms of transmission involved are still poorly understood. The principal cell types in human semen are spermatozoa, immature germ cells, and white blood cells. HIV can potentially be carried in any of these or in the seminal fluid. Some men with acute HIV infection may be particularly contagious as a result of abnormally elevated HIV-associated white blood cells or high levels of HIV RNA in semen. Most quantitative studies of HIV in semen have used commercially available HIV RNA assays to measure copy numbers of cell-free virions in seminal plasma. Even with current technological advances, it remains unclear whether transmitted strains of HIV originate as RNA virions or as integrated proviral DNA in infected seminal white blood cells. The HIV-1 species in semen often differ genetically from those in the peripheral blood of the same infected person, and the genetic sequences of cell-free HIV in semen differ from those of cell-associated HIV in semen. It, therefore, should be possible to determine whether the initial transmission event is mediated by a cell-free HIV or an HIV-infected cell. Mounting evidence from clinical, animal, and in-vitro studies indicates that HIV infected cells may be the critical vectors of transmission. However, the identification of the true source is complicated by the prevalence of cell-associated over cell-free HIV transmission, the risk factors associated with transmission, and the type and location of infected cells. In a search for the source reservoir of sexually transmitted HIV.

As stated, HIV is present in seminal fluid and white blood cells but HIV is not present in sperm. Through washing and the use of centrifugal force, sperm can be separated from the other components of semen and then injected into the woman's body or used for in vitro fertilization. In studies issued over the past decade, over 4500 fertilizations using treated sperm from HIV-positive men have been conducted worldwide without any infection of either mother or child. While the sperm washing is relatively cheap—roughly $200—fertility treatments can be expensive.

Saliva—Saliva contains few CD4+, macrophage, or monocyte cells, but it may contain antibodies to HIV. There continues to be some concern over the presence of HIV in saliva because of the exchange of saliva during deep kissing, the saliva residue left on eating utensils, and saliva on instruments handled by healthcare workers, especially in dentistry. Results of studies on hundreds of dental workers, many of whom have cared for AIDS patients, have shown no evidence of HIV infection. Studies by Fox (1991), Archibald (1990), Pourtois (1991), and Hasselrot (2009) showed that human saliva contains factors that inhibit HIV infectivity.

First Documented Kissing Transmission Case

In July 1997, the first documented case of HIV transmission via deep kissing was reported by the CDC. In this *one* case, the man was HIV positive, via IDU in 1988. Both he and his female partner had serious gum (periodontal) disease. His gums routinely bled with brushing or flossing. Investigators at the CDC believe that the HIV was transmitted via blood within the man's oral cavity due to oral lesions onto the mucous membrane of the woman (*MMWR*, 1997).

Breast-Feeding: Mother's Milk—The oral transmission of HIV from HIV-infected mothers to nursing infants is an unquestioned route of HIV infection. Breast milk contains CD4+, macrophage, and monocyte cells. Several studies have shown that HIV can be transmitted by breast-feeding. Van de Perre and coworkers (1993, updated) found that infection of babies via breast milk was most strongly correlated with the presence of HIV-infected cells in the milk, suggesting that infection might be cell-mediated. However, infection was also correlated with low levels of antibodies to HIV, suggesting that infection may be initiated by cell-free virus.

Prechewed Food—Aditya Gaur and colleagues (2008) reported that after ruling out other routes of transmission, such as breast-feeding, sexual abuse, blood transfusion, or needle stick injury, the investigators looked at caregivers and discovered that in two cases, HIV-positive mothers were in the habit of giving prechewed food to their infants. In one case, the child died of AIDS before the route of transmission was discovered, but the other child is receiving antiretroviral treatment. In the third case, a child was diagnosed with HIV at the age of 15 months in 1993. The infant's mother was HIV negative, and the strain of HIV carried by her HIV-positive partner was genetically dissimilar to the infant's strain, prompting the investigators to look elsewhere. They subsequently discovered that the child's great aunt had often looked after the child between the ages of 9 and 14 months and had given it prechewed food. The aunt died of AIDS in 1993. Most likely, the children received HIV through blood in the aunt's saliva. The CDC believes that in developing countries prechewed food may be more common due to the lack of prepared baby foods, so it may pose a greater risk in settings where HIV prevalence is high and oral health poor.

Notation—This is essentially a newly discovered route of HIV infection!

Dentist with AIDS Infects Patient During Tooth Extraction?

In July 1990, the CDC reported on the possible transmission of HIV from a dentist with AIDS to a female patient (*MMWR*, 1990a). This case, like no other before it, sent chills through many. But why this case? Because the vast majority of people go to dentists and they don't inject drugs and are not gay. This case, however, is difficult to resolve. For example, two years had elapsed from the time of the dental work to when the patient, Kimberly Bergalis, was diagnosed with AIDS. Both patient and dentist, David J. Acer of Stuart, Fla., were uncertain of exactly what happened. Some of the pertinent factors in this case are (1) review of dental records and radiographs suggest that the two tooth extractions were uncomplicated; (2) interviews with Bergalis and the dentist did not identify other risk factors for HIV infection. Bergalis, age 22, stated over national TV in 1990 that she was still a virgin. This point was disputed on June 19, 1994, during the TV program *60 Minutes* (with Mike Wallace). Yes, she did engage in sexual foreplay, but not intercourse. Yes, she was infected with the human papilloma virus, which can be sexually transmitted, but this is not at all uncommon in immune-suppressed AIDS patients with no history of sexual intercourse; (3) nucleotide sequence data indicated a high degree of similarity between the HIV strains infecting her and the dentist; and (4) the time between the dental procedure and the development of AIDS was short (24 months), and Bergalis developed oral candidiasis 17 months after infection. At this time, only 1% of infected homosexual/bisexual men and 5% of infected transfusion recipients develop AIDS within two years of infection.

Who Was David Acer?—David Acer, a bisexual, was diagnosed with symptomatic HIV infection in 1986 and with AIDS in 1987. He died on September 3, 1990. Since then, 1100 of his 2500 patients were contacted for HIV testing. In January 1991, the test results of 591 of these patients revealed that five were HIV positive: a 68-year-old retired school teacher, a middle-aged father of two, a 37-year-old carnival worker, an unemployed drifter, and a 19-year-old student. As with Bergalis, infection in these patients may have come from some other source. All six patients denied having sexual contact with the dentist or

with one another (*MMWR*, 1991a). If an absolute case can be made that Acer transmitted the virus to Bergalis, this will be the first documented case of a healthcare professional infecting a patient.

Bergalis died of AIDS on December 8, 1991. She was 23 years old and weighed 48 pounds.

How Did David Acer Infect His Patients?—There is no shortage of ideas as to how Acer might have infected his patients. For example, he could have used the same dental instruments on himself or his sexual partners that he used on his patients without sterilizing them.

The actual route of HIV transmission in the Acer-Bergalis case will most likely never be known. There have been suggestions that the dentist did not wish to die alone and chose certain people to infect. It was suggested that he may have attempted to infect still others, but was unsuccessful. A friend of the dentist said that he believed that Acer intentionally infected his patients to call attention to the HIV/AIDS problem in the United States. Acer felt that mainstream America was ignoring the problem.

A CDC estimate put the theoretical risk of HIV transmission from an HIV-infected dentist to a patient during a procedure with potential blood exposure at 1 chance in 260,000 to 1 chance in 2.6 million (Friedland, 1991).

(Read Denis Breo (1993). The dental AIDS cases—murder or an unsolved mystery? *JAMA*, 270: 2732–2734.)

Conclusion—Beginning 2013, two of the six, Lisa Shoemaker and Sherry Johnson, believed to have been infected by Acer have progressed to AIDS but are still alive; Kimberly Bergalis, Richard Driskill, John Yecs, and Barbara Webb have died. To date, the six people have received $10 million from Acer's insurance company.

Sexual Transmission of HIV: The AIDS Pandemic Signals the End of the Sexual Revolution in the United States

The predominant mode of global HIV transmission is through sexual contact. But, not all sexual practices are equally likely to result in HIV transmission (Table 8-5). HIV usually gains access to the immune system at mucosal or membrane lining surfaces. Such surfaces include the oropharynx (throat area), rectum, and genital mucosa. Mucosal surfaces are rich in Langerhans cells, dendritic cells that trap antigens and virus particles. In addition, lymphoid aggregates are found throughout the tissue immediately below the mucosal surface.

Sexual Behavior and Risk of HIV Infection

Sexual transmission of HIV occurs when infected blood, semen, or vaginal secretions from an infected person enter the bloodstream of a partner. This can happen during anal, vaginal, or oral penetration, in descending order of risk. Unprotected anal sex by a male or female appears to be the most dangerous, since the rectal wall is very thin. Masturbation or self sex is the safest. In general, a person's risk of acquiring HIV infection through sexual contact depends on (1) the number of different partners, (2) the likelihood (prevalence) of HIV infection in these partners, and (3) the probability of virus transmission during sexual contact with an infected partner. Virus transmission,

---

Table 8-5 Sexual Activity According to Degree of Risk for Transmitting HIV

Lowest Risk

1. Abstinence
2. Masturbating alone
3. Hugging/massage/dry kissing
4. Masturbating with another person but not touching one another
5. Deep wet kissing
6. Mutual masturbation with only external touching
7. Mutual masturbation with internal touching using finger cots or condoms
8. Frottage (rubbing a person for sexual pleasure)
9. Intercourse between the thighs
10. Mutual masturbation with orgasm *on,* not *in* partner
11. Use of sex toys (dildos) with condoms, or that are not shared by partners and that have been properly sterilized between uses
12. Cunnilingus
13. Fellatio without a condom, but never putting the head of the penis inside mouth
14. Fellatio to orgasm with a condom
15. Fellatio without a condom, putting the head of the penis inside the mouth and withdrawing prior to ejaculation
16. Fellatio without a condom with ejaculation in mouth
17. Vaginal intercourse with a condom correctly used and spermicidal foam that kills HIV and withdrawing prior to orgasm
18. Anal intercourse with a condom correctly used with a lubricant that contains spermicide that kills HIV and withdrawing prior to ejaculation
19. Vaginal intercourse with internal ejaculation with a condom correctly used and with spermicidal foam that kills HIV
20. Vaginal intercourse with internal ejaculation with a condom correctly used but no spermicidal foam
21. Anal intercourse with internal ejaculation with a condom correctly used with spermicide that kills HIV
22. Brachiovaginal activities (fisting)
23. Brachioproctic activities (anal fisting)
24. Use of sex toys by more than one partner without a condom and that have not been sterilized between uses
25. Vaginal intercourse without a condom and withdrawing prior to ejaculation
26. Anal intercourse with a condom and withdrawing prior to ejaculation
27. Vaginal intercourse with internal ejaculation without a condom but with spermicidal foam
28. Vaginal intercourse with internal ejaculation without a condom and without any other form of barrier contraception

Highest Risk

29. Anal intercourse with internal ejaculation without a condom

Source: Shernoff, 1988 Journal of Contemporary Social Work *updated.*

in turn, may be affected by biological factors, such as concurrent sexually transmitted disease (STD) infections in either partner. Behavioral factors, such as type of sex practice and use of condoms, or varying levels of infectivity in the source partner (for example, viral load) related to clinical stage of disease also increase the risk of HIV transmission/infection. Based on these factors, the risk for HIV infection is highest for an uninfected partner of an HIV-infected person practicing unsafe sex. In February 2001 researchers at the University of North Carolina, Chapel Hill reported that HIV could be transmitted via unprotected sex between 5 and 13 days after infection. Persons who have sex partners with risk factors for HIV infection or who themselves have multiple partners with high rates of injection-drug, "crack" cocaine, and methamphetamine use, prostitution, and other STDs are also at increased risk.

Danger of HIV Infection via Artificial Insemination

By early year 2010, 15 women were reported to have been HIV infected through the use of anonymous donor sperm to initiate pregnancy: one in Germany, two in Italy, four in Australia, two in Canada, and six in the United States. Thirty recipients of semen from HIV-infected donors refused to be HIV tested (Guinan, 1995 updated). All cases except Germany occurred *before* the availability of HIV antibody testing. But 31 years into the HIV/AIDS epidemic, the increasingly popular fertility business remains largely unregulated and unmonitored, even though it traffics in semen, long known to be one of the two main HIV transmission routes.

Only a few states (New York, California, Ohio, Illinois, and Michigan) require HIV testing of semen donors. There are no federal regulations.

Personal Choice—Personal Risks

Ray Bradbury wrote that "living at risk is jumping off a cliff, and building your wings on the way down." About 90% of the HIV infections that occur within the heterosexual noninjection-drug use population occur through one or more sexual activities. Some 90% of the HIV infections that

occur among gay males occur through anal intercourse. In any sexual activity, HIV is transmitted via a body fluid (see Figures 8-4 and 8-5, page 195 and Box 8.2, page 196).

Evidence That Prevention Is Working: First There Was the 80/20 Rule, Eighty Percent of New HIV Infections Come from Risky Behavior by Just 20 Percent of Infected People. Now It Is the 95/5 Rule. Stop Them and We Stop HIV Transmission?

The 95/5 Rule—Five of every 100 (5%) HIV infected will transfer HIV to another person in a given year. David Holtgrave (2004, 2009) of Emory University's Rollins School of Public Health found that transmission rates dropped during the 1980s from essentially 100% to about 5.49%. The rate fell again slightly at the beginning of the 1990s, then remained relatively stable at 4.0%–4.34%. Holtgrave believes this rate is surprisingly low. The drop indicates a real success of HIV prevention programs.

Following Holtgrave's findings, it means that in the mid-1980s virtually everyone who became HIV positive infected, in turn, someone else during any given year. With greater education and counseling, by the late 1990s the annual odds of someone passing his or her virus fell to 4.0% to 4.34%. And this would mean that at least 95% of persons living with HIV didn't transmit the disease to another person during any given year through 2012 (see Box 8.2, page 196).

FOLLOWING IS A PRESENTATION OF THE DIFFERENT BEHAVIORAL GROUPS AND HOW THEY PUT THEMSELVES AT RISK FOR HIV INFECTION AND TRANSMISSION.

Heterosexual HIV Transmission: Key Factors

Heterosexual HIV transmission means that the virus was transmitted during heterosexual sexual activities. As such, the proportion of HIV infection and AIDS cases among the heterosexual population in the United States is now increasing at a greater rate than the proportion of HIV infections and AIDS cases among homosexuals or IDUs. The key factors for persons at highest risk for heterosexually transmitted HIV infection include adolescents and adults with multiple sex partners, those with sexually transmitted diseases (STDs), and heterosexually active persons residing in areas with a high prevalence of HIV infection among IDUs. In 1985, fewer than 2% of HIV infections were in the heterosexual population. In 2010, about 38% of new HIV infections were in the heterosexual population, with 64% of these occurring in women!

Heterosexual HIV Transmission: Africa and Asia—Heterosexual intercourse is the most common mode of transmission of HIV in developing countries.

Africa: In Africa, over 80% of infections are acquired heterosexually, while mother-to-child transmission, unprotected sex between gay men, injection-drug use, and transfusion of contaminated blood account for the remaining infections.

Asia and Latin America: Heterosexual contact and injection-drug use are the main modes of HIV transmission in South and Southeast Asia. Studies in Haiti and other Caribbean and third-world countries indicate that HIV transmission is most prevalent among the heterosexual population. Globally, heterosexual transmission now accounts for over 90% of HIV/AIDS cases.

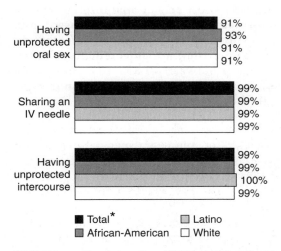

FIGURE 8-4   Knowledge about HIV Transmission: Percentages who say that HIV can be transmitted in the following ways . . . (Correct answers). National random sample of 2902 respondents age 18 and older. "Kaiser Family Foundation Survey (KFFS) of Americans on HIV/AIDS, Part Three—Experiences and Opinions by Race/Ethnicity and Age" (#7140), The Henry J. Kaiser Family Foundation, August 2004. The information was reprinted with permission from the Henry J. Kaiser Family Foundation. The Kaiser Family Foundation, a leader in health policy analysis, health journalism and communication, is dedicated to filling the need for trusted, independent information on the biggest health issues facing our nation and its people. The Foundation is a non-profit private operating foundation based in Menlo Park, California.

* The 2011 KFFS results were not significantly different than the 2006 data. (HIV/AIDS at 30, June 2011.)

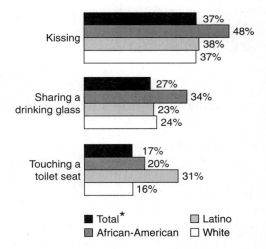

FIGURE 8-5   Misconceptions about HIV Transmission: Percentages who say that HIV can be transmitted in the following ways, or say they don't know . . . (Incorrect answers). National random sample of 2902 respondents age 18 and older. "Kaiser Family Foundation Survey (KFFS) of Americans on HIV/AIDS, Part Three—Experiences and Opinions by Race/Ethnicity and Age" (#7140), The Henry J. Kaiser Family Foundation, August 2004. The information was reprinted with permission from the Henry J. Kaiser Family Foundation. The Kaiser Family Foundation, a leader in health policy analysis, health journalism and communication, is dedicated to filling the need for trusted, independent information on the biggest health issues facing our nation and its people. The Foundation is a non-profit private operating foundation based in Menlo Park, California.

* The 2011 KFFS results were not significantly different than the 2006 data. (HIV/AIDS at 30, June 2011.)

HIV/AIDS ROULETTE

CASE I: THE WOMAN EXECUTIVE

I am a successful woman executive. A year ago I applied for life insurance. I was required to take an HIV antibody test. It came back positive.

I am not a prostitute or promiscuous. I am not and have never been an injection-drug user. I am not a member of a minority group, indigent or homeless, and I have not slept with a bisexual male (?).

I don't fit any of the stereotypes that people have designated for those infected with HIV. I got HIV from a man I love and have been seeing for five years. He is not homosexual or bisexual. He has never used injection drugs. He had no idea he was carrying the virus. He believes he may have been infected about six years ago by a woman with whom he had a brief, meaningless relationship. For that one indiscretion we will both pay the ultimate price.

CASE II: THE HIV-INFECTED MALE

A 21-year-old man walked into a sexually transmitted disease clinic and told the doctor he had "the clap," or gonorrhea, but he carried HIV.

When a counselor inquired about his sex partners, he told them about several, including a 12-year-old girl. The girl had gone elsewhere to be treated for gonorrhea and tested positive for HIV.

The man admitted to having sex with 27 women, including 13 teenagers. Ten of the partners couldn't be found. Of the 17 others, 12 tested positive for HIV.

The man has since died, and the clinic has not been able to track all of his sexual partners.

THE MESSAGE

There is a message to be found in these two cases: People with HIV are much more dangerous to a community than someone with AIDS. On average, the HIV infected are asymptomatic, on average, for 11 years. Those with AIDS and not treated are usually symptomatic. They are losing weight. They are sick. They have little or no sexual appetite. Those with HIV who are healthy and vigorous. That's where the sexual roulette begins.

Vaginal and Anal Intercourse—Among routes of HIV transmission, there is overwhelming evidence that HIV can be transmitted via anal intercourse. In vaginal intercourse, male-to-female transmission is much more efficient than the reverse. This is believed to be due to (1) a consistently higher concentration of HIV in semen than in vaginal secretions, and (2) abrasions in the vaginal mucosa (lining or membrane). Such abrasions in the tissue allow HIV to enter the vascular system in larger numbers than would occur otherwise, and perhaps at a single entry point.

That same reasoning explains why the *receptive* rather than the *insertive* homosexual partner is more likely to become HIV infected during anal intercourse. It appears that the membranous linings of the rectum, rich in blood vessels, are more easily torn than are those of the vagina. In addition, recent studies indicate the presence of receptors for HIV in rectal mucosal tissue.

Globally, most acts of anal intercourse are unprotected (condoms are not used), and an estimated 80% of those infected do not know they are infected. Anal intercourse is between 10 and 100 times more efficient in transmitting HIV than is vaginal intercourse.

Homosexual Anal Intercourse—Entering 2013, about 25% of homosexual men in San Francisco were/are HIV infected, probably the highest density of infection anywhere in the developed world. A gay activist said, "It colors everything we do out here. The gay community, to a large extent, is about addressing AIDS. It has to be, because it's literally a war: Your entire community is under siege."

In a single year, 1982, 21% of the uninfected gay male population became infected, and for some reason not yet known, many of those infected early died early. "Soon everyone, and I mean everyone, had a friend who was dying" (*Science in California*, 1993). During 1995 through mid-1997, three gay men died of AIDS each day. From mid-1997 through 2012, using aggressive anti-HIV drug therapy, daily deaths from AIDS have dropped to less than two per week (Conant, 1995 updated).

It appears that of all sexual activities, anal intercourse is the most efficient way to transmit HIV.

GAY MEN PUTTING THEMSELVES AT HIGH RISK FOR HIV INFECTION

Men having sex with men (MSM) between men is the most prominent mode of HIV transmission in nearly all Latin American countries, the United States, Canada, and some Western European countries.

Experts believe one reason risky behavior continues among the young is that they have not yet seen their friends die of the disease.

Another is simply the kind of risk-taking common among the young—the same impulse that prompts teenagers to drive fast or take up smoking. In three large American cities, 66% of gay men surveyed had *unprotected sex* in the last 18 months. *One in five* gay men in San Francisco and New York City said they had *unprotected sex* with an HIV-negative partner or with a partner whose HIV status was unknown. Linda Valleroy and colleagues at the CDC reported at the Eighth Conference on Retroviruses, February 2001, on testing and interview results of 2400 gay men ages 23 through 29. The men were from Baltimore, Dallas, New York, Los Angeles, Miami, and Seattle. Over 12% or 293 of the men were new HIV positives. *Twenty-nine percent* knew they were HIV positive before testing! Forty-six percent said they had unprotected oral sex during the previous six months. These data shocked the researchers.

On January 29, 1999, the *San Francisco Chronicle* carried a story about an $8 admission for a night of communal sex—the rules: no clothes, no condoms, no discussion of HIV. The article also covers an Internet link offering gay men the *extreme sex party* where becoming infected or HIV-infecting another is the erotic allure of the party. Still another twist is the *Russian Roulette Party* where noninfected men have sex with others, one of them being HIV positive!

Exit the Condom

During a health inspection of a gay sex club, the inspector felt something crunch underfoot. It was an empty blister pack of *Viagra*. The inspector, San Francisco's director of sexually transmitted disease prevention, began to wonder whether

Pfizer's impotence drug was contributing to unsafe sexual behavior and fueling an increase in HIV and other diseases. As a result of follow-up studies, he believes he has his answer. In the first three months of 2003, 43 new cases of syphilis and 14 new HIV infections have been diagnosed in Viagra users in San Francisco. Together these data imply that gay men are reverting to unsafe sex. And all this comes after the state and federal government have spent many millions of dollars on AIDS education and prevention.

Effect of Highly Active Antiretroviral Therapy (HAART) on Sexual Behavior and HIV Transmission (See Point to Ponder 8.1, page 198)

Recent studies on HIV-infected gay males in San Francisco revealed that the use of HAART reduced HIV transmission by 60%. However, the increase in unprotected anal sex rose from about 8% in 2000 to 25% in 2003 during the same time period. This behavioral change, going from protected to unprotected anal sex, has offset the beneficial effects of HAART. With the 2010 report showing that **pre-exposure prophylaxis (PrEP)** can prevent infection on exposure to HIV, it may mean that unprotected sex may increase in the coming years (see discussion of these 2010–2011 studies in Chapter 4, pages 83–102). This means that men and women will continue to have unprotected sex. For those who need it, being on HAART has taken away much of their fear, and the uninfected at-risk population no longer sees the pallid face of death in public places as in the past—they never developed the fears of yesterday, the days before HAART. For many with HIV/AIDS the time of disbelief and terror evolved into burnout and despair, which in turn has now become a time of recuperation and salvation. The newly infected mostly see salvation through HAART. They see magazine ads that show hot muscular men living life to the fullest thanks to HAART. Other ads show couples holding hands, sending messages that the road to true love and happiness is being HIV positive. Unlike the photos of buff men in the ads, most who are on drug cocktails are not having the time of their lives. They

SWISS EXPERTS SAY INDIVIDUALS WITH AN UNDETECTABLE VIRAL LOAD AND NO SEXUALLY TRANSMITTABLE DISEASES (STDS) WILL NOT TRANSMIT HIV DURING SEX

DOES UNDETECTABLE EQUAL UNINFECTIOUS?

Swiss HIV experts have produced the first-ever consensus statement to say that HIV-positive individuals on effective antiretroviral therapy—i.e., those with undetectable plasma RNA at less than 40 copies per milliliter of blood plasma—and without sexually transmitted infections are sexually noninfectious (Vernazza et al., 2008).

The statement says that "after review of the medical literature and extensive discussion," the Swiss Federal Commission for HIV/AIDS resolves that "an HIV infected person on antiretroviral therapy with completely suppressed viraemia (effective ART) is not sexually infectious, i.e., cannot transmit HIV through sexual contact." However, the Commission said, "it realizes that medical and biologic data available today do not permit proof that HIV infection during effective antiretroviral therapy is impossible, because the non-occurrence of an improbable event cannot be proven." The statement also discusses the implications of the consensus findings for doctors, for HIV-positive people, for HIV prevention, and for the legal system.

Bottom Line

The Swiss study implies that *undetectable* means *uninfectious*!

U.S. Investigators Disagree with Swiss Findings

The above Swiss findings that ART renders HIV infected people as "sexually non-infectious" immediately became a hotly debated topic that continues to be debated.

Seth Kalichman and colleagues (2008) reviewed 19 studies examining the relationship between the viral load found in blood versus that in semen. The bottom line of their review as it relates to the Swiss study is that semen that has an undetectable viral load is still potentially infectious and that cells in semen can contain HIV proviral DNA (HIV DNA embedded in the host-cell DNA) and can act as vehicles for the sexual transmission of HIV. Perhaps the real question is, has anyone shown a threshold below which people cannot transmit HIV?

Also, in 2009, at the 16th Conference on Retroviruses and Opportunistic Infections, several studies were presented that showed that HIV-infected males satisfying the Swiss criteria for becoming "sexually non-infectious" with undetectable viral loads in their blood plasma had measurable HIV RNA in their semen (Sheth et al., 2009; Marcelin et al., 2009; Butler et al., 2009). Earlier studies have shown that HIV is found in blood plasma cells of individuals even when they demonstrated undetectable blood plasma levels for HIV (Ibanez et al., 1999; Furtado et al., 1999). Further, current ART that suppresses the level of HIV in the blood does not stop HIV replication in the male or female genital tract. In short, the protection provided by ART is **NOT** absolute and ART is **NOT** absolutely predictable. And the disagreement continues.

Swiss Court Suspends Prison Sentence in Light of Findings to Set Aside 18-Month Prison Sentence for Exposing His Female Sex Partner to HIV in February 2009

In the first ruling of its kind in the world, the Geneva Court of Justice has quashed an 18-month prison sentence given to a 34-year-old HIV-positive African migrant who was convicted of HIV exposure by a lower court in December 2008, after accepting expert testimony from Professor Bernard Hirschel—one of the authors of the Swiss Federal Commission for HIV/AIDS consensus statement on the effect of treatment on transmission—that the risk of sexual HIV transmission during unprotected sex on successful treatment is one in 100,000. The prosecutor in the case asked that the charges be dropped because he was persuaded by the Swiss Federal Commission's findings of a risk of one in 100,000. The prosecutor said, "one shouldn't convict people for hypothetical risks."

Comments from the American Centers for Disease Control and Prevention

With the publication of the Swiss study, the CDC immediately released the following statement:

> An article recently published by Switzerland's Federal Commission for HIV/AIDS states that HIV positive individuals on effective antiretroviral therapy are not at risk for transmitting HIV to their sexual partners under certain circumstances. The Commission acknowledges that there are no scientific data that the risk of transmission in these circumstances is zero. The Centers for Disease Control and Prevention (CDC) underscores its recommendation

that people living with HIV, who are sexually active, use condoms consistently and correctly with all sex partners (February 2008).

The CDC statement was followed by similar statements from the WHO and UNAIDS.

UPDATE 2012—Two articles, one by Lambers-Niclot and colleagues (2012) and the other by Politch and colleagues (2012), report that HIV-infected men showing undetectable HIV in their blood simultaneously had detectable HIV in their semen. Although there is no doubt that ART significantly decreases the likelihood of HIV transmission, these data indicate that the risk for HIV transmission is not eliminated by suppressive ART. Shedding of virus in the male genital tract is not uncommon, even in men with consistently undetectable plasma HIV RNA. Furthermore, previous studies have shown no clear association between the presumed penetration of specific antiretrovirals into the genital tract and the likelihood of undetectable HIV in semen. Thus, despite the fact that the threshold level of genital-tract HIV necessary for transmission is not known, caution is warranted. Recommending safer sex practices for all HIV infected patients, even those with suppressed plasma or blood HIV-RNA, seems prudent. For more recent information on the use of ART and its effect on HIV transmission, see Chapter 4 SIDEBARS 4.3 and 4.4, pages 85–89 and 90–91.

spend mornings in the bathroom throwing up or suffering from diarrhea. They spend afternoons at doctor's appointments, clinics, and pharmacies. And they spend endless evenings planning their estates and trying to make ends meet because they are not well enough to support themselves and HAART. **The reality is, AIDS is not fun. It's not sexy or manageable. AIDS is a debilitating, deforming, terminal, and incurable disease. And the drugs used can bring on heart, kidney, and liver disease, cancer, and a host of daily discomforts, like never being able to stray too far from the nearest toilet.**

The Use of Methamphetamine (Crystal or Tina)

"Whenever I want sex, I want meth and whenever I am high on meth, I want sex." The use of crystal meth by gay and heterosexual men is not new; it is the sudden accelerated use of the drug among gay men that is of major concern.

Meth use and attendant HIV transmission has become such a concern across the nation that in New York City, Gay Men's Health Crisis, one of the nation's largest gay AIDS/HIV groups, has launched a major education campaign. The organization is putting up billboards, sending out mailings, sponsoring workshops, and dispatching counselors into the community to talk about meth abuse and HIV. Meth, a psychostimulant that

excites pleasure centers in the brain, makes users feel euphoric for hours. The drug impairs judgment, lowers inhibitions, keeps people awake for days, and can increase sexual arousal. They go from feeling like wallflowers to feeling like supermen, and safer sex messages are just forgotten. This drug has become almost normalized in the gay community. One gay male said, "It gives people a way to have sex for hours and hours and hours. It's the greatest euphoria you can ever feel."

Party and Play

Meth is so linked with this subculture of gay men engaging in anonymous sex with strangers that men advertise that they either have the drug or want it during sex in personal ads and on the Internet. Their notices carry the phrase "PnP" for "party and play," a euphemism for crystal methamphetamine and sex. For one gay male, his friends introduced him to crystal meth on a Thursday evening and he stopped using it on Monday morning. He lost count over the weekend when he hit having sex with 12 men. About a month later he developed a flu-like syndrome, got tested and he was HIV positive. In his mind he was thinking this was just one weekend. One weekend—and it will impact him for the rest of his life.

Circuit Parties—Circuit parties got their name from those who travel to various cities—the circuit—to attend several parties each year. The parties, which began in 1986, essentially are the gay version of raves, parties that are popular among some young people. There are two or three circuit party weekends a month. Among the cities where they are held: Montreal, San Francisco, Atlanta, Palm Springs, Miami, and Washington. The parties are not universally popular among gay men, although many say they have attended one. The parties generally attract professionals ages 21 to 35. The parties began with the intention of fundraising and community building. But somewhere along the way, the original intent of the party became diluted. Now, circuit parties have become weekend bashes. They attract thousands of mostly young gay men who dance until dawn and whose admission fees raise millions of dollars for AIDS prevention groups and gay charities. But, according to Ronald Johnson, an official of the circuit party organization, "It (circuit parties) became a social phenomenon above and beyond what (we) intended and beyond what (we) could control." Health officials say the parties have become a reflection of the risky behavior that is contributing to rising rates of HIV infection among gay men. Drugs are so prevalent at the parties that organizers often hire medical teams to treat overdoses. Troy Masters, publisher of a gay newspaper in New York, who now opposes these parties, said, "You wouldn't find the American Cancer Society throwing a smoking party." Gay Men's Health Crisis, which was founded in 1981 and serves 11,000 clients annually in the New York area, stopped holding its party in 1998 after it became known for drug use and sex. Two Philadelphia couples said they attend up to eight parties a year and usually take Ecstasy pills with a liquid shot of GHB or some ketamine, which can be liquid or powder. They agreed that "if you don't do drugs, you're not going to enjoy it as much."

Barebacking: Chasing the Bug—Intentionally Seeking HIV Infection

Bug chasing sounds like a group of children running around chasing crickets, butterflies, or grasshoppers. Enter Robert, age 30. He routinely hooks up with three to four men each week for unprotected sex—he hopes they are all HIV positive! For Robert, bug chasing is mostly about the excitement of doing something that everyone sees as crazy and wrong. Keeping this part of his life secret is part of the turn-on. That forbidden aspect makes HIV infection incredibly exciting for him, so much so that he seeks out sex exclusively with HIV-positive men. "This is something that no one knows about me, it's mine. It's my dirty little secret." He compares bug chasing to the thrill you get by "screwing your boyfriend in your parents' house," or having sex on your boss's desk. You are not supposed to do it, and that's exactly what makes it so much fun. When asked why he wants to become infected, his eyes light up as he says that the actual moment of transmission, the instant he gets HIV will be the "most erotic thing I can imagine." When asked whether he is prepared to live with HIV after that "erotic" moment, he dismisses living with HIV as a minor annoyance. Like most bug chasers, he has the impression that the virus isn't such a big deal anymore. "It's like living with diabetes. You take a few pills and get on with your life."

It has recently been observed that a minority of both HIV-positive and negative men have begun to consciously, willfully, and proudly engage in unprotected anal sex. This phenomenon is referred to as raw, skin-to-skin, or bareback sex. Such behavior in this group leads to the intentional transmission and reception of HIV! This form of barebacking is referred to as *"bug chasing"* or *"chasing the bug."* These HIV-negative gay men seek to become HIV infected. (See Point to Ponder 8.2, page 201.)

Brotherhood of the Infected: Bug Chasers and Gift Givers

According to Yvonne Abraham of the *Boston Globe Online,* and DeAnn Gauthier (1999), health professionals are seeing something unexpected in the gay community: a small group of men who want to contract HIV in the belief that it offers community and kinship. Increasing numbers of

RACIAL GAP SEEN IN HOMOSEXUAL HIV RATES AMONG MEN HAVING SEX WITH MEN (MSM): ON THE DOWN LOW AND LOOKING BACK ON THE DOWN LOW

In 2005, Frangiscos Sifakis, from Johns Hopkins Bloomberg School of Public Health in Baltimore, and colleagues with the National HIV Behavioral Surveillance system tested 1767 MSM at venues where they normally congregated, such as bars, clubs, and social organizations, in five different cities. Overall, 25% tested positive for HIV. However, the infection rate differed by race—46% among blacks, 21% among whites, and 17% among Hispanics. About half of those who tested positive were unaware of their HIV infection. Of those with unrecognized HIV infections, 64% were black, 18% were Hispanics, and 11% were white. Although most had undergone testing in the past, the researchers found that 58% with unrecognized infections had not been tested during the previous year. Stephanie Behel from the CDC in Atlanta said, "We know that persons who are aware of their HIV status take measures to seek treatment and reduce risk behaviors, which underscores the importance of annual HIV testing for MSM, particularly among black-American MSM."

FEAR, HATE, SECRETS, DENIAL, AND LIES: THE CLIMATE THAT KEEPS HIV TRANSMISSION GOING: ON THE DOWN LOW

The highest rate of HIV infection in the United States occurs among bisexual black men. And that has implications for black women, who are 19 times more likely to be infected than white women. That's because many black men have unprotected sex with other men but then conceal that fact and have unprotected sex with women. This behavior is called On The Down Low. These men are bisexual. They do not identify themselves as gay or homosexual. There are, of course, white bisexual men who pose the same threat to women as well. For example, the outing of former New Jersey Governor James McGreevey in 2004 makes the point that some closeted gay white men can or may expose their wives and girlfriends to HIV. Some sociologists believe that gay or bisexual black men are more afraid to come out of the closet than whites because they already face racial discrimination and are reluctant to take on the added burden of homophobia.

Although AIDS researchers have suspected for years that a culture of clandestine gay sex was helping to fuel the HIV epidemic, the "down low" syndrome has only recently become widely known. In 2005, J. L. King wrote a book, *On the Down Low: A Journey Into the Lives of "Straight" Black Men Who Sleep with Men*, about his secret life, and he appeared on the Oprah Winfrey TV show to discuss his sexual lifestyle, On The Down Low.

In 2006, Preeti Pathela and colleagues reported on a survey of 4193 men ages 18 and older in New York City. Four percent said they were homosexual, 91.7% said they were heterosexual, and 5% said they were bisexual. The study found that about 10% of the men who said they were heterosexual had slept with a man but not a woman in the previous year, and that such men were less likely to have had an HIV test than men who said they were homosexual. The study also found that 22% of men who had sex with men but who described themselves as heterosexual used condoms, compared with 55% of men who considered themselves gay. According to the researchers, the findings imply that physicians should not depend on a man's self-described sexual orientation when assessing his risk for contracting HIV or other sexually transmitted infections.

PERSONAL TESTIMONY OF A "NOT GAY" BISEXUAL

Never was, never will be. I can't claim to be something I was raised to hate. I'm just me, and I do what makes me feel good. Besides, my folks raised me as a Christian, and they would be really disappointed in me if I didn't live my life in the same steps that they were raised. So I'm not gay, even though I have sex with guys. And no, I'm not in denial. There are just some things about the lifestyle that I don't do. I don't club, I don't go to the Village, I don't do that Ball stuff, I don't geek over Beyonce, I just live my life—I do what I want to do. But I'm not gay.

LOOKING BACK ON THE DOWN LOW: ALSO KNOWN AS COMING OUT OF THE CLOSET

Robert Fullilove, Columbia University public health and HIV investigator, says that "Long before it was named 'down low,' we used to describe it as 'the behavior of bisexual black men who are in the closet.' It goes back to the dawn of time. The idea that it is completely new, and suddenly black men discovered they could have sex with other men, doesn't make sense." Keith Boykin writes in *Beyond the Down Low: Sex, Lies and Denial in Black America*, "One of the biggest lies we have told ourselves about the down low is that the story is new."

chat rooms and websites approach the subject of men who want to convert from HIV negative to positive. Marshall Forstein, medical director of mental health at Fenway Community Health Center in Boston, says some of the men feel lonely or shunned and believe that HIV will bring them attention from friends and caregivers. One California activist who stopped using condoms and later contracted HIV also noted, "When I was entering the gay community at the height [of the epidemic], I felt like I'd joined the war. And that somehow transformed HIV into this rite of passage as opposed to something to be reviled and avoided." Some websites even discuss conversion parties, where uninfected men can have unprotected sex with HIV-positive men to try to contract the virus. The groups refer to HIV infection as a rebirth and a way to bond with a new family. According to Gauthier, bug chasing as a form of bareback sex actually involves two categories of participants. There are the HIV-negative men who seek to become infected with the virus (bug chasers), and there are the *gift givers,* HIV-positive men who seek to share their gift of HIV with others. Chasers typically advertise for partners with statements such as: "Will let you _____ me raw only if you promise to give me all your diseases like AIDS/herpes, etc. Let's do it." Gift givers, on the other hand, typically make comments such as: "Attention neg men! Why stay locked in a boring world of sterile sex when you can join the ranks of the AIDS Freedom Fighters? Let me give you my gift and set you free." Becoming "bug brothers" may occur one-on-one but is just as likely to result at special marathon group sex parties that are held for the purpose of seroconverting as many HIV-negative participants as possible. That individuals would knowingly participate in such events is shocking not only to some members of the gay community, but also to the community at large (Gauthier, 1999).

The story of chasing HIV until infected is presented in a film, *The Gift.* It became available in 2003 and was shown nationally on the Sundance TV network on February 2, 2004. It is a powerful presentation of gay men in search of *The Gift,* HIV.

Gay Men Serosorting to Prevent HIV Infection

Many people living with HIV have based sexual and romantic choices on serostatus since the beginning of the epidemic. In recent years, an official term for this behavior was coined by prevention experts and is frequently used in the scientific literature: **serosorting.**

Serosorting is defined as "the practice of preferentially choosing sex partners, or deciding not to use condoms with selected partners based on their disclosed concordant (agreed with) HIV status." Matt Golden (2006) of the University of Washington, Seattle Center for AIDS and STDs (sexually transmitted diseases) looked at serosorting as a prevention activity adopted by gay men. Data from Golden's clinic found that HIV-positive patients were particularly likely to serosort. Forty percent and 49%, respectively, of his HIV-positive patients had unprotected receptive and insertive sex with HIV-positive partners but only 3% and 6%, respectively, with HIV-negative partners.

In November 2006, the San Francisco Department of Public Health began a highly visible print and web campaign featuring silhouettes of naked men embracing in erotic poses with their HIV status branded on their shoulders, with a caption reading, "Sero-Sorting is a Prevention Strategy."

Serodiscordant Couples

The term *serodiscordant* should not be confused with serosorting. Serosorting occurs mostly among gay men, as described above. *Serodiscordant* means one person of a sexual couple is HIV positive, the other negative; the term applies to *all* sexual couples in this situation. Such couples are sometimes referred to as "magnetic couples"— one positive, one negative. They do not necessarily seek each other out based on differing HIV status; many serodiscordant couples have come together through typical chance circumstances and were initially unaware of their respective statuses.

Moment of Truth?

Mark Milano believes that encouraging HIV-positive or negative gay men to ask strangers their HIV status is not only useless, it's dangerous. He says, "First, the information [exchanged] is arguably worthless. Someone you barely know has little motivation to be honest, since no personal or emotional bond exists. And even if someone thinks he's negative, he could be wrong. He may have been tested two years ago, or he may have been infected last week, in which case he would, most likely, have a high viral load, increasing the risk of infection. Relying on the self-reporting of someone you barely know when making a decision about safer sex is foolish at best. Recent studies have shown that a significant number of new infections occur during the window period—the time when someone who is newly infected still tests HIV negative." (See Chapter 7, Figure 7–1, page 159, for information on the window period.)

Heterosexual Anal Intercourse—A number of sexuality-oriented surveys of the heterosexual population indicate that between one in five and one in ten heterosexual couples have tried or regularly practice anal intercourse. Bolling (1989) reported that 70% to 80% of women may have tried anal intercourse and that 10% to 25% of these women enjoyed anal sex on a regular basis. He also reported that 58% of women with multiple sex partners participated in anal sex. James Segars (1989) reported that the highest rates of anal sex occur among teenagers who use drugs and older married couples who are broadening their sexual experiences.

Although it may increase the risk of HIV infection, it must be emphasized that anal intercourse is not necessary for HIV transmission among heterosexuals. In fact, most HIV-infected heterosexuals say they have never practiced anal intercourse.

Risk of HIV Infection, Number of Sexual Encounters—The risk of HIV infection to a susceptible person after one or more sexual encounters is very difficult to determine. In some cases, people claim to have become infected after a single sexual encounter.

In some reported transfusion-associated HIV infections, the female partners of infected males remained HIV negative after five or more years of unprotected sexual intercourse. Television star *Paul Michael Glaser* said that he had unprotected sexual relations with his wife Elizabeth for five years prior to her being diagnosed as HIV-infected. He was not HIV-infected. She received HIV during a blood transfusion, but was not diagnosed until after their firstborn child was diagnosed with HIV. Both have since died of AIDS. In other studies of heterosexual HIV transmission, many couples had unprotected sexual intercourse over prolonged periods of time with no more than 50% of the partners becoming HIV infected. There are many instances of heterosexuals and homosexuals who remained HIV negative after having repeated sexual intercourse with HIV-infected partners.

THE BIOLOGICAL FACTOR

The fact that not all who are repeatedly exposed become infected suggests that biological factors may play as large a role in HIV infection as behavioral factors. For biological reasons, some unknown (see Box 7.2, pages 173–174), some people may be more efficient transmitters of HIV; while others are more susceptible to HIV infection, that is, require a smaller HIV infective dose. Some people carry genes that may make them resistant to HIV infection (see "Mutant R-2 and R-5 Genes" in Chapter 5, pages 119–123). In addition, some men may be circumcised, have genital ulcers, or be in the early stage of HIV infection when viral loads are higher. (See more information on circumcision in Chapter 9, pages 261–264.)

Number of Sexual Partners and Types of Activity—One relatively large risk factor for HIV infection in both homosexuals and heterosexuals is believed to be the number of sexual partners. The greater the number of sexual partners, the greater the probability that one of the partners is HIV positive.

The scale of multiple-partnering during the late twentieth century and continuing into the twenty-first century is unprecedented. With over 7 billion people on earth ending 2013, an ever-increasing percentage of whom are urban residents; with air travel and mass transit available to allow people from all over the world to go to the cities of their choice; with mass youth movements advocating, among other things, sexual freedom; with a feminist spirit alive in much of the industrialized world, promoting female sexual freedom; and with 47% of the world's population made up of people between the ages of 15 and 44—there can be no doubt that the amount of worldwide urban sexual energy is unparalleled.

Knowing Your Sexual Partner—The amount of protection one actually obtains from limiting one's number of partners depends mainly on who those partners are. Having one partner who is in a high-risk group may be more dangerous than having many partners who are not. An example of this is seen in prostitutes, who may be more likely to be infected by their regular injection-drug-using partners than by customers who are not in a high-risk group. The risk status of a person who remains faithful to a single sexual partner depends on that partner's behavior: If the partner becomes infected, often without knowing it, the monogamous individual is likely to become infected (Cohen et al., 1989). See Point of Information 8.2.

POINT OF INFORMATION 8.2

HISTORY'S 10 MOST WELL-KNOWN HIV-POSITIVE CELEBRITIES

The list of famous people who have been open about their HIV diagnosis is a short one. Even among those known to us, most had their HIV status revealed either just before or after their deaths. While, sadly, many felt they had to hide their status, a few have used their influence to spread HIV awareness.

Rock Hudson, Died 1985. One of the most beloved movie stars of the 1950s and 1960s, Rock Hudson's death from AIDS was a shock to the world. In a move that is truly emblematic of the unparalleled stigma of HIV, his publicity team had covered up his illness by saying he had liver cancer.

Liberace, Died 1987. He was a pianist and entertainer who became a worldwide icon in the 1950s. He appeared in films and television shows and released numerous albums. He was the highest paid entertainer in the world for over a decade and was known for his opulent lifestyle.

Keith Haring, Died 1990. He was an iconic artist who rose to prominence during the 1980s. He was best known for his street murals and cartoonist figures.

Freddie Mercury, Died 1991. The lead singer of Queen, one of the top-selling rock bands of all time, Freddie Mercury was among the most recognizable faces of the 1970s.

Isaac Asimov, Died 1992. He was one of the most prolific authors of all time, best known for his science fiction novels and short stories. The cause of his death was kept secret for ten years!

Anthony Perkins, Died 1992. He was a film and stage actor who will always be remembered for his unforgettable turn as Norman Bates in Alfred Hitchcock's *Psycho*. He had a productive career that spanned nearly 40 years.

Robert Reed, Died 1992. He portrayed perhaps the most beloved father in the history of U.S. television. As Mike Brady on *The Brady Bunch,* he was the head of a highly traditional household. It was hard for some to believe that the man who played this almost puritanical character was in fact a gay man.

Arthur Ashe, Died 1993. He was the first black American man to win a Grand Slam title in tennis. Arthur Ashe broke down the color barrier. He was an accomplished champion and Hall of Famer.

Magic Johnson, Living 2013. Most people over the age of 30 won't soon forget the emotional public disclosure on November 7, 1991, from one of basketball's all-time greats. Magic's HIV diagnosis essentially ended a phenomenal NBA career, although he did make a few brief comebacks. His disclosure spurred a re-evaluation of safety in sports and was a watershed moment in HIV awareness. He has thrived since, leading some to believe he was somehow cured.

Greg Louganis, Living 2012. He was an Olympic diver who won multiple gold medals in the 1980s. He was one of the most recognizable faces in American sports during that decade. He tested positive in 1988, the same year he won two gold medals at the Seoul Olympics.

This list only covers ten of the most notable HIV-positive celebrities. There are many more famous people with HIV—some are out, but many are not, while there are others who might have HIV (or even died from HIV), but have never been tested.

The Effects of Sexual Partner Reduction in Uganda—In the mid-1980s Uganda had a 30% rate of HIV infection. Today it is less than 6%. A miracle? No, the bottom line was sexual partner reduction.

In 1986, the Uganda Ministry of Health started a vigorous HIV prevention campaign in which the slogans "Love Carefully," "Love Faithfully," and "Zero Grazing" (Uganda slang for "don't have sexual partners outside the home") were posted on public buildings, broadcast on radio and in speeches by government officials, teachers, and AIDS prevention workers across the country. Religious leaders scoured the Bible and the Koran for quotations about infidelity. Also, newspapers, theaters, singing groups, and ordinary people spread the message of abstinence. In short, Uganda promoted the A, B, C approach to lowering the HIV infection rates—**A** for abstinence, **B** for be faithful (stay with one sexual partner), and **C** if you fail A and B, use a condom. As a result of these prevention methods, in addition to sexual partner notification, the frequency of casual sex fell by 60% between 1989 and 1995. HIV-associated pregnancy rates fell by 50%. And there was a drop in the rate of HIV infection across Uganda. All of this was occurring at a time when condoms were not widely available. Some researchers have attributed Uganda's HIV prevention success to increased sexual abstinence among teenage girls, but statistics suggest that **partner reduction,** especially on the part of men, was far more important. Partner reduction has been an important factor in HIV prevention elsewhere as well. In Thailand, HIV infection rates declined steeply during the 1990s. Visits by men to sex workers also fell by 60%. Among gay men in America, HIV rates fell sharply during the 1980s. A significant part of this decline was attributable to the increased use of condoms, serosorting, and a reduction in sexual partners. In Zambia and northern Tanzania, where churches promoted faithfulness, HIV rates also declined. Meanwhile, in such countries as Botswana, South Africa, and Zimbabwe, condoms have been emphasized as the main method of prevention, and HIV rates have remained high.

Sexual Activities—In addition to a high-risk partner or a number of sexual partners, the types of sexual activities that occur are also significant (Table 8-5, page 193). Any sexual activity that produces skin, anal, or vaginal membrane abrasions (tears) prior to or during intercourse increases the risk of infection.

Orogenital Sex—Historically, it has been very difficult to establish the contribution orogenital sex makes to overall HIV transmission since few people engage solely in oral sex. (*Fellatio* is the technical or medical term used to describe oral contact with the penis, *cunnilingus* is used to describe contact with the vagina, and *anilingus* refers to oral-anal contact.) Instead, many people also have vaginal or anal sex, which are recognized routes of HIV transmission. although there have been a number of cases of apparent HIV transmission via orogenital sex, health professionals have tended to prioritize HIV prevention efforts in the areas of greatest risk. This strategy may have inadvertently downplayed the risks attached to orogenital sex, and left some individuals confused over risk reduction options. (See Snapshot 8.2.)

Orogenital Sex Is Not Risk Free: How Risky Is Orogenital Sex? The Question That Never Ends—This is one of the most frequently asked questions on HIV/AIDS hotlines. The question is difficult to resolve because most people do not limit themselves to a single sexual practice. Few people engage exclusively in oral sex! Orogenital sex may be a greater risk factor for becoming HIV infected than previously thought. The risk of transmission is related to the presence of HIV at the sexual sites (oral, vaginal, penile, and anal), the amount of HIV present, and whether there are physical openings such as tissue tears or open sores (Rothenberg et al., 1998; Kahn et al., 1998).

After reviewing over 100 research reports Sara Edwards and colleagues (1998) concluded that HIV can be transmitted through oral sex. In a very rigorous study, Beth Dillon and colleagues (2000) appear to have clearly pinpointed oral transmission in approximately 7%

TEENAGERS VIEW ORAL SEX AS LESS RISKY THAN SEXUAL INTERCOURSE!

Researchers surveyed 580 ethnically diverse ninth graders in two California public schools about their perceptions of oral sex and their chance of contracting HIV or any other sexually transmitted disease.

Results: About one in five ninth-graders report having had oral sex, and almost one-third say they intend to try it during the next six months. The teenagers, whose average age was 14$\frac{1}{2}$, also said that oral sex is less risky, more common, and more acceptable for their age group than vaginal intercourse. Girls and boys reported similar experiences and opinions about oral sex. Neither gender saw sex as a "big deal."

Also, in 2005, the National Center for Health Statistics released data from the most comprehensive survey of sexual behaviors ever provided by the federal government. The information released shows that just over half of U.S. teenagers ages 15 to 19 have engaged in oral sex, a proportion that increases with age to about 70% for those ages 18 to 19. It was also found that females and males reported similar levels of oral sexual experience. The findings are likely to intensify the debate over abstinence-only sex education. Supporters of these programs say they result in teens delaying intercourse, but opponents argue they have also led them to substitute other behaviors like oral sex. The new report tends to support this view, as it found that nearly one in four teen virgins has engaged in oral sex. In 2007, the survey results from two religious youth conferences, one in Florida and the other in Miramar, showed that 70% of 14- to 19-year-olds do not consider oral sex to be sex!

Clearly some of the teenage students who hear the abstinence-only message believe that they are engaging in abstinent behavior when they are having oral sex. In defense of these young people, it can be said that health educators are unclear. And why not? In 1998, President Clinton, in testimony about an affair with a White House intern, said, with great sincerity, that he had not had "sexual relations" but had engaged only in oral sex! It appears that even those elected as wise enough to lead our nation seem to be confused about what defines "sexual relations."

Public Health Laboratory Service, reported that oral sex may account for up to 8% of HIV infections among gay men. He said that oral sex leads to 30 to 50 new HIV infections annually in the United Kingdom. Evans states that the risk of HIV infection via oral sex is greater than previously thought.

Susan Buchbinder and colleagues in 2001 calculated that the odds of acquiring HIV from any single act of oral sex with an infected partner are roughly 4 in 10,000 (1 in 2500) compared with odds of 4 in 1000 (1 in 250) for anal sex with a condom.

It should also be recognized that one can get other sexually transmitted diseases from oral sex, such as gonorrhea, syphilis, chlamydia, and herpes. Even using antiretroviral therapy, which can lead to an undetectable viral load, there is still some risk. Ultimately, only you and your sexual partner can decide how much risk is acceptable.

Prostitution (Employment as a Sex Worker): United States

Sex Workers and Their Clients—A smartly dressed couple checks into a four-star city hotel armed with a bottle of champagne and condoms. In a building across the street, a couple who has just met is putting on a condom. In a parking lot of the local high school, in the backseat of a car, two young people, high on dope, are removing a condom after finishing sex. Out in the suburbs, a man puts one on before he has sex with his regular partner at his home. In a bathroom of a public transportation system, another man is performing oral sex on his male partner. No, these are not couples engaged in affairs. They are not people who have just met at a bar, nor teenagers after the school dance. They are certainly not long-time lovers. They are all people who are part of the sex industry, sex workers and their clients. (See Snapshot 8.3.)

Do Sex Workers Account for a Significant Transmission of HIV in the United States?—There is little if any evidence that prostitutes in the United States and most other developed

of primary infection cases. By mid-2000, strong evidence for at least 30 cases of oral HIV infection were reported in the United States (Dillon et al., 2000). In Britain, Barry Evans, director of

IF YOU DON'T TAKE A JOB AS A PROSTITUTE, WE CAN STOP YOUR BENEFITS

Because of the large unemployment rate in Germany, welfare reforms were instituted. One reform was the legalization of prostitution on the grounds that this would combat trafficking in women and cut links to organized crime. However, now that prostitution is no longer considered, by the law, to be immoral, there is really nothing but the goodwill of the job centers to stop them from pushing women into jobs they don't want to do, like prostitution! For example, a 25-year-old waitress who turned down a job providing sexual services at a brothel in Berlin faces possible cuts to her unemployment benefit under the new welfare reform laws introduced in 2005. Under Germany's welfare reforms, any woman under 55 who has been out of work for more than a year can be forced to take an available job, including one in the sex industry, or lose her unemployment benefits. The government had considered making brothels an exception on moral grounds, but decided that it would be too difficult to distinguish them from bars. As a result, job centers must treat employers looking for a prostitute in the same way as those looking for a dental nurse.

When the waitress looked into suing the job center, she found out that it had not broken the law. Job centers that refuse to penalize people who turn down a job by cutting their benefits face legal action from the potential employer. A lawyer from Hamburg who specializes in such cases said, "There is now nothing in the law to stop women from being sent into the sex industry. The new regulations say that working in the sex industry is not immoral anymore, so jobs cannot be turned down without a risk to benefits."

One woman who had worked in call centers had been offered jobs on telephone sex lines. At one job center in the city of Gotha, a 23-year-old woman was told that she had to attend an interview as a nude model and should report back on the meeting. Employers in the sex industry can also advertise in job centers. A job center that refuses to accept the advertisement can be sued. One woman who owns a brothel in central Berlin has been searching the online database of her local job center for recruits. She said, "Why shouldn't I look for employees through the job center when I pay my taxes just like everybody else."

the United States and other developed countries is that they tend to be seen as responsible for the spread of HIV—an attitude reflected in descriptions of prostitutes as reservoirs of infection or high-frequency transmitters. But the sex worker is only the most visible side of a transaction that involves two people: For every sex worker who is HIV positive there is, somewhere, the partner from whom she or he contracted HIV. Given the fact that the chance of contracting HIV during a single act of unprotected sex is not high, infection in a sex worker is likely to mean that she or he has been repeatedly exposed to HIV by clients who did not or would not wear condoms. The more accurate way of reading the statistics of HIV infection in prostitutes or sex workers is to view them as an indication of how strong a foothold the epidemic has gotten within a community.

Prostitution (Employment as a Sex Worker): Developing Countries

Do Sex Workers Account for a Significant Transmission of HIV in Developing Countries? The answer is YES—In a garbage-strewn alley in the city's red-light district, a 24-year-old prostitute slumps on a string bed, weak from tuberculosis and diarrhea. She knows she has AIDS but she has never heard of the multidrug cocktail that curbs the progress of the disease. Even if she had, she could never afford to buy it. Nobody wants the girls once they get sick, explains a health counselor who visits the alley each week. She says prostitutes with AIDS are shunned by many hospital doctors, brothel operators, and their own families. "We feel helpless; all we can do is comfort them and find them a place where they can go to die." This true vignette is happening in small towns, the suburbs, and every large city in developing nations. Many of the prostitutes are housewives out to make the difference between starvation and existence for their families. Many women knowingly risk exposure to HIV to economize the number of times they have to have sex with a stranger. They could make, say, the equivalent of $10 for one act of unprotected sex with one

nations play a large role in heterosexual HIV transmission (Cohen et al., 1989 updated).

A consequence of the attention prostitutes or sex workers have attracted in relation to AIDS in man, or they could make $10 for five acts of protected sex with five men. It is, for them, all about the money—a conscious choice, their only means of survival. The prostitutes sell their bodies for money or drugs to anyone who can afford their services. In some towns in Africa, Vietnam, and India between 50% and 90% of the prostitutes are HIV positive. Prostitution in developing countries is a large contributing factor to the spread of HIV/AIDS (see Figure 11-8, page 351).

India—In Chennai, India, mobile brothels manned by cell-phone toting operators are proving profitable. For those in the trade, running a mobile unit makes sound business sense as it cuts down on operational costs of renting a building and paying bribes. As for the client, it promises "pick and drop" sex workers at a place of his choice. More than 17 mobile units operate in the city, according to Chennai-based NGO Indian Community Welfare Organization (ICWO), which works with commercial sex workers (CSWs). According to estimates, there are 6300 women sex workers operating throughout the city. Thirty percent said they couldn't use condoms with regular clients. Another 30% said, at times, they would forget to have their clients wear condoms and 10% felt that condom usage would prolong sexual activity. Another 10% said some clients would object to it. As for reasons why they chose to be sex workers, 31% of respondents said they entered the profession due to family debts, and 29% said their husbands deserted them. About 29% said their lovers had ditched them.

Risk Estimates for HIV Infection During Sexual Intercourse in the Heterosexual Population— Estimates of the risk of HIV infection from a single heterosexual encounter depend on the following: (1) the probability that the sexual partner carries the virus; (2) if one of the sexual partners is HIV positive, the size of their viral load (suppression of viral load reduces the risk of HIV transmission); and (3) the reduction in risk by using condoms and spermicides.

Choosing a partner who is not in a high-risk group provides almost 5000-fold protection compared with choosing a partner in the highest-risk category (Figure 8-6).

In 2005 Perry Halkitis, director of the Center for Health Identity, Behavior and Prevention Studies, New York University, reviewed the literature on HIV transmission. From the data collected, he calculated the odds of HIV infection during sex in the absence of a condom (see Table 8-6).

Sexual connections as seen here are sometimes referred to as sexual networks. Such networks may involve (a) *serial monogamists*—persons who go from one relationship to another, one at a time, and (b) those involved in *concurrent relationships*—persons involved with more than one sexual partner in a given period who go back and forth between them. Both behaviors increase the possibility of infection/transmission because earlier sexual partners can be infected by later sexual partners.

Condoms are estimated to provide about 10-fold protection.

The implication of this analysis is clear: *Choose sex partners carefully and use condoms.*

Viral Load and Heterosexual Transmission

Recent data from two separate HIV investigations shed light on the issue of gender transmission. Thomas Quinn and colleagues (2000) reported that the lower the level of HIV in the blood, the less likely HIV-infected persons will transmit the virus to their heterosexual sexual partner. This research team studied 400 heterosexual couples over 2.5 years. In each couple, only one person was HIV positive (serodiscordant). No one with less than 1500 copies of HIV/milliliter of blood infected his or her partner. In those cases where one partner became infected, 80% of the time the viral load of the other partner was over 10,000. Such data confirm the benefit of lowering HIV levels in the blood via antiretroviral therapy. (Aspects of viral load are presented in Chapter 4, pages 94–96.) (See Point to Ponder 8.1, page 198.)

INJECTION-DRUG USERS AND HIV TRANSMISSION

While a number of drugs are ancient, the concept of injecting drugs is relatively recent.

Injecting oneself is mainly a twentieth century innovation because that is when (after 1960) cheap and disposable syringes became available. Experience from IDU transmission of HIV indicates that once HIV enters an injection-drug

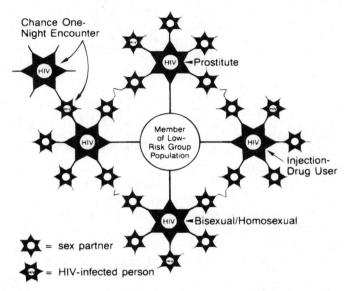

Risk Group Activities May Place You in the Middle of HIV Being Distributed Among Sexual Partners.

Chance One-Night Encounter

Prostitute

Member of Low-Risk Group Population

Injection-Drug User

Bisexual/Homosexual

= sex partner

= HIV-infected person

FIGURE 8-6   Risk Transmission of HIV. Sexual transmission can occur among homosexuals or heterosexuals. Prostitutes can be either male or female. The diagram shows possible bridges for transmission of HIV from high-risk groups into low-risk groups. In March 2008, New York Governor Eliot Spitzer, who gained national prominence relentlessly pursuing Wall Street wrongdoing, was caught arranging to meet with a high-priced prostitute. He later resigned from his position as governor. His visiting a prostitute placed him in an at-risk position. His wife, who said she had no knowledge of his activities, was placed at risk for contracting infectious diseases, including HIV, through Spitzer.

Then in 2009, Eldrick (Tiger) Woods revealed a series of extramarital affairs. Involved were prostitutes, nonprostitutes, and porn stars. The number of women involved, according to press releases and TV network news channels, was at least 14. Could he have possibly known of their sexual histories? The point here is, like Spitzer, Woods placed himself at risk for contacting or transmitting STDs, including HIV. According to reports, the mistresses claimed he had unprotected sex with them. Did he expose his former wife (they have divorced) Elin Nordegren or any of the other women to any of the STDs or HIV? And, what of other celebrities who disclosed their infidelities such as Reverend Jesse Jackson, Senator John Edwards, and Governor Arnold Schwarzenegger? Each fathered a child out of wedlock. Extramarital affairs without the use of condoms is risky at best with today's knowledge of STD and HIV transmission: How does one get those who supported these people from not following the leader?

Gaetan Dugas—an Air Canada flight steward identified as "Patient Zero" in Randy Shilts's *And the Band Played On*—showed just how large the chain or circle of transmission can be: at least 40 of the first 248 gay men diagnosed with AIDS in the United States had sex either with Dugas or with someone else who had. By contrast, heterosexual contact tracing resembles the spokes of a wheel: the wheel is so huge that it is practically infinite, with contacts leading linearly away from the index case. The transmission of HIV drew attention to a level of sexual activity among an exclusive group of individuals in a way that no other sexually transmitted disease had done at that point in time. To be safe, *you* must not become part of the chain.

Table 8-6 The Odds of Infecting Your Sexual Partner

If you're HIV positive and not using condoms and you are the:	Risk of your partner becoming infected:
Receptive partner of gay anal sex	1 in 1250
Insertive partner of gay anal sex	1 in 122
Receptive partner of straight vaginal sex	1 in 1,000,000
Insertive partner of straight vaginal sex	1 in 111,111
Receiver of penile oral sex	1 in 1250
Performer of penile oral sex	Negligible[1]
Receiver of vaginal oral sex	Negligible
Performer of vaginal oral sex	Negligible

Source: Jennifer Gong. POZ, *November 2005, copyright 2005 CM Publishing LLC.*
[1]Although the last three categories appear to be low risk, there are no guarantees.

use population, that country can expect a large and substantial HIV epidemic. IDU is a very efficient way of transmitting HIV, three times more efficient than through sexual intercourse.

HIV entered injection users during the mid-1970s and spread rapidly through 1983 largely unrecognized and unidentified. HIV transmission via IDU is the second most frequent risk behavior among adults/adolescents for becoming HIV infected in the developed world. Illicit drug injection has been reported in 151 countries. Ending year 2013, of 1.37 million cases of AIDS that will be reported to CDC, 493,000 (36%) will be directly or indirectly associated with injection-drug use. About half the females and about one-third of the heterosexual males who were diagnosed with AIDS had a sex partner who was an IDU (*HIV/AIDS Surveillance Report,* 1998 updated). It is estimated that half the estimated 56,000-plus new HIV infections in the United States, or 153 people per day in the year 2013, will be associated with IDUs. The epidemic among injection-drug users in New York City is an example of a very large, high-seroprevalence HIV epidemic. More than 100,000 injection-drug users have been infected with HIV, and over 50,000 cases of AIDS are reported among injection-drug users, their sexual partners, and their children in New York City (DesJarlais et al., 2000 updated).

UNITED STATES: HETEROSEXUAL INJECTION-DRUG USE (IDU)

Women and Injection-Drug Use

Over 90% of injection-drug users in the United States are heterosexuals. Thirty percent are women, 90% of whom are in their childbearing years. From 1988 to the beginning of 2013, female IDUs made up about 40% of all AIDS cases in women. Of the 41% of women infected by heterosexual contact, 38% were infected by having sex with a male IDU. During this same period over 8000 new cases of AIDS in children occurred—37% were from IDU mothers and 18% were from mothers whose sex partners were IDUs (*MMWR,* 1992; *HIV/AIDS Surveillance Report,* 2001 updated). Women IDUs and sexual partners of male IDUs represent the largest part (61%) of the estimated 100,000-plus HIV-infected women of childbearing age. Thus, there is a direct correlation between HIV perinatal transmission and pediatric AIDS cases and injection-drug use.

INJECTION-DRUG USE AND HIV INFECTIONS IN OTHER COUNTRIES

Sharing and reusing contaminated injection material is the easiest and most effective way to transmit HIV and other blood-borne diseases—particularly hepatitis C. Once in the bloodstream,

BOX 8.3

SPORTS AND HIV/AIDS: EARVIN "MAGIC" JOHNSON AND OTHER ATHLETES

HIV-INFECTED ATHLETES AND COMPETITION

The question regarding whether HIV-infected athletes should be allowed to compete has two facets:

1. Should these athletes be banned from competition to avoid the risk of spreading HIV infection?
2. Does the exercise that is demanded in competition accelerate the progression of HIV disease?

There is no hard, fast, scientifically supported answer to either question. However, as of the beginning of 2013, there has not been a single reported case of HIV transmission in any sporting event worldwide (Drotman, 1996 updated).

Magic Johnson: Professional Basketball Player, Los Angeles Lakers, HIV Positive

The first well-known HIV/AIDS-related name people became aware of in the United States was Rock Hudson, the famous movie star. He announced he had AIDS in July 1985 and died in October 1985. Rock Hudson's death from AIDS received international attention and was a major wake-up call to all Americans. The second well-known and respected personality to announce he was HIV infected was Magic Johnson, the National Basketball Association star. His announcement in 1991 came six years after Rock Hudson's. This shock was also felt around the world, especially in the United States and particularly in the black community. Now the U.S. community was forcefully aware of HIV/AIDs!

Earvin "Magic" Johnson said, "I thought the hardest thing I would ever have to do in life was try to beat fellow basketball greats Larry Bird and Michael Jordan on the basketball court. Instead the hardest thing was driving home from the doctor's office to tell my wife Cookie that I was HIV positive."

On November 7, 1991, Magic Johnson, age 32, appeared at a nationally televised press conference and said, "Because of the HIV virus I have obtained, I will have to announce my retirement from the Lakers today." He admitted having been "naïve" about AIDS and added, "Here I am saying *it can happen to anybody,* even me, Magic Johnson." He also assured the world that his wife, Cookie Kelly, two months pregnant, had tested negative for the virus.

Some Events Since Magic's Announced Retirement

June 4, 1992—Earvin III is born *without* antibody to HIV. As of August 14, 2012, Magic is age 54. His wife, age 58, and son, age 22, are HIV negative.

His 2012 checkup confirms he's still asymptomatic after 21 years. His one major regret is that he retired from basketball too soon.

Other Sports, Other Athletes—Basketball players are not the only athletes whose behavior may place them at risk for HIV infection. In 2012 there were at least 7131 professional athletes in the United States involved in boxing (4065), the National Football League (1854), National Hockey League (784), and National Basketball Association (428). Of these professionals, the CDC estimated 37 to be HIV positive.

John Elson (1991) wrote a revealing article for *Time* magazine just after Magic Johnson revealed his HIV status. Elson tells of groupies that follow athletes in all sports. They are usually college-age or older. Mainly they seek money, attention, and the glamour of associating with celebrated and highly visible "hard bodies." According to a 31-year-old who has had affairs with athletes in two sports, "For women, many of whom don't have meaningful work, the only way to identify themselves is to say whom they have slept with. A woman who sleeps around is called a whore. But a woman who has slept with Magic Johnson is a woman who has slept with Magic Johnson. It's almost as if it gives her legitimacy."

The Girls—Baseball players call them "Annies." To riders on the rodeo circuit, they are "buckle bunnies." To most other athletes, they are "wannabes" or just "the girls." They can be found hanging out anywhere they might catch an off-duty sports hero's eye and fancy, or in the lobbies of hotels where teams on the road check in. To the athletes who care to indulge them— and many do—these readily available groupies offer pro sports' ultimate perk: free and easy recreational sex, no questions asked. Recently, an HIV-infected female stated publicly that she had had sex with at least 50 Canadian ice hockey players. She could not recall their names. The sex may be free, but now there is a price for the lifestyle—HIV/AIDS.

Sports/Injuries/Blood—Concerns over the transmission of HIV are shared throughout sports, particularly those sports that cause blood-letting injuries—football, hockey, and boxing. In football Jerry Smith, a former Washington Redskin, died of AIDS in 1986; in December 2003, Roy Simmons, an offensive lineman for the New York Giants and Washington Redskins, revealed that he was HIV positive. He tested HIV positive in 1997 and has sex with other men.

In 2005, according to the *New York Times*, Trevis Smith, a seven-season veteran of the Canadian Football League's Saskatchewan Roughriders, was arrested

BOX 8.3 *(continued)*

on October 28 and charged with aggravated sexual assault. The police disclosed Smith's HIV-positive status to the public, saying such a warning was necessary. Team officials said they had been aware of Smith's status for about a year but privacy laws had prevented them from disclosing the information to his teammates. At a November 2 hearing, Smith was ordered by a judge to use condoms, disclose to his sexual partners that he is HIV positive, and give up his passport. The judge did not provide conditions on Smith's eligibility to continue playing in the CFL.

In 1996, the National Football League officials estimated that there was the *possibility* of one HIV transmission from body fluid exchange in 85 million football games played.

Boxing—In boxing, Esteban Dejesus, WBC lightweight champion, died of AIDS in 1989. Four other boxers are known to be HIV positive.

Tommy Morrison—In February 1996 Tommy Morrison, age 27, a heavyweight boxing title contender, said, on announcing that he was HIV positive, "I honestly believed I had a better chance of winning the lottery than contracting this disease. I've never been so wrong in my life. I'm here to tell you I thought that I was bulletproof, and I'm not."

Morrison had his sperm washed free of HIV and fathered a boy in late 2003.

ATTENTION: In March 2007 Tommy Morrison took a repeated series of HIV tests and was found to be HIV negative! He said, "I was kicked to the curb and lost more than ten years of my career because of a false positive. I was using steroids at the time. I believe that's why the test came back the way it did. But I've taken five or six different tests in the last three or four months, and I passed them all." It is believed that either the initial tests were improperly

run, his blood vial was mixed up in the laboratory, or the results were improperly interpreted. If someone truly tests HIV positive, they stay that way for life.

Ice Skating—In professional ice skating, the *Calgary Herald* and others reported that by 2007, at least 45 top U.S. and Canadian male skaters and coaches had died from AIDS (among them Rob McCall, Brian Pockar, Dennis Coi, Shaun McGill, and Nicole Lesh).

Swimming—In February 1995, Greg Louganis, the greatest diver in Olympic history, announced that he had AIDS. During the 1988 Olympics, he kept his HIV infection secret. He retired from swimming because of a fungal infection. He paid his hospital bill, in the thousands of dollars, in cash because he did not want his insurance company or the tabloids to learn his secret. Ending 2012, he is alive and well.

Tennis—Arthur Ashe died in 1993. He received HIV through a blood transfusion.

Baseball—Glenn Burke, outfielder, Los Angeles Dodgers/Oakland Athletics, died in 1995.

Race Car Drivers—It was reported in 1996 that Tim Richmond, race car driver, age 34, had died of AIDS. He won 13 Winston Cup races on the NASCAR racing circuit. One report states that Richmond may have infected up to 30 women (Knight-Tribune Service, March 27, 1996, A-1). His physician estimated that he was HIV positive for at least eight years. During this time, according to accounts of friends, he was sexually promiscuous. (Richmond actually died in 1989 but his story was kept silent until 1996.)

Ice Hockey—Bill Goldsworthy, five-time NHL All-Star, age 51, died of AIDS. He played 14 seasons in the NHL. He was diagnosed with AIDS in 1994. Goldsworthy said his health problem was caused by drinking and sexual promiscuity.

HIV spreads rapidly and relentlessly. When an HIV-positive injecting drug user shares a needle, transmission is pretty much guaranteed. One HIV-positive drug user can transmit the virus to thousands of people via contaminated equipment and into the general population through sexual contact with spouses and other intimate partners.

Injection-drug users (IDUs) remain largely hidden from public view because of associated stigma, discrimination, and imprisonment. Currently, 25 countries in the Asia-Pacific region impose the death penalty for offenses conected

with possession and abuse of drugs! Worldwide there are about 16 million injection-drug users. About 5 million are HIV positive. An estimated 80% live in developing countries. About 13.1 million live in Eastern and Central Europe and South and Southeast Asia. About 1.9 million live in North America and about 1 million live in Latin America. Eighty percent of IDUs are men. An estimated 3 to 4 million past and current injection-drug users are living with HIV/AIDS. Accordingly, in many countries, IDUs represent a significant proportion of those individuals who are in need of antiretroviral drugs. The dual epidemic of injection-drug use and HIV particularly affect resource-poor countries where there is limited access to HIV prevention measures such as needle and syringe exchange programs.

It appears that IDU is the major mode of HIV transmission in Russia, Kazakhstan, Malaysia, Vietnam, China, North America, Eastern and Western Europe, the Newly Independent States, and the Middle East. Additionally, it is becoming more of an issue in West Africa and Latin America. The greatest problem has been seen in the Newly Independent States, in Eastern Europe, and in China.

Outside of sub-Saharan Africa, almost one-third of all HIV infections stem from IDU.

To date, fewer than 10% of the IDUs received practical help to prevent the spread of HIV (Figure 8-7, below).

Eastern Europe and the Former Soviet Union

Five countries (China, Malaysia, Russia, Ukraine, and Vietnam) are characterized as mega-epidemics in terms of people who inject drugs. Taken together, these countries account for an estimated two to four million cases of HIV infection and constitute the largest concentration of injecting drug users living with HIV worldwide. In Eastern Europe and Central Asia the situation is particularly worrisome. Injection-drug users account for

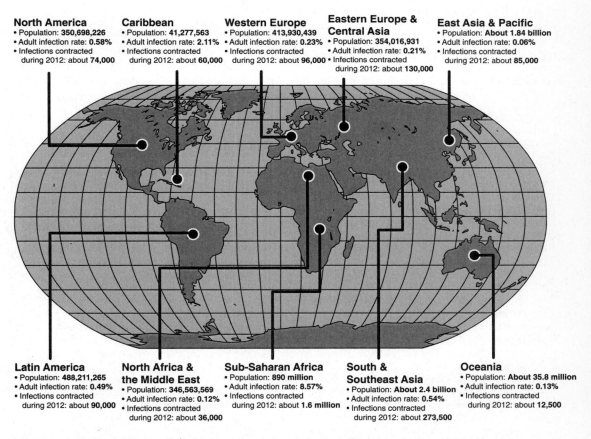

North America
- Population: **350,698,226**
- Adult infection rate: **0.58%**
- Infections contracted during 2012: about **74,000**

Caribbean
- Population: **41,277,563**
- Adult infection rate: **2.11%**
- Infections contracted during 2012: about **60,000**

Western Europe
- Population: **413,930,439**
- Adult infection rate: **0.23%**
- Infections contracted during 2012: about **96,000**

Eastern Europe & Central Asia
- Population: **354,016,931**
- Adult infection rate: **0.21%**
- Infections contracted during 2012: about **130,000**

East Asia & Pacific
- Population: **About 1.84 billion**
- Adult infection rate: **0.06%**
- Infections contracted during 2012: about **85,000**

Latin America
- Population: **488,211,265**
- Adult infection rate: **0.49%**
- Infections contracted during 2012: about **90,000**

North Africa & the Middle East
- Population: **346,563,569**
- Adult infection rate: **0.12%**
- Infections contracted during 2012: about **36,000**

Sub-Saharan Africa
- Population: **890 million**
- Adult infection rate: **8.57%**
- Infections contracted during 2012: about **1.6 million**

South & Southeast Asia
- Population: **About 2.4 billion**
- Adult infection rate: **0.54%**
- Infections contracted during 2012: about **273,500**

Oceania
- Population: **About 35.8 million**
- Adult infection rate: **0.13%**
- Infections contracted during 2012: about **12,500**

FIGURE 8-7 Global Impact of HIV/AIDS. About 38 million adults and children worldwide will be living with HIV/AIDS by the end of 2013, according to UNAIDS estimates. Estimated new infections for 2013, 2.5 million. *(UNAIDS; World Health Organization; U.S. Centers for Disease Control and Prevention; updated.)*

more than 60% of all HIV infections in Belarus, Georgia, Iran, Kazakhstan, Kyrgyzstan, Moldova, Russia, Ukraine, Tajikistan, and Uzbekistan.

Injection-Drug Use in Russia

Russian health officials estimate there may be as many as 4 million IDUs. About half are HIV infected. They say up to 60% of IDUs are between ages 18 and 30 with pre-college teenagers accounting for another 20%. Vadim Pokrovsky, head of the official AIDS prevention center, told a news conference broadcast on the Internet site www.presscentr.ru that "We are currently going through the peak of an epidemic among drug users. Currently about 90% of HIV infections are associated with IDU. In two or three years there will be another upsurge from sexual transmission of the disease."

Moscow—Change of Scene, Same Results

The hotbed of the disease has moved from the tiny Baltic enclave of Kaliningrad to Moscow and its suburbs. In some parts of Moscow, up to 5% of the young people are already HIV positive. If counted as a percentage of the population, Russia will reach U.S. levels. About 80% of the infected are aged 15 to 25. They will be lost in 10 years, just after they have finished their education. It means one gets infected at 20, graduates at 30, starts working, and dies. Murray Feshbach, a specialist in Russian demographic trends, estimates that 5 to 10 million people will die of AIDS in Russia after year 2015.

Current estimates are that 36,000 adults/ adolescents and 6600 babies are becoming HIV infected each year in Russia. The Russian federal government allocated about $300 million in 2012 for its HIV/AIDS programs.

Epidemic in the Ukraine

The Ukraine's HIV/AIDS epidemic, the worst of all the former Soviet Union nations, is causing alarm among Ukrainian physicians and other neighboring countries. In a nation of 50 million people, about 250,000 (5%) are HIV positive, and the level of infection continues to rise.

Figure 8-7 presents the estimated new HIV infections for 2012 across the globe.

POINT TO PONDER 8.3

COTROVERSIAL OPINIONS STATING THAT CRIMINALIZING DRUG USE MUST BE STOPPED BECAUSE IT PREVENTS HARM REDUCTION WITH RESPECT TO HIV TRANSMISSION

As delegates gathered for the XIX International AIDS Conference (AIDS 2012) in Washington, D.C., supporters of the 2010 Vienna Declaration, which urges governments to write evidencebased drug policies, launched an ad campaign calling on U.S. President Barack Obama and Republican presidential candidate Mitt Romney "to stop the spread of AIDS by ending the so called "war on drugs." British businessman Richard Branson; former president of Brazil Fernando Henriquc Cardoso; former president of Colombia Cesar Gaviria; Michel Kazatchkine, former executive director of the Global Fund to Fight AIDS, Tuberculosis and Malaria; Evan Wood, chair of the Vienna Declaration Writing Committee; and Julio Montaner, director of the BC Centre for the Excellence in HIV/AIDS, among others, have endorsed the declaration and the ad, which states, "You can't end AIDS unless you end the war on drugs. It's dead simple." Also at this conference, Mathilde Krim, founding chair of amFAR and a member of the board of the Drug Policy Alliance, and Ethan Nadelmann, founder and executive director the Drug Policy Alliance. wrote in the Huffington Post's "Politics Blog" that "Too many countries in the world have let their repressive and punitive drug policies get in the way of the public's health. The spread of HIV will not be stopped as long as drugs use remains criminalized and as long as people who inject drugs are given up for lost." In short, these delegates at AIDS 2012 said, "It is impossible to ignore an inconvenient truth: that drug war politics and policies in the United States and many other countries are severely jeopardizing the overall "fight against AIDS."

CLASS QUESTION—given that there are over 16 million injection drug users and millions of others who use a variety of other addictive drugs, do you think there will be a global decriminalization of drug use say in the next five years? 10 years? When? Present facts and figures to defend your choice. What is your opinion of the push for global decriminalization of drug use by the AIDS 2012 delegates listed above.

China

The lifting of a ban on AIDS-related reporting in 2000 in the state-run media appears to have fed a public panic through alarmist reports that China is on the verge of an epidemic. The government recently projected that the number of people infected with HIV could rise to 10 million by 2015 from an estimated 1 million now if preventive measures are not enforced. The current estimate provided by the Chinese health officials is believed, by the WHO and UNAIDS, to be several times that high. By 2001 HIV infections were found in every province with prevalence rates of 77% among injection-drug users, ages 20 to 29, and 11% among prostitutes.

Latin America

Latin America though 2012 had an estimated 2.02 million injection-drug users, of which about 20% are/were HIV positive (over 400,000). Ending 2013 there will be an estimated 1.82 million people living with HIV/AIDS in Latin America. More than 70% reside in the four largest countries in the region—Argentina, Brazil, Colombia, and Mexico. Brazil alone is home to more than 40% of the region's HIV/AIDS population (730,000 people).

Caribbean HIV/AIDS: Small Islands—Big Problems

The Caribbean region consists of 29 countries or territories with Spanish, Dutch, French, and British influences. The total population includes approximately 39 million individuals of African, European, and Asian descent, and indigenous groups. Approximately 20 million visitors travel to the Caribbean each year from the United States. Data from the CDC continues to indicate that the Caribbean is the largest contributor of new diagnoses of HIV infection in the U.S. foreign-born population in New York City, accounting for 38% of cases, with the total increasing to 55% if new diagnoses in individuals born in Puerto Rico are included.

In the Caribbean, an estimated 15,000 people die from AIDS annually and about 20,000 adults

---

SIDEBAR 8.2

JAMAICA: IT'S THE PEOPLE KILLING US, NOT AIDS!

Part of the Caribbean's susceptibility to HIV/AIDS is pervasive homophobia, which drives the epidemic underground, helping to spread infections and make education and outreach more difficult. In Jamaica, gay men have a 32% HIV infection rate and widespread homophobia amplifies the impact of HIV/AIDS. The "abominable act of buggery," as anal sex is termed in Jamaican law, is punishable by up to 10 years of hard labor. Popular dance music celebrates the murder of gay men, inciting and reflecting widespread acts of violence against gays. A religious context of homosexuality as a mortal sin compounds the contempt that checks any concern for gays. The reality in Jamaica is that men who have sex with men, for fear of being prosecuted and being found guilty under the sodomy law, pretend that they're not gay. They marry and fairly rapidly have children. And that is really a ticking time bomb. Gays—including those who have quite high levels of HIV viral load—are pressured to participate in heterosexual sexual relationships to prevent societal persecution and sometimes even criminal prosecution. "If it were AIDS that were killing us, I would use a condom," said a 20-year-old man in Kingston whose boyfriend was stabbed to death on the street for being gay. The same man had seen another close friend locked inside his parents' house by a crowd and burned alive. "It's people, not AIDS, that is killing us."

---

and children become infected. The total number of infected is about one million. In the Caribbean HIV infects 1% of the population, which means the Caribbean has the highest rate of HIV infection in the world after sub-Saharan Africa, and AIDS is already the single greatest cause of death among young men and women ages 25 to 44 years in this region. The rate of HIV infection in the Caribbean is about four times that of North America, Latin America, and South and Southeast Asia. The rate is 35 times that found in East Asia and the Pacific and almost 10 times the rate in Western Europe (Figure 8-7, pages 213). According to UNAIDS, if left unchecked HIV/AIDS will, by year 2020, cause 75% of deaths in the Caribbean. Such a scenario mimics what is happening in some parts of Africa. The disease has spread over the African continent through

PEOPLE DO STUPID THINGS—
THAT'S WHAT SPREADS HIV
(This was a headline in a
U.K. Guardian Newspaper, 2010)

Elizabeth Pisani, a 16-year veteran in HIV epidemiology, shared a story with her audience that sometimes people do stupid things for perfectly rational reasons. For example, she asked, "What is rational for an addict (injection drug user)?" To answer, she said,

I remember speaking to an Indonesian friend of mine, Frankie. We were having lunch and he was telling me about when he was in jail in Bali for drug injection. And it was someone's birthday, and they had very kindly smuggled some heroin into the jail, and he was very generously sharing it with all of his colleagues. And so everyone lined up, all the smack heads in a row. And the guy whose birthday it was filled up the fit, and he went down and started injecting people. So he injects the first guy, and then he's wiping the needle on his shirt, and he injects the next guy. And Frankie said, "I'm number 22 in line, and I can see the needle coming down towards me, and there is blood all over the place. It's getting blunter and blunter. And a small part of my brain is thinking, "That is so gross and really dangerous," but most of my brain is thinking, "Please let there be some smack left by the time it gets to me. Please let there be some left." And then, telling me this story, Frankie said, "You know, god, drugs really make you stupid." And you know, you can't fault Frankie for accuracy, but, actually, Frankie, at that time, was a heroin addict, and he was in jail. So his choice was either to accept that dirty needle or not to get high. And if there's one place you really want to get high, it's when you're in jail. Rational for the junkie—I need a fix, why not share a needle that you may or may not get a disease that may or not kill me in 10 years. I will probably die of something before that. Suddenly it becomes rational to share needles. Remember, there are as many ways to be rational as there are humans on planet earth!

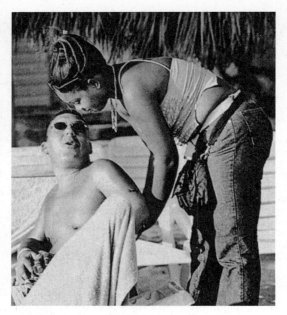

FIGURE 8–8 A Sex Worker Solicits a Tourist In Boca Chica, a Well-Known Beach for Prostitution about 20 Minutes from Santo Domingo. About 100,000 women in the Dominican Republic are engaged in sex work. Most sex workers will tell you they will not have sex without a condom, but sometimes clients think that insistence on using a condom is a bargaining tactic based on economics. Since its first appearance in the Caribbean, HIV/AIDS has been a mobile epidemic closely linked to the region's underground sex trade and has altered the economy in many regions of the Caribbean and Latin America. *(Photo by Hilda M. Perez/South Florida Sun-Sentinel.)*

mobility. Long-haul truck drivers having sex with prostitutes along their routes have brought it home to wives and girlfriends. Heterosexual sexual transmission accounts for 60% to 80% of infections. Likewise, throughout the Caribbean, tourists, truck drivers, shipmates, and soldiers have been important male agents of the spread of HIV (MSM about 10% to 15%), as is the use of injection drugs (6% to 10%). In Puerto Rico, for example, over half of 30,000 plus AIDS cases were/are associated with IDU. Between 35% and 50% of injection-drug users are HIV infected. According to the CDC, Puerto Rico has the fourth-highest HIV infection rate of American states and territories, behind Washington, D.C., New York City, and the U.S. Virgin Islands. Puerto Rico plays a special role as a global border town in the transmission of HIV because it is a central transportation and commerce hub for the Caribbean. It is a favorite location for both trafficking drugs and smuggling people, especially from the Dominican Republic. (See Sidebar 8.2 and Quicktake 8.1, page 216.) **Caribbean American HIV/AIDS Awareness Day, June 8 annually.**

The Sex Trade, Women and Children: Two Examples, the Caribbean and Southeast Asia

Overall, in the Caribbean, the majority of HIV infection is sexually transmitted (Figure 8-8, page 216). According to a 2000 UNAIDS report, the spread of HIV is partly driven by older men who have numerous sex partners and who seek out young women for sex and infect them. They in turn pass the virus on. If Caribbean women in general refuse unsafe sex and insist on the use of a condom, they often risk spousal abuse because it creates a suspicion of infidelity. Ten years ago there were seven times more infected men than women in the Caribbean. By 2003 that ratio had changed to 2 to 1. Aside from South Africa, the Caribbean is the only region where the proportion of women and girls living with HIV is higher than that of men and boys.

Southeast Asia, The Golden Triangle

There are no reliable statistics on the number of children working in the sex industry worldwide, but the lowest figure cited is 1 million. The United Nations Children's Fund estimates that one-third of sex workers in Southeast Asia are 12 to 17 years old. The smuggling of vast quantities of heroin and amphetamines from Myanmar and China through Thailand has given the region its infamous tag, "The Golden Triangle," but it's the explosion in the recruitment of girls into the lucrative Thai sex industry that has put this border town on the map. Every year, hundreds of young girls from Mae Sai, a town of 80,000 inhabitants on Thailand's northernmost border with Burma, are spirited away to brothels in Bangkok where they feed the insatiable appetite of the $20 billion commercial sex industry.

Drugs and Daughters—Mae Sai has two main trades, drugs and daughters. A nongovernmental organization in Mae Sai that works with local girls who are at risk of being sold estimates that of the village of Pa Tek's 800 families, 7 in every 10 have sold at least one daughter into the trade.

When a Burmese migrant in Pa Tek sold his 13-year-old daughter into prostitution for $114,

his wife had one regret—they didn't get a good price for her. She said, "I should have asked for $228. He robbed us." The mother earns about $100 a year selling bamboo bowls in the local market and lives in a thatched hut in Pa Tek village on the outskirts of Mae Sai. Prices vary from $114 to $913 per daughter: the latter figure is equal to almost six years' wages for most families. Parental bonds in impoverished households are easily broken. In fact, child prostitution is so established that many brothel agents live in the village and are often friends or relatives of the family from whom they buy the children. The director of the Child Protection and Rights Center in Mae Sai said, "Agents will come to the village with orders to fill so people in Bangkok, Thai men, and foreigners, mostly Europeans, can order girls like they order pizza. If they want a girl with thin hips and big breasts, the agents will come here and find her. They always deliver."

Caribbean Connection to America: South Florida

Five nations in the Caribbean with the highest infection rates have HIV infections in all segments of their populations. During the last 31 years about 350,000 Haitians have died of AIDS. UNAIDS estimates that Haiti, with 10% of the urban and 5% of the rural population infected (about 425,000; population 8.5 million), has the highest rate of HIV infection and 90% of all AIDS cases in the Caribbean. Next is the Bahamas at about 4% and 3% for Barbados. Guyana and the Dominican Republic are each at 2% with about 8% of their pregnant women HIV infected. (For data on Cuba, see Chapter 9, page 249.) **The Seventh National Caribbean American HIV/AIDS Awareness Day was celebrated June 8, 2011.**

The Connection

The cruise ships and planes that leave and return to Fort Lauderdale and Miami weekly depend on the allure of tropical beaches, exotic ports, and lusty streets in the islands. Discount department stores depend on shirts sewn in Haitian textile plants, and increasingly, much of the low- and high-tech workforce essential to South Florida comes from Haiti, the Dominican Republic, and other Caribbean countries. In short, there is no way that South Florida can be spared the effects of the HIV/AIDS calamity in the Caribbean. The region is so tightly linked through culture, race, ethnicity, and economics that any public health crisis in the islands is felt here. In a highly mobile, global age, there are few boundaries that cannot be crossed. The disease, carried unknowingly among tourists and workers every day throughout the region, respects no borders.

OTHER MEANS OF HIV TRANSMISSION

Other means of HIV infection have been documented. There has been a reported case of HIV transmission via *acupuncture*. It is believed that HIV-infected body fluids contaminated the acupuncture needles (Vittecoq et al., 1989). Unlicensed and unregulated *tattoo* establishments may also present an unrecognized risk for HIV infection to patrons. If the operator does not use new needles or needles that have been autoclaved (steam sterilized), the possibility exists that infection with HIV or a number of other blood-borne pathogens may take place. In addition, single-service or individual containers of dye or ink should be used for each client.

Organ/Tissue Transplants

On any given day, over 100,000 Americans are waiting for a transplant. About 15,000 organs are donated annually. Eighteen of those most in need die each day. There is a small but present risk of receiving HIV along with the transplant tissue. A CDC report revealed that a bone marrow transplant recipient became HIV-infected from an HIV-infected donor. HIV transmission has also occurred in the transplantation of kidneys, liver, heart, pancreas, and skin (*MMWR*, 1988). In May 1991, the CDC reported on 56 transplant patients who received organs and tissues from an HIV-infected donor in 1985. A transplantation service company supplied tissues to 30 hospitals in 16

states. All tissues came from a single young male who was shot to death during a robbery. He twice tested HIV negative before his heart, kidneys, liver, pancreas, cornea, and other tissues were removed for transplant. By mid-1991, three recipients of these tissues had died of AIDS and six others were HIV positive. As of mid-1991, 32 other recipients had been located, 11 of whom tested HIV negative. It is unknown whether the others have ever been tested.

In May 1994, the CDC published guidelines for preventing HIV transmission through transplantation of human tissue (*MMWR*, 1994b).

In January 2007, four transplant recipients received HIV- and HCV- (hepatitis C virus) contaminated organs in three Chicago hospitals. By November 2007, all four were HIV and HCV positive. The CDC is investigating whether the four people may, in turn, have transmitted those viruses to others before they learned they were infected. The organ donor, via a screening questionnaire, was known to have engaged in high-risk activity, but pretransplant tests were HIV negative, probably because the infections were too recent to generate antibodies. When organs are transplanted from such donors, the CDC recommends that the recipients be tested three months after their surgeries.

In 2009, a kidney transplant recipient contracted HIV from a living donor who tested HIV negative. This is the first confirmed case of HIV transmission through organ transplantation from a living donor reported since 1989 and the first such transmission documented in the United States since laboratory screening for HIV infection became available in 1985. The donor had reported a previous syphilis diagnosis and a history of male sex partners in his initial transplant evaluation. Testing 79 days before the procedure showed no evidence of HIV, hepatitis B, or hepatitis C infection. However, the investigation revealed he had had unprotected sex with one male partner of unknown HIV status during the one year before the transplant, including the time between his initial evaluation and surgery for organ harvesting. To prevent and screen for HIV in prospective living organ donors, CDC is now recommending the

SIDEBAR 8.3

HIV/AIDS TRANSPLANT ERROR

MEXICO

MEXICAN DOCTORS TRANSPLANT HIV-INFECTED KIDNEYS

In February 1999, Mexican health officials fired five physicians and warned two others for transplanting HIV-infected kidneys into two patients. One of the two patients has since tested HIV positive. According to the regional director of the state-run hospital, the physicians did not wait for the results of the HIV test on the kidney donor before making the transplant.

In April 2002, the unofficial estimate was that 150,000 Mexicans required access to HIV/AIDS care and treatment. The epidemic in Mexico is centered among gay men ages 15 to 44. The number of HIV-infected women is rapidly rising. (For current information on Mexico, see Chapter 10, pages 310–312).

ITALY

In February 2007, a 40-year-old woman died of a brain hemorrhage. With family consent, her organs were harvested and three of those organs, both kidneys and the liver, were separated and transplanted into three individuals. After the fact, it was found that the donor was HIV positive. All three organ recipients are on antiretroviral therapy.

TAIWAN

In August 2011, five transplant recipients received organs from a deceased HIV-infected donor due to a lapse in operating procedures, the Taipei-based National Taiwan University Hospital (NTUH) said that a transplant staff member believed he had heard the English word "non-reactive" during a briefing given over the telephone about the organ donor's HIV test. But "reactive," or HIV-positive, was in fact said. Information about the result was not double-checked as standard operating procedures require, NTUH said. "We deeply apologize for the mistake."

following: all living donor candidates should have their initial serologic HIV tests confirmed with a combination of an HIV serologic test and nucleic acid testing as close to organ donation as possible, but no longer than seven days prior. In 2012, about 90,000 people were on the kidney transplant list. Currently in the United States, the waiting time for a kidney is about 8 years.

According to CDC guidelines, "High risk patients should be excluded from organ and tissue donation unless the risk to the recipient of not performing the transplant is deemed greater than the risk of HIV transmission and disease." In other words, this is a risk–versus–benefits calculation.

Since 1981, at least 93 liver and kidney transplant cases have involved the use of human organs that were HIV positive. Of the 93 transplant cases, 71 of the patients were HIV negative prior to transplant and received organs that contained HIV. All became HIV positive. The average time for progression to AIDS was 32 months. The 22 people who were HIV positive prior to receiving an HIV-positive organ progressed to AIDS, on average, within 17 months (Horn, 2001). (See Sidebar 8.3.)

HIV/AIDS Patients and Organ Transplants

According to published reports, Larry Kramer, age 71, who cofounded the Gay Men's Health Crisis in 1981 and the AIDS Coalition to Unleash Power (ACT UP), suffered from end stage liver disease. After being rejected by other health centers, Kramer, who is HIV positive, received a new liver at the Thomas E. Starlz Transplantation Institute in Pittsburgh on December 21, 2001. As of December 2002, Kramer's liver transplant had cost Medicare about a million dollars and Empire Blue Cross about $500,000 for the medications he had to take, including $10,000 a month for Hepatitis B Immune Globulin, which he will receive for the rest of his life. Art Kaplan, director of the Center of Bioethics, said that the medical community has yet to debate the ethics of transplanting organs into people with HIV/AIDS. This is largely because centers like Starlz are just beginning to create possibilities. Beginning 2013, about 575 HIV-positive people have received transplants in the United States. (See Sidebar 8.3.) Between 2008 and 2012 at least 10 donor kidney transplants were made in South Africa between HIV-positive people. This has not yet been done in the United States. However, with the recent improvements in ART, transplant surgeons in the United States are considering it.

DISCUSSION QUESTION: Debate the ethics of giving an HIV-positive person an organ

transplant in light of the fact that thousands of young and old uninfected people die each year while waiting for a transplant.

INFLUENCE OF SEXUALLY TRANSMITTED DISEASES (STDS) ON HIV TRANSMISSION AND VICE VERSA

Sexual intercourse occurs more than 100 million times daily around the world. Results: 910,000 conceptions and over 600,000 cases of sexually transmitted disease/day. In the United States, according to the CDC, about 19 million new cases of sexually transmitted diseases occur each year. Over nine million (about 48%) of these cases occur in 15- to 24-year-olds. By age 21, about one in five people has received treatment for an STD. At current rates at least one American in four will contract an STD at some point in his or her life. Over 50 organisms that can cause an STD are transmitted through sexual activity (Hooker, 1996). Regardless of these facts, data from the CDC in 2001 revealed that one in four physicians do not screen their patients for STDs. In addition, a GayHealth.com online survey conducted in May 2001 found 4 in 10 gay and lesbian patients have physicians who don't ask about their sexual practices. Over 40% of the men surveyed said they have not been vaccinated against either hepatitis A or B, potentially fatal viral liver infections spread through sexual activity. Men who have sex with men are at higher risk than the general population for these diseases. The annual cost of STDs in the United States is in excess of $14 billion. The latest U.S. government information on STDs and their treatment can be found in the updated 2010 STD Treatment Guidelines published by the CDC in August 2012.

The Link Between Other STDs and HIV Infection: USA (April 2013 is the 18th STD Awareness Anniversary in the United States)

The publication of results from the Mwanza treatment study in 1995 provided convincing evidence that treating sexually transmitted diseases could slow HIV transmission (Grosskurth et al., 1995). These developments were the first important advances in biomedical prevention since the advent of an HIV test to screen blood for transfusion (1985). They also identified the first prevention interventions that did not require changing sexual or drug-use behavior. After these advances, treatment of sexually transmitted diseases and programs to prevent mother-to-child transmission became cornerstones of prevention programs.

STDs are linked with HIV in several ways. Because other STDs and HIV are spread by similar types of sexual activity, people who engage in behaviors that transmit HIV are also more likely to contract other STDs, and vice versa. Epidemiological evidence shows that populations and geographical regions in the United States with the highest STD rates also tend to have the highest rates of HIV. According to the CDC, "The geographic distribution of heterosexual HIV transmission closely parallels that of other STDs." In the past decade, high HIV incidence rates have shifted toward women infected through heterosexual activity, young adults, Black Americans, and people living in the southeastern United States, all populations with disproportionately high rates of STDs. (Point of Information 8.3)

Tissues Most Often Infected with an STD

Infection by sexually transmitted diseases usually occurs through the mucosal (membrane) surfaces of the male and female genital tracts and rectum. The mucosal route also accounts for a large percentage of heterosexual and homosexual transmission of HIV. It is known that STDs increase the number of T4 or CD4+ cells (HIV target cells) in cervical secretions, thereby increasing the chance of HIV infection in women.

Most AIDS researchers agree that treating STDs, which cures genital sores and reduces inflammation, can raise the body's barriers against HIV infection. According to a study by Grosskurth and coworkers (1995), researchers working in rural Tanzania saw the number of new HIV infections plummet by 42% after they improved STD health care.

Because HIV is sexually transmitted, the association between HIV and other sexually transmitted diseases can be in part attributed to the shared risk of exposure and shared modes of transmission.

Types of STDs Most Often Associated with HIV Transmission, Globally, and the USA, Specifically

STDs appear to increase susceptibility to HIV infection by two mechanisms. The first is genital ulcer diseases (e.g., syphilis, herpes, or chancroid), which result in breaks in the genital tract lining or skin. These breaks create a portal of entry for HIV. Additionally, inflammation that results from genital ulcers or non-ulcerative STDs (e.g., chlamydia, gonorrhea, and trichomoniasis) increases the concentration of cells in genital secretions that can serve as targets for HIV (e.g., the T4 or CD4+ cells).

Genital Ulcer Disease (GUD)—Signs of genital ulcer disease appear as open sores on the penis, vagina, other genital areas, and at times elsewhere on the body. The most widespread genital ulcer STDs are syphilis, genital herpes, and chancroid. About 60 million people (between 1 in 5 to 1 in 6) in America over age 12 have chronic genital herpes. There are about 1 million new herpes infections and 70,000 syphilis cases annually (Figure 8-9).

In early 1997, researchers from the University of Washington showed for the first time that herpes sores contain high levels of HIV, which they believe makes the virus especially easy to spread during sexual contact. Additional research by Timothy Schacker and colleagues (1998) also showed that HIV can be consistently found in herpes genital lesions of HIV-infected people. Such data suggest that genital herpes infection likely increases the sexual transmission of HIV.

Genital Nonulcerative Disease—The nonulcerative STDs include gonorrhea, about 650,000 new cases annually; chlamydia, about 3 million new cases annually; and trichomonal infections, about 5 million new cases annually (also called discharge diseases), and genital warts. There are over 30 million people in the United States infected with genital wart virus, with about 5 million new cases annually. There are about 100 types of genital wart viruses, the human papilloma virus or HPV. HPV is one of the most common sexually transmitted agents. Current estimates are that approximately 75% of the sexually active general population ages 15 to 49 years acquires at least one genital HPV type during their lifetime. Most individuals remain asymptomatic after acquiring the infection, and only about 1% will develop clinically or histologically recognizable lesions (Figure 8-10).

In most populations, the nonulcerative STDs are much more common than genital ulcer diseases. None causes the noticeable open sores that occur in the ulcer diseases, but they do cause microscopic breaks in affected tissue, and are associated with HIV transmission (Laga et al., 1993). The most common symptoms are warty growths on the genitals, discharge from the penis or vagina, and painful urination.

BOX 8.4

ASSAULT WITH HIV

Federal, state laws on criminalization

HIV criminalization laws began in 1990 when the federal Ryan White CARE Act passed. That law mandated that states criminalize intentional transmission of HIV in order to get funding for treatment and prevention programs.

Some states took it a step further than federal law required, defining intentional transmission as failing to disclose positive status to a sexual partner. The second time the act was reauthorized, in 2000, the requirement that states must criminalize intentional transmission was removed. The criminalization laws were put in place to protect the public—to prevent cases where someone with HIV knowingly exposed others to virus and did not disclose their HIV status before a sexual encounter.

The laws vary state by state. Some target those who have HIV/AIDS and fail to disclose their status to their partner before an encounter. At least 13 states have laws against HIV-positive people spitting or biting someone even though saliva does not transmit HIV.

Every state and territory has generic criminal statutes that could apply to conduct that exposed others to HIV. However, there is a growing frustration and fear about persons not revealing their HIV-positive status when they should (see the examples that follow).

Legislators around the country are passing an increasing number of laws intended to protect the public. This latest wave of legislation shifts the focus from earlier laws that protected the civil liberties of HIV-infected people to laws that seek to identify, notify, and in some cases punish people who intentionally place others at risk of contracting the virus. At least 36 states and two territories now make it a crime to knowingly transmit or expose others to HIV, with a third of those states enacting laws within the last five years.

In 2006, the California State Supreme Court ruled that constructive knowledge—when it is reasonably foreseen by a reasonably intelligent person that their actions could lead to harm—of the possibility that HIV transmission may occur is enough to allow for civil liability. However, this is the **first ruling anywhere in the world** to find that an undiagnosed individual may be criminally liable for HIV transmission.

According to a Missouri public health report in February 1998, Darnell McGee had sex with at least 101 females, including four whose ages were 13 or 14. It is reported that McGee infected 18 women but Missouri officials believe he infected 30 women.

Darnell "Bossman" McGee is just one of a number of men who recklessly and, in some cases, even willfully transmit HIV to their sex partners. Twenty-seven years ago it was Gaetan Dugas, or Patient Zero, a gay male who said he had sex with 2,500 people across North America and who knowingly infected an untold number (probably 50) of gay men across the United States. In 2012 David Dean Smith allegedly infected 3,000 people on purpose! He was arraigned and charged with two counts of "AIDS-sexual penetration with an uninformed partner." Both are HIV positive.

Selected Cases of HIV and Punishment

In 1997, there was Nushawn Williams, age 21, who in mid-1997 admitted to having unprotected sex with 50 to 75 women after he was told he was HIV positive. Most of them were teenagers ages 13 and up living in New York's Chautauqua County and in New York City. To date, 16 in Chautauqua are infected. The youngest was age 13; others were ages 15, 16, 18, and 21. In April 1999, Williams was sentenced to 14 years in prison. Only two women agreed to testify against him.

In February 2002, the San Francisco Superior Court Commissioner ordered a former San Francisco health commissioner to pay his ex-lover $5 million in damages for knowingly exposing him to HIV and lying about his HIV status. Also, in May 2002, a child molester with HIV in Kansas City, MO, was sentenced to three consecutive life terms, plus 52 years. He pleaded guilty in December to 13 counts, including statutory rape, sodomy, child molestation, and exposing others to HIV.

In January 2003, a 39-year-old Bronx, NY, second-grade teacher accused of sexually abusing students while HIV positive was sentenced to 10 years in prison.

In March 2004, in what may be the first verdict of its kind, a Cook County, IL, jury awarded $2 million to a woman who sued her fiancé's parents for allegedly covering up that he was dying of AIDS. The woman's lawsuit alleged his parents knew of his infection and lied to her when she asked about his deteriorating health.

In June 2005, a Massachusetts woman was charged with armed robbery and assault for allegedly stabbing a security guard with a syringe after he accused her of shoplifting. Witnesses say the 21-year-old then taunted customers asking, "Does anyone else want AIDS!?!" And in November, a former DC government worker who had known since 1996 that he was HIV positive was sentenced to a 21-year prison term for luring women and teenage girls into sexual relationships without telling them he was HIV positive.

In June 2007, a Kansas City, MO, man, who spent five years in jail for exposing his sexual partners to HIV, received a life sentence in prison for knowingly exposing at least 8 women to HIV, with three of them testing HIV positive.

BOX 8.4 *(continued)*

In 2008, the Ontario Superior Court sentenced a 32-year-old male to 18 years in prison for 15 counts of knowingly and secretly spreading HIV to his female sexual partners. Also in 2008, in Australia, a 36-year-old male received nine years in jail for knowingly and secretly endangering three female sexual partners. In May 2008, a Dallas, TX, court sentenced a 42-year-old HIV-positive male to 35 years in prison because he spit into the mouth and eye of a police officer during his arrest. The jury determined his saliva was a deadly weapon. In July 2008, a 43-year-old HIV-positive woman from Columbus, GA, was sentenced to three years in jail for spitting onto another woman's face. She said, "I hope you get AIDS, bitch."

In April 2009, a Canadian man who is thought to have recklessly transmitted HIV to seven women, two of whom subsequently died, has made legal history by becoming the first person to be convicted of first-degree murder for sexual HIV transmission. The case has reignited the criminalization debate in Canada, which has prosecuted more HIV-positive individuals per capita for sexual HIV exposure or transmission than any other country in the world. (See Point to Ponder 8.3, page 226 on the criminalization of HIV transmission.) Also, in May 2009, a 34-year-old HIV-positive man in Iowa was sentenced to 25 years in prison for not disclosing that he was HIV-positive to his sexual partner before having sex with him. In June 2009 a 53-year-old HIV-positive male in Texas was sentenced to 45 years in prison for "six counts of aggravated assault with a deadly weapon—his body fluids."

The Inspector for the U.S. Postal Service said there are at least two known cases in which people mailed HIV-tainted blood through the mail for malicious reasons. The most recent was an HIV-blood tainted letter sent to President Obama (2009).

In 2012, a federal judge upheld a 50-year sentence given by the Iowa Supreme Court to a man living with HIV who was found guilty of having unprotected sex with several female partners. He was convicted on four counts of criminally transmitting HIV for failing to disclose to female sexual partners that he carried HIV. He had been diagnosed with HIV and was taking medication for it at the time.

2011—Canadian Judge Rules That HIV Is Not A Death Sentence in HIV Criminalization Case

An Ottawa judge did the unexpected when he rejected attempted murder charges against a man accused of knowingly transmitting HIV, stating that HIV is no longer an automatic death sentence. He said, "In a country like Canada, where antiretroviral drugs of the highest quality are available to everyone free of charge, the likelihood anyone is going to die over the next 25 years from HIV is extremely remote. So the very notion that anyone could be charged with attempted murder today seems strange."

Between 1987 and 2013, at least 18 HIV-infected men and 3 HIV-infected women were incarcerated in 10 states because they **bit another person.** Two of the 18 bitten people became HIV positive. Prison terms varied from 18 months for reckless endangerment to 27 years for attempted murder. In nine cases within seven states, one HIV-infected woman and seven HIV-infected men went to jail for periods of one to five years for **spitting** on other people. At trial in the seventh of these cases in Texas, a court-recognized AIDS expert testified that HIV could be transmitted through the air! The man got a life sentence and an appeals court upheld the sentence. This man died in prison.

Sex and HIV: If you have the first without disclosing the second, you can go to prison. In some states sex crimes and sex work can be elevated to attempted murder if the perpetrator (criminal) is HIV infected. Disclosing one's HIV status to a sexual partner may exempt one from prosecution. But not telling—even if you do protect and don't infect—is still a crime in most states in America.

These cases represent just a few of the over 700 recorded cases through 2012.

DISCUSSION QUESTION: What is your response to these issues?

1. Is knowingly transmitting HIV an act of violence?
2. Should the reckless or intentional transmission of HIV be a crime? If yes, how severe the penalty?
3. Do the cases bolster arguments for more aggressive partner notification and contact tracing (see Chapter 9, pages 270–274)? Why?
4. Do HIV confidentiality protections help or hinder efforts to alter the course of the epidemic? Why?
5. Would more ready access to condoms have helped avert these tragedies? How?
6. Who is responsible when an HIV-infected person knowingly continues to have unprotected sexual relations with others? Should the infected person be warned another time, assuming that the educational message was not heard? If so, how many times should warnings go forth? Are public health officials responsible for protecting susceptible spouses or long-term lovers of those who are infected and knowingly refuse to use condoms? Should the police become involved if protective advice is not followed, or should confidentiality remain in effect while educational messages go out that untold persons in the community are infected and all should use condoms?
7. Do such incidents support calls for more sex education, or less? Or perhaps different approaches to sexuality education? What approach might work? Why?
8. Now read Point to Ponder 8.3, page 226.

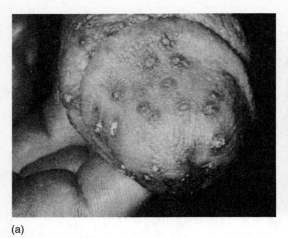
(a)

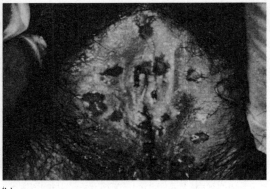
(b)

FIGURE 8-9 (a) Genital Herpes (HSV-2) Infection of the Glans Penis. Note these vesicles have crusted over, and thus, should no longer contain HSV-2. However, wearing a spermicide-treated condom, if involved in sexual activities at this stage, will help prevent possible transmission. (b) HSV-2 infection of the vulva. Note the large, superficial, ulcer-like areas on the labia. *(Photographs courtesy of the Centers for Disease Control and Prevention, Atlanta.)*

How Do Nonulcerative STDs Influence HIV Infection—For an example of how nonulcerative STDs may enhance HIV infection, an uninfected woman has about a 0.2% chance of being infected with HIV during vaginal intercourse with an HIV-positive partner. If her partner had gonorrhea instead, she would have a 50% to 70% chance of becoming infected.

Collectively, worldwide there are over 300 million cases a year of just seven major STDs: syphilis, herpes, and chancroid, which cause ulcers; and trichomoniasis, chlamydia, warts, and gonorrhea, which do not (Figure 8-11, page 227). They occur most frequently in those ages 20–24, followed by those ages 25–29, then ages 15–19.

HIV infection and other sexually transmitted diseases share the same risk factors. The major difference between HIV/AIDS and the other STDs is the degree of cell and tissue destruction and the mortality of HIV/AIDS.

PEDIATRIC TRANSMISSION

Children can acquire HIV from their mothers in several ways. A pregnant HIV-infected woman can transmit the virus to her fetus in utero (during gestation) as the virus crosses over from the mother into the fetal bloodstream (Jovaisas et al., 1985; St. Louis et al., 1993). At least 50% of newborn infections occur during delivery by ingesting blood or other infected maternal fluids (Scott et al., 1985; Boyer et al., 1994; Kuhn et al., 1994). If breast-fed, the newborn may also become infected from breast milk (Zigler et al., 1985; DeMartino et al., 1992; Van DePerre et al., 1993). In case reports, three women who contracted HIV by blood transfusions immediately after birth subsequently infected their newborns via breast-feeding. Other studies suggest that the risk of HIV transmission through breast-feeding is increased if the mother becomes HIV-infected during lactation (Hu et al., 1992).

The relative efficiency of these three routes of infection is unknown. However, the data on mothers' milk add to the urgency of learning more about mucosal transmission. The most likely explanation for HIV transmission through breast-feeding is that the virus penetrates the mucosal lining of the mouth or gastrointestinal tract of infants. If this occurs in newborns, then what of older children, adolescents, and adults? Does the mucosal lining change with development and become HIV resistant?

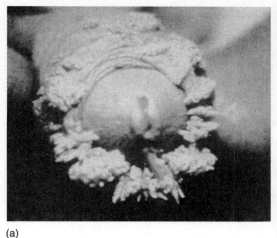

(a)

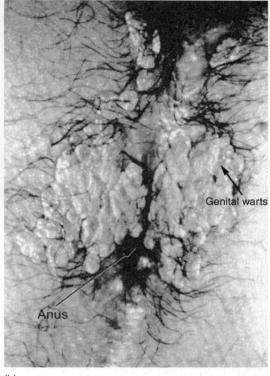

Genital warts

Anus

(b)

FIGURE 8-10 (a) **Genital Warts of the Male.**
Multiple warts or condylomas that are scattered around
the front edge of the foreskin and back along the penile
shaft. (b) **Genital Warts of the Female.** *(Photographs
courtesy of the Centers for Disease Control and
Prevention, Atlanta.)*

HIV-Infected Babies—One major problem in
perinatal transmission is how to determine
which babies are truly HIV infected as opposed
to just carrying the mother's HIV antibodies
(which would produce a false-positive test).
HIV transmission can occur during pregnancy
(in utero), as well as at the time of delivery
(intrapartum) and through breast milk. HIV transmission is more likely if virus can be cultured
from the mother's blood, or if she has later-stage
HIV disease, or if her T4 or CD4+ counts are
low; and is more likely to occur in the firstborn
than in the secondborn of twins. A baby automatically acquires the mother's antibodies and
may carry them for two or more years. Usually
by 18 months of age, most of the mother's antibodies will be gone. The babies may then begin
to show signs of clinical AIDS-related illness (see
Chapter 13 for a discussion of nucleic acid testing, page 398).

Although the rate of perinatal and breast milk
HIV transmission is unknown, evidence from
1986 into year 2013 indicates that over 90% of
pediatric AIDS cases acquired the virus in utero
from an HIV-infected mother after the first
trimester or during the birthing process. In 1990,
researchers concluded that a fetus can become infected as early as the eighth week of gestation
(Lewis et al., 1990). HIV has been isolated from a
20-week-old fetus after elective abortion by an
HIV-positive female and from a 28-week-old newborn delivered by cesarean section from a female
who was diagnosed with AIDS (Selwyn, 1986).

Probability of an HIV-Positive Mother Infecting Her Fetus

Reports on the probability of a fetus becoming
HIV infected when the *untreated* mother carries
the virus vary widely. Without antiretroviral

CRIMINALIZATION OF HIV TRANSMISSION

Criminalization herein refers to the application of criminal law to prosecute those who knowingly transmit HIV and/or expose others to HIV. What is criminal is the act of reckless endangerment, not the disease. Criminalization laws appear to be spreading and include much of the world, spanning Australia, Canada, Europe, and the United States (see Box 8.4, pages 222–223) into sub-Saharan Africa and Asia. Little research has been done on why policy makers pass such laws, or their effect, but they seem to go hand in hand with the frustration that, despite increasing access to treatment and nearly three decades of HIV prevention efforts, HIV continues to spread unchecked. While some people believe that criminalization can promote public health outcomes and improve HIV prevention efforts, it may also deter people from accessing voluntary counseling and testing services, discourage them from knowing their HIV status, and impede people from seeking appropriate care and support, which undermines prevention, treatment, and testing efforts. According to U.S. law, if you don't know you have HIV, you are less culpable should you pass it along to a partner. This provides a disincentive for people to know their HIV status. But, if people are unaware of their HIV status, they can't seek care for their disease. When people are aware that they have HIV and seek treatment, their viral load can be reduced, rendering them less infectious. Therefore, criminalization of HIV may lead to the spread of HIV.

Recently there has been an increased use of the law in relation to HIV, and new laws are also being introduced as part of national responses to HIV. Yet there is little evidence to suggest that the application of criminal law is effective in responding to HIV. In countries with a low or concentrated HIV epidemic, some governments see legislation as a method to stop it from becoming generalized. It may also be viewed as a vehicle to control the unacceptable behavior of some people. In countries with a high HIV prevalence, governments may need to show that they are now doing something proactive to address prevention fatigue.

Edwin Cameron, South Africa Supreme Court of Appeals Justice, wrote in an opinion piece in the *Korea Herald* that "In a misguided attempt to thwart the spread of HIV and AIDS, lawmakers in many parts of the world have passed criminal statutes that promote ignorance about the disease, punish its victims, and enhance the chances that the virus will infect new victims." He cites poorly drafted policies in Western and Central Africa that make HIV transmission a criminal offense, including mother-to-child transmission. Cameron continues that although there are rare and dramatic cases in which an HIV-positive person transmits the disease to another person with the intent to harm, there are existing laws criminalizing these actions that are more than adequate. Criminal laws targeting all HIV carriers, however, are counterproductive and inherently unjust because they make HIV-positive people, especially women, criminals.

A Major Issue Raising Doubt about Broad-Scale Criminalization of HIV Transmission

With improvement in ART, the infected may now almost reach expected life spans. Drug suppression of HIV to undetectable levels greatly lowers the risk of HIV transmission. Also, the results of the Swiss study (see Point to Ponder 8.1, pages 198–199 and chapter 4, Sidebar 4.3, pages 85–89) state that under certain conditions the HIV infected will not transmit HIV. The question should be asked, should such people with greatly reduced, that is, undetectable, viral loads be held accountable if they transmit the virus? And what of those who carry the virus but do not know? These people may, at the very least, expose their sex partners to possible HIV infection.

Global Criminalization Scan

The Global Network of People Living with HIV (GNP+) Global Criminalization Scan Web site, launched on December 1, 2008, is a living, growing document of laws, judicial practices, and case studies of criminalization worldwide. Data from over 150 jurisdictions in North America, Latin America, Europe, United States and Central Asia, and the Asia Pacific region are currently available, with more to come from Africa and the Caribbean sometime in 2012. Globally, 58 countries have laws to prosecute HIV transmission with 33 countries about to pass such laws. Atleast 32 of the 50 states in the United States have such laws.

According to data presented on the site, the ten countries which have seen the greatest number of prosecutions so far are (highest to lowest): Canada, United States, Sweden, Switzerland, Austria, Denmark, Australia, United Kingdom, Germany, and France.

CLASS DISCUSSION: What are your thoughts about the criminalization/prosecution of persons infected with HIV? Give examples to support your opinions, either pro or con.

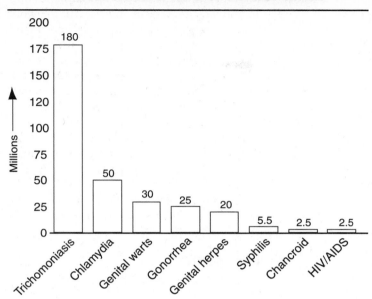

Annual Number of 8 STDs Worldwide

FIGURE 8-11 Global Incidence of Seven Sexually Transmitted and AIDS Disease, ages 15 to 49. According to the CDC, 50% of STDs in the United States are unreported and 50% to 90% of STDs worldwide are unreported.

drug therapy, the most often-quoted estimate in the United States is about 30%. With drug therapy and the use of cesarean sections, the risk to the fetus can be reduced to about 2%.

Other than viral load, there is little documented information on maternal factors that influence vertical transmission. As with other congenital infections, only one of a pair of twins may be HIV infected (Newell et al., 1990; Ometto et al., 1995; Bagasra, 1999). A mother's clinical status during pregnancy and the duration of her infection (stage of disease) may be important, but evidence remains circumstantial (see Chapter 11, pages 350–353, for update information). Studies to determine mother-to-fetus transmission relative to stage of disease are in progress.

According to the CDC classification, children under age 13 are considered pediatric AIDS cases. They make up about 0.8% of all AIDS cases in the United States. Cumulatively, through 2012, about 5% of reported pediatric male AIDS cases occurred due to blood transfusions, 3%

POINT OF INFORMATION 8.4

GET YOURSELF TESTED (GYT)

MTV, the Kaiser Family Foundation, and Planned Parenthood Federation of America unveiled GYT: Get Yourself Tested, for those under age 25. Data from the CDC show that 50% of all new STD infections occur in people under the age of 25 (ages 15 to 24). And by age 25, one in two sexually active young people will have an STD! Because many serious STDs produce few, if any, symptoms, most of those infected do not know it. Thus, the only way to be sure of your sexual health is to get tested. April 2012—The fourth annual **GYT: Get Yourself Tested** campaign kicked off with new initiatives on-air, online, and on the ground at college campuses and in more than 5,000 health centers across nation.

http://www.gyt09.org—The central hub of the campaign, gyt09.org, is a comprehensive information resource that includes facts about STDs; talking tips on how to discuss STD testing with partners, parents, and health care providers; and a testing location finder that connects users to local testing resources by entering a zip code. A wide range of other content, including all of the participating artists and celebrities, are also showcased on the site.

received HIV-contaminated blood factor VIII used in treating hemophiliacs, and in 2%, the cause was undetermined.

The largest numbers of pediatric AIDS cases through 2012 were in New York, Florida, California, and New Jersey, in that order. The highest incidence of all pediatric cases occurs in minority populations. Entering 2013, there were 10,000 pediatric AIDS cases in the United States. Blacks and Hispanics make up 13.6% and 16.3% of the United States population, respectively, yet make up 55% and 20%, respectively, of all pediatric AIDS cases. Thus 75% of pediatric AIDS cases occur within two minority populations.

Vertical Infection: HIV-Infected Childbearing-Age Women

Over 100,000 women of childbearing age are estimated to be infected with HIV in the United States. The majority of these women may not know they are infected; they are identified as infected only after their children are diagnosed as having an HIV infection or AIDS. It is not uncommon for untested HIV-infected women to go through several pregnancies before they express HIV disease. Also, there are women who become pregnant knowing they are HIV positive. They want to have a baby regardless.

Mother-to-fetus infection or **vertical infection** could be avoided by avoiding pregnancy, but this is possible only in cases where the female is aware of her infection and takes measures to prevent pregnancy (birth control or tubal ligation). In many cases, pregnancy occurred before the mother knew she was carrying the virus. In other cases, the mother has become infected after she has become pregnant. (See Chapter 11, pages 350–353, for more on HIV-positive pregnancies.)

Is It Possible to End Newborn HIV Infections?

Perhaps the greatest news to come out of this pandemic to this point in time is the fact that the HIV epidemic for newborns in the United States is about over! Newborn cases of infection are at less than 100 per year and falling. However, each year, about 400,000 children become infected with HIV through mother-to-child transmission, and 90% of these are in Africa. In the worst affected countries of sub-Saharan Africa, HIV infection rates between 10% and 30% are common among pregnant women, and much higher rates have been reported in many villages. Only a relatively small number of such women currently have access to preventive measures such as antiretroviral drugs for the protection of their babies. At the United Nations Special Session on HIV/AIDS in 2001, governments from 189 countries committed themselves to halving the rate of Mother to Child Transmission (MTCT) by 2010. This hoped-for reduction did not happen. Increased access to ART should make this happen by the end of 2013!

CONCLUSION

Although only one new route (prechewed food) of HIV transmission has surfaced over the last 31 years of this pandemic, many people still do not believe that's all there is. People still make the arguments that: (1) Scientists do not yet know enough about this disease to be certain there are no other routes of transmission; and (2) scientists know other routes exist but either are too frightened to tell the truth, or are under political pressure not to do so for fear of creating a public panic. Many thousands of people in the United States firmly believe that in a few years they will look back and say "I told you so: You can get HIV from HIV-infected people if they breathe on you or if you touch their sweat and so on."

DISCUSSION QUESTION: How do you get everyone to believe what medical and research scientists say? Should we get everyone to believe scientific dogma?

NATIONAL AIDS RESOURCES

AIDS Action Council	1-202-547-3101
Coalition for Leadership on AIDS	1-202-628-4160
Gay Men's Health Crisis	1-212-807-6655

Mothers of AIDS Patients	1-619-234-3432
National AIDS Information Clearinghouse	1-301-762-5111
National AIDS Network	1-202-546-2424
National Association of Persons with AIDS	1-202-483-7979
Project Inform (Alternative AIDS Info)	1-800-822-7422
Public Health Service Hotline	1-800-342-2437
Centers for Disease Control and Prevention Technical Information	1-404-639-2070
American Red Cross, National AIDS Education	1-202-639-3223
Guide to Social Security and SSI Disability Benefits for People with HIV Infection	1-800-772-1213

(You can write or call for this Social Security brochure: Social Security Administration, Public Information Distribution Center, P.O. Box 17743, Baltimore, MD, 21235.)

Summary

The World Health Organization began keeping records of AIDS-like cases in 1980. Beginning 2013, there were an estimated 65 million HIV/AIDS cases in 194 reporting countries and territories. About 28 million of these have died. About 2% of AIDS cases have occurred in the United States. At the end of 2013, of the 38 million living with HIV infection worldwide, about 4.3% or about 1,630,000 live in the United States. It has been reported that the first cases of AIDS entered the United States via homosexual men who had vacationed in Haiti in the late 1970s. However, there is evidence of AIDS cases in the United States as early as 1952. While testing West Africans for HIV infection, a second strain of HIV was discovered: HIV-2. Both are transmitted in the same manner and both cause AIDS. However, HIV-2 appears to be less pathogenic than HIV-1.

Nearly all Americans are aware that HIV can be transmitted through unprotected intercourse, the sharing of intravenous (IV) needles, and unprotected oral sex. Less than half, however, know that having another sexually transmitted disease (STD) increases a person's risk for HIV. In addition, even after years of public education, unwarranted fears of infection through casual contact persist. For example, about one in five Americans incorrectly believes that sharing a drinking glass can transmit HIV or is unsure about the risk of this activity. Sixteen percent believe that touching a toilet seat can transmit HIV or are unsure about the risk. Such views contribute to discrimination and stigma, which can interfere with public health efforts to encourage early testing and care.

There are two major variables involved in successful HIV transmission and infection. First is the individual's genetic resistance or susceptibility, and second is the route of transmission. Not all modes of HIV exposure are equally apt to cause infection, even in the most susceptible individual. There have been a number of studies and empirical observations that demonstrate that HIV *is not* casually acquired. HIV is difficult to acquire even by means of the recognized routes of transmission.

HIV is transmitted mainly via sexual activities involving the exchange of semen and vaginal fluids, through the exchange of blood and blood products, and from mother to child both prenatally and postnatally (breast milk). Besides cases of breast milk transmission and three cases of prechewed food, no other body fluids have as yet been implicated in HIV infection.

The current belief is that anal receptive homosexuals have a higher risk than heterosexuals of acquiring HIV because the membrane or mucosal lining of the rectum is more easily torn during anal intercourse. This allows a more direct route for larger numbers of HIVs to enter the vascular system.

Others at high risk for acquiring and transmitting HIV are injection-drug users. They infect each other when they share drug paraphernalia. Changes in sexual and injection-drug-use behavior can virtually stop HIV transmission among these people.

A major obstacle to reducing HIV transmission is that many people, one in five in the United States alone, don't know that they're infected, and may inadvertently be spreading the virus. The U.S. Centers for Disease Control and Prevention recommends that everyone between ages 13 and 64 be tested for HIV. The benefits of more frequent testing, perhaps every year for high-risk groups such as those who have unprotected sex with multiple partners or use injected drugs, are also being studied. Earlier detection would not only curb HIV transmission but might help those already infected, since there's evidence that patients who get early treatment tend to live longer than those treated later on.

CHALLENGE YOUR ASSUMPTIONS ABOUT THE HIV INFECTED

There is an Internet game called "POS OR NOT" that aims to increase HIV/AIDS awareness. The Web site, **posornot.com,** shows photographs and short biographies of men and women ages 21 to 30 and asks visitors to determine if each is HIV positive or not. The message from this exercise is that you can't judge someone's HIV status by looks, occupation, or taste in music.

PLAY THE GAME AND SEE IF YOU CAN TELL WHO IS HIV POSITIVE OR NOT.

Review Questions

(Answers to the Review Questions are on page 463).

1. True or False: Africa makes up the largest percentage of *reported* AIDS cases worldwide. Explain.

2. What evidence is there that HIV may have evolved in the United States and Africa at the same time?

3. Are HIV-1 and HIV-2 related? Explain.

4. True or False: HIV-1 and HIV-2 are transmitted differently and therefore are located in geographically distinct regions of the world. Explain.

5. True or False: HIV is *not* believed to be casually transmitted. Explain.

6. Name the routes of HIV transmission.

7. True or False: Deep kissing wherein saliva is exchanged is a direct route for *efficient* HIV transmission. Explain.

8. True or False: Insects that bite or suck have been claimed to be associated with HIV transmission. Explain.

9. True or False: Among heterosexuals, HIV transmission from male to female and from female to male is equally efficient. Explain.

10. True or False: If a person has unprotected intercourse with an HIV-infected partner, he or she will become HIV infected. Explain.

11. What is the percentage of risk that a developing fetus with an HIV-positive mother in America will be born HIV positive, with and without zidovudine therapy? With zidovudine and C-section?

12. Despite the warnings, groups that continue to engage in high-risk sexual activity include.

    A. high school students.
    B. black women.
    C. injection-drug users.
    D. prostitutes.
    E. all of the above.

13. True or False: Prior to 1985, use of blood component therapy put hemophiliacs at risk for contracting HIV.

14. True or False: Relapse to risky sexual behavior can be an important source of new HIV infection in the homosexual community.

15. True or False: The body fluids shown most likely to transmit HIV are blood, semen, vaginal secretions, and breast milk.

16. True or False: Participation in risky behaviors and not identification with particular groups puts an individual at risk of acquiring HIV infection.

17. True or False: Unprotected receptive anal intercourse is the sexual activity with the greatest risk of HIV transmission.

18. True or False: Women who are HIV infected always transmit the virus to their fetus during pregnancy or delivery.

19. True or False: A person infected with HIV can transmit the virus from the first occurrence of antigenemia throughout the rest of his/her life.

20. True or False: Women constitute the fastest-growing segment of the population with HIV infection.

21. True or False: The majority of HIV-infected women whose source of infection is known became infected through vaginal intercourse.

22. True or False: HIV infection in children is now a leading cause of death in children between the ages of one and four.

23. True or False: Sexual contact is the major route of HIV transmission among black Americans.

24. True or False: Urine is one body fluid that remains an unproven route of HIV transmission.

25. Which of the following is not a recognized mode of HIV transmission?

    A. Unprotected sex with an infected partner
    B. Mosquito bite
    C. Contact with infected blood or blood products
    D. Perinatal transmission

26. True or False: Only drug users and gay men need to worry about becoming infected with HIV.

27. You can become infected with HIV by

   A. sharing utensils with or drinking from the same cup as someone with HIV.
   B. mosquito bites.
   C. hugging someone with HIV.
   D. none of the above.

28. True or False: Using protection such as a latex barrier when performing sex (vaginal, oral, or anal) lowers the risk of HIV transmission.

29. HIV is not present in

   A. semen and vaginal secretions.
   B. sweat.
   C. blood.
   D. breast milk.

30. What major role do asymptomatic people with HIV disease play in the epidemiology of AIDS?

Preventing the Transmission of HIV

The best time to plant a tree is 20 years ago. The second best time is now.

African Proverb

CHAPTER HIGHLIGHTS

- An HIV/AIDS-free generation can begin with you.
- Prevention is today's virtual vaccine. Through 2012, prevention strategies in the United States have averted about 475,000 HIV infections.
- HIV transmission can be prevented; the responsibility rests with the individual.
- No new routes of HIV transmission have been found after 31 years.
- Safer sex essentially means using condoms and not knowingly having intercourse with an HIV-infected person.
- Eight questions to ask your sexual partner before having sex.
- Demand and supply of male/female condom, selected countries.
- Government-imposed warning labels on male condoms.
- Obstacles to condom education and distribution.
- The female condom (vaginal pouch) was FDA-approved in 1993; the second version, called FC2, was approved in 2009.
- Oil-based lubricants must not be used with latex condoms.
- Plastic male condoms are now available.
- Polymer gel condoms are being developed.
- Incorrect condom use is a common global problem.
- Microbicides, has their time come? First effective gel reported after 20 years of research.
- Circumcision for the prevention of HIV transmission.
- Universal test and treat has the potential to greatly reduce HIV infections.
- Pre-exposure prophylaxis (PrEP) studies show reduced HIV infection in HIV-negative men (MSM) and in heterosexual couples.
- Obama administration (2009) lifts ban reduced the use of federal money for needle exchange programs and reinstates the ban in 2012!
- Free syringe and needle exchange programs claim to help lower the incidence of HIV transmission. These exchange programs are available in 82 countries.
- About 4% of injection drug users, globally, are receiving antiretroviral therapy.
- Blood bank screening to detect HIV antibodies began in 1985. About 5 million people receive blood transfusions annually in the United States.
- Universal precautions and blood and body substance isolation are techniques to help health-care workers prevent infection.

- Universal precautions require certain body fluids from all patients to be considered potentially infectious.
- Blood and Body Substance Isolation (BBSI).
- Partner notification is a means of notifying at-risk partners of HIV-infected individuals.
- Five ways you can help prevent HIV/AIDS.
- Vaccines, the Holy Grail against disease.
- Vaccines are made from whole or parts of dead microorganisms, inactivated viruses, or attenuated (weakened) viruses, microorganisms, and naked DNA from these viruses and microorganisms.
- Experimental subunit vaccines are prepared using recombinant DNA techniques.
- There is no effective vaccine for prevention of HIV infection. All experimental vaccines to date have failed.
- Russian and Indian scientists believe they will have an effective HIV vaccine in the next 10 to 15 years.
- Global AIDS vaccine trial sites.
- Results from the world's largest and longest HIV vaccine trials show a modest (?) first-ever success!
- Are time and money being wasted on HIV vaccine research?

Don't walk in front of me, I may not follow. Don't walk behind me, I may not lead. Just walk beside me and be my friend.

Albert Camus

The first major HIV/AIDS benefit song was "That's What Friends Are For."

Carole Bayer Sager
Sung by Dionne Warwick,
Radio City Music Hall,
New York City, March 17, 1990

An HIV/AIDS-free generation can begin with you! LEARN: EDUCATE–DONATE–PARTICIPATE:VOLUNTEER

THE AIDS GENERATION: "I KNEW EVERYTHING ABOUT IT, AND I STILL GOT IT!"

The "magic bullet" to cure or prevent HIV infection has not been found, and too many people with or affected by HIV/AIDS are isolated by cultural, geographic, and economic barriers. HIV is a preventable disease, and the first step in preventing disease is the transformation of information into knowledge and getting people to use that knowledge. For example, the slogan "Practice Safer Sex" is now as common as "Buckle Up for Safety" and "Just Say No to Drugs," but HIV infections among age groups over 12 continue at an alarming pace.

Most people in the United States know how HIV is spread and what to do about it, but nevertheless, they get carried away and ignore precautions in the heat of passion. As it is written, "Hormones will always trump neurons." A teenager who was told her drug-addicted boyfriend was HIV positive said, "I know he loves me and would never do anything to hurt me." In the face of such emotional responses, what chance do precautions or prevention have in succeeding?

Some scientists have convinced themselves that AIDS is not caused by HIV but by antiretroviral drugs. Worse yet, they have succeeded in convincing politically powerful figures, setting back HIV/AIDS control programs for years as in the case of South Africa. That country's leaders have changed their views, but the damage has been done. (See Chapter 2, pages 30-37 for a discussion on AIDS dissidents.)

Nothing can be more important to a state than its public health; the state's paramount concern should be the health of its people.

Franklin Delano Roosevelt
32nd President of the United States

PREVENTION, NOT TREATMENT, IS THE LEAST EXPENSIVE AND MOST EFFECTIVE WAY TO REDUCE THE SPREAD OF HIV/AIDS. HOWEVER, WHEN FACED WITH DISCRIMINATION, ALIENATION, AND MARGINALIZATION, PEOPLE WILL NOT DISCLOSE THEIR RISK FACTORS, USE CONDOMS, GET TESTED FOR HIV, SEEK TREATMENT, OR TALK OPENLY ABOUT HIV/AIDS.

How we define the problem determines our solution.

Jonathan Mann
Former head of the World
Health Organization's Global
Program on AIDS, deceased.

Thirty two years into one of the worst health disasters in human history, the HIV/AIDS pandemic continues to grow exponentially, outstripping prevention efforts and treatment programs;

every day it kills about 6000 people and infects about 7000 more. The global effort is inadequate to check its spread or stop the deaths. Currently, prevention services reach about 14% of individuals at risk for HIV worldwide (see Table 9-1). Antiretroviral therapy (ART), entering 2013, has been made available to about 8 million people, leaving about 15 million who need these drugs now. Expansion of prevention services could avert over half the new infections estimated to occur by 2015, and save about $24 billion in costs for ART (Merson et al., 2008 updated).

The HIV/AIDS pandemic is almost, if not actually, incomprehensible in size and scope. And in the developing world, this pandemic may only be at mid-stage! Two things are now clear: the first is that treatment can, if the majority of the infected receive ART, affect the transmission or spread of HIV, and second, treatment as prevention (TasP) is not an either/or choice—both are vital. But, what can be done now that will change the course of this pandemic? Something has to be done! What can be done and by whom? The world must engage in the largest possible dissemination of HIV, prevention strategies and antiretroviral drugs, and it must develop a vaccine.

Table 9-1 Percentage of Individuals at Risk with Global Access to HIV Prevention Services

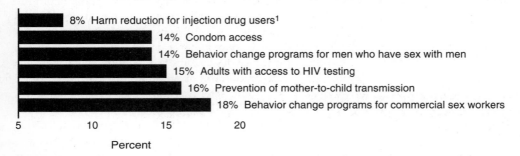

8% Harm reduction for injection drug users[1]
14% Condom access
14% Behavior change programs for men who have sex with men
15% Adults with access to HIV testing
16% Prevention of mother-to-child transmission
18% Behavior change programs for commercial sex workers

Percent

[1] Harm reduction refers to a range of practical and evidence-based approaches toward reducing the negative consequences associated with drug use, especially injection drug use.

Source: Global HIV Prevention Working Group, 2007; WHO/UNAIDS/UNICEF, 2007—Adapted and updated.

Prevention Efforts Will Not Eliminate HIV Transmission

Of the many mysteries posed by HIV/AIDS, perhaps the deepest and most damaging is a human one: why have we failed to stop its transmission? Most people with HIV in the world, including a vast majority of the 45.7 million who are infected in sub-Saharan Africa, caught it from a sexual partner. Despite billions of dollars spent to slow this form of transmission, only a few countries have had significant success—among them Thailand, Uganda, and Zimbabwe—and their achievements have been unreplicable, poorly understood, and short-lived as new HIV infections are once again on the rise in these countries. We know that abstinence, sexual fidelity, and consistent condom use all prevent the spread of HIV. But various prevention programs have not persuaded people to act accordingly.

HIV Prevention Begins with Knowing One's Own Risk, but Many Know Less Than They Think!—During the 2011 51st Interscience Conference on Antimicrobial Agents and Chemotherapy (ICAAC), an abstract presentation entitled "Human Immunodeficiency Virus Risk Perception and Interest in Pre-Exposure Prophylaxis among Persons Visiting a Sexually-Transmitted Infection Clinic in Chicago" was presented by physicians at Rush University Medical Center and the Ruth M. Rothstein CORE Center in Chicago, Illinois. They conducted an anonymous survey of 494 people at a sexually transmitted infection (STI) clinic in Chicago. The most surprising finding was that 84% (301) of the high-risk participants in this urban STI clinic perceived themselves as having no or low risk for HIV. Despite the participants having high levels of knowledge about HIV transmission risks, their rate of consistent barrier protection (condom) use for vaginal, oral, and anal sex was extremely low (<20%). And they showed a lack of interest in the use of ART (PrEP) to prevent their receiving or transmitting HIV. The authors concluded that despite having knowledge of HIV transmission risk, the majority of participants in this survey who exhibited high-risk behavior/environment did not recognize their own risks. Additionally, condoms were not consistently utilized. Together, low education level and low-risk perception of HIV transmission risk may impact future PrEP use. Explanation of PrEP is presented in Chapter 4, pages 84–86.

PRIMARY GOAL OF PREVENTION

The primary goal of HIV prevention is to prevent as many infections as possible. This requires allocating HIV prevention resources according to cost-effectiveness principles: Those activities that prevent more infections per dollar are favored over those that prevent fewer. This is not current practice in the United States, where prevention resources from the federal government to the states flow in proportion to reported AIDS cases. Although such allocations might be considered equitable, more infections could be prevented for the same expenditures were cost-effectiveness principles invoked. The downside of pure cost-effective allocations is that they violate common norms of equity. In 2013 the federal government allocated about $900 million for HIV prevention programs in the United States (see Figure 14-8, page 446).

GLOBAL PREVENTION

> I think we have to divide the world as we would like it to be from the world as it is.
>
> Thomas R. Frieden
> Health Commissioner,
> New York City, 2002

When it comes to HIV/AIDS, there is no first world or third world. This is one global pandemic that requires a commitment to science-based methods of prevention and therapy to address the biologic process of infection and disease. Because we live in a global village, the public health of Africa, Asia, and elsewhere affects the public health of the United States. As there is one global economy, there is one global public health. Prevention of infectious diseases in any country is prevention for all. In each of the years

Table 9-2 Approaches to HIV/AIDS Prevention

- Identifying and tracking new HIV infections to access prevention interventions
- Education, behavior modification, and community interventions
- Partner services, identification, and notification and linking to medical care
- Condoms and other barrier methods
- Use of pre- and post-HIV infection antiretroviral drugs (PrEP/PEP)
- Treatment/prevention of drug/alcohol abuse
- Clean syringes (needle exchange programs)
- Interruption of transmission from mother to child
- Pre-, during-, and post-prophylactic HIV infection antiretroviral therapy (testing and treatment)
- Screening and treatment of other sexually transmitted diseases
- Topical microbicides
- Circumcision
- Vaccination

from 1998 through 2012, on average, an estimated 1.5 million people died from AIDS. Worldwide by the end of 2013, about 30 million people will have died of AIDS. About 80% of these deaths will be in Africa. While waiting for an effective vaccine, how can the out-of-control spread of HIV be slowed? How can people everywhere be saved from HIV infection? In a word, *prevention* is the only hope short of a vaccine. (See Table 9-2, above.)

Stop, listen, and learn all you can about HIV/AIDS. Prevention and life—it's your choice!

Investing in Prevention Because Prevention Works!

The transmission of HIV can be prevented by not having sex, not using contaminated syringes and not getting transfusions of tainted blood or blood products, Experts have pointed out these absolute measures work for some, but not all people are at risk. Failing total abstinence, definitive scientific studies have shown that the risk of transmission can be greatly lessened by other preventive measures such as using antiretroviral drugs, circumcision, condoms, clean syringes and screened blood products. Other successful prevention strategies include reducing other STD"s, TB and malaria.

Prevention Works: After over three decades of experience with HIV in the United States, we know that prevention works. Our national investment in HIV prevention has contributed to dramatic reductions in the annual number of new infections since the peak of the epidemic in the mid-1980s, and an overall stabilization of new infections over the past decade. Given continued increases in the number of people living with HIV, this stabilization is in itself a sign of progress. Other important signs of progress include dramatic declines in mother-to-child HIV transmission and reductions in new infections among injection drug users and heterosexuals over time.

Globally, over the past 12 years, HIV infections have decreased by an estimated 20%. The estimated new infections remain somewhat stable at about 2.5 million people. This is down from about 3.3 million in 2000.

Investing in Prevention: HIV prevention has generated substantial economic benefits. For every HIV infection that is prevented, an estimated $355,000 is saved in the cost of providing lifetime care and HIV treatment, resulting in significant cost savings for the health care system.

Spending money on prevention is a smart investment. For example, in America, the CDC's goal is to lower the HIV infection rate from its estimated 56,000 each year to 28,000. A 2003 study by HIV economists at Emory University estimated that preventing 50% of new HIV infections yearly would save about $11 billion in medical costs annually. The potential for HIV prevention interventions to save lives and dollars emphasizes the need to spend money now rather than later, and to maintain consistent, if not increasing, funding to protect those at high risk. At the 2002 14th International AIDS Conference, Michael Saag reported that in the United States, health care for each patient in the advanced stages of AIDS costs an average of $34,000 a year. The cost of treating the average patient with HIV is about $14,000. The average of $14,000 and $34,000—$24,000—times 1.6 million people living with HIV/AIDS in America comes to over $38 billion! Estimates are that about 900,000 people in 2012 received some measure of care for their HIV infection. The amount of federal money to be spent on HIV/AIDS for 2013 HIV/AIDS cases is $28.4 billion (see Figure 14-8, page 446). The HIV/AIDS prevention budget for 2013 is near $1 billion. The bottom line is, governments and their people must invest more in prevention.

Ending 2013, globally about 8 million people will be receiving antiretroviral drugs, but each year between two million and three million people become newly infected—so, for every case that goes into treatment, two or three more people join the back of the line that will require therapy. **Question: Are the prolonged care and costs of therapy sustainable over the next 20 to 50 years even if a vaccine is found?**

ANTIRETROVIRAL DRUGS HAVE AN IMPACT ON PREVENTION, BUT WE CAN'T TREAT OUR WAY OUT OF THIS PANDEMIC

Drug Therapy Does Benefit Prevention

There is a variety of evidence supporting HAART's beneficial effect on HIV prevention, both in preventing HIV infection of HIV-negative persons and in the transmission of infection from HIV-positive persons to others.

Some Examples:

- **First,** the provision of antiretroviral treatment to HIV-infected women and their infants around the time of delivery has been shown to significantly reduce mother-to-child transmission. By 2015, it is believed that few if any such transmissions will occur.
- **Second,** follow-up of healthcare workers exposed to HIV through needle stick injuries or other accidental contact with body fluids found that persons taking antiretroviral post-exposure prophylaxis (PEP) were less likely to become infected compared to those who did not. The concept has now been extended to the general public. (See Chapter 4, pages 90–91, for discussion.)
- **Third** (this point is a bit less direct), HAART can dramatically reduce the levels of virus in the blood. The lower blood levels of HIV lower the chance of HIV being sexually transmitted.
- **Fourth** is the value antiretroviral therapy has in promoting HIV testing. A precondition of reducing your risk is knowing your HIV status. With the availability of antiretroviral therapy and its ability to extend lives, people now have reason to be tested.
- **Fifth,** increasing use of antiretroviral drugs, by high-risk people prior to engaging in sexual activities, has been shown to prevent infection via pre-exposure prophylaxis (PrEP)—see Chapter 4, pages 85–89, for discussion.

One of the most important preventive measures available is for people to get tested to learn their HIV status. This information (a) helps those infected to seek proper care and (b) helps the infected to protect their sexual partners. Drug therapy, HIV testing, and risk prevention are a dynamic trio. (See Chapter 13, pages 385–416, on HIV testing.)

Can Drug Therapy Counteract Prevention Efforts?

Increases in sexual risk behavior in recent years have led to heated discussion on the role of treatment in HIV transmission. In other words, ART has dramatically improved the length of survival and the physical well-being of persons living with HIV/AIDS and thus has increased their opportunity to transmit HIV to others.

CONCLUSION—The trade-offs between the potential benefits of ART in reducing the likelihood of HIV transmission and the potential harm resulting from increased risk behavior are very complex and involve moral, ethical, and economic considerations. (See the Concept of Test and Treat, Box 9.1, pages 262–263.)

Prevention Is a Matter of Choice

> Being a man or a woman is a matter of birth. Being a person who makes a difference is a matter of choice.
>
> Byron Garrett

Prevention is a hard sell. It is easier to get thousands of dollars to rescue a baby down a well than it is to get a few hundred dollars to cover old wells.

The fact that there is no cure for HIV/AIDS, no vaccine in the immediate future, and that drugs are costly and cause severe side effects makes prevention crucial. CDC researchers reviewed 83 studies from 1978 through 1998. They found that as soon as prevention education began in the early 1980s, the rate of new HIV infections plummeted and that it has remained relatively stable, at about 56,000 new infections a year.

The means of preventing HIV infection exist. They must be used effectively to make an impact on this escalating pandemic. **HIV prevention does not have to be perfect to be effective.** The existing methods of HIV prevention are presented in this chapter.

Prevention—Is Anyone Listening?

Why do people knowingly engage in sexual behavior that can lead to a slow and painful premature death? Why don't the best-intentioned HIV prevention programs often have a greater impact? (See Point of View 9.1, page 239.)

Robert Smith of HIV Edmonton, Canada, and Michael Yoder, chairman of the Canadian AIDS Society, reported at the 14th International AIDS Conference that North American prevention programs are failing. They believe it's back to the drawing board for the AIDS community that has discovered, to its horror, that no one seems to care

about safer sex anymore. (Safer sex means any sexual activity that helps prevent HIV or other STDs within semen, vaginal fluid, or blood from entering the bloodstream of another person. Generally this means using a condom.) People are not listening: **Too few are getting tested.** After 31 years of being bombarded with safer sex messages, you'd think everyone in North America would know how to protect themselves from HIV and other sexually transmitted diseases. As health professionals are becoming increasingly aware, they have come to realize getting the facts out is one thing—doing it in a way that changes people's behavior is another.

Among the depressing reports out of the 2002 International AIDS Conference in Spain is a study showing that most of the young, gay, HIV-positive men in major U.S. cities are unaware that they're infected. More than half the HIV-positive men who didn't know they had the virus considered themselves at low risk of HIV infection and nearly half of them reported they didn't use condoms. They concluded that in North America, young people seem to be fed up with hearing about AIDS. These data remain true through 2012.

Internationally, it seems, there is similar skepticism. At the same conference, the Joint United Nations Program on HIV/AIDS (UNAIDS) quoted grim statistics on a pandemic still in its early stages, with no stabilization of the epidemic in Africa and with exploding epidemics in Eastern Europe and Central Asia. Although the conference was full of stories about how prevention programs across the world are making a difference, the overall message focused on the staggering numbers of people living with HIV and the need for prevention and improved care. This message has been repeated at every International AIDS conference since 2002. However, in 2010, the World Health Organization (WHO) announced that new infections had dropped worldwide by 19%. Progress is being made, although slowly.

A Virtual Vaccine to Prevent HIV/AIDS: Education

With regard to HIV infection, there is no available vaccine against the virus, but there is a

WHY ARE THE EXPERTS SAYING THAT CURRENT PREVENTION METHODS ARE INSUFFICIENT AND THAT NEW PREVENTION MESSAGES MUST BE BROUGHT OUT WITH RENEWED VIGOR?

The global approaches to HIV/AIDS prevention are working, but are not sufficient. How else do we account for the annual two to three million people who will become infected with HIV and the two million others who will die? This latter figure may not register very well, but it is the equivalent of about twenty 747s, fully loaded, crashing every day into a mountain. Unless we address the underlying causes of HIV/AIDS, society can look ahead to an expansion of the pandemic over the next 20 years, especially in countries like China, India, and Russia. Some epidemiologists forecast 100 million people infected by 2025, mostly through sexual transmission and nearly all in poor countries. (And add to this scenario that many millions of HIV-negative people are and will be impacted by this disease.) To escape that fate, all countries must support measures that help women achieve an equal place in society and must seriously underwrite social and economic progress. Strong support for community-driven structural interventions is desperately needed now to turn back this pandemic, which threatens the health and stability of women in many poor countries, and by extension, the whole world.

IS THERE SOMETHING WRONG WITH WHAT IS BEING DONE?

Globally, for decades HIV/AIDS program planners have been developing prevention interventions to modify the behaviors that put people at risk. Typically, they have been limited in scope and duration. Efforts focus on prostitutes and their clients, homosexual men, and intravenous drug users, each group with its own label and built-in potential for stigma and discrimination. Promotions of abstinence, being faithful, or using condoms (ABC) are now common in many programs. But the same behavior change strategies don't work for everyone, especially the millions of women who have no risk factor other than being married. Studies in communities across Africa and Asia reveal that as many as three out of four HIV-positive monogamous women are infected by their husbands. For 22 years, HIV/AIDS mainly affected men. Over the next eight years, half the people in the world living with HIV were women and, in some areas, as many as 60% are women. In short, the main factors that make women, especially young women, more vulnerable to HIV/AIDS are widespread gender inequality, i.e., their low social status, combined with the effects of severe poverty. These structural factors explain why HIV/AIDS prevention interventions that focus on behavior and risk alone will, in the long

run, fail. Designing prevention interventions without aggressively addressing the structural factors of inequality and poverty is essentially akin to applying Band-Aids to a hemorrhage, or believing that you can change the global tides by running your tap water down your drain.

UNITED STATES

Progress in the diagnosis and prevention of HIV in the United States has stalled. Over the past 31 years more than 640,000 Americans have died of HIV/AIDS. But, while mortality rates decreased by a remarkable 75% with the advent of antiretroviral therapy, there has been no improvement in stopping new HIV infections. What is the current reality? New HIV diagnoses are slightly rising. Late diagnoses are common, as is high-risk behavior. Partner notification is rare, as is counseling of HIV-positive patients to avoid transmission of the disease. Put it all together and you have about 56,000 new cases of HIV each year, with about 5% of the infected causing about 95% of the new infections, and 40% of these will exhibit AIDS within one year of their very late diagnosis. Yet, it is estimated that one-half to two-thirds of all of these new cases are preventable. In New York City, where one in every six HIV/AIDS patients lives, only one-third of adults with three or more sexual partners in the past year had been tested for HIV in the prior 18 months. A New York study of more than 4000 HIV patients revealed that less than 20% of partners had been notified, and less than 5% of partners had been tested. Yet, studies indicate that risky behavior declines by half in those who know they are HIV positive.

The United States Goes Quiet on HIV/AIDS Messages: Does This Mean Prevention Messages Have Lost Their Punch?

Perhaps it is the success of drug therapy, the large decrease in annual AIDS-related deaths, or the fact that AIDS, once considered a death sentence, is now viewed as more of a manageable ailment that has brought about an alarming complacency toward HIV infections in the United States. But make no mistake, HIV/AIDS continues to devastate families and friends across America. The domestic challenge cannot be ignored. In his March 2009 column, "America Has Gone Quiet on HIV/AIDS," the Kaiser Family Foundation's President and CEO Drew Altman gives a preview of selected findings from a survey conducted by the foundation on Americans' awareness of HIV/AIDS.

The data from this survey are presented in Fig-ures 9-1 and 9-2. They suggest a state of relatively lessened concern about HIV/AIDS, despite the fact that in August 2008, the CDC announced that the number of new HIV infections each year in the United States is 40% higher than previously thought. The CDC also underscored that the epidemic continues to be concentrated in familiar higher-risk groups: gay and bisexual men, black Americans, and young adults.

APRIL 2009: THE CENTERS FOR DISEASE CONTROL AND PREVENTION (CDC) LAUNCHES THE "ACT AGAINST AIDS" (AAA) TO RENEW THE NATION'S FOCUS ON HIV/AIDS IN AMERICA

The CDC announced a new five-year, $45 million prevention communication campaign, Act Against AIDS, which aims to combat complacency about the HIV crisis in the United States. The campaign—which highlights the alarming statistic that every 8.5 minutes another person in the United States becomes infected with HIV—features targeted messages and outreach to the populations most severely affected by HIV, beginning with black Americans. Targeted communications are designed to encourage HIV testing among the two groups of black Americans most severely affected—men who have sex with men (MSM) and women—and increase knowledge about HIV and AIDS in black American communities. Over the course of the multi-year campaign, additional phases will be launched for other populations at increased risk, including Latinos and other groups of MSM, women, and injection-drug users. The CDC also announced the Act Against AIDS Leadership Initiative, a partnership with 14 of the nation's leading black American organizations to integrate HIV prevention

Percentage of Americans Who Say They Have Heard a Lot about AIDS Has Fallen Since 2004

Percentage of Americans saying that they have seen, heard, or read a lot/some about the problem of AIDS in the past year...

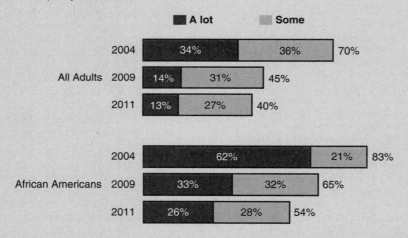

FIGURE 9-1   Public Information about HIV/AIDS Has Fallen Significantly. The drop-off in attention to HIV/AIDS in the United States could partly be a response to the current focus on the economy, but related findings suggest it's a longer-term trend. Figure 9.2 shows that the percentage of the overall public and of African Americans naming HIV/AIDS as the most urgent health problem facing the nation has declined since 1995.
(Adapted from the Kaiser Family Foundation, March 2009 and June 11, HIV/AIDS at 30 and their July 2012 survey.) From this survey, three-quarters of Americans could not name an individual who stands out as a national leader in the fight against HIV/AIDS, and no person who was mentioned makes it into double digits.

Americans Naming HIV/AIDS as Most Urgent Health Problem Facing the Nation

Percentage of Americans naming HIV/AIDS as the most urgent health problem facing the nation in an open-ended question...

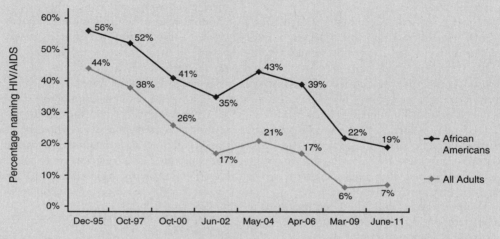

FIGURE 9–2   Percentage of Americans believing HIV/AIDS is the most urgent problem facing the United States, surveyed from December 1995 through March 2009. *(Adapted from the Kaiser Family Foundation, March 2009 and June 2011 and July 2012 survey.)*

into each organization's outreach programs. (CDC materials on AAA can be found at the organization's Web site, at *http://www.cdc.gov/hiv/aaa*.)

CAVEAT: This campaign will do little to identify the 300,000 people who live with HIV but do not know it. (See Point of Information 10.2, page 319.)

UPDATE 2012

On January 1, 2012, the CDC began a new 5-year HIV prevention funding cycle with health departments in all 50 states, eight cities, the District of Columbia, Puerto Rico, the U.S. Virgin Islands, and the 6 Pacific Island jurisdictions. Almost $340 million will be awarded to individual health departments on an annual basis according to a formula that better matches resources of the geographic burden of HIV, as measured by the number of people reported living with HIV in each jurisdiction. This new funding approach ensures that many areas with heavier HIV burdens receive urgently needed funding increases. By March

2012, the CDC awarded an additional $20 million to health departments as part of this funding cycle to implement innovative HIV prevention demonstration projects.

A UNIVERSAL APPROACH TO HIV/AIDS PREVENTION?

A universal approach to prevention could include early partner notification, risk-education counseling, comprehensive quality care, including mental health and substance abuse treatment, CD4 level monitoring and reporting, drug resistance monitoring, and mandatory HIV testing. As has recently been suggested by the CDC, it could also include routine HIV testing for those between ages 13 and 64, to allow population surveillance and treatment. Is this feasible on a global basis? Probably not. But it could be accomplished in the developed nations, especially the United States, if HIV/AIDS were treated like any other sexually transmitted disease. (CLASS DISCUSSION, PRO/CON.)

virtual vaccine (meaning a procedure as effective as a preventive vaccine): *education.* Thus, the leading primary preventive is education: teaching people how to adjust their behavior to reduce or eliminate HIV exposure. Because the vast majority of HIV infections are transmitted through consensual acts between adolescents or adults, the individual has a choice as to whether to risk infection.

Despite widely supported educational efforts at both institutional and street levels, a large number of gay males, drug abusers, and heterosexuals continue to participate in *unsafe sexual practices.* Unsafe sex is defined as having sex without using a condom. This allows the exchange of potentially infectious body fluids such as blood, semen, and vaginal secretions. Unsafe sex most often occurs among gay men and with injection-drug users, by bartering sex for drugs, and by having sex with multiple partners. The sharp increase in the use of crack cocaine and methamphetamine and their connection to trading sex for drugs has led to a dramatic rise in almost all sexually transmitted diseases.

Safer Sex

Some would argue that the reason prevention efforts are not optimally effective is because sex inherently celebrates recklessness, carelessness, or simply the abandonment of reasonable, rational, intelligent, and sensible behavior in the pursuit of pleasure. Yes, safer sex does require some restrictions and responsibility. But, safer sex can be just as rewarding and much healthier over the long term. Those spontaneous moments that lead to sex but not safer sex can be life threatening or can leave one with diseases that require expensive and sometimes painful medical treatment. Safer sex provides an opportunity to be open and honest about what risks there are in a sexual relationship before it happens and how you and your partner want to handle those risks.

Sexual behavior typically does not occur in public, making it difficult to motivate people to use protection when potential transmission occurs and making it almost impossible to verify reports of what people say they have or have not done.

Safer sex is a cerebral concept that sounds good. Yet it is not the cerebrum, but some other part of the body that takes over at the sight of a good-looking, sexy man or woman beckoning in the direction of his/her car. The need for safer sex has never in history fared well in the face of raw lust.

The idea of *safer sexual practices* began with Richard Berkowitz in 1979 and now refers almost exclusively to the use of a latex or plastic condom with or without a spermicide. It should be remembered that for many generations of people in the United States, unsafe sex was the norm, but since HIV, people are asked to make safer sex practices the norm.

Among the severely drug addicted, concerns about personal safety and survival are secondary to drug procurement and use. Thus, their range of unsafe behaviors leads to random sex and sex without condoms. These behaviors are in part responsible for the increased incidence of HIV and other sexually transmitted diseases (Weinstein et al., 1990).

Comparing HIV/AIDS Prevention to Cancer

AIDS prevention is, in a sense, more essential than, say, cancer prevention. Preventing one HIV infection now will not simply prevent one death from AIDS, as preventing one incurable cancer would prevent one cancer death. Preventing an HIV infection now will help break the chain of transmission, averting the risk that the infected person will knowingly or unknowingly pass the virus on to others who in turn might infect a still wider circle of people.

ADVANCING HIV PREVENTION: NEW STRATEGIES FOR A CHANGING EPIDEMIC

In April 2003 the Centers for Disease Control and Prevention (CDC), in partnership with other U.S. Department of Health and Human Services agencies, other government agencies, and nongovernment organizations (NGOs) decided to change their *primary* prevention strategy, in use for the past 24 years—preventing HIV infection among the at-risk uninfected, to the former *secondary* prevention strategy of preventing HIV transmission by those who are infected and their sexual partners. The former secondary prevention mission involves a large federal monetary investment in initiatives that offer HIV testing and counseling to the HIV infected. This marks a substantial shift in priorities. At stake is some $90 million that the federal government provides to community groups for HIV prevention each year.

The new strategy, now in place, is aimed particularly at the estimated 320,000 people who have HIV but do not know it and may be passing it to others unwittingly. The major reasons for this shift in prevention strategy are (1) that efforts to reduce the number of annual HIV infections in America have either, depending on one's point of view, stalled or failed. New infections dropped to about 40,000 cases each year in 1988 and then at least from 2002 through 2010 *increased* to about 63,000 and dropped to about 56,000 new infections per year; and (2) the advent of antiretroviral drug therapy in 1995 and its continued success at prolonging the lives of the HIV infected has made a significant increase in numbers of healthy HIV infected who, along with those who do not know they are infected, continue the transmission of HIV.

Global Prevention Concerns—It is not certain that other countries, even if they have the ability, will follow the prevention strategy shift occurring in the United States. Most countries, at least through 2012, stayed with the original primary prevention strategy. It is estimated that in order for the secondary strategy to be effective globally, it will require some $15 billion to $20 billion a year for at least the next 10 years. Where will that money come from? This money does not include the additional monies needed for medical care and living facilities, etc.

DISCUSSION QUESTION: Do you agree with the strategic shift in prevention by the CDC? Support your decision with known data/facts that can be found within this book or from other sources (see Box 14.2, pages 449–451, AIDS Programs: An Epidemic of Waste?), **and ask yourself if the CDC is using expanded testing/counseling to dodge the criticism it has received from conservative politicians about funding "safe sex" programs. Do you hold much hope for a successful prevention program in developing countries? Why?**

PREVENTING THE TRANSMISSION OF HIV

The News Is Mostly Bad

We are now into the 32nd year of a pandemic that has touched—directly or indirectly—virtually every person on the planet. We know so much about the virus, yet despite our knowledge, our only option is to *prevent* the initial infection. Prevention is foremost because there is no vaccine, no cure, and, even using the best HIV/AIDS drug cocktails available, long-term survival for most of the infected remains questionable, even for those who can tolerate and afford the drugs. As the world faces this realization, alarming statistics continue to emerge about the spread of HIV infection.

The Hard Questions

How can reputable HIV/AIDS scientists explain to the public that the world is being consumed by a disease that is preventable and have it make sense?

The political, social, cultural, economic, and biological factors that have led to the HIV pandemic seem overwhelming. How can a drug user be persuaded to use clean needles to prevent an infection that may kill him in 10 years, when he faces an immediate struggle in a violent environment every day? How can condom use be promoted in countries with inadequate supplies of condoms or resources to provide even basic immunizations? Why should young women on the streets of New York, San Francisco, New Delhi, or Bangkok who depend on the sex industry for daily survival care about safer sex when it might lead to rejection by their customers and an end to their livelihood?

DISCUSSION QUESTION: How would you answer the hard questions?

Gender Power

In many societies, there is a large power differential between men and women. Socially and culturally determined gender roles bestow control and authority on males. The subordinate status of women is reinforced by the fact that men in many countries are the main or only wage earners in the majority of families. This is compounded further by age differences: In most heterosexual relationships, the man is the older partner.

Wives in many cultures are expected to tolerate infidelity by their husbands, while remaining totally faithful themselves. But HIV/AIDS has raised the price of such tolerance, as it puts women at great risk of infection by their husbands. Many women feel powerless to ask their husbands to use condoms at home. Even when they can do this, their need to protect themselves may conflict with a social or personal imperative to have children.

Is There Hope?

Hopelessness threatens reason, but there is reason to believe that education may reduce the number of new HIV infections. In San Francisco, gay men organized grassroots efforts to educate themselves about HIV transmission, and the results are impressive: Less than 1% of the gay male population was infected with HIV after 1985, compared to 10% to 20% in the preceding years. People can change their behavior when educated about the risks of transmission.

Educators Given the Job of Prevention: Spread Knowledge, Not HIV

HIV has just as much potential to kill someone infected in 2013 as it did in 1981, but today's sixth graders and older are hearing much less about HIV/AIDS than did students from the late 1980s through the early 2000s. The great irony is that our fear of HIV now stands in inverse proportion to the damage it does. HIV/AIDS is killing millions of people a year—"but those people are in Africa and Asia, so they don't count." To dismiss HIV or AIDS as someone else's or some other country's problem is to deny the fundamental reality: Sex is one of the few things that can link you to anyone else on this planet. Remember the 1990s bromide, *If you have sex with someone, you're having sex with everyone they ever had sex with*? It's still true. (See Point of Information 8.3, page 220.)

Current Success of Education Prevention Programs

What HIV/AIDS Prevention Method Lasts a Lifetime?

Education (See Figure 9-3)

A growing number of countries have documented the success of their education prevention efforts through careful program evaluations and well-designed surveys. There should be no doubt in anyone's mind that education prevention

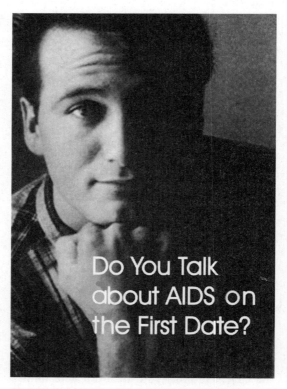

FIGURE 9-3 Do You Talk About AIDS on the First Date? *(Courtesy of the Centers for Disease Control and Prevention, Atlanta.)*

programs can reverse a major epidemic, as has been seen in Uganda and Zambia; can contain an emerging epidemic as has occurred in Thailand and Brazil; and can avoid an epidemic altogether, as has been well documented in Senegal.

Complacency: The Success of Highly Active Antiretroviral Therapy—HAART

The success of HAART is good news for the people living longer, better lives because of it, but the availability of treatment may lull people into believing that preventing HIV infection is no longer important. This complacency about the need for prevention adds a new dimension of complexity for both program planners and individuals at risk. **First,** while the number of AIDS cases is declining, the number of people living with HIV infection is growing. This increased prevalence of HIV in the population means that even more prevention efforts are needed, not fewer. For individuals at risk, increased prevalence means that each risk behavior carries an increased risk for infection. This makes the danger of relaxing preventive behaviors greater than ever. **Second,** past prevention efforts have resulted in behavior change for many individuals and have helped slow the epidemic overall. However, many studies find that high-risk behaviors, especially unprotected sex, are continuing at far too high a rate. This is true even for some people who have been counseled and tested for HIV, including those found to be infected. **Third,** the long-term effectiveness of HAART is unknown. HIV develops resistance to these drugs. If the development of drug resistance is coupled with a relaxation in preventive behaviors, resistant strains can be and are being transmitted to others and spread widely. It is very important to note that society must not let the advances in ART over the past 18 years make us complacent about the global pandemic. Prevention ultimately remains the answer to significantly reducing this epidemic. (See Figure 9-4.)

Grim Reality

Steven Findlay (1991) wrote that burying those who have died from AIDS has become

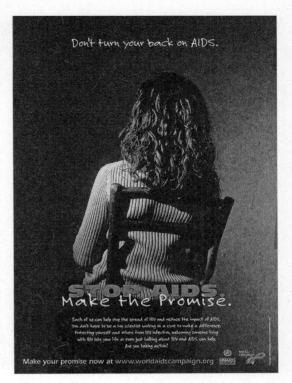

FIGURE 9-4   Prevention Can Work. The world must face the problem: The HIV/AIDS pandemic. *(Source: United Nations Program on AIDS.)*

almost routine. With a 31-year death toll estimated at about 655,000 ending year 2013, most Americans are indeed becoming accustomed to HIV/AIDS-related deaths. But how many will have died, say, ending in the year 2020 or 2030 in America or worldwide? Will therapeutic vaccines be produced? Will our healthcare system become swamped and ineffective? The best guess by scientists is that no effective vaccine will be found in the near future. Through the year 2013 it is projected that worldwide about 30 million people will have died of AIDS.

What We Know

Based on over 30 years of intensive epidemiological surveys, scientific research, and empirical observations, it is reasonable to conclude that HIV is not a highly contagious disease. HIV transmission occurs mainly through an exchange of body fluids via various sexual activities, HIV-contaminated blood or blood products, prenatal events, and in some cases postnatally through breast milk. Since 1981, only one new route of HIV transmission has been discovered, giving babies prechewed food. (See Chapter 8, pages 187, 191, for discussion.)

HIV Is a Relatively Fragile Virus: Life Span of HIV in Different Environments

The virus is fragile and, with time, self-destructs outside the human body.

The most recent data show that HIV remains active for up to five days in dried blood, although the number of virus particles (titer) drops dramatically. But it is dangerous to assume that there are no infectious viruses remaining in the dried blood or stored body fluids from an HIV/AIDS patient. In cell-free tissue culture medium, the virus retains activity for up to 14 days at room temperature (Sattar et al., 1991). According to a recent study, HIV was found to survive between two and four days in glutaraldehyde, a lubricant used to clean surgical instruments. This finding has serious implications for instruments too delicate to be autoclaved (high-pressure steam sterilization), such as endoscopes (Lewis, 1995).

Joseph Burnett (1995) reported that HIV can survive 7 days storage at room temperature, 11 days at 37°C (98.6 degrees Fahrenheit) in tissue culture extracellular fluid, and can still be infectious in refrigerated postmortem cadaver tissue for 6 to 14 days. Nadia Abdala and colleagues (1999 updated) reported that HIV recovered in the blood from used syringes can remain active up to at least six weeks. The bottom line is HIV is more resistant to the environment than originally believed.

SEXUAL RISK TAKING DEPENDS ON SEXUAL ACTIVITY

People can't control their partners' sexual practice decisions, but they are in charge of what sexual practices they themselves engage in.

Choosing sexual practices that are less dangerous can help minimize their risk of STDs and HIV. Below is a list of common sexual behaviors ranked in order from least risky (6) to most risky (1):

6. Protected oral sex, using a condom or dental dam

5. Protected vaginal sex, using a male or female condom

4. Protected anal sex, using a male or female condom

3. Unprotected oral sex

2. Unprotected vaginal sex

1. Unprotected anal sex

Sexual transmission accounts for the majority of HIV infection in the developing world, but this is the most difficult type of transmission to prevent. The use of condoms, reducing numbers of partners, and abstinence remain the mainstays of preventing sexual transmission of HIV, but they will not be enthusiastically adopted just because health authorities tell people to do so.

Sexual behavior has changed in many populations: among gay men in San Francisco, among injection-drug users in Amsterdam and New Haven, CT, and among sex workers and their clients in Nairobi, to name a few. In most of these examples it is not clear how the behavioral change took place. Even so, success stories in HIV/AIDS prevention seem to have some elements in common, including consistent and persistent intervention measures over a period of time, a clear understanding of the realities of the target population, and involvement of members of that population in prevention efforts. Successful interventions do far more than provide information: They teach communication and behavioral skills, change perceptions of what is *preventive behavior,* and ensure that the means of prevention, such as condoms or clean needles, are readily available.

Table 9-3, page 247 provides a number of recommendations for preventing the spread of HIV. These recommendations place the responsibility for avoiding HIV infection on both adults and

Table 9-3 CDC Guidelines for Prevention of HIV Infection

I. For the General Public:

1. Sexual abstinence
2. Have a mutual monogamous relationship with an HIV-negative partner (the greater the number of sexual partners, the greater the risk of meeting someone who is HIV infected).
3. If the sex partner is other than a monogamous partner, use a condom.
4. Do not frequent prostitutes—too many have been found to be HIV infected and are still "working" the streets.
5. Do not have sex with people who you know are HIV infected or are from a high-risk group. If you do, prevent contact with their body fluids. (Use a condom and a spermicide from start to finish.)
6. Avoid sexual practices that may result in the tearing of body tissues (for example, penile-anal intercourse).
7. Avoid oral-penile sex unless a condom[a] is used to cover the penis.
8. If you use injection drugs, use sterile or bleach-cleaned needles and syringes and *never* share them.
9. Exercise caution regarding procedures such as acupuncture, tattooing, ear piercing, and so on in which needles or other unsterile instruments may be used repeatedly to pierce the skin and/or mucous membranes. Such procedures are safe if proper sterilization methods are employed or disposable needles are used. Ask what precautions are being taken before undergoing such procedures.
10. If you are planning to undergo artificial insemination, insist on frozen sperm obtained from a laboratory that tests all donors for infection with the HIV virus. Donors should be tested twice before the sperm is used—once at the time of donation and again six months later.
11. If you know you will be having surgery in the near future and you are able to do so, consider donating blood for your own use. This will eliminate the small but real risk of HIV infection through a blood transfusion. It will also eliminate the more substantial risk of contracting other transfusion blood-borne diseases, such as hepatitis B.
12. Don't share toothbrushes, razors, or other implements that could become contaminated with blood with anyone who is HIV infected, demonstrates HIV disease, or has AIDS.

II. For Healthcare Workers:

1. *All* sharp instruments should be considered potentially infective and be handled with extraordinary care to prevent accidental injuries.
2. Sharp items should be placed into puncture-resistant containers located as close as practical to the area in which they are used. To prevent needle stick injuries, needles should not be recapped, purposefully bent, broken, removed from disposable syringes, or otherwise manipulated.
3. Gloves, gowns, masks, and eye coverings should be worn when performing procedures involving extensive contact with blood or potentially infective body fluids. Hands should be washed thoroughly and immediately if they accidentally become contaminated with blood. When a patient requires a vaginal or rectal examination, gloves must always be worn. If a specimen is obtained during an examination, the nurse or individual who assists and processes the specimen must always wear gloves. Blood should be drawn from all patients—regardless of HIV status—only while wearing gloves.
4. To minimize the need for emergency mouth-to-mouth resuscitation, mouthpieces, resuscitation bags, or other ventilation devices should be strategically located and available for use where the need for resuscitation is predictable.

III. For People at Risk of HIV Infection:

1. See the recommendations for the general public.
2. Consider taking the HIV antibody screening test.
3. Protect your partner from body fluids during sexual intercourse.
4. Do not donate any body tissues.
5. If female, have an HIV test before becoming pregnant.
6. If you are an injection-drug user, seek professional help in terminating the drug habit.
7. If you cannot get off drugs, do not share drug equipment.

IV. For People Who Are HIV Positive:

The prevention of transmission of HIV by an HIV-infected person is probably lifelong, and patients must avoid infecting others. HIV-seropositive persons must understand that the virus can be transmitted by intimate sexual contact, transfusion of infected blood, and sharing needles among injection-drug users. They should refrain from donating blood, plasma, sperm, body organs, or other tissues. HIV-infected people should:

1. Seek continued counseling and medical examinations.
2. Not exchange body fluids with sex partners.

(continued)

Table 9-3 *(continued)*

3. Notify former and current sex partners, and encourage them to be tested.
4. If an injection-drug user, enroll in a drug treatment program and do not share drug equipment.
5. Do not share razors, toothbrushes, and other items that may contain traces of blood.
6. Do not donate any body tissues.
7. Clean any body fluids spilled with undiluted household bleach.
8. If female, avoid pregnancy.
9. Inform healthcare workers on a need-to-know basis.

V. Practice of Safer Sex:

Safer sex is body massage, hugging, mutual masturbation, and closed-mouth kissing. HIV-seropositive patients must protect their sexual partners from coming into contact with infected blood or bodily secretions. Although consistent use of latex condoms with a spermicide can decrease the chance of HIV transmission, condoms do break. (Also see 1 through 6 under "For the General Public" in this table.)

[a] Tests show that HIV can sometimes pass through a latex condom. Experts believe that natural-skin condoms are more porous than latex and therefore offer less effective protection. Never use oil-based products such as Vaseline, Crisco, or baby oil with a latex condom because they make the latex porous, causing latex deterioration and breakage, thus nullifying the protection the condom provides against the virus.

adolescents. **Lifestyles must be reviewed, choices made, and risky behavior stopped.** The Public Health Service and the CDC have established guidelines that, if followed, will prevent HIV transmission while still allowing individuals to be somewhat flexible in their personal behaviors (*MMWR*, 1989).

Eight Questions to Ask a New Sexual Partner

Because most routine HIV tests only detect the virus after about 12 to 16 weeks (or later) after infection, it's useful to know your partner's sexual history for the past six months to one year or more. Although it may be embarrassing to engage in this conversation, answers are needed: your life may depend on how you react to what you hear. Of course, there is always the question of truth in what you are hearing. However, not to ask is to give up before you start. At the very least, the conversation about past sexual activities gives you a chance to gauge or judge the veracity of what is being said. Here is a list of eight questions you can ask before engaging in sexual activities. These questions need to be asked before a relationship gets to the point of sexual intimacy. These questions are not all-inclusive, but a suggested beginning.

1. Have you ever tested positive for a sexually transmitted disease (STD)? If so, were you treated?
2. How many sex partners have you had since your last STD test?
3. Have you had any STDs in the past six months to a year?
4. If you have been diagnosed with herpes or genital warts, are you having outbreaks? Are you on treatment now? Is it working?
5. Have you had an HIV test recently? How recently?
6. How did your latest test turn out?
7. Have you done anything to put yourself at risk for HIV in the past six months to a year?
8. Do you have any objection to using a condom? If yes, we cannot have sex!

Quarantine

With few exceptions, proposals to quarantine all individuals with HIV infection have virtually no public support in the United States. Given the civil liberties implications of quarantine, its potential cost, and the realization that alternative, less repressive strategies can be effective in limiting the spread of HIV infection, quarantine proposals in most countries have been dismissed. Despite claims that HIV/AIDS is similar to other diseases for which quarantine has been used, public health officials have insisted on distinguishing between behaviorally transmitted infections and those that are airborne. HIV/AIDS is not airborne.

Cuba—The Next-Door Neighbor

To date, the power to quarantine, for any disease, has rarely been used in the United States. In fact, only one country, Cuba, officially used the power of quarantine in 1986 and free healthcare to stem the spread of HIV. Data to date indicate that the use of quarantine of HIV-infected and AIDS persons in Cuba had been very effective. Cuba has a 0.0001% (1 in 10,000) rate of HIV infection. Cuba had 17 sanitoriums holding some 900 persons, of which about 200 had AIDS. Cuba stopped the quarantine of HIV-infected persons in mid-1993.

At the beginning of 2013, about 20% of Cuba's HIV/AIDS population, by choice, live in the remaining 14 sanitoriums. The rest live outside and receive care at a few specialty centers. A key criterion for living outside the sanitoriums is disclosure to one's sexual partners and providing evidence to health authorities that one is sexually responsible. The authorities actively pursue contact tracing and HIV testing of sexual partners, strategies borrowed from their TB program. There is also mandatory HIV testing of pregnant women, soldiers, and blood donors, but anonymous testing is available for the general public. From 1986 through 2012 only 38 babies were born with HIV infection. Last year, over 1 million HIV tests were done in Cuba, out of a population of 11.4 million. From 1985 through 2012 about 25 million HIV tests have been taken by the Cuban population. Meticulous identification of every HIV-positive individual in Cuba allowed the tracking of HIV transmission to its source.

Cuba has screened all blood donors for HIV since 1986. Jorge Perez, who diagnosed the country's first AIDS patients and helped shape the policies of the Santiago sanatorium as its director for 14 years, said, "The Cuban point of view is that you have the right to be sick, but not to transmit it to anyone else." Currently, Cuba has the distinction of having one of the smallest HIV infection rates (0.1%) in the world in a region with one of the highest.

NEW RULES TO AN OLD GAME: PROMOTING SAFER SEX—NOBODY HAS A BODY TO DIE FOR!

The use of barrier methods is one of the few behavioral strategies that individuals can adopt to protect themselves against sexually transmitted diseases. Male, and in some countries female, condoms are currently the only barrier methods widely available. However, there are many cultural, gender, economic, and service-delivery barriers that impede the wide-scale and consistent use of barrier methods for preventing the transmission of HIV and other sexually transmitted diseases.

Barriers to HIV Infection

The two most effective barriers to HIV infection and other sexually transmitted diseases are **(1) abstinence,** which can be achieved by saying *no* emphatically and consistently; and **(2) forming a no-cheating relationship with one individual, preferably for life.** These solutions to the danger of HIV and STD infections may not be "cool," but they do work. These two apparently safe approaches are endorsed by the surgeon general as the preferred methods. For those who do not practice abstinence, barrier methods are necessary to prevent HIV infection/transmission.

Other Barrier Methods

Other barrier methods used to prevent HIV infection are the same methods used to prevent other sexually transmitted diseases and often conception or pregnancy. They include diaphragms, latex condoms, plastic condoms (new in 1995), and latex dental dams used in conjunction with a spermicide. Barrier dams, or dental dams, are thin sheets of latex or similar material placed over the vagina, clitoris, and anus during oral sex. (Ask your dentist to show you a dental dam.) **Spermicides** are chemicals that kill sperm. These same chemicals have also been shown to kill some bacteria and inactivate certain viruses that cause STDs. Spermicides are commercially available in foams, creams, jellies, suppositories, and sponges. Use of these products may provide protection against the transmission of STDs, but the only recommended barrier protection against HIV infection is a condom. National Condom Week is February 14–21. National Condom Day is always on Valentine's Day.

Diaphragms—There's good data from a variety of different sources to indicate that the cervix is the most vulnerable site for HIV infection. This does not mean that all infection occurs at the cervix, but probably most. Because of this fact, researchers hypothesized that the diaphragm (a latex or silicone dome forming a barrier to the cervix) would protect women fitted with one against HIV. The result of the diaphragm studies, however, showed that diaphragms did not protect against HIV infection.

Condom—A Medical Device?

Condoms are classified as medical devices. Every condom made in the United States is tested for defects and must meet quality control guidelines enforced by the federal Food and Drug Administration (FDA).

From the CDC: Sexually Transmitted Diseases, Including HIV—Latex condoms, when used consistently and correctly, are highly effective in preventing the transmission of HIV, the virus that causes AIDS (Figure 9–5, below). In addition,

Relative Risk for Transmission from a Person Living with HIV: Why it's so important to always practice safer sex.

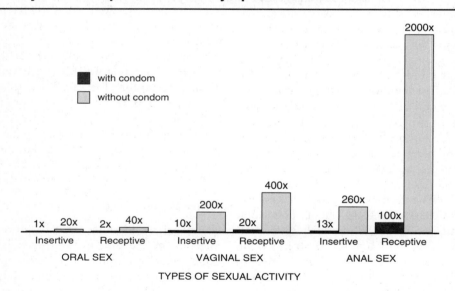

FIGURE 9-5   Decisions about Sexual Activity and Condom Use Have a Major Effect on the Risk for HIV Transmission. This chart shows how the relative risk for a person living with HIV transmitting HIV to a person without the disease varies according to sexual activity and condom use. For example, insertive oral sex with a condom has a low risk for HIV transmission. But receptive anal sex without a condom is 2000 times riskier. Not having sex is the best way to protect against the transmission of HIV. But if you are having sex, it's important to know that all sex is not the same when it comes to transmitting HIV. *(Courtesy of the Centers for Disease Control and Prevention, Atlanta.)*

correct and consistent use of latex condoms can reduce the risk of other sexually transmitted diseases (STDs), including discharge and genital ulcer diseases. While the effect of condoms in preventing human papillomavirus (HPV) infection is unknown, condom use has been associated with a lower rate of cervical cancer, an HPV-associated disease.

Choosing the Condom: Manufacturers, Colors, and Shapes

Condoms are intended to provide a physical barrier that prevents contact between vaginal, anal, penile, and oral lesions and secretions and ejaculate.

At least 50 brands of condoms are manufactured in the United States. There are colored condoms—pink, yellow, and gold; flavored condoms; and condoms that are perfumed, ribbed, stippled, and glow in the dark. This assortment of condoms exposes the user and his partner not only to rubber but also to a variety of different chemicals—some that can cause allergic skin reactions **(contact dermatitis).** One to two percent of people are sensitive to latex rubber and demonstrate contact dermatitis.

Condoms have many colloquial or slang terms: they are also called rubbers, prophylactics, bags, skins, raincoats, sheaths, French letters, Hazmat suits, and love gloves. They can be lubricated or not, have reservoir tips or not, and can contain spermicide.

Condom Size

Most brand-name condoms are made in four different lengths and widths (sizes). There is no standard length for condoms, though those made from natural rubber will stretch if necessary to fit the length of the man's erect penis. The width of a condom can also vary. Some condoms have a slightly smaller width to give a closer fit, while others will be slightly larger. Condom makers have realized that different lengths and widths are needed and are increasingly broadening their range of sizes. An Internet retailer now advertises 95 sizes of "They Fit" condoms whose length ranges from 3 inches to 10 inches.

History of Condoms

Condom use can be traced back to 1000 B.C. when Egyptian men used linen sheaths or animal membranes as a sheath to cover their penises (Barber, 1990). Animal intestines were flushed clean with water, sewn shut at one end and cut to the length of the erect penis. In 1504, Gabrielle Fallopius designed a medicated linen sheath that was pulled on over the penis to prevent syphilis infection. A Japanese novel written in the 10th century refers to the uncomfortable use of a tortoise shell or horn to cover the penis.

It is interesting to note that condoms were used far more often throughout history as protection against STDs than as contraceptives. For example, an 18th-century writer recommended that men protect themselves against disease by placing a linen sheath over the penis during intercourse.

The term "condom" came into common usage in the 1700s. According to accounts in the early 1700s, condoms were sold and even exported from a London shop whose proprietress laundered and recycled them in a back room (Barber, 1990). Condoms became more widely available after 1844. The latex condom was first manufactured in the 1930s.

Condoms have been available in the United States for about 150 years, but have never been as openly accepted as they are now. Their sale for contraceptive use was outlawed by many state legislatures beginning in 1868 and by Congress in 1873. Although most of these laws were eventually repealed, condom packages and dispensers until only a few years ago continued to bear the label "Sold only for the prevention of disease," even though they were being used mainly for the prevention of pregnancy.

After the advent of non-barrier methods of contraception during the 1960s (mainly the use of the birth control pill) there was an ensuing epidemic increase in most sexually transmitted infections. Condoms once again are being marketed for the prevention of disease (Judson, 1989).

Safer Sex, the Choice of Condom

Although a variety of preventive behaviors have been recommended (Table 9-3, pages 247–248), the responsibility of safer sex, with a condom, is a personal choice. If one decides to use a condom, then the choice is what kind, and whether to use a spermicide.

THE MALE CONDOM

The average American-made condom most often sold is made of latex, is about 8 inches long, and in general, one size fits all. About 500 million condoms are sold annually in the United States. Ten to 15 billion are sold annually worldwide but about 30 billion more are needed, most of them in Asia (Grimes, 1992 updated). Regardless of what appears to be a large number of condoms sold worldwide, globally, consistent male condom use remains a minority strategy because of moral objections, limited consumer acceptability, or logistic reasons. The costs of condom use—including financial, interpersonal, aesthetic, and social costs—are too high for most people. Instead, many people in different settings adapt their sexual practices in ways that do not include male condoms, often with unknown or only marginal benefit for HIV or STD prevention.

Intact latex condoms provide a continuous mechanical barrier to HIV, herpes virus (HSV), hepatitis B virus (HBV), *Chlamydia trachomatis,* and *Neisseria gonorrhoeae.* A recent laboratory study indicated that latex and *polyurethane condoms (plastic)* are the most effective mechanical barriers to fluid available, containing HIV-sized particles (0.1 μm in diameter; the width of a human hair is 860 × wider). The male polyurethane condom is thinner than the latex condom, which makes them more agreeable in feel and appearance to some users. However, they also break more easily during use. (See Sidebar 9.1 and Snapshot 9.1, page 253.)

Three prospective studies in developed countries indicated that condoms are unlikely to break or slip during proper use. Reported breakage rates in the studies with latex condoms were 2% or less for vaginal or anal intercourse (*MMWR,* 1993; Spruyt et al., 1998).

SIDEBAR 9.1

TWO ANECDOTES ON CONDOM USE IN SOUTH AFRICA

Women in South Africa are brought up to be subservient to men. Especially in matters of sex, the man is always in charge. Women feel powerless to change sexual behavior. Even when a woman wants to protect herself, she usually can't; it is not uncommon for men to beat partners who refuse intercourse or request a condom. "Real men" don't use them, so women who want their partners to use a condom must fight deeply ingrained taboos.

Anecdote One

A nurse in Durban, South Africa, coming home from an AIDS training class, suggested that her mate should put on a condom as a kind of homework exercise. He grabbed a pot and banged loudly on it with a knife, calling all the neighbors into his house. He pointed the knife at his wife and demanded: "Where was she between 4 P.M. and now? Why is she suddenly suggesting this? What has changed after 20 years that she wants a condom?"

Anecdote Two

This schoolteacher is an educated man, fully cognizant of the AIDS threat. Yet even he bristles when asked if he uses a condom. "Humph," he says with a snort. "That question is nonnegotiable." So despite extensive distribution of free condoms, they often go unused. Astonishing myths have sprung up. If you use one, your erection can't grow. Free condoms cannot be safe: They have been stored too long, kept too hot, kept too cold. Condoms fill up with germs, so they spread AIDS. Condoms from overseas bring the disease with them. Foreign governments that donate condoms put holes in them so that Africans will die.

Choice—The best choice for preventing STDs and pregnancy is condoms that are made of *latex* or *polyurethane* and contain a *spermicide.* The spermicide is added protection in case the condom ruptures or spills as it is taken off. Although some laboratory evidence shows that some spermicides can inactivate HIV, researchers have found that these products cannot prevent a person from becoming HIV infected.

NEW YORK CITY AND WASHINGTON, DC UNVEIL OFFICIAL CONDOMS

NEW YORK CITY

In February 2007, health officials in New York City and Washington, DC unveiled their cities' official condoms as part of their efforts to curb the spread of HIV and other sexually transmitted diseases. Each city presents its own packaging. New York City's packaging is black with **NYC/CONDOM** placed in multicolored circles. The Washington, DC packaging carries messages printed in English and Spanish. Experts believe packaging is very important to acceptance/normalizing condom use.

New York City hopes to distribute at no cost to recipients 20 million NYC condoms annually, at a cost to the city of about $720,000. The condoms can be obtained online or at many businesses throughout the city. In 2008, 39 million condoms were given out! Also in 2008, New York City redesigned the condom package to say "Get Some." The goal for 2011 forward is to distribute 52 million condoms annually.

Reaction to NYC Condom Campaign

In a joint statement, Cardinal Edward Egan, head of the Archdiocese of New York, and Bishop Nicholas DiMarzio of Brooklyn criticized the distribution program, calling it an immoral "anything goes" policy that degrades society. The cardinal and bishop said, "Our political leaders fail to protect the moral tone of our community when they encourage inappropriate sexual activity by blanketing our neighborhoods with condoms." They added, "By their actions, they ignore that truth and degrade societal standards."

QUESTION: This question acknowledges that condom use globally and in the United States can be a very moral and sensitive issue for some, for others a volatile issue. In defense of their use, this question is not meant to lessen differing points of view on the issue of condom use. However, the question is: **CAN ANYONE INVOKE THE MORAL HIGH GROUND IF THAT BELIEF PERMITS UNNECESSARY HIV INFECTION AND LOSS OF LIFE? YOUR RESPONSE IS?**

In December 2010 the Catholic Pope partially relented on the church's stand against the use of condoms. Catholics may now use condoms to prevent HIV infection in some cases.

WASHINGTON, DC

Washington, DC distributed about four million city-branded condoms in 2010, 2011, and 2012 at no

cost to recipients. The condoms cost the city about $40,000. Distribution was similar to that in New York City.

In 2010, 2011 and 2012, DC made 500,000 female condoms available in beauty salons, convenience stores, and high schools. Their goal is to make female condoms available anywhere male condoms are available.

During the 13th International AIDS Conference held in Durban, South Africa, July 9–14, 2000, researchers from the Joint United Nations Program on AIDS (UNAIDS) presented the results of a study of a product that contains nonoxynol-9 (N-9). The study found that the spermicide N-9 did not protect against HIV infection and may have increased the risk of transmission. Women using N-9 gel became infected with HIV about 50% more often than women who used the placebo gel.

Buying Male Condoms—Women are taking a more active role in buying condoms. In 1985, women bought about 10% of the condoms sold. Now they purchase 40% to 50%. According to surveys, most women buying condoms are single, and their concern is about HIV infection rather than pregnancy. The fact that more women are willing to buy condoms is evidence that HIV education is working to some degree.

Many condoms are purchased from vending machines. The FDA recommends the following guidelines when purchasing condoms from a vending machine:

1. Is the condom made of latex or polyurethane?

2. Is the condom labeled for disease prevention?

3. Is the spermicide (if any) outdated?

4. Is the machine exposed to extreme temperatures or direct sunlight?

In mid-1992, the first drive-up "Condom Hut" opened in Cranston, RI. With each purchase the customer receives a brochure on safer sex.

It is generally recommended that condoms be stored below 25°C (77° Fahrenheit; room temperature is 72°F or 22.2°C). The packaging should be impermeable to both sunlight and gas. If air, which includes ozone, enters the package, it will affect the condom very quickly—ozone is like rust to a condom. Latex is a natural product—it will go bad if you don't treat or store it properly.

Condoms in Prisons

Entering 2013, condoms are available in state prisons in Vermont and Mississippi and in urban jail systems in New York City, Philadelphia, Los Angeles, San Francisco, and the District of Columbia. A number of additional states and cities are now considering making condoms available in their prison systems. Condoms have been available in most European prisons for more than 10 years.

Condoms in Public Schools?

Condoms are now being dispensed without charge in most college and university and public health clinics, and in over 400 high school health offices in the United States. Some cities in Canada have been providing access to free condoms in high schools since 1984.

In December 1999, the American Medical Association (AMA) adopted a policy that advocates handing out condoms in schools and minimizes the value of abstinence-only sex education. While some doctors and groups have called the policy medically irresponsible, it is supported by the U.S. surgeon general. The policy, based on studies, concluded that safer sex programs are effective in delaying sex in teenagers, and that abstinence-only programs have limited value. (For more information on abstinence in the USA see Point of Information 12.4, page 376.)

Are Policies or Studies Reality?

Regardless of educational programs on safer sex and condom usage, recent studies indicate that adults and teenagers still refuse to use condoms. What they know is not equal to what they do! Based on their findings, the researchers said information-oriented school- and community-based AIDS prevention programs will not succeed in getting some adults and adolescents to use condoms because there is no association between knowledge and preventive behavior.

Equally discouraging is a recent study in the United States. A 2004 online survey by the American Social Health Association of 1155 people ages 18 to 35 indicated about 84% believed they adequately protected themselves against HIV and other STDs, but nearly half engage in unprotected sex. Approximately 47% of the respondents never used protection for vaginal sex, 82% never used protection for oral sex, and 64% never used protection for anal sex. The survey showed that 93% believed their current or most recent partner did not have an STD, yet one of three people have never discussed HIV or STDs with their partner, while 68% did not think they would contract HIV or an STD. (See Point of Information 9.1, page 255.)

Food and Drug Administration (FDA) Requires a Warning Label on Condoms

In 2006, the FDA stated that all latex condom manufacturers must include the following information on their condom packages: "Condoms Greatly Reduce, But Do Not Eliminate the Risk of Pregnancy and HIV Infection When Used Correctly during Sexual Intercourse." Manufacturers had one year to comply. They did!

Polyurethane (Plastic) Condoms—For the 1% of the general population that is sensitive to latex and for those who have a variety of other reasons not to use a latex condom, there is now a clear, thin, FDA-approved polyurethane (plastic) condom for sale in the United States. The condoms are colorless, odorless, and can be used with any lubricant. The current cost is about $1.80 each. A report by Ron Frezieres and colleagues (1999) states that although polyurethane and latex condoms provide equivalent levels of contraceptive protection, the polyurethane

CLARIFYING THE ISSUES OVER CONDOM USE

Two major issues surface in the debate over advocating condom use in the prevention of HIV infection: One concerns the concept of efficacy, the condom's ability to stop the virus from passing through, and the other, the fear that making condoms available will encourage early sexual activity among adolescents and extramarital sex among adults.

EFFICACY (DO THEY WORK?)

No public health strategy can guarantee perfect protection. For instance, the influenza vaccine is only 60–80% effective in preventing influenza, but thousands of deaths could be prevented annually through the wider use of this less-than-perfect vaccine. The real public health question is not whether condoms are 100% effective, but rather how can we more effectively use condoms to help prevent the spread of disease?

All condoms are not 100% impermeable; they are not all of the same quality. Investigators using different testing methods have reported that latex condoms are effective physical barriers to high concentrations of Chlamydia trachomatis, Neisseria gonorrhoeae, the herpes and hepatitis viruses, cytomegalovirus, and HIV (Judson, 1989). But for maximum effectiveness condoms must be properly and consistently used from start to finish (Table 9-4).

Because the condom covers only the head and shaft of the penis, it does not provide protection for the pubic or thigh areas, which may come in contact with body secretions during sexual activity.

Norman Hearst and colleagues (2004) used computerized searches of peer-reviewed scientific literature, and other publications of national and international organizations, to determine the most likely probability that condoms will prevent HIV transmission. Hearst determined that if a condom was used properly, it was 90% effective in stopping the transmission of HIV.

In 2005, the American Foundation for AIDS Research (AMFAR), a well-respected AIDS organization, issued an analysis of the effectiveness of male and female condoms in preventing the transmission of HIV. The analysis revealed that when used consistently and correctly, male condoms are 80% to 95% effective in reducing the risk of HIV infection, while female condoms are 94% to 97% effective in reducing the risk. AMFAR's analysis concludes that the scientific evidence does not support recent governmental policy changes that stress a lack of condom efficacy in pre-

venting HIV transmission. Thus, AMFAR concludes that condoms are "highly effective" in blocking HIV infection/transmission. These data are sure to fuel the ongoing debate. In spite of the argument, pro and con on the use of condoms, next to abstinence, condoms are about the only mechanical device available for safer sex. The bottom line is that condoms reduce some of the risks in preventing the transmission of HIV and other STDs, thus condoms are used for safer sex but they cannot guarantee safe sex.

INCORRECT CONDOM USE IS A COMMON GLOBAL HEALTH PROBLEM

A study by international researchers found 14 common usage errors with condoms that hamper their efficacy against STDs and pregnancy. The analysis of 50 studies of sex workers, STI clinic attendees, monogamous married couples, university students,

---

Table 9-4 Proper Placement of a Condom on the Penis[a]

---

1. Open the packaged condom with care; avoid making small fingernail tears or breaks in the condom.
2. Place a drop of a water-based lubricant inside the condom tip before placing it on the head of the penis. Be sure none of the lubricant rolls down the penis shaft as it may cause the condom to slide off during intercourse.
3. Hold about half an inch of the condom tip between your thumb and finger—this is to allow space for semen after ejaculation. Then place the condom against the glans penis (if uncircumcised, pull the foreskin back).
4. Unroll the condom down the penis shaft to the base of the penis. Squeeze out any air as you roll the condom toward the base.
5. After ejaculation, hold the condom at the base and withdraw the penis while it is still firm.
6. Carefully take the condom off by gently rolling and pulling so as not to leak semen.
7. Discard the condom into the trash.
8. Wash your hands.
9. Never use the same condom twice.
10. Condoms should not be stored in extremely hot or cold environments.

---

[a]Males should practice putting on and removing a condom prior to engaging in sexual intercourse.

and adolescents spanning 14 countries between 1995 and 2011 revealed problems such as:

1. Late applications
2. Early removal
3. Failure to fully unroll the condom
4. Incorrect storage
5. Condom reuse
6. Completely unrolling before applying to the penis rather than unrolling on the penis
7. Failure to leave space for semen collection
8. Inside-out application that is then reversed
9. Exposure to sharp objects (like teeth) during package removal
10. Not checking for damage before use
11. Breakage
12. Slippage
13. Leakage
14. Not using water-based lubricants

According to lead researcher Stephanie Sanders and colleagues (2012) of Indiana University's Kinsey Institute for Research in Sex, Gender and Reproduction, closing the gap between typical and perfect condom use is essential to greatly reducing the epidemics of STIs and unintended pregnancies.

Condoms used in the study were Durex and SSL (Seton Scholl London).

DO CONDOMS ENCOURAGE SEXUAL ACTIVITY?

Many persons assert that those who promote condom use to prevent HIV infection appear to be condoning sexual intercourse outside of marriage among adolescents as well as among adults. In 2006, Natalie Smoak and colleagues presented an overall assessment of 174 studies published on whether condoms encourage sexual activities; beginning sex at an earlier age, having sex more frequently, or having more sexual partners. Bottom line, they report that **condoms do not promote any of these sexual behaviors. Administrators of these studies feel that condoms no more cause sexual activity than umbrellas cause rain.**

ANECDOTE: HUMOR

Presenting facts without understanding won't work. Here is a simple story to emphasize the point: "A minister, following his custom, paid a monthly call on two spinster sisters. While he was standing in their parlor, holding his cup of tea, engaged in their usual chit chat, he was startled by something that caught his eye. There on the piano was a condom! 'Ladies, in all the years we've known each other I have never intruded into your private lives, and never felt the need to. But now I am forced to ask what is that thing doing there?' One of the ladies replied, 'Oh, that's a wonderful thing, pastor, and they really work!' The minister was agitated: 'I'm not talking about their value or effectiveness. I just want to know what that thing is doing on your piano.'"

"'Well, my sister and I were watching television. We heard this lovely man, the surgeon general of the whole United States. He said that if you put one of those on your organ, you'll never get sick. Well, as you know we don't have an organ, but we bought one and put it on the piano, and we haven't had a day's sickness since!'"

condom's higher frequency of breakage and slippage suggests that this condom may confer less protection from sexually transmitted infections than do the latex condoms.

THE FEMALE CONDOM OR FEMIDOM (VAGINAL POUCH)

The female condom was FDA-approved in May 1993 and has become available to the general public. Before giving the condom final approval, the FDA asked that two caveats be put into the labeling. First, the agency required a statement on the package label that male condoms are still the best protection against disease, and second, that the label compare the effectiveness of female condoms with that of other barrier methods of birth control. Both conditions were met to the FDA's satisfaction. According to the FDA, in a study of 150 women who used the female condom for six months, 26% became pregnant. The manufacturer contends that the pregnancy rate was 21%—and only because many women did not use the condom every time they had sex. With "perfect use," company officials say, the rate is 5%, in contrast to 2% for male condoms.

Design of the Female Condom

The female condom is now called the **vaginal pouch.** However, the female condom is being used by gay men for anal sex. A report from gay men using this condom says that they are having problems with the condom's design and experience usage difficulties. In short, of the gay men interviewed, none believe the female condom will replace their use of the male condom for anal sex.

Description of the Female Condom

The female condom is 17 cm (about 6-3/4 inches) long and consists of a 15 cm poly-ure-thane sheath with rings at each end (Figure 9-6, page 258). The closed end fits into the vagina like a diaphragm. The outer portion is designed to cover the base of the penis and a large portion of the female perineum (the area of tissue between the anus and the beginning of the vaginal opening) to provide a greater surface barrier against microorganisms. Studies of acceptability, contraceptive effectiveness, and STD prevention are currently underway. *Potential advantages* of this product are: (1) it provides women with the opportunity to protect themselves from pregnancy and STDs; (2) it provides a broader coverage of the labia and base of the penis than a male condom; (3) its polyurethane membrane is 40% stronger than latex; and (4) it is more convenient; it can be inserted hours before sexual intercourse. *Disadvantages* are the female condom (1) is not aesthetically pleasing and (2) can be difficult to insert and remove.

Because of the nitrile rubber used to make it, the female condom is both strong and durable. No special storage arrangements have to be made because polyurethane is not affected by changes in temperature and dampness. The expiration date on the female condom is 60 months (5 years) from the date of manufacture.

Global Use of the Vaginal Pouch (Female Condom)—Female Health Company (FHC) of Chicago is the sole manufacturer of the female pouch. Under agreement between UNAIDS and FHC the female pouch is sold for between 50 cents and 90 cents in the developing world to encourage its use and provide greater access to women. It is also marketed in the Americas and Europe for about $2.50. In March 2002, France unveiled its first female pouch (condom) machines, blue for men and pink for women. Currently about **14 million** female condoms are distributed on an annual basis to women in developing countries. By comparison, between **6 and 9 billion** male condoms per year are distributed to men! Female condoms were distributed in 88 countries in Africa, Asia, and Latin America. Distribution began in India in early 2004. They cost third-world governments 12 cents each. Male condoms cost 3 cents each! UNAIDS hopes to get the female condom into all developing nations. In March 2009 the FDA approved the Female Health Company's new FC2 (Female Condom 2ndVersion) female condom. The new condom is made softer and is quieter during use, in response to a complaint with the initial version in use in 77 nations. The new material should also lower the condom's cost. The FC2 condom became available in the United States in 2009. The cost is about $6.50 to $7.00 for a three-pack.

Redressing the Balance of Power

The symbolic importance of the female condom should not be understated: It is the first woman-controlled barrier method officially recognized as a means for the prevention of sexually transmitted disease. The female condom allows women to be able to deal with the twin anxieties—HIV/AIDS and unwanted pregnancy—with a method that is under their own control.

Many women become HIV-infected not because of their own behavior, but because of their partner's. Because of the nature of gender relations, women may have little influence over their partner's sexual behavior.

Commentary: Positive messages for women have been spread worldwide on the advantages of using the female condom. But convincing women, in large numbers, to use this relatively new device may not be so easily accomplished. For example, it took 17 years before women in developed countries accepted and began to routinely use the tampon.

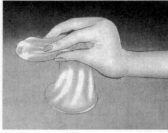
(a)

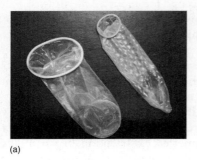

1. The outer ring covers the area around the opening of the vagina. The inner ring is used for insertion and to hold the sheath in place during intercourse.

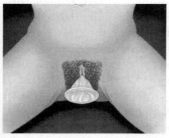

2. Hold the sheath at the closed end, grasp the flexible inner ring and squeeze it with the thumb and middle finger so it becomes long and narrow.

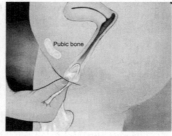

3. Choose a position that is comfortable for insertion – squat, raise one leg sit or lie down. Gently insert the inner ring into the vagina. Feel the inner ring go up and move into place.

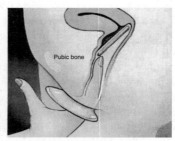

4. Place the index finger on the inside of the condom, and push the inner ring up as far as it will go. Be sure the sheath is not twisted. The outer ring should remain on the outside of the vagina.

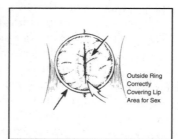

5. FC2 female condom is now in place and ready for use with your partner.

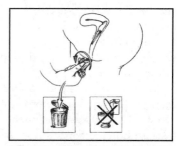

6. The FC2 material is designed to adhere to the vaginal walls and transfer heat. However, extra lubricant may be added to the inside of FC2.

7. To remove the condom, twist the outer ring and gently pull the condom. Wrap the condom in the package or in a tissue and throw it in the garbage. Do not put in the toilet.

(b)

FIGURE 9-6 (a) The female condom, or vaginal pouch, compared in size to the male condom. (b) The 7-inch female condom or vaginal pouch is made of lightweight, lubricated nitrile rubber and has two flexible rings (1), one at each end. It is twice the thickness of the male latex condom. The inner ring (2) is used to help insert the device and fits behind the pubic bone. The outer ring remains outside the body. Unlike the diaphragm, the vaginal condom protects against the transmission of HIV, which can penetrate the vaginal tissues. The pouch can be inserted anytime from several hours to minutes prior to intercourse. The vaginal pouch is inserted like a diaphragm and removed after sex. FC1 was FDA-approved in 1993; second generation FC2 was approved in 2009. *(Courtesy of Female Health Co., Chicago.)*

Condom Lubricants

It has been demonstrated that petroleum or vegetable oil-based lubricants should not be used with latex condoms. Latex condoms exposed to mineral oil for 60 seconds demonstrated a 90% decrease in strength (Anderson, 1993). There are a number of water-based lubricants that do not adversely affect latex condoms; these should be the lubricants of choice.

DISCUSSION QUESTION: Reaching this point in the text and having just read the section on male and female condoms, do you think that the advantages of using condoms outweigh their disadvantages? Do you think the danger for life, with respect to HIV and other life-threatening STDs, is high enough that condoms should be as familiar to everyone as are toothpaste and toilet paper, and also as available? Defend your view with credible information.

AN ALTERNATIVE TO CONDOMS: VAGINAL MICROBICIDES (MI-CRO-BA-CIDES) AND CIRCUMCISION (CIR-CUM-CI-SION)

Microbicides

Twenty two ago, a Ugandan woman, a peer educator in her community, stood up at the 1991 AIDS Prevention Conference and asked, "If they can put a man on the moon, why can't they make something we can use to protect ourselves from HIV?" Since then, researchers and advocates have tried to answer her call. In a world where most new HIV infections occur among women and where a young African girl is now much more likely to get HIV than an African boy, finding new, effective methods of HIV prevention has never been more urgent.

One of the answers may be found in **microbicides.** Microbicides are substances that can prevent HIV (and possibly other sexually transmitted infections) from spreading. Some are designed for vaginal use and some for rectal use. They may take the form of gels, creams, suppositories, films, lubricants, or even a sponge or vaginal ring. In 2011 the National Institutes of Health funded the first ever vaginal ring trial.

The dapivirine-maraviroc ring is the first combination microbicide to enter clinical trials. It is also the first vaginal microbicide containing an entry inhibitor. The belief is that combining the two drugs, which act at different points in the HIV life cycle, may provide greater protection against HIV than a single drug alone. A report from these trials is expected by the end of 2013.

Compared with gels that must be applied daily or immediately before sex, vaginal rings' major advantage is that they provide slow, continuous delivery of a drug or multiple drugs to cells inside the vagina over a period of weeks or months. The rings, which will be worn inside the vagina for 28 days, are made of silicone and are about 2.25 inches in diameter and are a quarter of an inch thick. (For more information on microbicides, visit www.global-campaign.org.)

The term *microbicide* is a generic term applied to anything (for example, the delivery of drugs) designed to prevent infection by HIV and other sexually transmitted pathogens when applied in the vagina or rectum. Because HIV and STI (sexually transmitted infection) pathogens can attack the body in multiple ways, an effective microbicide will have to stop this attack at one or more stages in the infection process. Microbicides are designed primarily to provide protection to receptive sex partners, be they male or female, HIV positive or HIV negative. The first generation of microbicides (those that are farthest along in the clinical trials and likely to come to market first) are designed for vaginal use. But researchers and developers clearly recognize that both men and women have anal intercourse and that rectal microbicides are needed. Many of the candidate microbicides now in development are likely to be bi-directional—that is, capable of disabling HIV in both semen and vaginal secretions. These would give HIV-positive women a way to reduce their male partner's risk of infection even if he chooses not to use condoms.

The Ideal Vaginal Microbicide: A Woman-Controlled Protection

An ideal vaginal microbicide would be safe and effective, and also tasteless, colorless, odorless, nontoxic, stable in most climates, and affordable. It must be pointed out that like condoms, microbicides will not protect injection-drug users.

It will take generations to change male sexual behaviors, and women, especially in the under-developed nations, do not have generations—they are dying now in very large numbers 24 hours a day, seven days a week, 365 days a year! The idea that women will have a way of re-asserting control over their own sexuality, the idea that they will be able to defend their bodily health, the idea that women will have a course of prevention to follow that results in saving their lives, the idea that women may have a microbi-cide that prevents infection but allows for conception, the idea that women can use micro-bicides without bowing to male dictates, the idea that men will not even know the microbicide is in use—these are ideas whose time has come.

It has been estimated that if used by only 30% of women, microbicides could save 6 million lives over five years. These data are based on a microbicide that is 60% effective. But, the first generation of vaginal microbicide is not ex-pected to receive FDA approval until 2013.

The High-Tech Microbicides

The new high-tech microbicides incorporate already developed or very new and experimen-tal anti-HIV drugs. Some even have a systemic effect, meaning that they block HIV infection sometime after application by protecting cells against HIV rather than by acting as a simple barrier. One trial already incorporates a cur-rently available HIV drug into a microbicide. Tenofovir is under investigation in gel form as a possible vaginal microbicide. The highest tech end of microbicide research is starting to look at what could be topical vaccines that actually incorporate anti-HIV antibodies. To date, some 60 microbicides are under investigation. Cer-tain of these trials will have ended in 2010. An effective microbicide could be available sometime in 2012. To date, 11 microbicide trials have failed. (Quick Take 9.1)

THE CAPRISA 004 STUDY RESULTS

For the first time (after 20 years of research and failures), a vaginal gel has proved capable of blocking HIV: It cut in half a woman's chances of getting HIV from an infected partner in a South African study.

Scientists called it a breakthrough in the long quest for a tool to help women whose partners won't use condoms.

However, the results of the CAPRISA 004 study need to be confirmed in other studies. Also, that level of protection may not be enough to win approval of the microbicide gel in the United States. But they are optimistic it can be improved.

"It's the first time we've ever seen any micro-bicide give a positive result" that scientists agree is true evidence of protection, said Anthony Fauci, director of the U.S. National Institute of Allergy and Infectious Diseases.

The gel, spiked with 1 percent antiretroviral drug tenofovir, cut the risk of HIV infection by 39% overall and by 54% in women who used the gel consistently (highly adherent).

To be licensed in the United States, a gel or cream to prevent HIV infection may need to be at least 80% effective. That might be achieved by adding more tenofovir or getting women to use it more consistently. In the study, women used the gel only 60% of the time; those who used it more often had higher rates of protection. The gel also cut in half the chances of getting HSV-2, the gen-ital herpes virus.

The same drug, tenofovir, used in the micro-bicide reported on in 2010 was also used as a pre-exposure prophylactic (PrEP) taken by HIV-negative gay and bisexual men and transgender women. It reduced the risk of HIV infection by 44% in those less adherent and by about 70% in those who were at least 70% adherent (see Chapter 4, pages 85–89, Sidebar 4.3 on PrEP and the PreExposure Prophylaxis Initiative [iPrEP study results]). For an excellent review of PrEP, PEP/ Universal Test, and Treat: Strategic Use of Antiretro-viral Drugs, see the report by Jonathan Weber and colleagues 2010 (it should be noted that this article appeared before the iPrEP work was published).

MICROBIDES: TOPICAL PREVENTION AGAINST HIV

Current microbicide development is focused on the use of antiretroviral drugs that inhibit key stages in HIV replication: viral entry, reverse transcription, integration, and maturation. HIV entry into target cells represents the first point at which microbicides could interrupt initial transmission events. Although much is known about the HIV life cycle, far less is known about initial events in the mucosa of the genital tract and rectum that must be prevented or aborted to ensure protection from HIV infection. Microbicides have a relatively short window of opportunity for blocking infection. Increasing evidence from animal models suggests that infection is established relatively quickly at the mucosa after exposure to HIV. In a nonhuman primate (NHP) model, a 30- to 60-minute exposure to SIV/HIV is sufficient to establish infection. That is most likely the time frame required for viral attachment to target cells and the optimal window for prevention of initial infection by entry inhibitors. HIV has been found to primarily target T4/CD4 and effector memory populations within mucosal tissue, which express high levels of CCR5. Viruses in the initial infection, founder viruses appear to show low macrophage tropism. Tracking of labeled viruses in explant models and NHP studies has shown that the virus can penetrate shallow layers of stratified epithelium and come in contact with potentially susceptible T cells and Langerhans cells within these epithelial surfaces. Microbicides, such as topical pre-exposure prophylaxis (PrEP) products, gels, capsules, tablets, films, and intravaginal rings (IVR), are designed to be delivered around the time of sexual intercourse or (in the case of IVR) over a prolonged period. One of the advantages of microbicides is their ability to be delivered to virally exposed surfaces without causing longer-term toxicity in otherwise healthy but at-risk individuals. Several factors that are important to microbicide development include safety and efficacy in real-world situations, affordability, acceptability, entry point for drug delivery, potential for resistance, and the ability to prioritize the best-in-class products for testing in large scale clinical efficacy trials. Key issues in microbicide development include viral entry, inhibition of co-receptor interaction, reverse transcriptase, and viral integration and viral maturation. Emerging research areas, include developing formulation strategies, examining resistance to antiretroviral microbicides, developing combination microbicides, and studying microbicides in relation to other HIV prevention technologies, such as condoms. A number of Phase III trials of microbicides are currently under way including trials of tenofovir gel and a dapivirine IVR (Shattock et al., 2012).

CIRCUMCISION AND THE PREVENTION OF HIV TRANSMISSION

As summarized in an editorial authored by Daniel Halperin of the University of California, San Francisco, and Robert Bailey of the University of Illinois at Chicago in a recent issue of *The Lancet,* the highly vascularized foreskin (fold of skin covering the end of the penis) contains a higher density of Langerhans cells—the primary target cells for sexual transmission of HIV—than cervical, vaginal, or rectal mucosa (Helperin et al., 1999). They also note the foreskin is more susceptible to traumatic epithelial disruptions (tears) during intercourse, which allows additional vulnerability to blood, ulcerative STDs, and HIV.

A summary on the Technical Meeting on Male Circumcision—Global held in Washington, D.C., in September 2002 states that a synthesis of 28 studies shows that circumcised men are 50% less likely to be infected by HIV than noncircumcised men.

It is estimated that if male circumcision became routine across sub-Saharan Africa, 6 million new HIV infections and 3 million deaths could be prevented over the next 20 years. Currently, the results of the three randomized controlled trials conducted in Kenya, South Africa, and Uganda showed that circumcision does protect males from HIV and STD infections. The three studies showed that circumcision reduced the risk of HIV infection by 60% (Gray et al., 2007; Wawer et al., 2007). Data from the 2011, 6th International AIDS Society Conference support these studies.

Male Circumcision Doesn't Affect Women's HIV Risk

In two recent reports on the effect of male circumcision as it relates to HIV infection in women of HIV-positive circumcised partners, there did not appear to be any benefit to the women. These studies were conducted in Uganda and Zimbabwe (Turner et al., 2007; Wawer et al., 2008; Tobian et al., 2008).

The World Health Organization (WHO) and the UNAIDS Secretariat convened an international expert consultation to determine whether male circumcision should be recommended for the prevention of HIV infection. Based on the evidence presented, which was considered to be compelling, experts attending the consultation recommended that male circumcision now be recognized as an additional important intervention to reduce the risk of heterosexually acquired HIV infection in men. Currently, it is estimated that 665 million men or about 30% of men worldwide have been circumcised. In the United States about 79% of the current male population has been circumcised.

Warnings—The UN agencies emphasize that male circumcision does not provide complete protection against HIV infection. It should never replace other known effective prevention methods and should always be considered to be part of a comprehensive prevention package, which includes correct and consistent use of male or female condoms, reduction in the number of sexual partners, delaying the onset of sexual relations, and HIV testing and counseling. In other words, although circumcision is effective, people cannot circumcise their way out of this pandemic.

Problems—The circumcision operations in the studies were done in state-of-the-art clinics and they were done well, but real-world application may be different. There can be complications. And there are a finite number of those complications. The operation takes about 20 to 30 minutes with moderate to severe side effects and costs are $65–$95 per procedure. In most cases it takes up to 30 days to heal, and the after-effects, such as infections, of the operation can be very serious and painful. Add to this the cultural and religious aspects of having this operation.

Lastly, extrapolating the African needs to the U.S. epidemic is difficult. There is little information on the effectiveness of circumcision for heterosexual males as a method of HIV prevention in the United States. This is partly because the United States has a low HIV prevalence (about 0.6%), because most American men are circumcised (79%), and also because the epidemic is concentrated in men who have sex with men, in whom the protective effect of circumcision is less clear (Warner et al., 2009; Gray et al., 2009, reports from the 2009 Prevention Conference in Atlanta, Georgia). While the African trials dealt with heterosexual men, in the United States the highest risk groups are men who have sex with men (MSM), drug injectors who share needles, and women who have sex with high-risk men. Thus, the United States AIDS epidemic is unlike the one in Africa. So far, there has been no rush of U.S. men seeking circumcision.

Because Botswana health officials believe the evidence/benefits for the use of circumcision is overwhelming, they have begun a campaign to circumcise about 500,000 men. They believe this will prevent about 70,000 new HIV infections by 2025.

UNAIDS and PEPFAR at the December 2011 16th International Conference on AIDS and Sexually Transmitted Infections (STIs) in Africa (ICASA) launched a five-year action framework to accelerate the scale-up voluntary medical male circumcision (VMMC) for HIV prevention. The framework, developed by the World Health Organization (WHO), UNAIDS, PEPFAR, the Bill and Melinda Gates Foundation and the World Bank in consultation with national Ministries of Health, calls for the immediate roll-out and expansion of VMMC services in 14 priority countries of eastern and southern Africa. Reaching 80% coverage of adult VMMC in the 14 priority countries would entail performing approximately 20 million circumcisions on men aged 15–49 by the year 2015.

A review of 9 recent articles on VMMC revealed that 67% of men in sub-Saharan Africa are circumcised, that circumcision is very cost effective with one HIV infection prevented for every 5 to 15 circumcisions performed.

INJECTION-DRUG USE (IDU) AND HIV TRANSMISSION: THE TWIN EPIDEMICS

About 25% of the estimated 2.3 million (ending of 2013) U.S. HIV/AIDS cases recorded since 1981 were transmitted through injection-drug use. They represent about 12% of annual HIV infections and 19% of people living with HIV/AIDS. About 75% of all people with IDU-related HIV/AIDS are either black (50%) or Latino (24%).

Outside Africa, a huge part of the HIV/AIDS pandemic involves people who were infected through IDU. In Russia, 83% of infections in which the origin is known come from needle sharing. In Ukraine, the figure is 64%; Kazakhstan, 74%; Vietnam, 52%; China, 44%. Shared needles are also the primary transmission route for HIV in other parts of Asia.

Both injection-drug use and HIV infection are on the increase. They are twin epidemics in the United States and Europe because the virus is readily transmitted by injection-drug users and then from infected drug users to their non-infected sexual partners. Stopping injection-drug-associated HIV transmission in theory is easy—just avoid injection-drug use. But that is a difficult proposition for most of the estimated 16 million IDUs worldwide of whom about 3 million are HIV positive. The number of countries reporting IDU in 1989 was 80; in 2008, 148. IDUs will remain a major HIV connection to the homosexual, bisexual, heterosexual, and pediatric populations.

HIV PREVENTION FOR INJECTION-DRUG USERS

Public attitudes toward drug users are usually hostile, not only because users are engaging in an illegal activity but also because such behavior is deemed morally suspect. Assumptions that drug users are more likely to engage in criminal and delinquent behavior also fuel public fears, and injecting drug users are thus isolated and shunned. Stigma and fear of arrest discourage millions from contacting health and social services, no matter how great their need. The response to HIV in people who inject drugs has been especially poor in many of the countries in which harm-reduction measures are needed most. About 4% of the IDUs currently receive ART.

Regardless of whether one uses injection drugs, there are practical reasons why everyone should be concerned with HIV within the drug injection community. Most obvious is that injection-drug users have sex with nonusers, and the virus can spread to their partners and children.

What can be done and what is being done to prevent HIV transmission by this population? Available drug rehabilitation programs are far too few. It is estimated that only 15% of injection-drug users in the United States and less than 1% in developing countries are receiving treatment at any given time. Many addicts want to quit their habit but may become discouraged because of having to wait so long before getting treatment because of lack of money and treatment centers. Even if there were a sufficient number of treatment centers, there will always be the hard-core IDUs who will not enter a program (Figure 9-7).

IDUs have an economic motive to share equipment. Most syringes now being used by IDUs stay in circulation from 1 to 24 days! At the beginning of 2013, studies continue to show that about 35% of IDUs share equipment and over 60% have unprotected vaginal sex. Perhaps the most important obstacle may be that IDUs have little interest in health care or changing their behaviors. In addition, there is always the problem of legality. IDU is illegal throughout the United States and in most if not all other countries.

IDUs know this and fear incarceration without the possibility of a "fix." A catch-22 situation also exists for those who want to help make injection-drug use safer: Many U.S. governmental agencies and law enforcement officers interpret the intention of making drug use safer as advocating drug use. They believe that giving

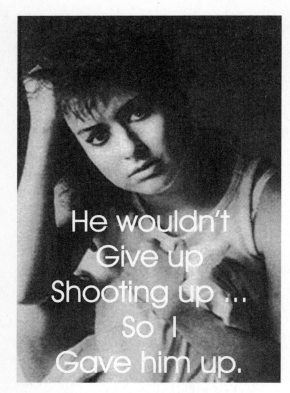

FIGURE 9-7 He wouldn't give up shooting up . . . so I gave him up. *(Courtesy of the Centers for Disease Control and Prevention, Atlanta.)*

about 10% of injecting drug users worldwide enjoyed access to HIV prevention services of any kind, while substitution therapy—i.e., offering users methadone instead of heroin—is permitted in only 70 countries, and needle and syringe exchange programs are available in only 82 countries. **(Note: From this point forward, NEP stands for** *needle exchange programs* **and involves a needle and a syringe.)**

The Needle Exchange Program (NEP) Strategy: One Needle, One Syringe, Each Time

The idea of syringe-needle exchange programs is based on the established public health policy of eliminating from any system potentially infectious agents or, where possible, carriers of infectious agents. The rationale of NEPs is similar, wherein active injection-drug users exchange used, potentially contaminated syringes for new, sterile syringes (Figure 9-8). In general, these exchanges are done on a one-used-needle-and-syringe for one-new-needle-and-syringe basis, although some programs will add an additional number of needles and syringes on top of those already exchanged. NEPs also provide other paraphernalia and supplies including cotton, cookers, water, and sterile alcohol prep pads. In addition, NEPs offer a variety of other services to IDUs including education, HIV testing and counseling, referrals to primary medical care, substance abuse treatment, and case management.

The world's first NEP on record began in 1984 in Amsterdam, The Netherlands. It was started by an IDU advocacy group called the Junkie Union.

Jon Parker is believed to be the first person in the United States to distribute free drug injection equipment publicly. He did so in North Haven, CT, and in Boston in November 1986.

The Problem—A needle exchange is *not* going to be a welcome neighbor. All the assurances in the world about security and policing and good neighbor agreements can't remove fears of noise, crime, and disorder. Even though an exchange may be needed, the neighbors have a right not to face associated problems. Yes? No?

syringes/needles to IDUs is like giving matches to a pyromaniac (someone with an impulse to start fires). As a result, many proponents of safer drug use have avoided becoming involved in the issue. The 2000 Kaiser Family Foundation National Survey of Americans showed that 58% of those polled were in favor of syringe-needle exchange programs. In December 2009, the 24-year ban on the use of federal money to fund needle exchange programs (NEPs) was lifted. But, in 2012 the ban was reinstated!

Peter Lurie and colleagues (1998) state that each year, over 1 billion syringes [now it is about 2 billion] would be required for IDUs to have a sterile syringe for each injection. Despite the fact that injecting drug use has led to the widespread transmission of HIV worldwide, the provision of HIV prevention, treatment, and the care services to IDU populations remains low. In 2012, only

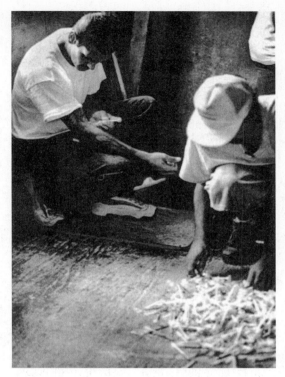

FIGURE 9-8 Getting a Fix. An injection-drug user shoots up in a shooting gallery in the La Perla neighborhood of Old San Juan, Puerto Rico. Another man sorts used syringes to be exchanged for new. *(Photo by Enrique Valentin/South Florida Sun-Sentinel.)*

Evaluation of Needle Exchange Programs

Unlike with sexual transmission, there is a proven prevention solution here: needle exchange programs, which provide drug injectors with clean needles, usually in return for their used ones. Needle exchange is the cornerstone of an approach known as *harm reduction:* making drug use less deadly. Clean needles are both tool and lure—a way to introduce drug users to counseling, HIV tests, treatment and rehabilitation, including access to opioid-substitution therapies like methadone. Needle exchange is HIV/AIDS prevention that works. While no one wants to have to put on a condom, most drug users prefer injecting with a clean needle. In 2003, an academic review of 99 cities around the world found that cities with needle exchange saw their HIV rates among injecting drug users drop 19% a year; cities without needle exchange had an 8% increase per year. Contrary to public fear, needle exchange has not led to more drug use or higher crime rates. Studies have also found that drug addicts participating in needle exchanges are more likely to enter rehabilitation programs. Using needle exchange as part of a comprehensive attack on HIV is endorsed by virtually every relevant United Nations and United States government agency. However, the majority of IDUs worldwide do not have access to needle exchange programs.

Needle Exchange Programs in the United States

Entering year 2013, over 220 NEPs operating in all 50 states and the District of Columbia were exchanging about 40 million syringes annually. It is unclear how many of these programs receive federal funding. In 2012 state and local government funding for NEPs came to over $16 million. An IDU makes over 1000 drug injections each year (*MMWR,* 1997). The San Francisco AIDS Foundation operates the largest NEP in the United States. There are too many NEPs to list, but a few are presented here.

Tacoma, Washington—Its NEP began in August 1988. It began as a one-man program by Dave Purchase, a 20-year drug counselor.

The NEP in Tacoma held the HIV infection rate to under 5% over a five-year study period (1988–1992). During that same five-year study period, the prevalence of HIV infection among IDUs in New York City, with few syringe exchange programs, increased from 10% to 50%! About 1.5 million syringes are exchanged annually.

New York City—In November 1988, after many delays, New York City began its NEP. The program was canceled in early 1990—the reason: because over 50% of NYC's 240,000 IDUs were HIV infected, the program was offered too little too late to have an impact. IDUs make up about 38% to 40% of NYC AIDS cases. The NEP was resumed in 1992. In 1998 there were at least five NEPs operating in New York City. In May 2000, New York State passed a law making it legal to buy needles without a prescription, the forty-third state to do so. About 3 million syringes are exchanged annually.

New Haven, Connecticut—Its 16-year-old program has demonstrated that NEPs dramatically slow the rate of infection without encouraging new injection-drug use. Some indicators even suggest that the program has been responsible for a decrease in both crime and the amount of drugs used illegally. These results have enabled policymakers elsewhere to call for NEPs.

After the passage of a 1992 law permitting pharmacies to sell syringes without a prescription, syringe sharing has dropped 40% in the state of Connecticut. Seventy-five percent of HIV/AIDS cases in Connecticut occur among IDUs, their sex partners, and their children.

California—Each year about 8000 Californians are infected with HIV, and injection-drug use is the second leading cause of those infections. In October 1999 a law was passed that would allow cities and counties to establish NEPs. Entering 2013 at least 15 cities and 17 counties had funded NEPs. About 4 million syringes are exchanged annually.

Hawaii—In 1990, Hawaii became the first state to legalize a statewide NEP. The state legislature felt it was necessary to stem the rate of HIV infection in women and newborns. About 1 million syringes are exchanged annually.

Beginning 2008, all 50 states have some type of NEP system in place.

Puerto Rico—In 2009 Puerto Rico began using vending machines for after-hours addicts. Using a special card in the vending machine, they can obtain syringes, cookers, cotton filters, gauze, and sterile water to prepare their drugs for injection.

Needle Exchange Programs in Other Countries

There are an estimated 16 million IDUs worldwide. And, over 3 million are HIV positive. Many countries are now involved in NEPs to lower the spread of HIV.

Needle exchange program results from England, Austria, The Netherlands, Sweden, and Scotland, presented at the Fourth International AIDS Conference (1988), suggest that the European programs attracted IDUs who had no previous contact with drug treatment programs; and that IDUs were drawn from NEPs into treatment programs, thus the decrease in drug use. There was no indication in these studies of an increase in injection-drug use in cities with exchange programs. Where HIV testing had been done, the rate of HIV infection showed a marked decline after the introduction of NEPs (Raymond, 1988; Hagen, 1991).

Some of the 82 countries with active NEPs are: Canada, England, France, Ireland, The Netherlands, Australia, New Zealand, Italy, China, and Russia. Russia will stop financing *its* NEPS beginning 2013.

Injection Treatment Centers or Drug Consumption Rooms

Some countries, instead of offering NEP, offer IDU treatment centers. Switzerland is currently providing IDUs with heroin three times a day in 18 treatment centers across the country. So far Swiss health authorities say the program, which began in 1986, has reduced criminal activity among the participants by about 60%. The program also reduced their rate of homelessness from 12% to zero and their death rate by 50%. Entering 2013, following Switzerland's lead, Germany, The Netherlands, Spain, Portugal, Australia, Luxembourg, Norway, and Vancouver, British Columbia (the site of North America's first consumption room) have implemented consumption or injection rooms for the legal use of heroin. In 2012 Dar es Salaam, Tanzania, opened its first heroin consumption room. There are about 50 legal heroin consumption rooms or clinics in nine countries, worldwide. Requests for heroin consumption rooms in Austria and the United States have been denied.

DISCUSSION QUESTION: The United States has zero tolerance for such activities and will not become involved in what the

Swiss term "an innovative program." Do you think the United States should, based on the Swiss data, offer heroin to the addicted in a controlled environment similar to the Swiss? Present credible reasons/data to support your stand.

Summary

Entering 2013, 85% of IDUs in Glasgow, 83% in Lund, 85% in Sydney, 74% in Tacoma, and 88% in Toronto reported they had changed their behavior in order to avoid HIV/AIDS. The most commonly mentioned specific behavior change: reduced sharing of injection equipment. There were about 300,000 IDUs living with HIV/AIDS in the United States at the end of 2012.

PREVENTION OF BLOOD AND BLOOD PRODUCT HIV TRANSMISSION

A combined fear of disease and lawsuits has led most wealthy developed nations to adopt a zero tolerance policy regarding HIV contamination of the blood supply. However, 10% of all new HIV infections in developing countries are due to transfusions of tainted blood. In the early 1980s, 1 of every 50 bags of blood collected in San Francisco contained HIV. The chance of acquiring either HIV or hepatitis C from a blood transfusion in America is now about 1 in 1 million.

Blood Donors

In the United States, there are at least 52 medically related restrictions for donating your blood. Thirteen of these reasons place a person on permanent restriction from donating blood—for example, being HIV positive, having multiple sclerosis, being a hemophiliac, being a man who has had sex with other men since 1977 (even once), having used injection drugs (even once), or having had a stroke.

There should be no risk in the United States or in other developed nations of contracting HIV by donating blood if blood centers use a new, sterile needle for each donation. Yet a 2005 survey revealed that 25% of those polled believed that they could become HIV infected by *donating blood*.

IN 2011 The United Kingdom dropped its policy against gays donating blood. The United States may also drop the same policy in 2013.

Blood Collection and Screening Blood for HIV

Testing blood for infectious diseases began with syphilis screening in the 1940s. Hepatitis B antibody screening was added in the 1970s, HIV antibody screening in 1985, the hepatitis B-core antigen in 1986, HTL V-I and II-antibodies in 1988, and hepatitis C antibodies in 1990. Inclusion of the HIV antigen (p24) test in 1996 provided detection of HIV infection sooner than antibody testing. At least eight tests for infectious diseases are now routinely performed on each unit of blood collected.

No Blood Purchases for Transfusion—All blood transfused in the United States comes from volunteer donors. Blood from paid donors is used for pharmaceuticals such as Rh Ig (type g immunoglobin), albumin, and intravenous immunoglobulins. Under the current standards for blood banks and transfusion services of the American Association of Blood Banks, all units must be clearly labeled volunteer, paid, or autologous (donated for self-use).

U.S. FDA Approves Blood Screening Test for HIV—Blood screening for HIV and HIV-testing procedures are presented in Chapter 13, page 399. The risk of becoming HIV infected from a blood transfusion has dropped by more than 99% from 1983 to 2003. Regardless, a male living in Durango, TX., received contaminated blood during heart bypass surgery in August 2000. In 2002, two people became HIV infected from blood transfusions in Florida and one in Colorado in 2008. Tracing the infectious blood back to its donor source revealed that, in each incident, the donors were in the **window period;** they were infected but the blood test failed to detect the virus. About five million people receive blood transfusion annually in the United States.

Blood Transfusions Worldwide—Twenty-six years after the industrialized world began to screen all blood used in transfusions for HIV, about 1 in 10 people in developing countries are still being infected through this route.

A combination of the lack of screening with high levels of infected donors turns transfusion into a form of roulette. As 2013 began, blood transfusions accounted for 5% to 10% of HIV infections worldwide.

Blood Safety—From 1985 into 2013, over 600 million units of blood or plasma have been screened for HIV antibody in the United States. By excluding those who test HIV positive and by asking people from high-risk behavior groups not to donate blood, the incidence of HIV transmission from the current blood supply is relatively low. With faster and more accurate testing procedures now in use, the risk is becoming even lower. However, the probability or risk of receiving HIV-contaminated blood will never be zero. The reason a small risk still exists is because some people infected with HIV may donate blood during their window period. During that period, a person may be infected with HIV, but the test cannot yet detect the infection. And, second, the test is not 100% accurate.

INFECTION CONTROL PROCEDURES

With no cure or vaccine for HIV/AIDS, prevention of infection is of paramount importance. With the advent of the HIV/AIDS epidemic, healthcare workers and others who are occupationally exposed to body fluids, especially blood, are understandably concerned about the risk of becoming HIV infected. However, when precautions are observed, the risk is very small, even for those treating HIV/AIDS patients.

Two sets of infection control procedures are in use in hospitals, medical centers, physicians' offices, and units that deal with people in medical emergencies. One is called **universal precautions,** the other is **blood and body substance isolation.**

Universal Precautions (UP)

Universal precautions are standard practices that workers observe on the job to protect themselves from infections and injuries. These precautions or safety practices are called *universal* because they are used in all situations even if there seems to be no risk. Universal precautions had their beginnings in 1976 when barrier techniques were first recommended for the prevention of hepatitis B infection. Precautions required the use of protective eyewear, gloves, and gowns, and careful handling of needles and other sharp instruments.

Under universal precautions, the blood and certain body fluids of all patients are considered potentially infectious for HIV, hepatitis B virus (HBV), and other blood-borne pathogens.

Universal precautions are intended to prevent parenteral (introduction of a substance into the body by injection), mucous membrane, and broken skin exposure of healthcare workers (HCWs), teachers, or any other person who may become exposed to blood-borne pathogens. In 1987, the CDC also published a report that got the immediate attention of most, if not all, informed healthcare workers. The report stated that three health-care workers who were exposed to the blood of AIDS patients tested positive for HIV. What was so startling was that until that time, needle punctures and cuts were thought to be the only dangers in a clinical setting. These three cases appeared to involve only skin exposure to HIV-contaminated blood. One of the three cases involved a nurse whose chapped and ungloved hands were exposed to an AIDS patient's blood.

The second case involved a nurse who broke a vacuum tube during a routine phlebotomy on an outpatient. The blood splashed on her face and into her mouth. A blood splash was also involved in the third case. The worker's ungloved hands and forearms were exposed to HIV-contaminated blood (Ezzell, 1987).

An Important Wake-Up Call

These three cases of HIV infection informed healthcare workers in the most dramatic way that they were all vulnerable. Perhaps these three cases produced a fear among healthcare workers out of proportion to the actual risk of their becoming infected. Although calculations show that the risk of HIV infection after exposure to blood from an HIV/AIDS patient is about 1 in 200, if you are that one, probability is meaningless.

Who Is Affected by Universal Precaution Mandate?

The universal precautions as published by the CDC currently apply to some 5.3 million healthcare workers at 620,000 work sites across the United States and another 700,000 Americans who routinely come in contact with blood as part of their job, for example, people in law enforcement, education, fire fighting and rescue, corrections, laboratory research, and the funeral industry.

In summary, the concept of universal precautions assumes that all blood is infectious, no matter from whom and no matter whether a test is negative, positive, or not done at all. Rigorous adherence to universal precautions is the surest way of preventing accidental transmission of HIV and other blood-borne pathogens.

Blood and Body Substance Isolation (BBSI)

An alternative, and some believe superior, approach to the CDC's universal precautions in areas of high HIV prevalence is the system referred to as *body substance precautions or Blood Body Substance Isolation (BBSI)* (Gerberding, 1991).

In practice, these precautions are similar to universal precautions, in that prevention of needle stick injury and use of barrier methods of infection control are emphasized. Philosophically, however, the two are quite different. Whereas universal precautions place a clear emphasis on avoidance of blood-borne infection, body substance precautions take a more global view. **Blood body substance isolation (BBSI) requires barrier precautions for all body substances (including feces, respiratory secretions, urine, vomit, etc.) and moist body surfaces (including mucous membranes and open wounds).** BBSI is designed as a system to reduce the risk of transmission of all nosocomial (hospital-associated) pathogens, not just blood-borne pathogens. Gloves are worn for any anticipated or known contact with mucous membranes, nonintact skin, and moist body substances of all patients.

SEXUAL PARTNER NOTIFICATION: DISCLOSURE

One of the most controversial issues in HIV prevention is *contact tracing, partner notification, or disclosure* of sexual contacts mostly because HIV/AIDS is considered an incurable disease with a great deal of stigma attached to the infected. Disclosure can cause an increase in stigma and discrimination, but it is also, paradoxically (contrary to common sense, yet is perhaps true), an essential step in fighting stigma and discrimination.

Partner notification is the practice of identifying and treating people exposed to certain communicable diseases. The term "partner notification" rather than disclosure is used by the CDC and some healthcare providers because it more comprehensively describes the process by which the physician, other healthcare workers such as Disease Intervention Specialists (DIS, someone who is specially trained in STD work), and the infected person may provide information to at-risk partners and sometimes to family, friends, or care providers.

Why Partner Disclosure Matters

Every disclosure is unique, with specific risks and benefits. One benefit of disclosure is that it can be a practical means of getting support and referrals. You'll also reduce the risk of HIV transmission to others, and you may help keep others close by allowing them to share your worries and triumphs. Also, by informing a sex partner (former or current), he or she can decide to get tested.

How Does One Communicate in Partner Notification: Disclosure?

There are two very different approaches to informing unsuspecting third parties about their potential exposure to medical risk.

Each approach has its own history, including a unique set of practical problems in its implementation, and provokes its own ethical dilemmas. The **first** approach, involving the moral *duty to warn,* arose out of the clinical setting in which the physician knew the identity of the person deemed to be at risk. This approach provided a warrant for disclosure to endangered persons without the consent of the patient and could involve revealing the identity of the patient. The **second** approach—that of contact tracing—emerged from sexually transmitted disease control programs in which the clinician typically did not know the identity of those who might have been exposed. This approach was founded on the voluntary cooperation of the patient in providing the names of contacts. It never involved the disclosure of the identity of the patient. The entire process of notification was kept confidential (Bayer et al., 1992).

THE U.S. FEDERAL GOVERNMENT HAS NOW ADOPTED PARTNER NOTIFICATION AS ITS CORNERSTONE IN ITS EFFORT TO HELP CONTROL THE SPREAD OF HIV

A major reason for the federal government's push for partner notification is that it is a more efficient and focused way to test for HIV. Studies show that routine testing and counseling among the general population typically turns up new infections in less than 1% of those tested. But among the sexual partners of HIV-positive people, infection rates are around 20%. Partner notification concentrates on a group most likely to have previously undetected infections.

It should also be noted that between one in four to one in five HIV-positive people in the United States do not know they are infected. Ending 2013, the number of people living with HIV/AIDS is estimated at 1.62 million. This means that there are between 324,000 and 405,000 infected who do not know of their infection! They can't disclose, but they do place others at risk.

History of Sexual Partner Notification

The concept of partner notification was proposed in 1937 by Surgeon General Thomas Parran for the control of syphilis (Parran, 1937). By tracing and treating all known contacts of a syphilitic patient, the chain of transmission could be interrupted. According to George Rutherford (1988), contact tracing has been successfully used for a number of STDs beginning in the 1950s. It is still used in cases of syphilis, endemic gonorrhea, chlamydia, hepatitis B, STD enteric infections, and particularly in cases of antibiotic-resistant gonorrhea.

In 1985, when the HIV antibody was first used in screening the blood supply, notification of blood donors and other HIV-infected individuals and their contacts became possible. The strategy in HIV partner notification is the same as that used for the other STDs: to identify HIV-infected individuals, counsel them, and offer whatever treatment is available. In asymptomatic HIV-infected people only counseling is given. (See Box 9.1, page 271.)

Partner Notification Depends on Cooperation

Partner notification depends on HIV-positive people to give the names of their partners; but they may be reluctant to do so fearing that their identification may result in physical abuse and loss of jobs and housing. For a review of partner notification read the article by Kevin Fenton et al. (1997). Those who oppose the use of partner notification call the investigators "sex police."

Examples in the Use of Sexual Partner Notification/Contact Tracing

One—In April 1993 an incarcerated male asked for an HIV test. The diagnosis was positive. Contact tracing turned up a network of 124

BOX 9.1

CHELSEA GULDEN, AGE 27, MOTHER AND PREVENTION DISCLOSURE ADVOCATE

Chelsea Gulden is a 27-year-old HIV-positive mother and prevention/disclosure advocate (Figure 9-9). She was diagnosed in 2003 while she was a student in the University of North Carolina system. "My boyfriend and I tested positive in 2003. The first thing that came to mind was I couldn't have kids. But I had only two or three days to stress out. I went back to the doctor and I learned I was five weeks pregnant. I didn't know much about HIV. I kept asking myself what it meant for my quality of life and immediately became concerned about my pregnancy. I had to stop and make sure that my motives for wanting a child were the right ones. For instance, was I really ready for a baby? Was I in a place where I could take care of a child both emotionally and physically?"

CHELSEA'S BIG DECISION

After discussions with her physician and learning as quickly as possible all that she could about HIV/AIDS, Chelsea decided to keep her pregnancy. After her decision, her pregnancy, delivery, and newborn were labors of love. Her cherished son, who is HIV negative, is now five and a half years old and without a doubt the greatest joy in her life.

HER MAJOR FEARS

She worries that her health and economic budget may not last long enough for her to mother her son through college. She would like more children if she can find the right person, but again she fears that she may not be there in the long run. Another concern is how other children may treat her son when they find out his mother is HIV positive.

POST-DIAGNOSIS ADVENTURES

Since diagnosis, Chelsea has worked on spreading awareness and HIV education across the Carolinas and abroad. She is currently responsible for implementing programs for HIV-infected youth in the Charlotte area. This effort was started to assist with keeping a continuum of medical care and support as these youth learn to cope with their diagnosis. Her presentations have taken her many places. She has spoken at many HIV/AIDS gatherings and conferences. In October 2006, an appearance in *HIV Plus* and on the *Oprah Winfrey Show* boosted Chelsea's speaking career. In 2007, Chelsea made the cover of *POZ Magazine*. Her speaking circuit has taken her

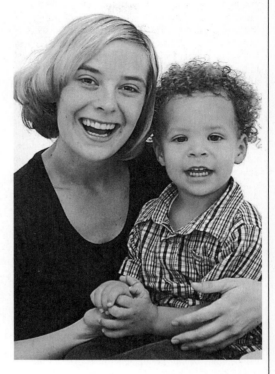

FIGURE 9-9   **Chelsea Gulden.** Going into her senior year of college, Chelsea unexpectedly found out that she was HIV positive. She had such faith that the HIV test would be negative, she did not return for her test results. A disease intervention specialist located Chelsea and told her she tested positive. Chelsea said, "My whole world collapsed, my heart dropped to my feet." Several days later she learned she was five weeks pregnant.
(With appreciation to Chelsea Gulden who provided the information used herein and to Emile M. Knight who granted permission and the photograph of Chelsea and her son.)

across the United States as an AIDS awareness speaker for the Safe Haven Project, as well as teaching sexual health at the University of North Carolina–Charlotte. As a devoted advocate for HIV/AIDS awareness prevention and disclosure, she first makes time to be a devoted and responsible mother. (See Point of View 9.2, page 272.)

HIV-POSITIVE PEOPLE CARRY THE BURDEN OF DISCLOSURE: DO I HAVE TO KISS AND TELL?

The advantages and disadvantages of self-disclosure must be carefully weighed, especially if the impact is likely to be so stressful as to diminish all anticipated benefits. The most important aspect influencing an individual's extent of disclosure must be how it will impact the person in question, those around them, and the community. The extent of the existing stigma in the community can greatly influence the way, and to whom, disclosure is made.

For example, one woman (granddaughter) said that her grandmother called and said, "your grandfather has bone cancer." A couple of months later she called again and said, "he has lung cancer." Several months later the granddaughter found out that her grandmother had lied—grandfather had AIDS.

TELLING SOMEONE YOU ARE HIV POSITIVE— FIGURE 9–10

In an ideal world, everyone would recognize that sexual safety and health is an obligation and responsibility of all parties involved. Asking about HIV and STD status and being prepared for safer sex would be expected of everyone. Unfortunately, because so many people are uneducated about HIV, STDs, and safer sex, the ideal world doesn't exist. HIV-positive people carry the burden of assessing the level of risk they engage in and/or subject others to.

Telling someone that you're HIV positive is rarely easy. If the person you're telling is a potential sex partner it can become even more challenging. When you disclose your HIV-positive status to a potential sex partner, you run the risk of rejection. A lot depends upon the person that you are disclosing to and your relationship with them. Because of the stigma that comes with the HIV infection, people may reject you, gossip about you, openly or secretly discriminate against you or your family, or even threaten you. Revealing your status to someone else can be scary, isolating, and overwhelming. For those who are in denial about their HIV-positive status, it will be difficult to admit it to someone else or to disclose to or protect a sexual partner.

Don't Ask, Don't Tell

Others who are bound by fear, shame, and distrust may even lie about their status. Some HIV-positive people believe in the "don't ask, don't tell" policy—if your partner doesn't ask, then you don't have to tell. Your only obligation is to do everything in your power to keep him or her safe. Others pick and choose those whom they feel that they can trust with this information.

Do Ask, Do Tell

Still others are open about their status and disclose to family, friends, and sexual partners with little hesitation.

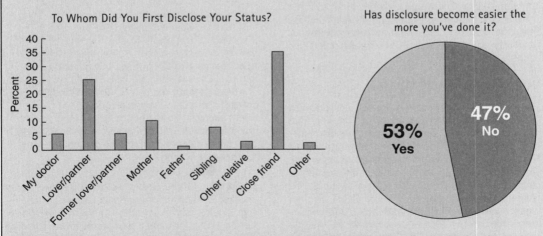

To Whom Did You First Disclose Your Status?

Has disclosure become easier the more you've done it?

53% Yes   47% No

FIGURE 9–10   Ninety-three Percent of People Who Disclosed Their HIV Status to Someone within the First Year after Diagnosis. *(From* POZ Magazine *September 2011, March 2011 Survey. Reprinted courtesy of Smart + Strong/POZ.)*

persons; all were linked by syringe sharing and syringe sharing with sex. One hundred twenty-one were contacted and offered an HIV test; 118 accepted the test; 44 were positive. One hundred thirteen of the 124 lived in the same county. The estimated cost for partner notification in this network was $13,969 (*MMWR*, 1995).

Two—During a five-month period (February through June 1999) seven young people were diagnosed with HIV in a small rural town in Mississippi. The CDC, working with the Mississippi Health Department through partner contact investigation, defined a social network of 122 people. Persons in the network had a median age of 21 (range: 13 to 45 years). Of the 78 people tested for HIV infection, five women (median age, 16 years) and two men (median age, 25 years) were infected, all through heterosexual sex. Results of the interviews of the infected and noninfected people indicated a serious lack of HIV/AIDS prevention knowledge (*MMWR*, 2000a).

Three—At the 2004 11th Conference of Retroviruses and Opportunistic Infections investigators said they found the number of new HIV infections in men from 37 southern colleges has risen rapidly in just a few years. In 2000 there were 6; in 2001, 19; in 2002, 29; and in 2003, 30. Of that total of 84 new infections, 73 were in blacks and 11 in whites. Sixty-three percent reported having sex with men only, 33% with both men and women, and 4% with women only. They attended 33 colleges in North Carolina, two in South Carolina, one in Georgia, and one in Florida. The outbreak was identified in time for the authorities to ask North Carolina's colleges to include safer sex messages during Fall 2004 orientation sessions. Stories about the outbreak that appeared in campus newspapers, contact tracing or partner notification, and free HIV testing helped reveal and tie this minor college epidemic together.

Conclusion

In January 2003, two separate studies, one by Patricia Kissinger and colleagues and the other by Tamara Hoxworth, reveal that previously held conceptions on the negative aspects of partner notifications are wrong. Their findings reveal that partner notification rarely damages relationships or promotes violence and that, if anything, exposure to partner notification contributes to safe behaviors. Partner notification did not lead to more relationship breakups among HIV-positive individuals, in comparison to syphilis-infected persons.

DISCUSSION QUESTION: With current life-sustaining and preventive antiretroviral treatments available, is there an overwhelming excuse not to use partner notification—especially when so many HIV/AIDS experts promote the "hit early" approach to therapy?

What is your response to the reasons for partner notification and to the opposition's point of view?

The Duty to Warn

The **duty to warn** may extend to nonpatient third parties in other contexts, based on the provider's primary duty to the patient. Thus, healthcare professionals have a duty to inform patients that they have been transfused with HIV-contaminated blood, and this duty may extend to third parties. A physician in one case failed to inform a teenager or her parents that she had been transfused with HIV-contaminated blood. When the young woman's sexual partner tested positive for HIV, the court upheld his claim against the physician based on the physician's failure to inform the patient. Similarly, courts have upheld that a healthcare professional's duty to inform the patient of his or her HIV infection may extend to those the patient foreseeably puts at risk, such as a spouse or family member caregiver. On the other hand, courts have ruled that disclosure is wrongful in cases in which the third party, such as a family member, is not at actual risk of infection, or the physician has no knowledge that the patient has failed to disclose to the partner (Gostin et al., 1998).

Entering 2013, at least 39 states in the United States have enacted partner notification laws that provide for penalties that range from a misdemeanor (a crime less serious than a felony, which is a serious crime) to attempted murder for anyone who does not reveal to a sexual partner that he or she is HIV positive. At least 44 states passed laws requiring or permitting workers (mostly healthcare workers or public safety employees) to be notified of potential exposure of HIV. In some cases, the laws allow testing of the source patient. To date, Arkansas and Missouri are the only states that require patients to notify healthcare providers of their HIV status before receiving care. All 50 states are now somewhere in the process of establishing the capacity for contact tracing at the request of a patient.

DISCUSSION QUESTION: If a law were passed that made persons who practiced high-risk behaviors and who contracted HIV/AIDS pay for their own care and treatment or forgo medical help—do you think these people would continue to engage in high-risk behaviors? Would this law be an effective means of HIV transmission prevention? Present examples to support your position. (Can you relate this scenario to those who smoke and develop cancer?)

For a detailed report on partner notification published by the WHO and UNAIDS see: http://www.who.int/asd/knowledge/rptngdiscl.html.

VACCINES

Imagine having the ability to eliminate a disease—not just to alleviate its symptoms, but to erase it completely, as if it had never existed. This is the promise of vaccines. Humankind has benefited from more than 200 years of successful vaccine use. One hundred years ago, parents worried most about their children contracting diphtheria, and 50 years ago they worried about polio; today, the most serious childhood infections have largely disappeared from the developed world. Moreover, the World Health Organization officially declared the global eradication of smallpox in 1980. In addition, vaccines are now available to combat adult diseases such as cervical cancer and shingles. Yet there are three major 21st century scourges that still demand efficacious vaccines: HIV/AIDS, tuberculosis, and malaria.

THE FIRST HUMAN VACCINE: THE IMPACT OF VACCINES ON INFECTIOUS DISEASES

The first human vaccine was developed in 1796 by Edward Jenner to prevent smallpox. With the exception of clean drinking water, no other human health intervention has had the impact of vaccination on reducing infectious diseases.

THE JOURNEY TOWARD AN HIV/AIDS VACCINE NOW IN ITS 30th YEAR (1983–2013)

It's clear that treatment and prevention efforts alone can't end the HIV/AIDS pandemic. Treatment delivery fails to meet the global need, and more people than ever before are living with HIV. But a vaccine—preventive and/or therapeutic—has eluded scientists for nearly 30 years.

Every year in the United States, vaccines prevent about 3 million deaths and save about a million children from disabilities caused by infectious diseases. Vaccines have been documented to be the most cost-effective means of improving human health. No human vaccine is 100% effective, but most vaccines protect between 70% and 95% of those vaccinated against the targeted disease.

According to the CDC, over the past 20 years, the number of diseases prevented by vaccines has doubled and their is great promise for new vaccines in the 21st century.

Some Key Points about Vaccines

1. A vaccine teaches the immune system how to defend itself against a disease-causing agent, known as a pathogen.
2. A vaccine is designed to prevent one specific disease or pathogen; therefore, a vaccine matches a certain disease.
3. A preventive vaccine is meant for people who have not been infected with the pathogen that the vaccine is designed to protect against.
4. A preventive vaccine is not a treatment or cure for someone who is already infected with the specific pathogen. (See Point of Information 9.2.)

HIV VACCINE DEVELOPMENT AND ITS ROLE IN PREVENTION

In the spread of any contagious disease, each act of infection has two parties: one who already has the disease and one who does not. Vaccination works by treating the uninfected individual to prevent his or her infection. Since it is impossible to say in advance who might be exposed, that means vaccinating everybody. The alternative is to treat the infected individual, stopping him or her from being infectious. For this to curb an epidemic would require an enormous public-health campaign of the scale used to promote vaccination. But this campaign would be of a different kind. It would have to identify all (or at least almost all) of those infected. It would then have to persuade them to undergo not a short, simple vaccination, but rather a drug regimen that would continue indefinitely.

> Several lines of evidence indicate that development of an effective vaccine for HIV is going to be, at best, extremely difficult. The inability to solve fundamental scientific questions is the root cause for why a successful vaccine is not currently within our grasp. A renewed, organized, focused effort is needed to overcome these scientific obstacles. The immediate prospects for hitting on a worthwhile HIV vaccine would possibly be like hitting a baseball blindfold.

> Ronald C. Desrosiers, 2007
> Immunologist, New England
> Primate Research Center

Despite the effectiveness of antiretroviral therapy (ART) and considerable success in reducing the price of the drugs in resource-poor settings, the relentless spread of HIV continues to overwhelm all efforts to contain it. Like a horse without a rider, ART can't go the distance alone. HIV/AIDS cannot be stopped without an effective means of preventing future infections. Unfortunately, the quest for a vaccine continues to elude our best scientific efforts. The new vaccines that looked so promising a few short years ago have produced disappointing results. Some scientists argue that there is no guarantee we will ever have a vaccine, while others are more optimistic but recognize that HIV presents a uniquely difficult challenge. Yet even if a perfect vaccine were created today, it would take roughly 10 years to provide it to all those who need it. It is difficult to overstate the damage that another 10 years without a vaccine will do. To better understand what a vaccine is, how they have been made and used, and why we do not have a vaccine for HIV, the following information on vaccines is presented.

The Holy Grail

A vaccine is considered the Holy Grail in the battle against disease. The Holy Grail of HIV/AIDS prevention is a single-dose, safe, affordable oral or injectable vaccine that gives lifelong protection against all subtypes of HIV.

It is always better to prevent disease than to treat it. Vaccines protect against those disease-bearing agents that come into contact with un-vaccinated individuals.

Historically, vaccines have provided a safe, cost-effective, and efficient means of preventing illness, disability, and death from infectious diseases through the use of vaccinations.

It is now abundantly clear that no pharmacologic agent, no educational efforts directed to safer sex (regardless of how vigorously implemented), and no nutritional modification will stop or prevent this pandemic from continuing. Halting the spread of HIV requires an effective vaccine. Ending 2013, an estimated 68 million people will either be living with HIV or will have died from it.

Vaccine—Its Impact on Prevention

An effective HIV vaccine cannot take the place of HIV-prevention efforts, any more than prevention efforts can take the place of a vaccine. The best way to address the HIV pandemic is using multiple interventions at multiple levels. The protective power of a vaccine, if one is found, will be of enormous benefit in HIV prevention. But there have been increases in sexual risk behavior in men who have sex with men (MSM) since the advent of ART. There is concern that when a vaccine becomes available there could be similar increases in risk behavior among people who receive the HIV vaccine because they feel they can't become infected with HIV.

Dispelling What Vaccine Scientists Thought They Knew about Creating Vaccines for Disease Prevention

One benefit from all of the HIV-vaccine research to date is that scientists found out that they know far less than they thought they knew about producing specific prevention vaccines. Almost all previously developed vaccines were made empirically (based on observations). From smallpox to measles, most FDA-approved vaccines have been developed through trial and error: substitute, kill, attenuate, fragment, mix, and test for the one that works. For example, scientists believed that vaccines work simply by producing antibodies, right? Well, probably not. This misconception coupled with basic ignorance of how they do work is stalling the urgent quest for an HIV/AIDS vaccine. No one yet has found out how highly successful vaccines like polio, measles, and hepatitis B actually protect people from disease. Phillippe Kourilsky, director of the Pasteur Institute, said, "We've had many successful vaccines

over the past decades but we've missed a chance to see how these vaccines work. Each time a vaccine works the scientific community wanders off and leaves it to the public health workers to use it—and fails to invest in the research to understand how and why it really works. If we had done that we would have been in a much better position to tackle the AIDS [HIV] vaccine problem." Scientists are, for the first time, learning about the mechanisms of viral-host pathologies necessary to produce preventive vaccines.

What Is a Vaccine?

It is a substance that teachers the body to recognize and defend itself against agents/organisms that cause disease. The substance is a suspension of whole microorganisms, or viruses, or a suspension of some structural component or product of them that will elicit an immune response after entering a host. In brief, vaccines mimic the organisms, virus, or other agents that cause disease, by alerting the immune system to their presence. Because of this advance warning system, when the real organism or virus invades the body, the immune system marshals a response before the disease has time to develop. That is, the immune system, by previous exposure, has learned or been trained to defend itself against a disease-causing agent.

Ideally, the body will make **neutralizing antibodies** (antibodies that prevent infection by neutralizing—cancelling out—HIV's ability to cause infection; an effective neutralizing antibody is the "Holy Grail" of preventing HIV infection) that bind to and disable the foreign invader **(humoral immunity)** and trigger white blood cells called T cells to organize **attack cells** in the body to destroy those cells that have been infected by viruses **(cellular immunity).** Once the immune system's T cells and B cells are activated, some of them turn into **memory cells.** The more memory cells the body forms, the faster its response to make antibody the next time the same agent is recognized in the body. (See Chapter 5, pages 105–132, for a discussion of the human immune system.) To date all successful vaccines prevent disease through the production of neutralizing antibodies. (See Point of Information 9.3)

THE GOAL OF DEVELOPING AN HIV VACCINE

PAST PRESIDENT CLINTON SETS A VACCINE GOAL

Speaking to the graduating class at Morgan State University on **May 18, 1997**, President Clinton invoked the legacy of John F. Kennedy's 1960s race to the moon and set a national target of developing an AIDS vaccine within the next 10 years (2007). This was **the first annual Vaccine Awareness Day in America.** The president said, "We dare not be complacent in meeting the challenge of HIV, the virus that causes AIDS." He then announced the creation of a research center at the National Institutes of Health in Bethesda, MD, to complete the task. However, Clinton's goal for a preventive HIV vaccine by year 2007 failed.

In June 2001, Health and Human Services Secretary Tommy Thompson told scientists at a Geneva gathering that an HIV vaccine would be available within three to five years. There was a collective audible groan from his audience as they must have recalled a similar comment by Margaret Heckler on April 23, 1984.

With the failure of a third human HIV vaccine, in which there was so much hope (see POV 9.3, pages 280–281), there is a real fear that there may never be an acceptable HIV vaccine! However, it must be cautioned that historically, it has taken decades and more setbacks than advances from the discovery of a virus or bacterium until an effective vaccine is licensed. Typhoid was discovered in 1884 but there was no vaccine until 1989, over 100 years later. The measles vaccine took 42 years to develop. Malaria was discovered in 1893 but still has no vaccine. In the 1930s, two experimental polio vaccines failed because they were determined to be unsafe, and polio vaccines were almost abandoned. At the time, we understood how to prevent infection by sanitation and avoiding public swimming areas, just as we know how to stop HIV infection today. We needed new tools then, and we need them now.
May 18, 2012—The Fifteenth Vaccine Awareness Day—has passed.

Predictions Continue for an HIV/AIDS Vaccine

Now the date for a vaccine has been pushed to 2020 at the earliest, some 40 years following the announcement by the CDC of a new and baffling disease affecting gay men in the United States. It is important to understand that even if an HIV/AIDS vaccine is found now, the vaccine will have no impact on the approximately 24 million new infections estimated to occur by 2020. Because there are no current prospects for a medical cure for HIV/AIDS, the only remaining strategy for slowing the next 24 million infections is through treatment prevention efforts.

JULY 2010—NIH-Led Scientists Find Antibodies that Prevent Most HIV Strains from Infecting Human CD4+ Cells

Almost everyone infected with HIV makes some neutralizing antibodies to it. But, while neutralizing antibodies have been known to occur since the earlier years of this pandemic, none of these antibodies have the properties to serve as a cornerstone around which an HIV vaccine could be made. However, two publications by Zhou et al., 2010 and Wu et al., 2010 reported in the July issue of *Science* may change the seemingly impossible task of creating an HIV vaccine into the possible. In the 1990s an antibody was found that neutralized about 40% of known HIV strains. Then in 2009 antibodies PG 6 and PG 9 were found. They neutralized 73% and 79% of known HIV strains, respectively. In 2010, lead by a team from the NIAID Vaccine Research Center (VRC), scientists found two naturally occurring antibodies called VRC01 and VRC02 in the blood of a 60-year-old black, gay male (Donor 45) who is defined as a slow progressor (for a discussion of individuals who naturally progress to AIDS at a much slower pace than others, see Box 7.2 on pages 173–174).

Antibodies VRC01 and VRC02 are produced by memory-specific B cells. B cells producing these two antibodies are extremely rare. Using flow cytometry, the team isolated just 29 of these cells from among the 25 million cells they screened.

Ironically, Donor 45's antibodies did not protect him from HIV infection, perhaps because HIV had replicated in large numbers before he could produce necessary antibodies. There is evidence that his immune system took from many months to perhaps years to produce these antibodies. He is alive and living with HIV for 21 years.

In August 2011, Xueling Wu and colleagues reported discovering antibodies similar to VRC01 in the blood of two HIV infected Africans known as donor 74 and donor 0219. The researchers further discovered that these VRC01-like antibodies all bind to the same spot on HIV in the same way. This suggests that an

HIV vaccine should contain a protein replica of this spot, known as the CD4 binding site, to elicit antibodies as powerful as VRC01. The CD4 binding site is one of the few parts of the continuously mutating virus that stays the same across HIV variants worldwide, and the virus uses this site to attach to the cells it infects. The scientists now aim to create proteins they can deliver through a vaccine to serve as signposts that direct the development of B-cell DNA to produce VRC01-like antibodies.

HOW THESE TWO NEUTRALIZING ANTIBODIES WORK

The two antibodies strongly bind to HIV's gp120 spike (see Figure 3-3 on page 53 or Figure 4-2 on page 77). HIV uses its gp120 spike to link up with the CD4 cell's receptor. The antibody and gp120 bind to each other in such a way that HIV is stopped from entering the CD4 cell. What is so significant about these two antibodies is that they bind to a virtually unchanging part of HIV. Regardless of the number of HIV mutations or the vast number of HIV strains worldwide, the gp120 site remains open to these neutralizing antibodies! This would appear to be the first real Achilles heel of HIV. And this has created a great deal of excitement among vaccinologists working on the creation of an HIV vaccine.

BREAKTHROUGH—Later in 2010, scientists at NIH successfully cloned one of the two VRC antibodies to HIV. Produced in large enough quantities, the cloned antibody can be injected. Testing is scheduled to start sometime in 2012. But, even if this approach works, injecting manufactured antibodies won't be an immediate practical solution. A gram of the antibody (necessary per injection) is estimated to cost $100. Perhaps 100 million people would need to be injected once a month! Just to inject one million people is prohibitively expensive. The greater hope is that the body, once exposed to the antibody, will take on the job of producing that antibody providing sustained protection.

The Use of Weakened or Inactivated Agents to Trigger Humoral and Cellular Immunity

Some vaccines, such as those against smallpox, polio (Sabins), measles, mumps, and tuberculosis, contain genetically altered or weakened organisms or viruses that are reproduced in the body after being administered but do not generally produce disease. Yet since the virus or bacterium is still active, there is a small risk of developing the disease.

Whooping cough, cholera, and influenza vaccines are made of inactivated whole organisms and viruses or pieces of them. Because killed organisms and inactivated virus do not replicate inside the recipient, the vaccines confer only humoral immunity (the production of antibody), which, in some cases, are short-lived, and booster vaccine shots are required.

What Then Is the Goal of an HIV Vaccine?

The goal of an HIV vaccine is to teach the immune system new and hopefully better ways to win the battle against the invading agent. Currrent HIV vaccines exploit the side of the immune system that is learned (acquired) by providing information to cells in new ways in hopes of enhancing their learning and making them more effective fighters. Why the human immune system cannot learn to make neutralizing antibodies against HIV from the current group of vaccines in clinical trials is the "billion dollar question." At the beginning of 2012 there were over 30 clinical trials ongoing, using about 40 different vaccines, in four continents involving 24 countries. The most advanced vaccine trial that got under way in 2005, the adenovirus-5 vector vaccine, failed. (See Point of View 9.3, page 280–281.)

Types of HIV Vaccines

Scientists are attempting to design three types of HIV vaccines: (1) a **preventive** or **prophylactic vaccine** to protect people from becoming HIV infected. Historically, primary vaccine prevention has most often been referred to with the term *sterilizing vaccine,* which confers 100% immunity. In reality vaccines do not achieve 100% disease prevention; (2) a **therapeutic vaccine** (this is not a true vaccination, but a postinfection therapy to stimulate the immune system. A therapeutic vaccine would drastically shorten the time one had to take antiretroviral therapy (ART). This would free up large amounts of the drugs which could be used to greatly reduce the number of people on waiting lists of AIDS drug assisted programs (ADAP) across the United States—some 90,000 entering 2013. Think what this could mean globally! The term "vaccination" is reserved for preventive strategies) for those who are already infected with HIV to prevent them from progressing to AIDS; and (3) a **perinatal vaccine** for administration to pregnant HIV-infected women to prevent transmission of the virus to the fetus.

What Is an Effective Viral Preventive Vaccine?

An effective preventive viral vaccine usually blocks viral entry into a cell, but vaccines are generally *not* 100% effective. For example, measles vaccine is 95% effective, tetanus 90%, hepatitis B 85%, and influenza 50% to 70%. Vaccine researchers attending the Seventh Conference on Retroviruses and Opportunistic Infections in February 2000 said that they may have to lower their sights regarding an HIV vaccine and settle for one that does not completely prevent HIV infection. Based on recent calculations, it has been estimated that a vaccine that is only 30% effective against HIV can begin to eradicate the virus if it is widely administered and accompanied by prevention education.

Why Is There No Preventive HIV Vaccine?

Because HIV, once inside the cell, is capable of integrating itself into the genetic material of infected cells, a vaccine would have to produce a constant state of immune protection, which not only would have to block viral entry to most cells, but also would continue to block newly produced viruses over the lifetime of the infected person. Such complete and constant protection has never before been accomplished in humans, but it has been accomplished in cats

that are vaccinated against the feline leukemia virus, also a retrovirus. Perhaps more pertinent explanations for why there is still no HIV vaccine nor is one likely to be available soon are the facts that scientists lack sufficient understanding of HIV infection and the biology of HIV disease/AIDS is very complex.

Scientists know that the body defends itself against HIV in the early years of infection. But the great mystery has always been why it cannot neutralize HIV completely. One possibility is that the body has trouble seeing all the variant viruses. Like a Stealth fighter plane, some HIV may have hidden parts that do not show up on the immune system scanner. As a result, the immune system may not produce the right kind of antibody to neutralize all the variant HIVs. (See discussion of Original Antigenic Sin, Chapter 5, page 121.)

Requirements for an HIV-Specific Vaccine

Scientists agree that blocking an infection requires the production of neutralizing antibodies. This is how standard vaccines work: They show the immune system a protein that is unique to the virus or bacterium. If they ever get into the body, the defenses will quickly make antibodies that latch onto that protein, blocking and destroying it. HIV, however, presents a changing target. It mutates so fast that it constantly changes the proteins on its surface. So a vaccine that triggers an attack against one strain of HIV may be powerless against another (recall the discussion of "Original Sin" in Chapter 5). Furthermore, the virus covers its surface with sugar (called glycosylation), forming a glycan shield which hides its proteins from antibodies. (See Point of View 9.3, pages 280–281.)

TYPES OF EXPERIMENTAL HIV VACCINES

To make vaccines, scientists use either **dead microorganisms** and **inactivated** or "killed" **viruses** (examples are influenza and rabies) or **attenuated viruses** (examples are measles,

MUCH ACCOMPLISHED, MUCH TO DO

At the 2008 annual American Association for the Advancement of Science (AAAS) meetings, AAAS President David Baltimore (Figure 7-7, page 175) said, "Scientists are no closer to developing an HIV vaccine now than they were when vaccine research began." But, he said, "I want to take an optimistic stance and say this is too important to give up on." Baltimore told his audience that the HIV-vaccine development community is depressed after recent failed attempts to develop a vaccine but said that will not halt HIV vaccine research. The HIV-vaccine community needs to begin thinking about vaccine development in a very different way, he said, adding that "scientists are beginning trendy and difficult research involving gene therapy, immunotherapy, and stem cell therapy." He also said that researchers are trying to design vectors that can carry genes that will be of therapeutic advantage.

No Way Out—Antiretroviral therapy (ART) for those infected with HIV or who have developed AIDS is critical, but no one should forget that there is no way out of the AIDS epidemic without a vaccine. There is no way to stop unprotected or unsafe sex, sharing needles by injection-drug users, or childbearing and breast-feeding by HIV-infected women.

FAILURE OF HIV VACCINES AND RESULTING IMPACT

Between 2001 and 2008, three candidate HIV vaccines failed to benefit those participating in the vaccine trials: the 2001 ALVAC canarypox vector vaccine, the 2003 VaxGen or AIDSVAX (a modified version of an earlier Genentech rgp 160 vaccine), and the 2004 Merck adenovirus-based vaccine (MRKad-5 HIV-1 gag/pol/nef trivalent vaccine). (The ad-5 trial, called the STEP trial, was stopped in September 2007 because it was not effective in preventing HIV infection or stopping viral load increase in human test subjects.) The adenovirus is a common cold virus. The shell of the adenovirus was used as a vector (means) to carry or deliver three pieces of HIV-DNA taken from HIV's Gag, Pol, and Nef genes (discussed in Chapter 3, pages 57–63). The resulting product is unable to replicate, so that while it initially infects a CD4 cell, it can't produce new HIV. However, it was hoped it would stimulate a cellular immune response that would destroy HIV after infection. This was a major setback!

Several candidate vaccines that are modeled on the ad-5 system have now been postponed or canceled. For some scientists this has been the failure of a specific product but not of the concept. For other scientists this failure spells doom for vaccine research as it is currently practiced. Currently, about $1 billion is spent each year on HIV vaccine research, but there is not likely to be a useful product any time soon. The estimated cost for the ALVAC vaccine and trials was $130 million; for the AIDVAX, it was $185 million and for the Merck ad-5, $200 million.

Is Time and Money Being Wasted on HIV Vaccine Research?

You have read what David Baltimore thinks current vaccine research has to offer—very little. "We need to go back to square one and begin thinking in a different way."

Ronald Desrosiers (2008) of the New England Primate Research Centre at Harvard University and Neal Nathanson of the University of Pennsylvania have eloquently condemned the current approach to HIV vaccine research. Both argue that researchers must return to basic science instead of generating similar pipeline products to be tested in wasteful and expensive human trials. Desrosiers said that the enormous genetic diversity of HIV, its ability to replicate unrelentingly despite everything the immune system can throw at it, the fact that the immune system cannot protect against superinfection, and the fact that we do not currently know what constitutes an immune response to HIV all persuaded him that at the current time an effective HIV vaccine "is not feasible." Agreeing with Baltimore's views, Desrosiers urged a return to basic discovery research and to work being done with artificial viral vectors that generate broadly neutralizing antibodies against HIV (beginning to be recognized as essential in a vaccine) themselves, instead of trying to stimulate the body to make them.

Neal Nathanson (2008) basically agrees. He said that he and other researchers had long ago defined HIV as a virus that defies vaccination. He, too, urged a return to basic science, such as the devising of genetic assays to search for broadly neutralizing antibodies, and said that the marginal effects seen so far in lowering HIV viral load in human volunteers did not justify further large human studies as currently proposed. For example, the $130 million PAVE (a consortium of government-funded agencies involved in HIV vaccine research) 100 trials (similar to ad-5 trials) were to begin in January 2008. They have been postponed. A smaller trial began in mid-2010.

In June 2008, the National Institute of Allergy and Infectious Diseases (NIAID) created an HIV Discovery Branch to promote synergy between basic HIV researchers and vaccine designers. This new branch will build bridges between the two groups and monitor HIV developments in multiple fields related to HIV vaccine discovery. In mid-2008, Russian and Indian scientists announced that they should have an effective HIV vaccine in the next 10 to 15 years.

mumps, and rubella) and **microorganisms.** Attenuated (at-ten-u-ate-ed) means that viruses and other microorganisms are modified; they are capable of reproducing and invoking the immune response but lack the ability to cause a disease.

Use of Attenuated HIV Vaccine—In 1997 data from several labs revealed that a vaccine made from weakened or attenuated SIV-HIV's simian analog can cause AIDS-like symptoms in adult monkeys. These findings have worried some investigators about attempting to use an attenuated HIV vaccine in humans. Robert Gallo, director of the Institute for Human Virology, believes that a live HIV vaccine is too dangerous. He said that "live, low-replicating retroviruses almost always cause disease; that's been our experience in all animal systems. If those vaccinated do not get the disease in three years, it will not tell you what will happen in 10 years or 30 years."

Use of Whole Inactivated or "Killed" Viruses

To inactivate viruses for use in vaccines, the viruses are treated with formalin (for-mah-lin, a strong disinfectant) or another chemical. There is a danger in using inactivated viruses—*they may not all be inactivated.* Inactivated virus vaccines have been made against hepatitis B, rabies, influenza, and polio (Salk vaccine). Salk's first vaccine killed a number of recipients in the late 1950s because not all the polio viruses were destroyed; that is, some could still replicate.

Subunit Vaccines

Subunit vaccines are made from antigenic fragments of an organism or virus most suitable for evoking a strong immune response. Specific subunits can be mass produced and used in pure form to make a specific vaccine. Vaccine against hepatitis B is made from a subunit of the hepatitis B virus and produced in quantity in yeast.

In the United States, researchers are currently basing their vaccine strategies on the use of subunit proteins, gag/pol and nef gene products of HIV. (See Chapter 3 for discussion of the nine genes of HIV, pages 57–59.)

DNA VACCINE

What Is a DNA Vaccine?

To make a DNA vaccine, a gene (or length of DNA) that is responsible for making a protein in the infectious virus or organism is inserted into a bacterial plasmid (a circular length of DNA that can replicate by itself inside a bacterial cell). Plasmids carrying the gene of choice are replicated in trillions of bacteria; the bacteria are then broken open and the trillions of plasmids, each carrying a copy of the gene, are purified. The purified genes/DNA are then given to a patient. Cells of the person take up the DNA and begin to make the exact protein the gene made while it was in the virus or microorganism from which it was taken. Such a protein is considered an antigen by the body, and the immune system mounts a defense against it. Entering 2013, there are at least nine DNA vaccines in human trials.

PROBLEMS IN THE SEARCH FOR HIV VACCINE

In retrospect, in the movie *Rocky,* Rocky Balboa had it easy. Downing raw eggs at 5 A.M., sprinting through the streets of Philadelphia, pummeling sides of raw beef, and pumping out one-armed pushups prepared him to go the distance against world heavyweight champion Apollo Creed. Brute force was what it took. He eventually won! With regard to developing an HIV/AIDS vaccine, brute force is just one of the ingredients essential to winning.

HIV poses some unique problems for making a human vaccine. **First** is the problem of HIV establishing latency, the ability to hide inside host cells; its capacity to adapt to host defenses via its ability to mutate or change; its ability to avoid human immune responses; and its capacity to destroy or disable critical immune system cells.

Second, scientists have not established what immune responses are crucial for protecting the body against HIV infection. Studies over the last couple of years have shown that the cell-mediated arm of the immune system may be more important than the HIV antibody response. If this turns out to be true, investigators will have to regroup with respect to producing an HIV vaccine—most vaccines in field trials now are geared toward producing sustained HIV antibody responses.

Third, predictably, money—or rather, lack of it—is an important obstacle. Even though vaccines are among the most cost-effective medical interventions ever devised, they are not big money-makers. **Drug companies are traditionally reluctant to invest in any form of vaccine development that carries high costs, low profits, and big risks of costly legal suits should accidents occur.** Their current analysis of the state of HIV/AIDS vaccine research is particularly bleak. Of the estimated **$30 billion to $40 billion spent globally each year** on HIV/AIDS research, care, and prevention, about **$1 billion** goes into vaccine research.

Fourth, the science is very tough. Animal models used to test HIV vaccines have severe limitations; no researcher has successfully demonstrated which immune responses correlate with protection from HIV.

Fifth is time. All of the preceding items require enormous amounts of time to accomplish: the process of scientific discovery, raising money, or creating an animal model. Linking together all of the people necessary to achieve success in vaccine research is much like linking together all of the people necessary to build the old cathedrals. Linking the builders of these cathedrals took generations of time. It was considered an honor to contribute one's work on that cathedral, a piece at a time, even though one knew it would not be finished in their lifetime or perhaps one's children's lifetime. The Washington Cathedral in Washington, DC was started in 1907. It was completed in 1990—83 years of progress to success. Similarly, vaccine researchers are progressing, one piece of information at a time, toward a successful vaccine.

The obstacles to a successful vaccine are scientific and political. These obstacles will be overcome.

Current Costs for Vaccine Development

In 2005 through 2012, the U.S. federal government and private corporations spent about $800 million annually. AIDS vaccine investigators estimate that this is between 1% and 10% of monies spent on all other aspects of the HIV/AIDS pandemic. The pharmaceutical sector estimates a cost of $50 million to $100 million, just to get to the point of identifying an effective vaccine. To build a production plant could cost between $100 and $200 million. How much it then costs to make the vaccine and deliver it is probably going to vary, depending on the size of the manufacturing plant and the type of vaccine that's made. Before a successful vaccine is found, produced in mass quantity, and made available to the market, the price will be several billion dollars.

The Journey Toward an HIV Preventive Vaccine

Vaccine programs in the United States and in other nations are led by some of the most talented and dedicated scientists in the world. One must admire them and the dedicated public and private teams developing each vaccine candidate. Together they recognize that a preventative vaccine is our best long-term hope to control the pandemic, although it will not be a magic bullet replacing other preventive interventions.

SEPTEMBER 2009—NEWS BROKEN THAT A PARTIALLY EFFECTIVE HIV VACCINE WAS FOUND!

After years of failure and frustration, a major breakthrough was announced in HIV/AIDS vaccine development: For the first time ever, a vaccine has been found to be safe and at least partly effective in protecting humans from HIV.

A U.S. military HIV/AIDS Research Program funded a study of 16,400 people (ages 18 to 30) in Thailand. The study showed that a two-stage "prime-boost" vaccine, also known as RV 144, a combination of two vaccines, neither of which worked when tested in humans before, appeared to reduce HIV risk by 26.4% in a relatively low-risk, primarily heterosexual population. (The intent of using two vaccines— prime-boosting—is that the combination of vaccines MAY induce different types of immune responses that will enhance the overall immune response—a response that would not occur if only one of the vaccines was used.) That is, admittedly, only a modest benefit, and it's also worth noting that the vaccine was not designed to protect against every strain of HIV. However, the news that this vaccine had any benefit at all is nonetheless extremely welcome and has powerful implications for the long journey we still need to take to discover a vaccine that will be useful. RV 144 was designed to test the vaccine strategy's ability to prevent HIV infection, as well as its ability to reduce the amount of HIV in the blood (viral load) of those who became infected after they enrolled in the study. **The vaccine failed to reduce viral load.** Nelson Michael and colleagues reported at the 2010 Conference on Retroviruses and Opportunistic Infections that the effectiveness (efficacy) of the RV144 vaccine dropped over the first year of the trials. Michael said, "It is very likely that this vaccine only worked for a short period of time." And its protection is only temporary, requiring six shots spaced months apart. But this vaccine may prove to be a landmark, a significant beginning on the way forward to finding a commercially effective vaccine. The full results of this study have been published by *The New England Journal of Medicine:* www.nejm.org (October 20, 2009).

Beginning in 2013, there are three HIV vaccines advancing in the pipeline. Scientists are very hopeful that 2013 will be an exciting year toward producing an effective HIV vaccine!

QUESTION—Should a vaccine with such modest impact (31%) be brought to market?

Disclaimer: The author of this book cannot be held responsible for any inaccuracies found in the inclusion of information by any organization, treatment, therapy, or clinical trial. The use of their information is not an endorsement of their facts or data. Any information found within this textbook should always be used in conjunction with professional medical advice.

For additional information about the search for an HIV/AIDS vaccine, the following literature is recommended.

AIDS Vaccine Research
Flossie Wong-Staal and Robert C. Gallo, Eds.
Marcel Dekker, 2002

Shots in the Dark: The Wayward Search for an AIDS Vaccine
by Jon Cohen
W.W. Norton, 2001

HIV and Molecular Immunity: Prospects for the AIDS Vaccine
by Omar Bagasra
Eaton Publishing, 1999

The Search for an AIDS Vaccine: Ethical Issues in the Development and Testing of a Preventive HIV Vaccine (Medical Ethics Series)
by Christine Grady
Indiana University Press, 1995

These addresses will list most of the important vaccine Internet addresses and serve as linkage to others.

Summary

We should be winning HIV prevention. There are effective means to prevent every mode of transmission; political commitment on HIV has never been stronger, and financing for HIV programs in low- and middle-income countries increased over eightfold between 2001 and 2011. However, while attention to the pandemic, particularly for treatment access, has increased in recent years, the effort to reduce HIV incidence is faltering. For every patient who initiated antiretroviral therapy in 2012, two or three other individuals became infected.

The numbers become so large that the individuals suffering and the personal, societal, and economic losses become impossible to measure or to even attempt to estimate. While there have been successes in slowing the epidemic in some communities and dramatic advances in survival in developed countries due to combination antiretroviral therapy, it is very important that people do not become complacent and focus on false beliefs that the pandemic is declining, that individuals are becoming less infectious, or that HIV control will be much better in the twenty-first century. If anything, the limited success in prevention should encourage a continued effort to work harder at educating more people about how best to prevent further transmission through safer sex practices, antiretroviral therapy during pregnancy, treatment of STDs, provision of condoms, screening of the blood supply, the use of sterile needles, or many of the other avenues that can help to slow the pandemic until a vaccine can be developed.

Historically, most prevention programs were designed to address the needs of persons who were at risk for contracting HIV. During the first decade of the epidemic, fewer prevention programs focused on persons living with HIV. Then in 2001, CDC introduced the Serostatus Approach to Fighting the HIV Epidemic (SAFE), which defined a framework for improving the health of persons living with HIV and preventing transmission to others. In 2003, CDC implemented the Advancing HIV Prevention (AHP) initiative, which formally adopted prevention measures for persons living with HIV as a core element of a comprehensive approach to HIV preventions. Despite considerable success, many prevention challenges remain. Racial/ethnic disparities have increased during the past 30 years, especially among black men and black women. HIV prevalence remains high among MSM overall.

The key to stopping HIV transmission lies with the behavior of the individual. That behavior, if the experience of the past 31 years can be used as an indicator, has proven to be very difficult to change. Behavioral prevention can only achieve so much. Safer behaviors are *not* sustainable 100 percent of the time.

Changing sexual behavior and using a condom is referred to as **safer sex practice.** The latex and nitrile rubber condoms are the only condoms believed to stop the passage of HIV, and a spermicide should be used with the condoms. Oil-based lubricants must not be used because they weaken the condom, allowing it to leak or break under stress. Water-based lubricants are available and should be used. There is at least one female condom, called a vaginal pouch, approved by the FDA and sold worldwide. It is inserted like a diaphragm. It offers protection to both sexual partners.

An HIV test developed in 1985 to screen all donated blood in the United States has reduced the risk of HIV transfusion infection. But blood bank screening has reduced the size of the blood donor pool. Many hospitals are encouraging people who know they might need an operation to donate their own blood for later use—autologous transfusion.

In September 2009, the results of a six-year HIV vaccine study appeared to show a weakly effective protection against HIV infection. The results of this study have created heated debate.

Entering 2013, the only FDA-approved HIV vaccine trials have failed. In late 2009 a U.S. military HIV/AIDS research program funded a vaccine RV 144 that demonstrated a short-term, low-impact efficacy, not useful for commercial purposes. In mid-2010 two highly effective neutralizing antibodies were found. They may lead the way to a successful HIV vaccine. Many top HIV/AIDS scientists have ruled out the use of an attenuated HIV vaccine. Inactivated whole virus vaccines are also being held back because there is no 100% guarantee that all HIV used in the vaccine will be inactivated.

Even if a vaccine does well in Phase III trials, will it be effective against all the HIV mutants in the HIV gene pool? Can the threat of vaccine-induced enhancement of HIV infection be overcome? How are vaccine testing agencies going to handle the ethical question of vaccine seroconverting normal subjects to positive antibody status? The social repercussions may be devastating for those who, when tested, test HIV positive even though they are HIV-free.

There are some 5.3 million healthcare workers in the United States. It is crucial that they adhere to the Universal Protection Guidelines set down by the CDC, as a significant number of them are exposed to HIV annually. The risk of HIV infection after exposure to HIV-contaminated blood is about 1 in 200.

Some states have implemented HIV partner notification; other states are beginning to experiment with HIV partner notification or contact tracing programs. It is too early to tell how successful locating and testing high behavioral risk partners will be, or the cost-to-benefit ratio. If these programs are to be successful, they will have to ensure confidentiality to those who are traced. Partner notification or contact tracing continues to work well for other sexually transmitted diseases.

In short, considerable success in the prevention of HIV infection in the United States has been achieved. HIV testing and donor deferral have markedly increased the safety of the nation's blood supply. Perinatal transmission of HIV has been greatly reduced. Reductions in needle sharing have resulted in a substantial decrease in HIV transmissions associated with injection-drug use. These and other prevention successes have reduced the incidence of HIV infection from more than 150,000 cases per year in the mid-1980s to about 56,000 cases per year in 2010.

FIVE WAYS YOU CAN HELP PREVENT HIV/AIDS

1. Become informed.
2. Share your information.
3. Have an HIV test and get treatment if called for.
4. Encourage others to take the HIV test/treatment.
5. Become socially and politically active in the fight against HIV/AIDS.

Review Questions

(Answers to the Review Questions are on page 463.)

1. Which is the better condom for protection from STDs, one made from lamb intestine or one made from latex rubber? Explain.

2. Which lubricant is best suited for condom use? Explain.

3. Briefly explain safer sex.

4. True or False: If a person has unprotected intercourse with an HIV-infected partner, he or she will become HIV infected. Explain.

5. True or False: If injection-drug users (IDUs) were given free equipment—no questions asked—this would stop the transmission of HIV among them. Explain.

6. What is the current risk of being transfused with HIV-contaminated blood in the United States?

7. What do you think should happen in cases where a person who knows he or she is HIV positive lies at a donor interview, and donates blood?

8. Why do most scientists wish to avoid using an attenuated HIV vaccine or an inactivated HIV vaccine?

9. What is the advantage of using recombinant HIV subunits in making a vaccine?

10. What are universal precautions? Who formulated them?

11. True or False: Latex condoms eliminate the risk of HIV transmission.

12. True or False: Partner notification is usually performed by the infected individual or a trained and authorized health department official.

13. True or False: The Centers for Disease Control and Prevention estimates that as many as 1 in 100,000 units of blood in the blood supply may be contaminated with HIV.

14. True or False: The three types of vaccines that scientists are interested in developing are preventive, therapeutic, and perinatal vaccines.

15. True or False: Used disposable needles should be recapped by hand before disposal.

16. True or False: Prompt washing of a needle stick injury with soap and water is sufficient to prevent HIV infection.

17. True or False: The FDA approved the first vaccine for broad-scale testing in the United States in 1997.

18. HIV/AIDS is not curable, but it is preventable. Write a short essay on the best methods of prevention.

19. True or False: Using latex barriers when performing vaginal, oral, or anal sex lowers the risk of HIV transmission.

20. True or False: In September 2009, a somewhat successful vaccine against HIV was created.

21. True or False: MSM receive a 180-day supply of Truvada.

22. True or False: The iPrEX study involved only HIV-negative gay males.

Prevalence of HIV Infections, AIDS Cases, and Deaths among Select Groups in the United States and in Other Countries

---

CHAPTER HIGHLIGHTS

- XIX International AIDS Conference, Washington, DC, July 2012: "An AIDS Free Generation"
- HIV/AIDS is a new plague.
- UNAIDS defines a generalized epidemic.
- The meaning of prevalence, incidence, and rates for HIV/AIDS are presented.
- Worldwide, ending 2013, heterosexuals will continue to make up about 95% of people living with HIV/AIDS.
- Worldwide, 50% of new HIV infections are in people under age 25.
- Worldwide, about 7000 new HIV infections occur daily.
- Worldwide, women represent about 55% of all HIV-infected adults and about 50% of AIDS deaths.
- In sub-Saharan Africa, 59% of the HIV infected are women.
- AIDS is the world's leading cause of death by an infectious disease.
- AIDS is ranked sixth in causes of death worldwide.
- Prevalence of HIV/AIDS by global region is presented.
- In the United States, men make up an estimated 74% of all AIDS cases; 26% are women.
- The majority of people with HIV/AIDS can be associated with certain lifestyle behaviors.
- HIV/AIDS can be associated with single or multiple exposure behaviors.
- HIV/AIDS cases can be separated by sex, age group, race, ethnicity, and sexual preference.
- Risk is strongly tied to social behavior.
- At-risk groups include homosexual and bisexual men, transgender women, injection-drug users (IDUs), hemophiliacs, transfusion patients, and the sex partners of these people.
- HIV infection is strongly associated with injection-drug use and men having sex with men.
- Men having sex with men (MSM) make up the invisible world of HIV/AIDS cases in this pandemic.
- The CDC recommends testing of men having sex with men (MSM) every three to six months.
- At least 85 countries have laws prohibiting men having sex with men.
- About 54% of new HIV infections occurred in the black population.
- About 17% of new HIV infections occurred in the Latino population.

- All military personnel are tested for HIV.
- Two per 1000 college students are HIV infected.
- Ending 2008, all states reported the HIV infected by name.
- High rates of HIV infection have been found among prisoners.
- The greatest HIV threat to healthcare workers is syringe-needle stick injuries.
- All 50 states and U.S. territories must report all HIV and AIDS cases.
- The CDC continues to update U.S. HIV surveillance estimates in 2012.
- Ending 2013: **Reported** AIDS cases in the United States will reach 1.41 million, of which about 665,000 will have died.
- Ending 2013, there will be an estimated total of 2.36 million HIV infections in the United States.
- People do not always tell the truth when completing questionnaires, especially with regard to sexual behavior.
- By the end of 2013, an estimated 68 million people worldwide will have been HIV infected and about 30 million of them will have died of AIDS.
- Some HIV/AIDS statistics on Canada, Mexico, and the United Kingdom are provided.
- HIV/AIDS information for India, China, and Russia is presented.
- A global distribution of AIDS cases is presented.
- See the Interactive HIV/AIDS map by Emory University Rollins School of Public Health (AIDSVu.org).

The World Trade Center (WTC) and the Pentagon were attacked on September 11, 2001. No one expected to see commercial airliners hijacked and flown into crowded skyscrapers and government buildings. Likewise, in the early 1980s, no one expected the sudden appearance of a deadly new disease spreading across the cities of America. Only a few years earlier some prominent scientists had declared that the fight against infectious disease was over. The horrible damage caused by fuel-laden airliners crashing into buildings and exploding into a fiery inferno was all but beyond our imagination. Equally beyond our imagination was this new disease that appeared 31 years ago. It was a disease that appeared without warning and seemed to lead to a painful, agonizing death in just a few weeks for some, a few months for others. The depth and scope of human destruction was so unprecedented that only a few people were quick to recognize the horror that was to come. On September 11, while the image of the jetliners with their passengers exploding into the World Trade Center was still painfully fresh, we were further stunned to see these seemingly invincible structures collapse, crushing almost 3000 men, women, and children in a vast cloud of toxic dust, rubble, and fire. A week earlier, no one would have believed that such pillars of concrete and steel could possibly collapse, let alone from the top down. In the tragedy that began to unfold in the beginning of the 1980s, scientists were puzzled and bewildered as they watched a disease that led to the collapse of the human immune system, so to speak, also from the top down. Working from the inside out, here was a diabolically clever virus that destroyed the very system that was otherwise designed to defeat it. The beginning of AIDS in America in 1981 is the greatest plague in history to cross the globe, and the 2001 attack on the WTC and the Pentagon, the largest attack on the United States, caused the greatest loss of life on U.S. shores since the Japanese attack on Pearl Harbor. The two have much in common. Both tragedies have appeared over and over again on television. Both require the best in people to set them right—to save lives. The United States and the world must not let terrorists or HIV determine our way of life. Both require acts of heroism and research. Both require sacrifice, resolve, and the determination to overcome. Both have placed America and the world in a race against time.

The News Media: The Result of Omission

When AIDS isn't visible in the media, it doesn't exist for many communities that rely on media to tell them what matters most. This is true not only in the West, but in Africa and in other developing nations, where stigma and discrimination against HIV/AIDS sufferers is deeply entrenched, and where silence and denial still drive many governments to cover up their frightening levels of HIV infection. Often the young people who most need to know how to protect themselves have few programs directed their way. At the same time, there are many stirring and effective responses led by unsung young heroes whose stories could inspire a greater mobilization. But who is going to tell these stories if the media doesn't? HIV/AIDS will surpass the bubonic plague or "Black Death" of Asia and Europe in the fourteenth century unless a vaccine is found. That plague killed about 40 million people. By the end of 2013, about 30 million will have died from AIDS. Each day HIV/AIDS kills over twice the number of people who died September 11, 2001, in New York City and at the Pentagon. No terrorist attack, no war or force of nature in our lifetime has ever killed 30 million people and threatened 38 million more with premature deaths in just over a quarter of a century! HIV is a virus of mass destruction. (See Box 10.1, page 290.)

A WORD ABOUT HIV/AIDS DATA

As most college students might say, nothing could be more boring than statistics and numbers. Regardless, if you're reading or hearing them with regard to the HIV/AIDS pandemic, the use of statistics is one of the better ways to understand the dimensions of this pandemic. It's important to get a grasp of the numbers of

people with HIV and AIDS so that an informed policy on economic, social, and political issues can be made that will eventually change the scope of this pandemic.

The term *HIV/AIDS* refers to three categories of diagnoses collectively: (1) a diagnosis of AIDS (new infections); (2) a diagnosis of HIV; and (3) a concurrent diagnosis of HIV infection and AIDS.

The UNAIDS defines a generalized epidemic as "high-level—where adult HIV prevalence (the number of people living with HIV at some point in time) among the general adult population is at least 1% and transmission is mostly heterosexual." A concentrated epidemic is defined as "low-level—where HIV is concentrated in groups with behaviors that expose them to a high risk of HIV infection."

All HIV/AIDS data, including data from the Centers for Disease Control and Prevention (CDC), Joint United Nations Program on HIV/AIDS (UNAIDS), World Health Organization (WHO), and other organizations should be treated as broadly indicative of trends rather than accurate measures of HIV/AIDS incidence or prevalence. A large number of HIV/AIDS cases in developing countries, in particular, are underreported due to a lack of adequate medical and administrative personnel, the stigma associated with the disease, or the reluctance of countries to incur the loss of trade, tourism, and other losses that such revelations might produce.

Morbidity (Disease) and Mortality (Death)

Because morbidity and mortality of HIV/AIDS cases are multicausal, diagnosis and reporting can vary significantly, thereby distorting comparisons. The WHO and other international entities are dependent on such data despite its inaccuracy and are often forced to extrapolate or build models based on relatively small samples, as in the case of HIV/AIDS. Changes in methodologies, moreover, can produce differing results; for example, the ranking of AIDS mortality ahead of TB mortality. This is partly due to the fact that HIV-positive individuals dying of TB

BOX 10.1

XIX INTERNATIONAL AIDS CONFERENCE, WASHINGTON, DC. JULY 22–27, 2012
TURNING THE TIDE TOGETHER (AIDS 2012)

BRIEF HISTORY OF THE INTERNATIONAL AIDS CONFERENCE

The International AIDS Conferences began in 1985 and were held yearly through 1994. Because the conferences became so large in attendance, it was decided to hold them every other year beginning in 1996 (See Table I-2, page 9, for a list of conferences). The conferences have provided a unique global venue for the struggle against HIV/AIDS. The latest meeting took place in Washington, DC, in July 2012 **(AIDS 2012).** It has been 22 years since the United States hosted the International AIDS Conference, which is convening in the United States for the first time since 1990, after a travel ban on HIV positive individuals was overturned by U.S. lawmakers in 2008 and signed into law in 2009. However, over 25,000 people living with HIV/AIDS advocates, policy makers, activists, researchers, and media representatives from nearly 200 countries attended the conference that highlighted the latest scientific advances and strategies for treating and preventing HIV. There are four main goals to any AIDS conference. **First** is to call the world's attention to truly focus in on this pandemic and appreciate the many challenges this disease presents. **Second** is to share essential information globally and to learn from each other. **Third** is to inspire and to invigorate each other, to renew a global commitment to defeating this disease. And **fourth** is to raise money, lots of money!

ATTENDANCE AND PRESENTATIONS

There were about 194 sessions involving scientific reports, oral presentations, and poster exhibitions. And yes, there were AIDS activist demonstrations. This time was like the last time because the United States was not giving enough money for global HIV/AIDS. This was the largest of the International AIDS meetings in its 22-year history.

HIGHLIGHTS FROM THE 2012 INTERNATIONAL AIDS CONFERENCE, WASHINGTON, DC

The theme of the conference was "Turning the Tide Together." The meeting's theme was intended to emphasize the need for a global commitment to end the HIV/AIDS pandemic. Together, presenters, from senior government officials and heads of international organizations to civil society leaders and scientists, all echoed that for the first time in the history of AIDS

that an end to the pandemic is on the horizon. However, speakers cautioned that there are still numerous challenges that must be addressed before the international community reaches zero new HIV infections and zero AIDS-related deaths.

Throughout the conference, much attention focused on global HIV/AIDS targets agreed upon in June 2011—in particular, the goal of eliminating new HIV infections among children, reducing all sexual transmission of HIV by 50%, and getting 15 million people on HIV treatment by 2015. Representatives of both international organizations and civil society stressed that unless investments in the HIV response are increased, the goals will not be realized.

Follow the Money

All AIDS conferences are about the money. This one, more than most, was also about questions. There are now far more ways to profitably spend money on HIV/AIDS prevention and treatment than in the past. And the benefits of spending more—which most countries are not eager to do—are bigger than ever. Questions: Is it worth spending $7 billion more per year to speed the decline of new infections? Is there justification for providing HIV prevention drugs to uninfected Americans when those infected in other countries are going without? Should pregnant women be put on treatment before men in order to prevent the heartbreak and expense of orphan children? Is being able to get a viral load test in an unelectrified village worth the cost of the hand-held device that makes it possible, and can the world come up with enough money to provide the essential drugs to all who need them, for life? Those are just a few of the questions emerging from five days of conversations at the 19th International AIDS Conference. Also emerging from the AIDS 2012 meetings was questions about where all the money is going and how wisely it is being spent at home (United States) or in other countries. The answer, not wisely at all, not in the United States or in foreign countries. Critics argue that progress shown in the United States should not have cost over a half trillion dollars and rising rapidly, nor is there true accountability for the $50 to $60 million the United States has spent on the President's Emergency Plan for AIDS Relief (PEPFAR) to just 15 countries. And why does the United States continue to give millions of dollars to countries like China and Russia to help with their HIV/AIDS problems? The broader feelings expressed

BOX 10.1 *(continued)*

about so much money being spent on this one disease were that it is better to pay now and not forever! Right now, over eight million people are on anti-HIV drugs at a cost of about $18 billion per year. If all HIV-infected were on treatment, the cost is estimated at $86 billion per year! Where will the money come from? Who can clearly afford their own HIV/AIDS programs? But, the presentations that drew the largest audiences were those that stressed the OPINION offered by Secretary of State Hillary Rodham Clinton some five months prior to the AIDS 2012. Her opinion became the single message that pervaded the meetings, the message being **that we can have an "AIDS-free generation."** Her statement then, and followed up on by some scientists prior to AIDS 2012, set the stage for an unprecedented optimism at AIDS 2012 toward learning how science and society would bring about the **"End of AIDS."** This movement began in part following three years of prevention break-throughs. Collectively, these prevention studies gave rise to talks about but not promises (by recognized HIV/AIDS scientists) that there would be a **CURE** for HIV/AIDS. The studies showed that optimally treated patients are un-likely to transmit HIV.

Other studies showed that those who are HIV-negative (uninfected) could take antiretroviral drugs like Truvada to prevent their becoming HIV infected. Thus emerged the belief in the ability of scientists to procure an AIDS-free generation. The problem is, to different people, the term "AIDS-free generation" has different meanings. Does it mean no child will be born with HIV infection? The adults living with HIV will not progress to AIDS? That the incidence of HIV infection will drop to near zero? That combination prevention will stop HIV transmission? That the HIV infected will not transmit or become ill and lead happy AIDS-free lives? A consensus on just what the term means is not yet available. For some, if not many or most, it means there will be a **CURE** and soon! But cure is a slippery term, for just as AIDS does not necessarily mean illness (just a low T4 or CD4 cell count), cure does mean health. Timothy Brown (Figure 4.1, page 72) has been declared cured, but he is by no means healthy. He has sustained significant neurological damage from the treatment that cured him of HIV and has other disabilities. Further, if this "cure" is to come from treatment, the drug treatments themselves are harmful to patients. Research has provided some of the tools necessary and a window into finding a cure. However, according to the best HIV/AIDS scientists, a cure is at least 10 years away. Steven Deeks, University of California, San Francisco, said, "The enthusiasm is not that we are going to have a cure any time soon. The enthusiasm is that it is now possible and there is a

group effort aimed in this direction. No one thinks that this is going to be easy, but that it is possible, and now there is global buy-in. It could take decades unless we get really lucky. This is going to be a trial of errors and is probably going to require combination therapy—but we have gotten lucky before."

The AIDS 2012 meetings at best suggest that science may have brought this disease to a tipping point wherein one can see a light at the end of a tunnel that has been very dark until now. Still, there is a very wide gap that separates where we are in ending AIDS from where we want to be in ending AIDS.

SOCIAL MEDIA NETWORKS DURING AIDS 2012

One of the great ironies of the International AIDS Conference is that people affected by HIV are those most unlikely to attend. For citizen journalists at the conference, being able to send emails and use Twitter bypassing mainstream media offers a great opportunity to have a real influence on the reporting and dissemination of HIV-related issues. From July 21st through the 27th about 100,000 tweets went out tagged #AIDS 2012. In addition, the Kaiser Family Foundation, the official Webcaster for AIDS 2012, sent out over 60 webcasts about conference events. It has been suggested that the power of social networks can drive necessary changes in moving toward that "AIDS-Free Generation." Currently, there are about 175 million Facebook users and 125 million Twitter users in the United States. Women make up about 70% of social network users.

SUMMARY

The XIX International AIDS Conference (AIDS 2012) closed without the physical presence of President Obama but with a full cast of other high-profile U.S. politicians who expressed their commitment to ending the disease.

Call it a triple win for fighting the AIDS pandemic: treating people with HIV early keeps them healthy, treatments cut their chances of infecting others, and now research shows it's also a good financial investment. Getting treatment to the world's 38 million people with HIV is key to curbing this pandemic, but it's not going to cure or bring about an AIDS-free generation in the next ten years.

THE END OF AIDS: This phrase was heard many times for the five days of the meetings. There were hundreds of sessions on the latest scientific HIV research, thousands of posters pointing to new tools to use against HIV, and inspiration came from numerous plenary speakers, leaders in their fields of research,

—————— BOX 10.1 *(continued)* ——————

science, advocacy, and policy, who told everyone the tide is turning on HIV/AIDS. But is it? Despite the developments of recent years, serious problems remain. There are approximately 56,000 people who become infected with HIV each year in the United States. This number has remained unchanged for nearly the past ten years. Serious adjustments need to be made in our prevention methodologies. Phil Wilson, President and CEO of the Black AIDS Institute, said, "I charge everyone who attended this Conference to ask this one important question, was it all worth it? Was it worth your time, energy, and expense to come to Washington for a week or more? When we leave DC, where do we go from here?" He said, "We are done with the sessions and the lessons. Now we must move on and out beyond DC and back to our families and our communities, where we must spread the news from AIDS 2012. It's now up to us—each and every one of us has an obligation to take what we have learned back into our communities, to our local leaders, our nontraditional partners, to our policy makers at every level." However, according to the observations of some conference delegates, the session presenters mostly assumed their audiences were experts in the areas of academia, research, and politics, and were clearly not presenting to an audience of actual HIV-affected or infected people. There were but a few sessions that offered innovative community based models of care or strategies to overcome barriers. The exclusion was felt by many of delegates and members of the HIV community, who were led by Housing Works activists in a series of actions under the slogan of "Nothing about us, without us," a demand for the science field and policy makers to not only include people living with the virus in the discussions, but to position them at the core of all decision making processes. Protesters brought light to the fact that the only inclusive space for the (non badge holding) community at large was down in the basement, contrasted with the pharmaceutical brands, which were hosted in a super security-lined exhibition space on the top level. Protesters later changed their slogan to "Nothing about us, without us. We are coming out of the basement!" At the end of AIDS 2012, the conference was handed over to officials representing the organizing committee of the XX International AIDS Conference, which will be held in Melbourne, Australia, in 2014.

CLASS QUESTION: Is the end of the AIDS pandemic truly in sight? Yes or no? Support your answer with factual statements supported by research published information.

were included in the AIDS mortality category in the most recent WHO survey. Another example is the global data on those living with HIV/AIDS. The WHO/UNAIDS global data said there were about 33.2 million such people at the end of 2007, but this estimate results from a low estimate of 30.6 million and a high estimate of 36.1 million—recognizably a large margin for error. Such data come from using a relatively simple equation that calculated low- and high-risk populations with the crude adult death rate and the HIV-infected survival rate, along with variables including the start date of HIV for that country and the demand for risky sex. The bottom line is that estimates are just that—estimates. However, estimates can prove to be very useful in predicting what is occurring now and what lies ahead.

In early 2007, epidemiologists (those who study the spread of disease in a population), analysts, and heads of AIDS programs from 124 countries began to refine and improve country HIV/AIDS estimates. These data for 2007 became available in early 2008, and have been updated through 2012.

YEAR 2013

As we begin this thirteenth year of the new millennium and enter into the early years of the fourth decade of AIDS, it is evident that the small epidemic recognized among a handful of homosexual men in 1981 is quite different from the global pandemic of today. For developed countries, current antiretroviral regimens are allowing HIV-infected individuals to live longer, healthier lives. However, the use of these regimens may be associated with complacency and a relapse to unsafe sexual practices resulting in sustaining the HIV epidemic, as will be discussed. For developing countries the problem is far more complex. The infrastructure to support the use of antiretroviral drugs is not in place, the cost of the drugs is too high, and the vast majority of HIV-infected people do not even know they are infected. Education and condom distribution campaigns have had

limited success, but they remain the primary avenues of prevention.

Developed Countries: Is the HIV/AIDS Crisis Over?

In the developed nations, too many people think the HIV/AIDS crisis is over. Think again. It is estimated that by the end of 2013, about 68 million people will have been HIV infected, with about 38 million of them alive. About 90% of infections are in developing nations that hold about 10% of the world's wealth. There is still neither a cure nor an effective vaccine.

Entering year 2013 there does not appear to be an immediate end to either the spread of HIV infection or the devastation caused by HIV/AIDS. Who would have imagined in the mid-1980s that HIV would eventually spread to every country of the world? And the global HIV/AIDS pandemic is not expected to peak for another 10 to 15 years (2014 to 2023).

Reporting and Underreporting AIDS Diagnosis and AIDS Deaths

Many countries have a long history of reporting AIDS cases and in some—including the United States, Canada, and much of Africa—reporting of all AIDS cases is compulsory. A problem with AIDS case reporting is that different countries have different definitions of what actually constitutes AIDS. While a definition of AIDS is becoming standardized, there is still the problem that some resource-poor areas lack HIV testing facilities, and therefore they have to diagnose AIDS (and thus HIV) on the presence of several marker conditions such as the presence of tuberculosis (TB). Another problem is that people in many countries without the proper AIDS diagnosis resources die of AIDS, but are not counted as an HIV infection or an AIDS death.

Antiretroviral treatment has made it difficult to interpret trends in AIDS diagnoses and AIDS deaths in countries where most people have access to the drugs. Also, in countries where AIDS is highly stigmatized, government policy is not to record AIDS as a cause of death. Also, doctors may be inclined to spare shame to a family by misrecording the cause of an AIDS death. Such underreporting occurs worldwide!

The Statistical Politics of This Pandemic

For over a decade the former director of UNAIDS, Peter Piot, sounded the alarm of the quickly moving and horribly devastating modern-day plague, the HIV/AIDS pandemic. In 2007 he said, "the pandemic and its toll are outstripping the worst predictions. It is now one of the make or break forces of this century." The developed nations responded with AIDS funding at $10 billion a year. Regardless, this was considered insufficient funding. Organizers at the WHO, UNAIDS, and other HIV/AIDS organizations insisted that many billions of dollars more will be required each year just to catch up to the growing need of funding. And then, something happened on the way to securing greater amounts of money.

What Happened?

In November 2007, the WHO along with UNAIDS published its "AIDS Epidemic Update '07." Indeed this report presented some surprising information about this global pandemic. At first glance it appeared that the pandemic was fast fading with the devastating number of estimated HIV/AIDS cases of 2006 in free-fall. In 2006, it was reported that 39.5 million people were living with HIV/AIDS. The number dropped to 33.2 million in 2007. And new HIV infections fell from 4.3 million in 2006 to 2.5 million in 2007—a drop of 42% in one year! What happened? Were the new prevention methods, new drugs preventing infections, abstention, and education finally showing huge results?

Not Exactly

What happened is that WHO and UNAIDS admitted that their numbers had been greatly overstated initially. Stephen Lewis, former special UN envoy for HIV/AIDS in Africa, stated that these organizations "had clearly been using inflated numbers for years." He accused the WHO and UNAIDS of irresponsibility.

Much more on this subject can be found at the beginning of this book. Because of the 2007 AIDS Epidemic Update Report, all global HIV/AIDS numbers have been reduced accordingly.

Estimates by UNAIDS

Currently, UNAIDS reports that each day about 7000 people become newly infected with HIV, or 5 men, women, and children per minute. Eleven percent of the newly infected people are under age 15. Over 50% of new infections are now occurring in people between ages 15 and 24, primarily due to sexual transmission. Worldwide, women now represent 50% of all people over age 15 living with HIV infection. At the end of 1998, UNAIDS reported that AIDS had become the world's most deadly infectious disease. It reached this level of human devastation in just 18 years. Of all causes of death worldwide, AIDS has moved up to sixth place. These data are a bit ironic because as Peter Piot, former executive director of UNAIDS, said, "The pandemic is out of control at the very time when we know what to do to prevent its spread."

As shocking as these numbers are, they do not begin to adequately reflect the physical and emotional devastation to individuals, families, and communities coping with HIV/AIDS, nor do they capture the huge deleterious impact of HIV/AIDS on the economies, on the security of nations, and on entire regions.

What About Reported HIV Infections?

Each positive HIV test means one person is infected. This method of looking at an epidemic can give a very clear picture in terms of people who have been infected. But most countries only report their AIDS cases. They do not have the means to test for HIV. As a result, most countries grossly underestimate the number of HIV-infected people. However, even in developed countries, one in every three or four people living with HIV has never been tested. And for those tested, not all test results are reported.

Another point to remember is that looking at the years in which people tested HIV positive does not say when they were infected—the HIV test itself may come many years after infection occurred. When looking at HIV statistics, it's important to keep in mind that there might be more than one reason for trends in the data. An increase in diagnoses might not mean that more people are becoming HIV infected than in previous years. It might mean that HIV testing has become more easily available than in recent years, or that stigmatization of people with HIV has declined, so more people are willing to be tested.

Overwhelming Numbers of HIV/AIDS Cases in the United States

It is easy to be overwhelmed by statistics in reporting on HIV infections and AIDS cases and to lose track of the human faces of the pandemic. But certain numbers, like the first half-million documented AIDS cases reported in October 1995 and 665,000 dead ending 2013, take on a compelling quality of their own. Therefore, within this chapter there are many statistics presented on all facets of the HIV/AIDS pandemic. **After reading this chapter one will have gained a deeper insight into the spread of HIV and those who are affected by HIV: those who have it, and those who don't—those who will suffer and those who won't. In reality we are all impacted by this disease in one way or another.**

Prevalence/Incidence/Rate
How Many People Are HIV Positive?

The **prevalence** of a disease refers to the percentage of a population that is living with that disease at a given point or date in time. **HIV or AIDS prevalence = the number of people living with HIV or AIDS in a population at some point in time.** For example, if 200 specific high-risk males are tested for HIV and 20 of them are found to be HIV positive, the results mean that within this population the HIV prevalence is 10% ($20 \div 200$ ($20/200$) $\times 100 = 10\%$).

The **incidence** means the number of times an **event occurs** in a given time frame or

period in a specific population, for example, the number of new AIDS cases or new HIV infections that occur each month or each year (events that occur within a specified period of time), expressed as a percentage of the total population being studied. The two terms are similar. However, changes in HIV incidence statistics can give a better idea of whether prevention strategies are succeeding in reducing the number of new infections. A society that shows regularly declining incidence figures is one that is experiencing fewer new HIV infections.

The **rate** is the number of HIV or AIDS cases divided by the population in each group, multiplied by 100. The rate of HIV transmission represents the annual number of new HIV infections per 100 persons living with HIV. It is calculated by dividing HIV incidence for a given year by HIV prevalence for the same year and multiplying this number by 100. Put simply, the transmission rate compares the annual number of new infections to the number of persons living with HIV, and indicates the likelihood that an HIV-infected individual will transmit HIV to others. In this way, it provides a better means to assess the effects of public health efforts to promote changes in risk behavior, as well as the preventive effects of HIV diagnosis and treatment. Researchers found that the HIV transmission rate has declined dramatically since the early days of the epidemic. In the early 1980s, for example, the transmission rate was 92%, meaning there were 92 transmissions per 100 persons living with HIV at the time. With the implementation of HIV testing and other prevention efforts, transmission rates declined to about 5% (Hall et al., 2008).

NOTE: The incidence of HIV infection in the United States has never been directly measured. In the early 1990s, back-calculation models using AIDS incidence data and the probability distribution of the incubation period from HIV infection to AIDS diagnosis provided historical trends of HIV incidence, but these models could not provide timely data on current transmission patterns. The development of laboratory assays that differentiate recent versus long-standing HIV infections now makes it possible to directly measure HIV incidence. (See Point of Information 10.1, page 316 and Chapter 13 for additional information on the use of this laboratory technique, called STARHS pages 383–385.)

The higher the transmission rate, the greater the burden or impact of HIV/AIDS on each community. This burden can be directly compared across countries and racial/ethnic groups of different population sizes, because the rate assumes that each group has exactly the same population. The current transmission rate in the United States is between 4% and 5%. (Four to five in every 100 HIV-infected people will transmit HIV to someone else.)

FORMULA FOR ESTIMATING HIV INFECTIONS

A formula proposed by the CDC for use in determining the number of HIV-infected persons in a given city is as follows:

National Number of Persons Living with HIV/AIDS (2012)   Number of PLW HIV/AIDS in Your City (2012)

$$\frac{258,000}{900,000} \times \frac{(e.g.,)\ 1000}{x} = 258,000$$

(Estimated national number of HIV-infected persons)

$$x = 900,000,000$$

$$x = \frac{900,000,000}{258,000}$$

$$x = 3488$$

(About 3488 persons in this sample city are estimated to be HIV infected.)

Single or Multiple Exposure Categories

In Table 10-1, page 296, the number of AIDS cases estimated ending 2013 is presented with respect to adult/adolescent single or multiple exposure categories. For example, under *Single Mode of Exposure,* heterosexual contact accounts for 10% of all AIDS cases. Under *Multiple Modes*

Table 10-1 Total Adult/Adolescent AIDS Cases by Single and Multiple Exposure Categories, Estimated Ending 2013, United States

	AIDS Cases	
Exposure Category	No.	(%)
Single Mode of Exposure		
1. Men who have sex with men	613,404	(44)
2. Injection-drug use	320,643	(23)
3. Hemophilia/coagulation disorder	13,941	(1)
4. Heterosexual contact	153,351	(11)
5. Receipt of blood transfusion	13,941	(1)
6. Receipt of transplant of tissues/organs	45	(0)
7. Other/undetermined	200	(0)
Single Mode of Exposure Subtotal	**1,115,820**	**(80)**
Multiple Modes of Exposure		
1. Men who have sex with men; injection-drug use	92,480	(6.8)
2. Men who have sex with men; hemophilia	180	(0)
3. Men who have sex with men; heterosexual contact	27,200	(2)
4. Men who have sex with men; receipt of transfusion/transplant	3,715	(0)
5. Injection-drug use; hemophilia	185	(0)
6. Injection-drug use; heterosexual contact	59,850	(4.4)
7. Injection-drug use; receipt of transfusion	1,610	(0)
8. Hemophilia; heterosexual contact	110	(0)
9. Hemophilia; receipt of transfusion/transplant	820	(0)
10. Heterosexual contact; receipt of transfusion/transplant	1,610	(0)
11. Men who have sex with men; injection-drug use; hemophilia	60	(0)
12. Men who have sex with men; injection-drug use; heterosexual contact	13,600	(1)
13. Men who have sex with men; injection-drug use; receipt of transfusion/transplant	610	(0)
14. Men who have sex with men; hemophilia; heterosexual contact	26	(0)
15. Men who have sex with men; hemophilia; receipt of transfusion/transplant	43	(0)
16. Men who have sex with men; heterosexual contact; receipt of transfusion/transplant	261	(0)
17. Injection-drug use; hemophilia; heterosexual contact	90	(0)
18. Injection-drug use; hemophilia; receipt of transfusion/transplant	45	(0)
19. Injection-drug use; heterosexual contact; receipt of transfusion/transplant	1,120	(0)
20. Hemophilia; heterosexual contact; receipt of transfusion/transplant	45	(0)
21. Men who have sex with men; injection-drug use; hemophilia; heterosexual contact	15	(0)
22. Men who have sex with men; injection-drug use; hemophilia; receipt of transfusion/transplant	16	(0)
23. Men who have sex with men; injection-drug use; heterosexual contact; receipt of transfusion/transplant	170	(0)
24. Men who have sex with men; hemophilia; heterosexual contact; receipt of transfusion/transplant	10	(0)
25. Injection-drug use; hemophilia; heterosexual contact; receipt of transfusion/transfusion	28	(0)
26. Men who have sex with men; injection-drug use; hemophilia; heterosexual contact; receipt of transfusion/transplant	9	(0)
Multiple Modes of Exposure Subtotal	**209,115**	**(15)**
Risk Not Reported or Identified	**69,705**	**(5)**
Total AIDS Cases	**1,394,100**	**(100)**

(*Source: For exposure categories.* CDC HIV/AIDS Surveillance Report *(updated estimate through 2013)*)
Pediatric AIDS cases = 10,900 (Total adult AIDS cases about 1,405,000−10,900 (pediatric) = 1,394,100)

of Exposure, 5% of AIDS cases occurred among injection-drug users who also had heterosexual contact. Table 10-1 lists the numbers and percentages of all reported AIDS cases broken down into seven categories of people who contracted HIV/AIDS from a single risk mode of exposure and 26 categories of people who contracted HIV/AIDS from multiple risk modes of exposure. Note that of the total number of adult/adolescent AIDS cases, 80% occurred from single risk modes of exposure. Of these, 44% occurred among men who had sex with men and about 23% among injection-drug users.

A composite representation of all AIDS cases by exposure category estimated beginning 2013 is shown in Chapter 8, Figure 8-1, page 183.

2009 U.S. HIV/AIDS Atlas Shows Graphic Representation of HIV Rates by County

If one thinks of the AIDS pandemic as a global wildfire, the way that you fight wildfires is to identify the hot spots. The United States now has an exciting way to identify those hot spots: a brand-new online "HIV/AIDS Atlas" created by the National Minority Quality Forum. (www .nmqf.org). The atlas shows a graphic representation of HIV rates by county in all 50 states, Washington, DC, Puerto Rico, and the U.S. Virgin Islands. It promises to provide HIV advocates and policymakers with a powerful new tool in their efforts to fight HIV/AIDS in the areas of the United States that are most in need of services, such as urban areas and specific sections of southern states. (HIV/AIDS Atlas: www.maphiv.org/maphiv/).

BEHAVIORAL RISK GROUPS AND STATISTICAL EVALUATION

Behavioral Risk Groups and AIDS Cases

As the pool of AIDS patients grew in number during 1981–1983, individual case histories were separated into **behavioral risk groups.**

The early case histories of AIDS patients clearly separated people according to their social behavior and medical needs. AIDS patients were placed into the following six risk behavior categories: (1) homosexual and bisexual men; (2) injection-drug users; (3) hemophiliacs; (4) other blood transfusion recipients; (5) heterosexuals; and (6) children whose parents are at risk. Each of these groups is considered to be at risk of HIV infection based on some common behavioral denominator. That is, those within these groups represented a higher rate of AIDS cases than people whose needs or behaviors excluded them from these groups. However, because there is some mixing between individuals in behavioral risk groups, HIV infection has gradually spread to lower-risk behavioral groups. Over time the behavioral risk groups have been aligned and defined according to age, exposure category, and sex (see Table 10-1 for a ranking in the United States).

A review of AIDS cases by sex/age at diagnosis, and race/ethnicity in the United States, shows that white, black, and Hispanic males between the ages of 20 and 44 make up 79% of all male AIDS cases. Between ages 20 and 59, they make up 97% of all male AIDS cases. People between the ages of 25 and 44 make up about 35% of the nation's 82 million workers.

Statistical Evaluation of Selected Risk Behavioral Group AIDS Cases

Adult/Adolescent AIDS Cases—On October 31, 1995, the United States reached a half-million (501,310) reported AIDS cases. Ending 2013, an estimated 1.41 million AIDS cases and about 665,000 AIDS-related deaths will be reported to the CDC. Cumulative through 2012 about 14% of AIDS cases have occurred among the heterosexual population, 24% occurred among injection-drug users, and 58% occurred in the male homosexual/bisexual and IDU populations. In 2004, for the first time since the United States AIDS pandemic began, more blacks were diagnosed with AIDS (40.2%) than whites (39.8%). Table 10-2, page 298 presents

Table 10-2 Adult/Adolescent Behavioral Risk Groups, Race and Sex: Percentages of Total AIDS Cases—United States, Estimates for 2013

HIV/AIDS	No. of Cases[a]	% of Cases
Exposure Group		
Men who have sex with men	14,000	40
Injection-drug user (IDU)	5075	14.5
Homosexual/IDU	2100	6
Hemophiliac	15	0
Heterosexual contact	7700	22
Transfusion related	35	<0.1
None of the above	6090	17.4
Total		100%
Race/Ethnicity (all cases)[b]		
White (non-Hispanic)	10,850	31
Black (non-Hispanic)	16,450	47
Hispanic	7000	20
Other	700	2
Sex (adults only)		
Male	26,600	76
Female	8400	24
Age Group (yrs)		
13–19	175	0.5
20–24	1260	3.6
25–29	4970	14.2
30–39	16,030	45.8
40–49	9100	26
50–59	2555	7.3
60 and above	910	2.6

[a]Cumulative estimated total = 35,000 adult/adolescent plus 60 pediatric = 35,060 = 100% of cases for 2013.

[b]About one-third of the U.S. population (estimated 320 million ending 2013) or about 90 million are black and Hispanic. Blacks make up about 13.6% and Hispanics about 16.3%. *(Adapted from AIDS Surveillance Report, December 2009, updated.)*

the total estimated number of new AIDS cases for 2013 and their distribution based on race, sex, and exposure group.

Figure 10-1, page 299 shows that the percentage of AIDS cases for ethnic-related adult/adolescent groups. Estimating through year 2013, whites made up 67.5% of the population and represented 41% of adult/adolescent AIDS cases. Blacks made up 13.6% of the population but

represented 39% of the adult/adolescent AIDS cases. At some point in their lives, about 1 in 16 black men will be diagnosed with HIV. For black women the rate is 1 in 30. Hispanics made up about 16.3% of the population but represented about 19% of the adult/adolescent AIDS cases.

According to estimates, ending 2012, black Americans made up about 54% of all new AIDS cases and Latinos 20%. Together blacks and Latinos represent about 74% of all new AIDS cases, but make up about 29.9% of the population. The two populations also represent 85% of all pediatric AIDS cases. In 2012, black women made up about 65% of new AIDS cases reported among females. White women made up 15% and Latino women 20% of new AIDS cases.

There are myriad factors contributing to the spread of HIV among blacks. Information about the threat of AIDS has not been disseminated widely or effectively enough, particularly among those under 21 who feel they are invulnerable. An official with the New York AIDS Coalition tells a story about a 15-year-old girl who said: "Don't tell me nothin about no AIDS cause that won't impact me. And if I was to get it, all I'd have to do is take a pill in the morning and I'll be O.K." In 2004, Cynthia Davis, a leading AIDS activist in Los Angeles, wrote to leaders of 300 black churches inviting them to a summit on the worsening problem of HIV/AIDS in the black community. She received a response from five!

Figure 10-2, page 299 is a U.S. map of estimated AIDS cases through 2013. Note that the highest incidence of AIDS cases occurs along the coastal regions.

Behavioral Groups At Greatest Risk: Gay and Bisexual Men, Blacks, and Hispanics/Latinos and Percentages of HIV-Infected People

The point of placing people in behavioral risk groups is not to offend them but to provide a warning that certain behavior might make them more vulnerable to HIV infection. It is not race or ethnic group that places people at high or low risk for infection, it is their behavior.

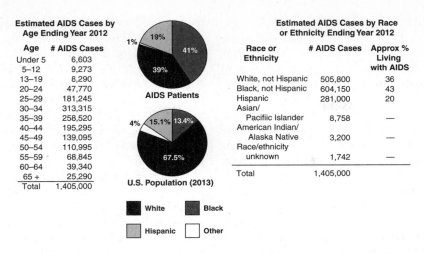

Estimated AIDS Cases by Age Ending Year 2012

Age	# AIDS Cases
Under 5	6,603
5–12	9,273
13–19	8,290
20–24	47,770
25–29	181,245
30–34	313,315
35–39	258,520
40–44	195,295
45–49	139,095
50–54	110,995
55–59	68,845
60–64	39,340
65 +	25,290
Total	1,405,000

AIDS Patients

U.S. Population (2013)

White   Black

Hispanic   Other

Estimated AIDS Cases by Race or Ethnicity Ending Year 2012

Race or Ethnicity	# AIDS Cases	Approx % Living with AIDS
White, not Hispanic	505,800	36
Black, not Hispanic	604,150	43
Hispanic	281,000	20
Asian/ Pacifiic Islander	8,758	—
American Indian/ Alaska Native	3,200	—
Race/ethnicity unknown	1,742	—
Total	1,405,000	

FIGURE 10–1 Estimated AIDS Cases by Age and Racial and Ethnic Classification. Adults AIDS cases show a disproportionate percentage among blacks and Hispanics. About 58% to 60% of reported AIDS cases occur among racial and ethnic minorities. The figures reflect higher rates of AIDS in black and Hispanic injection-drug users and their sex partners. Percentages of the population are based on the numbers of AIDS cases in the United States estimated ending year 2013. U.S. population is about 320 million. Prevalence of HIV infection among adults ages 18–49 in noninstitutionalized household population in the United States is about 0.47%.

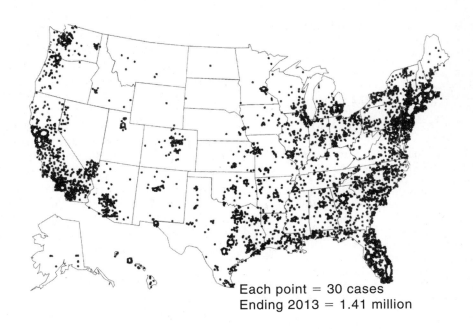

Each point = 30 cases
Ending 2013 = 1.41 million

FIGURE 10–2 United States: Estimated Cumulative AIDS Cases and Approximate Location Ending 2013. *(CDC, Atlanta Surveillance Branch.)*

Keep in mind that because a group of people is at risk for HIV does not mean that these people are predestined to become infected. People are placed within these groups because of their social behavior, a behavior that has been associated with a high, medium, or low risk of becoming HIV infected. Essentially, there is no zero-risk group because a scenario can always be formulated to show that under certain circumstances one or more members of that group could become HIV infected. (See Box 10.2.)

The fact that AIDS was first identified in 1981 in seemingly well-defined behavioral groups (homosexual men, injection-drug users, hemophiliacs, Haitian immigrants) probably contributed to a false sense of security among people who did not belong to any of these groups. However, as information about HIV and AIDS accumulated, it became clear that HIV was transmitted in body fluids. This had grave implications for all social groups. It is highly probable that in the different behavioral risk groups there are lifestyle or medical history factors that increase the efficiency with which the virus is transmitted.

Men Who Have Sex with Men (MSM)—The term *men who have sex with men* (MSM) was first used in 1994 to reduce stigma. It refers to all men who have sex with other men regardless of how they identify themselves (gay, bisexual, or heterosexual). The CDC estimated, in 2010, that MSM made up 4% of the U.S. male population ages 13 and older. In the United States, HIV and AIDS have had a tremendous impact on MSM. In 1981, almost 100% of all AIDS cases reported to the CDC occurred in MSM. In the 1980s, the infection rate among gay men in San Francisco was over 60%. For the 2000s it dropped to about 27% per year.

Recent studies show that a significant percentage of gay men who had originally adopted safer sex behaviors are relapsing to unsafe sex. For example, in 2004 the CDC reported an 8% increase in new HIV cases among gay men. And in a study of gay men ages 15 to 29 by Duncan MacKellar of the CDC (2005), 10% of 5600 men tested HIV positive but 77% of them were unaware they were infected. *Before being tested* the majority of these men thought they were at low risk of being HIV positive, and half of them had unprotected sex during the previous six months. A 2007 CDC report states that about 46% of black gay men in the United States may be HIV positive.

The data presented at CDC's 2010 National STD Prevention Conference found that the rate of new HIV diagnoses among MSM is more than 44 times that of other men and more than 40 times that of women. By risk group, gay and bisexual men of all races remain the population most severely impacted by HIV. MSM account for over half of all new HIV infections in the United States each year (53%), as well as nearly half of people living with HIV (48%). While new HIV infections have declined among both heterosexuals and injection drug users, infections among MSM have been steadily increasing since the early 1990s. In addition to the data, CDC's National Behavioral Surveillance System 2010 report gave the following data about MSM in the United States.

1. One in five MSM is HIV positive (20%).

2. The highest infection rate, 28%, was found among black MSM. Eighteen percent of Hispanic MSM were infected, as were 16% of white MSM.

3. Lower levels of income and education were associated with higher rates of HIV infection.

BOX 10.2

THE HIV/AIDS SCENARIO

HIV/AIDS is unstoppable in the short term. Because it takes an HIV infection so long to develop into AIDS, virtually all the AIDS cases that occur during the next 5 to 20 years will be the result of existing infections. Therefore, the epidemic cannot be materially reduced in this time frame by any reduction in new HIV cases. Worldwide, millions of HIV infections will progress into AIDS into the next decade. Will some of your friends and associates *still* regard HIV/AIDS as someone else's problem? HIV/AIDS has invaded all segments of society worldwide. To some degree, it **is everyone's problem!**

The Coalition for National HIV Awareness Month pronounced July 2012 as the first annual National HIV Awareness Month.

---

4. Among MSM with HIV, 59% of blacks were unaware of their infection, compared to 46% of Hispanics and 26% of whites.

5. MSM under age 30 had lower HIV prevalence than older men. However, 63% of HIV-positive MSM ages 18 to 29 were unaware of their infection, compared to 37% of HIV-positive MSM age 30 and older.

6. Among HIV-positive MSM younger than 30, 71% of blacks were unaware of their infection, compared to 63% of Hispanics and 40% of whites.

7. MSM make up about of 46% of those living with HIV/AIDS.

8. In June 2011, the CDC changed its recommendation of yearly testing of MSM to testing every three to six months. Of 7000 men who thought they were HIV negative, 9% were, in fact, HIV positive.

9. MSM make up about of 53% of 1.4 million U.S. AIDS cases through 2013.

September 27: National Gay Men's HIV/AIDS Awareness Day: At Least 85 Countries Have Laws Prohibiting MSM; Eight of These Countries Impose a Death Penalty for Homosexual Acts

Demographic Changes of HIV-Infected Men in the Gay Community

HIV/AIDS is not, and never was, a gay disease. But HIV/AIDS has had a catastrophic impact on gay communities throughout the world. HIV risk is actually increasing among gay men in many countries, including much of Europe.

Data compiled by the CDC and reported in June 2001 reveals a striking change in the disease's demographics in America (HIV/AIDS Surveillance Report, 2001). Year-end data shows that 74% of HIV/AIDS cases in white Americans, 37% in black Americans, and 42% in Latino Americans resulted from homosexual contacts. Ending 2013, of the estimated 746,000 MSM living with HIV/AIDS in America, 34% will be white, 46% black, and 20% Hispanic. About 380,000 of the 746,000 are progressing to AIDS (Wolitski et al., 2001; Catania et al., 2001 updated). About 400,000 gay men will have died of HIV/AIDS through 2013.

According to Patrick Sullivan and colleagues (2009), the annual HIV incidence of infection among gay men is about 2.2%. About a third of the gay men surveyed knew they were HIV infected.

According to Jessie Juusola and colleagues (2011), at the present rate of HIV transmission, there will be 539,000 new infections in MSM by year 2030.

Overall, of the 30 million AIDS deaths worldwide ending year 2013, about 2.8 million will be gay men. These data overwhelmingly make this global pandemic a heterosexual pandemic.

February 7, Thirteenth National Black HIV/AIDS Awareness Day: HIV/AIDS in the Black Community

To be inclusive of all blacks in the United States who are represented in national HIV surveillance data and HIV prevention efforts, the term *blacks* as used in this book includes African Americans, Caribbean Americans, Africans, and other persons of black race who may not self-identify as African American.

In July 2009, over 5000 people—the largest number in recent history—attended the centennial convention of the National Association for the Advancement of Colored People (NAACP), an *Act Against AIDS Leadership Initiative* (AAALI) partner. The convention's theme "Bold Dreams, Big Victories" was echoed by speakers ranging from President Barack Obama and Attorney General Eric Holder to Speaker of the House Nancy Pelosi and other congressmen and senators, to Reverend Al Sharpton, Reverend Jesse Jackson, NAACP Chairman Julian Bond, and other icons of the civil rights movement. The NAACP convention presented an HIV/AIDS educational session entitled "The Great Silence: The Impact of HIV/AIDS on African American Women."

In March 2010, Jamie Foxx and Ludacris partnered with the CDC to promote "i know," a new social media effort to amplify the voices of black American young adults ages 13 to 29 years in the fight against HIV/AIDS. As a new element of CDC's Act Against AIDS campaign, "i know" will get the facts about HIV/AIDS out far and wide to this hard-hit population through social media

HIV EPIDEMICS IN 2012 ARE SEVERE AND EXPANDING IN MEN HAVING SEX WITH MEN (MSM) GLOBALLY IN BOTH LOW-INCOME AND HIGH-INCOME COUNTRIES

Despite evidence of a disproportionate burden, HIV in MSM continues to be understudied, under-resourced and inadequately addressed. In July of 2012, investigators published six articles in Lancet about the immediate need to mobilize and engage gay men in order to lower their rates of HIV infection. In general, the articles in combination say that "despite decades of research and community, medical and public health efforts, HIV remains uncontrolled in MSM in 2012. This reality demands reinvigorated effort, new approaches grounded in biology and epidemiology, and concerted effort to reduce the structural risks that aid and abet HIV's spread among MSM." The researchers reported that HIV prevalence among MSM is 15% or higher in the United States, Spain, Chile, Thailand, Malaysia, South Africa, and several other nations in Africa and the Caribbean. Central to HIV's disproportionate impact on MSM is the greater transmission risk associated with unprotected receptive anal sex—a 1.4 percent probability, which the authors said is 18 times higher than for penile-vaginal intercourse. Amphetamines and deliberate avoidance of condoms also pay a role. If the transmission probability or receptive anal sex was similar to that associated with unprotected vaginal sex—cumulative HIV incidence in MSM would be reduced by 80–98% within five years. The study, "Global Epidemiology of HIV Infection in Men Who Have Sex with Men," was published in the Lancet (2012;doi:10.1016/S0140-6736(12)60821-6) as part of a series of articles called "HIV in Men Who Have Sex with Men." Also, in July of 2012, the HIV Prevention Trials Network (HPTN) released the results of their HPTN 061 study. Their data shows disturbing rate of new HIV infection occurring among black gay and bisexual men in the U.S., particularly young black MSM. The HPTN 061 study showed that the overall rate of new HIV infection among black MSM in this study was 2.8% per year, a rate that is nearly 50% higher than in white MSM in the U.S. Even more alarming, HPTN 061 found that young black MSM—those 30 years of age and younger—acquired HIV infection at a rate of 5.9% per year, three times rate among U.S. white MSM. The overall infection rate among black MSM in this U.S. study is comparable to the rate seen in the general populations of countries in sub-Saharan Africa hardest hit by the HIV epidemic. HPTN 061 was a large multi-site study of HIV and black MSM conducted in six U.S. cities, and the first to determine the rate of new HIV infection among such a large prospective group of U.S. black MSM.

platforms such as Facebook, Twitter, a new website, and text messages aimed at sparking conversation. Kevin Fenton, director of CDC's National Center for HIV/AIDS, Viral Hepatitis, STD, and TB Prevention said, "At CDC, we have the science, but it is their voices that will make the difference."

The latest number for new HIV infections in the United States, estimated by the CDC for 2007, is 63,230. This number dropped to 56,000 from 2010 through 2012. Therefore, the numbers provided for the black community are based on estimates of 56,000 cases for years 2012 and 2013. Black Americans have been disproportionately affected by HIV/AIDS since the epidemic's beginning, and that disparity has widened over time. Blacks account for about 561,000 AIDS cases, of which about 286,000 have died. The epidemic has also had a disproportionate impact on black women, youth, and men who have sex with men, and its impact varies across the country. Ending 2013 there will be approximately 1.63 million people living with HIV/AIDS in the United States, including an estimated 674,000 who are black. Analysis of national household survey data found that 2% of blacks in the United States were HIV positive—a higher rate than for any other racial/ethnic group.

A Brief Synopsis of the HIV Epidemic among Blacks

- Although black Americans represent only 13.6% of the U.S. population, they account for half of AIDS cases diagnosed. Blacks also account for a disproportionate share of HIV/AIDS diagnoses in states/areas with confidential name-based HIV reporting.

- The AIDS case rate per 100,000 among black adults/adolescents is more than nine times that of whites. The AIDS case rate for black men (82.9) was the highest of any group, followed by black women (40.4). By comparison, the rate among white men was 11.2.

- Of newly infected men, the percentages are: blacks 45%, of whom 46% are gay; whites 35%, of whom 35% are gay; Latinos 19%, of whom 19% are gay.

- HIV-related deaths and HIV death rates are highest among blacks. Blacks account for 56% of deaths due to HIV, and their survival time after an AIDS diagnosis is lower on average than it is for other racial/ethnic groups. Black men had the highest HIV/AIDS death rate per 100,000 men aged 25–44, at 39.9; it was 5.5 for white men. The HIV/AIDS death rate among black women aged 25–44 was 23.1, compared to 1.3 for white women.

- HIV/AIDS is the fourth leading cause of death for black men and the third for black women aged 25–44, a ranking higher than for their respective counterparts in any other racial/ethnic group.

- HIV prevalence among blacks exceeds 5% in nine separate zip codes in Detroit. In New York City's Manhattan borough, 17% of black middle-aged men are living with HIV/AIDS—a level approaching the HIV prevalence rate in South Africa.

- A 2010 CDC report estimates that 1 in 16 black men and 1 in 32 black woman will get HIV in their lifetime (See Snapshot 10.1, page 304).

Black Women and Black Young People

- Black women and black young people account for the majority (66%) of new AIDS cases among women; white and Latina women account for 17% and 16% of new AIDS cases, respectively.

- Black women represent more than a third (36%) of AIDS cases diagnosed among blacks (black men and women combined). By comparison, white women represented 15% of AIDS cases diagnosed among whites.

- Although black teens (ages 13–19) represent only 16% of U.S. teenagers, they account for 69% of new AIDS cases reported among teens. A similar impact can be seen among black children.

The Latino Community—USA

The eleventh annual National Latino AIDS Awareness Day, an observance sponsored by the Latino Commission on AIDS, will be held on October 15, 2013, the last day of Hispanic Heritage Month, in 200 cities and 45 states. Latino leaders sponsor activities that respond to the state of AIDS among Latinos in their communities. In recognition of the surging number of new infections among Latinos and young Latinos, organizers will use the day to promote and sponsor prevention activities, alert religious leaders and public officials to the need to reduce new infections, and care for Latinos infected with the virus.

The rate of infection among Latinos in the United States reflects an increasingly dire situation. Latinos represent about 16.3% of the total population. Ending 2013 Latinos will represent an estimated 19% of new HIV/AIDS cases in America. About 275,000 Latinos are currently living with HIV/AIDS. The CDC estimates that 81% of HIV infections among Latino men occur in the gay/bisexual population with the majority of these infections occurring in men age 30 and under. The rate of HIV infection among Latino

ACROSS THE UNITED STATES: WASHINGTON, DC

In February 2006, National Public Radio (NPR) examined the state of HIV/AIDS in the nation's capital. According to NPR, the rate of new AIDS cases reported each year in the district is 10 times the national average. Of the district's more than 600,000 residents, an estimated one in 50 is living with AIDS and one in 20 is HIV positive. Cornelius Baker, former executive director of the Whitman-Walker Clinic in the district, said several factors contribute to the high HIV prevalence rate in the city. The city has a small population, with a large gay community and a majority black population that is being ravaged by HIV. In addition, there is a poor healthcare infrastructure, inadequate primary care, and high rate of drug addiction. The city's high rate of incarceration also contributes to the number of HIV/AIDS cases. Marsha Martin, the senior deputy director of the district's HIV/AIDS Administration, said HIV/AIDS has fallen "off the radar screen" in the city.

From 1997 through 2006, almost 70% of AIDS patients received an HIV diagnosis within one year of their AIDS diagnosis and of those, 53% were tested one month before their AIDS diagnosis! In mid-2006 Martin made condoms available in all public places that serve alcohol and has expanded the city's needle exchange program, targeted prevention messages at sexually active teenagers and college students, offered HIV testing in more physicians' offices and emergency departments, and required mandatory HIV testing of inmates during the prison intake and discharge process. Also, in June 2006, Martin launched an unprecedented city-wide campaign for routine HIV testing of every person between ages 14 and 84. The campaign targeted 450,000 people to be tested. Ending this campaign about 45,000 had been tested with 1200 being HIV positive. A prevalence of about 3%! The slogan to begin the HIV testing campaign was "Come Together D.C., Get Screened for HIV." Washington, DC has the highest rate of new AIDS cases in the United States at 179 per 100,000 people. Martin wanted every DC citizen to know his or her HIV status by year 2010. It did not happen!

In November 2007, a new 120-page national report appeared, entitled "We're the Ones We've Been Waiting For: The State of AIDS in Black America and What We Are Doing about It!" The data is about blacks living in Washington, DC. A summary of the major findings in this report is:

- Black men have an HIV infection rate of 6.5%, followed by Hispanic men at 3% and white men at 2.6%.
- Although black American residents account for 57% of the District's population, they account

for 81% of new reports of HIV cases. Black American women constitute 58% of the District's female population, but account for 90% of all new female HIV cases in the District.

- Homosexual contact in the District is the leading mode of HIV transmission, accounting for 37% of newly reported infections; heterosexual contact accounts for 28% and IDU accounts for 18%.
- The District's rate for newly reported AIDS cases is higher than rates in Baltimore, Philadelphia, New York City, Detroit, and Chicago.
- The majority of newly reported cases was among residents ages 30 to 49.
- Among residents ages 40 to 49, 7.2% have HIV/AIDS.

(These data do not differ significantly. Found in the District of Columbia Annual 2010 Report.)

For those wishing to read more about the HIV/AIDS tragedy unfolding in our nation's capital, read the "District of Columbia HIV/AIDS Hepatitis, STD and TB 2010 Annual Report." The capital has a 3.2% infection rate—three in 100 DC residents are living with HIV/AIDS. This rate is second only to sub-Saharan Africa!

Black AIDS Institute Executive Director Phill Wilson said that "[the U.S.] response to the epidemic in black America stands in sharp contrast to our response to the epidemic overseas." The report found that more blacks in the United States are living with HIV than in Botswana, Ethiopia, Guyana, Haiti, Namibia, Rwanda, and Vietnam—7 of the 15 countries targeted in the President's Emergency Plan for AIDS relief. Wilson also said that "infection levels among blacks in DC are higher than in 28 African countries." The Black AIDS Institute is the policy center dedicated to reducing HIV/AIDS health disparities by mobilizing black institutions and individuals in efforts to confront the epidemic in their communities. Their motto describes a commitment of self-preservation: "Our People, Our Problem, Our Solution." It is a nonprofit charitable organization based in Los Angeles, California (www.blackaids.org).

Test and Treat: Pilot Program for DC

In 2009, the World Health Organization (WHO) proposed that the HIV epidemic can be significantly curtailed through annual, voluntary HIV testing and immediate antiretroviral treatment for individuals who test positive for HIV infection. In 2010, the National Institute of Allergy and Infectious Diseases (NIAID), the

CDC, and the D.C. Department of Health began several studies designed to answer whether implementing a combined strategy of expanding HIV testing, diagnosing infection early, and providing more HIV-infected patients with medical care and treatment was feasible. The results of the project will be analyzed to determine the cost effectiveness of the test-and-treat approach. The project will run through 2012.

The DC area receives about $45 million in annual Ryan White funds (see Box 14.1, Life of Ryan White, pages 429–430). In March 2010, the city of Washington, DC became the first city in the United States to distribute free female condoms. (See Figure 9-6, page 258.) The initiative made 200,000 free female condoms available in beauty salons, convenience stores, and high schools.

UPDATE 2012—The DC Department of Health reported that new HIV infections and AIDS cases have fallen by 50% from 2010 through 2012—that's the *Good News,* but for Latino men living in the district, HIV infections are rapidly increasing. It is now estimated that one in 36 Latino men in the district will become infected.

FEBRUARY 2011 A group called Prevention-Works has been distributing free needles in DC for more than 12 years. It provided about one-third of the free needles in the city, distributing about 100,000 sterile syringes to 2200 people in 2010. Michael Rhein, president of the board of PreventionWorks, said dwindling private donations, delays in city funds, and high turnover of top managers at the nonprofit agency in recent years were among the

factors that led to the decision to close in February. PreventionWorks used a retrofitted medical van that traveled to 12 locations across the city. It also did HIV/AIDS testing and provided condoms and referrals for drug treatment. In many ways, Rhein said his group was often the only access that drug users on the street had to health and medical services. "We worked with our clients without judgment, even though their activities may be illegal. We met with them where they're at, to improve their health." It is important to keep in mind that syringe exchange prevents the spread not just among users, but between users and their sexual partners and unborn children. It also cleans the alleys, parks, and garbage cans of used syringes to prevent needle sticks. With over 26% of women and 18% of all people living with HIV/AIDS in the District reporting contracting the disease from injection drug use, it's a public health imperative to ensure that injection drug users have the tools and information they need to inject more safely. Comparisons to syringe distribution volume in other DC urban areas suggest that they are far from meeting the demand for sterile syringes in the District.

According to David Holtgrave and colleagues (2012), given the lifetime medical cost of HIV, estimated at $367,134 per infected person, and the effort's first-year free female condom distribution cost of $414,186, the 23 HIV infections prevented represented more then $8 million in savings. Because of these results, the District now plans to distribute 250,000–300,000 female condoms annually.

men is three times greater than the infection rate found among white, non-Hispanic men. Similarly, women and children in the Latino community have rates of infection that are four to seven times greater than the rates found among white women and children.

AIDS is the fourth leading cause of death for Latinos ages 25 to 34, and third among those ages 35 to 44. Since 1981, about 110,000 Hispanic/Latinos have died from HIV/AIDS through 2013.

There are about 48 million to 50 million Latino/Hispanic people in America. The rate of new AIDS cases among Latinos is about four times the rate among white Americans but about three times lower than the rate for black Americans. According to the AIDS Healthcare Foundation, 45% of Latinos have never tested for HIV and 40% have never talked with a doctor about HIV/AIDS.

About 88% of Latinos living with HIV/AIDS live in nine states and Puerto Rico. New York, California, and Puerto Rico top the list.

The CDC reported that one in 52 Latinos would contract HIV during his or her life-time compared to one in 170 whites and one in 22 blacks.

Injection–Drug Users USA—According to the CDC, as many as 25% of the nation's estimated 1.9 million injection-drug users may be HIV infected. This behavioral risk group contains the nation's second largest group of HIV infected and AIDS patients. An association between injection-drug use and AIDS was recognized in 1981, about two years before the virus was identified. AIDS in IDUs and hemophiliacs offered the first evidence that whatever caused AIDS was being carried in and transmitted by human blood. Of IDUs, 74% listed IDU as their only risk factor for HIV infection; 26% were also homosexual/bisexual. It is estimated that through 2012 40% of infected women and 22% of infected men were infected through IDUs.

IDU AIDS cases have been reported in all 50 states and the District of Columbia. Among the adult/adolescent heterosexual AIDS cases, over half had sexual partners who are/were IDUs.

About 55% of all IDU-associated cases were reported in the Northeast, which represents about 20% of the population of the United States and its territories. The South reported 20% of IDU-associated AIDS cases, 5% from the Midwest, and the West reported the remaining 20%.

The rate of IDU-associated AIDS continues to be higher for blacks and Hispanics than for whites. Except for the West, where rates for whites and Hispanics were similar, this difference by race/ethnicity was observed in all regions of the country and was greatest in the Northeast. Since 1981, about 200,000 IDUs will have died of HIV/AIDS through 2013. (See QuickTake 10.2, page 306)

Heterosexuals—The spread of HIV in the general population is relatively slow. The CDC estimates there are about 170 million Americans without an identified at-risk behavior.

Data from the CDC for years 2004 through 2012 indicate that about 15% of all the AIDS cases and about 35% of all new HIV infections in the United States occurred through heterosexual contact. Most of the heterosexual AIDS cases occurred in persons or the sexual partners of individuals with another identified behavioral risk. The number of heterosexual HIV/AIDS cases in the general population is only a fraction of 1%.

Global HIV/AIDS Cases and Heterosexuality

Worldwide ending year 2013, there will be an estimated 11 million people living with AIDS and about 30 million will have died of AIDS. According to the Worldwatch Institute, South

---

QUICKTAKE 10.2

QUICK FACTS OF HIV INFECTION AMONG INJECTION DRUG USERS, USA 2012

For the first time in more than a decade, the CDC has conducted a large-scale survey of HIV seroprevalence and risk behaviors among injection-drug users (IDUs). More than 10,000 IDUs in 20 large U.S. cities participated. Overall, 9% of study participants were HIV infected. Prevalence was higher among Hispanics (12%) and non-Hispanic blacks (11%) than among non-Hispanic whites (6%); it was also higher in the Northeast and South (12% and 11%) that in the Midwest and West (5% and 6%). Nealy half of the IDUs who tested positive for HIV infection (45%) were unaware of their serostatus. In an analysis that combined these individuals with those who were HIV negative, high-risk behaviors were found to be very common: 69% of the individuals reported unprotected vaginal sex, 23% reported unprotected anal sex, and 34% reported needle sharing. On the plus side, 72% reported being tested for hepatitis C virus (HCV) infection, and 89% reported having an HIV test. But, only 4% of people living with HIV who inject drugs and are eligible for treatment receive ART.

Comment: The prevalence of HIV infection in this survey (9%) was substantially lower than the prevalence documented in the last national survey of IDUs, conducted in the 1990s among those entering drug treatment (18%). Unfortunately, more than 40% of those found to be HIV infected in the current survey were unaware of their infection, and high-risk behaviors were common (CDC, 2012).

Africa's HIV pandemic is perhaps the worst on the globe. It has engulfed the country, and "barring a medical miracle, one of every five adults will die of AIDS over the next 10 years." This unprecedented social tragedy is also translating into an economic disaster. The working-age population is being lost to HIV/AIDS. In Zimbabwe, state morgues have extended their hours to cope with the soaring death rate, mostly as a result of AIDS. An estimated 2000 people now die every week in that southern African country; nearly 70% of them from HIV/AIDS-related illnesses. The main hospital in Harare has opened its morgue around the clock, and other hospital and mortuary facilities have extended closing time by four hours. At the University of Durban Westville in

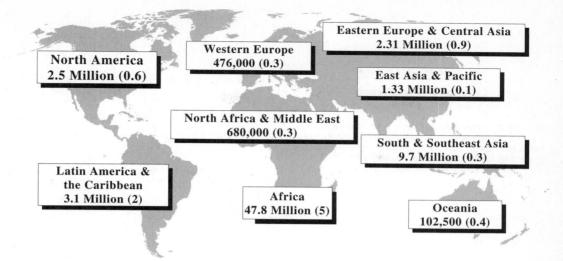

Region	Infections
North America	2.5 Million (0.6)
Western Europe	476,000 (0.3)
Eastern Europe & Central Asia	2.31 Million (0.9)
East Asia & Pacific	1.33 Million (0.1)
North Africa & Middle East	680,000 (0.3)
South & Southeast Asia	9.7 Million (0.3)
Latin America & the Caribbean	3.1 Million (2)
Africa	47.8 Million (5)
Oceania	102,500 (0.4)

Estimated: Global Total 68 Million HIV Infections Ending 2013 and HIV/AIDS Prevalence Rates (%). Global Prevalence Rate (0.8%)

FIGURE 10–3 Estimated Number of Global HIV Infections Projected Using Data from United Nations AIDS Program and World Health Organization. Of the estimated 68 million HIV-infected persons, about 38 million **are living** in some state of HIV/AIDS illness. Over 4 million of these are children. Of 209 countries reporting to the WHO and UNAIDS,194 have reported AIDS cases. World population rates will reach over 7 billion ending 2013 *(World Population Web site).* All numbers have been rounded off and may not add up to 68 million.

KwaZulu-Natal, 14% of students tested HIV positive in 1997; in 2001 it was about 40%.

Worldwide, ending 2013, *heterosexuals* will make up about 87% of the estimated 38 million living HIV-infected people. About 65% of these infected people live in sub-Saharan Africa. North America, Latin America, South and Southeast Asia, and Africa account for about 93% of global HIV infections (Figure 10-3, page 307). Of the 2013 estimated 38 million living HIV-infected people worldwide, about 95% live in nonindustrial nations.

An update on UNAIDS estimates is that, on average, 2.5 million new HIV infections occurred annually from 1997 through 2012. The AIDS death toll for these 15 years is estimated at 28 million, of which about 11 million were women and 5.5 million were under age 15 (Table 10-3). The

Table 10-3 Leading Cause of Death Worldwide from 1998 Estimated through 2013

Infectious Diseases	All Diseases
1. **HIV/AIDS**	1. Heart diseases
2. Diarrheal disease	2. Cerebrovascular diseases
3. Childhood diseases	3. Lower respiratory diseases
4. Tuberculosis	4. Obstructive pulmonary diseases
5. Malaria	5. Diarrheal diseases
6. STDs excluding HIV/AIDS	6. **HIV/AIDS**
7. Meningitis	7. Tuberculosis
8. Tropical diseases	8. Perinatal conditions

(Data Courtesy of the World Health Organization, 1998 updated.)

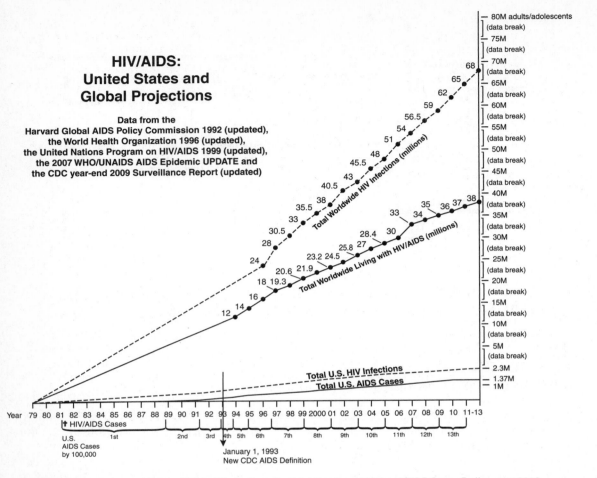

HIV/AIDS:
United States and
Global Projections

Data from the
Harvard Global AIDS Policy Commission 1992 (updated),
the World Health Organization 1996 (updated),
the United Nations Program on HIV/AIDS 1999 (updated),
the 2007 WHO/UNAIDS AIDS Epidemic UPDATE and
the CDC year-end 2009 Surveillance Report (updated)

FIGURE 10–4 Estimated U.S. and Global Projections for Total Number of HIV and AIDS Cases. Ending year 2013, about 1.41 million U.S. AIDS cases will be reported to the CDC. Estimated total U.S. HIV infections through 2013 is 2.3 million. Worldwide the total number of people living with HIV/AIDS is expected to reach about 38 million ending 2013 (30 million dead and about 10.5 million living with AIDS). Through the year 2013, about 2% of all HIV infections and 2.8% of total AIDS cases will have occurred in the United States. William Hazeltine, AIDS researcher formerly at the Dana Farber Institute, and now with Human Genome Sciences, Inc., said that if prevention does not work or a cure is not found, some *1 billion* people could be HIV positive by the year 2025. *(Source: Harvard Global AIDS Policy Commission 1992 and World Health Organization 1993, 1994, National Census Bureau 1998, and projected data.)*

NOTE: *The true data would not give rise to the linear increments as shown, but the true data per year for HIV infections and persons living with HIV/AIDS globally are guesstimates or at least best estimates because of underreporting, wrongful reporting, case overlap, errors and, through 2013, the lack of complete mandatory reporting of AIDS cases or HIV infections worldwide.*

United States will have about 1.41 million AIDS cases ending 2013—worldwide there will be about 29 times that number (Figure 10-4, page 308).

Worldwide, it is estimated that 6 in every 100 sexually active people aged 15 to 49 is HIV infected. Ending 2012, there will be an estimated 38 million people living with HIV infection. There are over a dozen countries whose population is not equal to 38 million people!

American Military The incidence of HIV infection can be measured best in groups that undergo routine serial testing. Because active duty military personnel and civilian applicants for the service are routinely tested for HIV antibody, there is a unique opportunity to measure the incidence of HIV infection in a large, demographically varied subset of the general population.

Beginning 2004 the military began HIV testing of all personnel every two years. The current infection rate among all military personnel is about 0.02% or two per 10,000.

College Students A study was conducted by the CDC with the American College Health Association (Gayle, 1988). At five campuses the rate of HIV-positive blood was 2 per 1000. In contrast, the rate of HIV in the general heterosexual population was 0.2/1000.

The question is why college students have a rate of HIV infection about 10 times higher than the general heterosexual population. Are college students less informed than the general heterosexual population?

Surveys indicate that college students are well educated about HIV/AIDS. Why, then, the higher rate of infection? Perhaps it's the age-old dilemma of information versus behavior. **They know what to do but they don't do it.** College students have always had information on drug use, alcoholism, pregnancies out of wed-lock, and sexually transmitted diseases, but this knowledge has not appreciably reduced at-risk behaviors. STDs are at an all-time high in teen-age and college students.

Prisoners The United States has the highest incarceration rate in the world followed by Russia. Anne Spaulding and colleagues (2002) estimated that about 25% of all people living with HIV infection have passed through a correctional facility in the United States. Beginning 2013, the nation's prison population is at an all-time high, over 2.3 million adults contained in 1300 state and 71 federal prisons. Ninety percent of prisoners are men.

According to the U.S. Bureau of Justice Statistics, 1% of these people or 20,000 are HIV positive and of these, 25% have AIDS (Rubel et al., 1997 updated). The total number of *prisoners, parolees,* and *probationers* in 2012 was about 6.5 million with an HIV-positive rate of about 0.8% or about 50,000 being HIV positive (DeGroot et al., 1996 updated). Entering 2013, over 6000 adult inmates in U.S. state and federal prisons and jails had died of AIDS.

Currently, two states, Alabama and South Carolina, continue to segregate HIV/AIDS prisoners into designated HIV/AIDS units. And, about 25 states test all inmates for HIV at admission or at some point while in custody. Forty-seven states and the federal system reported testing inmates if they have HIV-related symptoms or if they requested an HIV test. Forty states and the federal system test inmates after they are involved in an incident in which an inmate is exposed to a possible HIV transmission, and 16 states and the federal system test inmates who belong to specific high-risk groups. Missouri, Alabama, Florida, Texas, and Nevada test all inmates for HIV upon their release.

Condom and Needle Syringe Distribution in Prisons The number of U.S. prisoners living with HIV is alarmingly high—it is estimated at two to five times that of the general population. As recently reported by the federal government, the rate of AIDS cases is three and a half times as great. The same risky behaviors occur inside as on the outside. Although prohibited by state laws, sex and substance use do happen in correctional facilities—and they happen in the absence of condoms and sterile syringes, both of which are considered contraband in most U.S. jails and prisons. Only one state, Vermont, and five cities—Los Angeles, San Francisco, New York, Philadelphia, and Washington, DC—regularly distribute condoms to inmates. Mississippi does so for prisoners receiving conjugal visits from their spouses. The majority of prison systems throughout Europe and Canada permit condom distribution. To date, no prison system inside the United States distributes or permits the use of injection-drug-use equipment (Sylla, 2008). However, such programs do exist in prisons outside the United States. The first prison needle and syringe program was set up in Switzerland in 1992; since then, such programs have been started in more than 50 prisons in 12 countries in Europe and central Asia.

AGING WITH HIV/AIDS: THE HIDDEN SIDE OF THIS CRISIS IN THE UNITED STATES

The Fastest-Growing Group of People Living with HIV/AIDS in the United States The face of AIDS has changed dramatically from the 1980s into the new millennium. HIV/AIDS cases among men, in particular gay men, and IDUs predominated in the 1980s. But, there have always been older people with HIV and from the 1990s onward the numbers of HIV/AIDS cases among the elderly, women, and people of color increased significantly. **The senior citizens of today did not grow up in the age of HIV/AIDS—they did not have sex and HIV or AIDS in the same thought.**

Recently at a senior center in New York City, volunteers were passing out condoms. An 82-year-old woman, with a smile on her face, said, "You're giving us condoms, who is going to give us a guy?"

SEPTEMBER 18: ANNUAL NATIONAL HIV/AIDS AGING AWARENESS DAY

Two phenomena are driving the aging of the HIV epidemic in the United States. Infected people are living longer because of ART, and the number of older individuals becoming HIV infected is increasing. It is estimated that by 2015 over half of all people living with HIV/AIDS will be older than age 50.

Research on Older Adults with HIV (ROAH)—In 2006, key findings of ROAH, the nation's first comprehensive study addressing the aging HIV/AIDS population, conducted by the AIDS Community Research Initiative of America (ACRIA), was released. Prior to this study, many saw the face of AIDS in New York City as that of an age 50 or younger, white, homosexual male—the media archetype of the 1980s.

Yet in New York City and other urban centers, the face of HIV/AIDS is now that of a heterosexual-identified person over the age of 50 who is a person of color and increasingly likely to be female. In San Francisco ending 2013 about 55% of AIDS cases will be of people age 50 and older. The study showed that one decade after the introduction of highly active antiretroviral therapy (HAART), a dramatic decrease occurred in mortality rates, and life expectancy increased among people living with HIV/AIDS. With new HIV infection rates remaining stable, the net result is an HIV-positive population that is both aging and growing. The AIDS Community Research Initiative of America states that about 35% of all people living with HIV/AIDS in the United States are over age 50. That is about 567,000 people! And 70% (over one million) are over age 40. A large percentage of these people were infected prior to age 50 but are surviving because of ART. Ending 2013, they will make up about 20% of all AIDS cases, 18% of new HIV/AIDS diagnosis, 28% of those living with HIV/AIDS, and make up about 38% of all deaths due to HIV/AIDS. Currently, about 16% of AIDS cases in those ages 50 and older occur due to IDU (www.nia.nih.gov and www.hivoverfifty.org).

Florida—In Florida, a state with a large retired population, the number of recorded AIDS cases among those over age 50 rose from 6 in 1984 to over 20,000 in 2012, or about 20% of the state's cases. In Dade County, Florida, a popular destination among retirees, about 20% of people with HIV/AIDS are seniors. Forty-four percent of women over 50 in Florida with AIDS and 18% of Florida men over 50 with AIDS are known to have become infected through heterosexual sex. These numbers are predicted to grow as the more sexually liberal baby boom generation ages.

Many seniors feel that HIV infection is just a problem for young people, homosexuals, and injection-drug addicts. Now, the use of Viagra compounds the problem. With the use of Viagra, seniors are more sexually active, and few practice safer sex. The manufacturer of Viagra is trying to incorporate safer sex messages into its advertisements.

Baltimore—In August 2011, the Greater Baltimore HIV Health Services Planning Council released the results of a survey that found two-thirds of the region's HIV/AIDS victims were age 45 to 64. The last time the group conducted this study, just seven years ago, the majority of HIV cases were among those who were 25 to 44.

The rapidly changing dynamic of the epidemic due to the aging of the HIV/AIDS population requires an equally dynamic change in the way older people think about the disease. Until recently, people in their 50s and 60s believed they were at little risk of contracting the virus. But that's no longer a safe assumption.

Healthcare Workers—Healthcare workers are defined by the CDC as people, including students and trainees, whose activities involve contact with patients or with blood or other body fluids from patients in a heathcare setting. They represent about 7.7% of the U.S. labor force. **The risk of HIV transmission from healthcare worker to patient during an exposure-prone invasive procedure is remote. There is a greater and well-documented risk of transmission from an infected patient to a healthcare worker.**

According of the CDC, through December 2001, there were 57 documented cases of occupational HIV transmission to healthcare workers in the United States. Only one reported case has been confirmed since 2001.

Ruthanne Marcus and colleagues (1988) reported that, across the board, healthcare workers exposed to HIV-contaminated blood have about a 1 in 300 chance of becoming infected. Other more recent reports place the risk of HIV infection at 1 in 250.

Needle Stick Injuries—Healthcare workers are in a quandary about the possibility of becoming HIV-infected via needle sticks. Articles such as "Needle-stick Risks Higher Than Reports Indicate" and "The Risk of HIV Transmission via Needlesticks Is Low" convey conflicting viewpoints.

Needle sticks and penetration of sharp objects account for about 80% of all healthcare workers' exposures to blood and blood products. There are about 800,000 needle stick injuries from contaminated devices in healthcare settings each year. Of these, about 16,000 devices are contaminated with HIV (Miller et al., 1997).

ESTIMATES OF AIDS CASES AND HIV INFECTION

In 1987, Otis Bowen, then secretary of Health and Human Services, said "AIDS would make Black Death pale by comparison."

As long as the number of newly infected people each year exceeds the number who die, the pandemic will continue to build.

Who Reports AIDS Cases and to Whom? United States

AIDS cases are reported to the CDC through the SOUNDEX system, which involves translating names into specific sets of numbers and letters. While the resulting codes are not unique, when they are combined with other information, such as birthdates, individual cases can be followed without revealing names.

AIDS Reporting Systems

Reporting AIDS cases reveals past HIV infections. When an AIDS case is reported, it is like looking at a 10- to 12-year-old photograph of the infection date (average time, without drug therapy, from infection to AIDS diagnosis is 10 to 12 years). AIDS became reportable in all 50 states, the District of Columbia, and U.S. territories to the CDC in Atlanta in 1986.

By the end of 1993, all 50 states, the District of Columbia, and four territories (Guam, Pacific Islands, Puerto Rico, and the Virgin Islands) reported adult/adolescent cases. The CDC also reported the numbers of adult/adolescent/pediatric AIDS cases per 100,000 population by state. For the 10 leading metropolitan areas of at least 500,000 population for AIDS ending year 2012, see Table 10-4. Ending year 2012, the 10 states reporting the highest incidence of AIDS cases for adults/adolescents can be seen in Table 10-5 and Figure 10-5, page 313.

Table 10–4 Ten Metropolitan Areas Reporting Highest Number of AIDS Cases through Year 2012, Estimated

Metropolitan Area	Number of AIDS Cases/ 100,000 people
Miami	37.2
Baton Rouge	30.6
New York City	27
Washington, DC	26.6
Atlanta	18.7
San Francisco	18.3
Houston	15.1
Philadelphia	11.3
Chicago	11.2
Los Angeles	10.3

Table 10–5 Ten States Reporting Highest Number of AIDS Cases through Year 2012, Estimated

States	Number of AIDS Cases	Approximate # Living with AIDS
New York	250,765	101,250
California	216,044	81,000
Florida	139,850	64,395
Texas	94,519	42,525
New Jersey	75,229	24,300
Georgia	42,371	21,870
Pennsylvania	41,473	21,465
Illinois	40,508	20,250
Maryland	36,650	17,820
Massachusetts	27,000	11,745
	964,480 or 70.4% of all AIDS cases in America (1.37 million)	405,082 or about 42% of 964,480 AIDS cases

Names-Based HIV Reporting

In mid-2005, the CDC urged all state health departments toward names-based reporting. The CDC wanted a single accurate system that would provide national data to monitor the scope of HIV infections nationally (all other illnesses are reported by name). All states used names-based reporting ending 2008.

It is expected that HIV reporting will provide a more accurate view of recent transmission trends. The information will also help direct money to the most effective programs and could affect allocations for HIV patient care. The decision of states to report HIV cases was most influenced by the development of successful treatment, which allows many people with HIV to live healthier longer. But that progress has made it hard for statisticians to calculate backward to estimate time of infection. AIDS case reporting now has become much more of an indicator of who is getting treated, who is not getting tested early, and how effective their therapy is.

SHAPE OF THE HIV PANDEMIC: UNITED STATES

There is a common misconception that the AIDS pandemic is under control in the developed world. While the mortality rate associated with HIV has been sharply reduced because of behavioral changes and antiretroviral drugs, they are imperfect solutions. Drug therapies are expensive, often toxic, and not a cure. AIDS education programs have impeded but have not stopped the epidemic. The United States has the highest rate of HIV infection among the world's most highly industrialized countries, in spite of the fact that it serves as a leader in AIDS education and prevention. About one in 140 people in the United States has been HIV infected. The ratio in some sub-Saharan countries is one in five, and in some African villages the ratio is one in two in women of childbearing age.

It is estimated that there were about 19,000 people HIV infected in 1977, and ending 1982, 190,000. Prior to 1981, 32 were believed to have died of AIDS (Table 10-6).

HIV infections reached their peak ending 1982 and then rapidly declined. Ending 1982 there were an estimated 529,000 people infected in the United States. No one can say exactly which factors have been responsible for bringing the HIV infection rate down from some 190,000 people in 1982 to about 50,000 each year from 1988 through 2001. From at least 2002 through 2009 there were about 60,000 to 63,000 new infections per year and from 2010 through 2012 about 53,000 to 56,000 new infections per year. For a breakdown of new HIV infections, see Figure 10-6, page 315. These

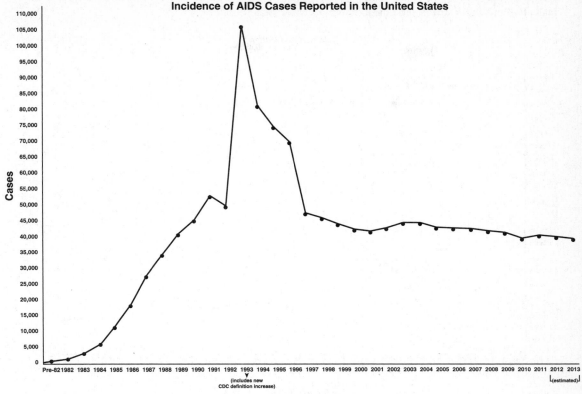

Incidence of AIDS Cases Reported in the United States

Cases (y-axis): 0 to 110,000

Date of Diagnosis (x-axis): Pre-82 1982 1983 1984 1985 1986 1987 1988 1989 1990 1991 1992 1993 1994 1995 1996 1997 1998 1999 2000 2001 2002 2003 2004 2005 2006 2007 2008 2009 2010 2011 2012 2013

(includes new CDC definition increase)

(estimated)

FIGURE 10-5 Incidence and Estimates of AIDS in Persons 13 and Older by Year of Diagnosis—United States, pre-1982 through 2013. The total for 1995 reflects a 9% reduction in AIDS cases from 1994 due to a drop in the backlog of persons to be identified as AIDS cases according to the 1993 definition of AIDS. AIDS cases reported in 2002 increased for the first time in 10 years, about a 2.2% rise over 2001. Data for years 2002 through 2007 reflect an increase, from the low number in 2001, in AIDS cases resulting from therapy failure and increases in gay males. Throughout the American pandemic, about 84% of persons with AIDS were/are ages 20–49.

figures are estimates with new cases of HIV infection now reportable by federal law, and will change over the coming years. (See Point of Information 10.1, page 316.)

The Newly HIV-Infected Populations—USA

For the 50,000 to 60,000-plus new HIV infections occurring as far back as 1999, or earlier, through 2012 annually, the CDC estimated, on average, that 67% of the infected were men. Of these men, 42% were infected via homosexual sex, 25% through IDU, and 33% through heterosexual sex. Of these men, 54% are black, 26%

are white, and 20% are Hispanics. Black American men make up 75% of new HIV infections among heterosexual cases. A small percentage are members of other racial/ethnic groups. Of the estimated 16,065 new infections among women in the United States annually for 2002 through 2012, the CDC estimated that approximately 75% of women are infected through heterosexual sex and 25% through injection-drug use. Of newly infected women, approximately 64% are black, 17% are white, 17% are Hispanics, and a small percentage are members of other racial/ethnic groups. The CDC estimates that over the next four years, about 120,000 people under the

Table 10-6 AIDS Deaths in the United States

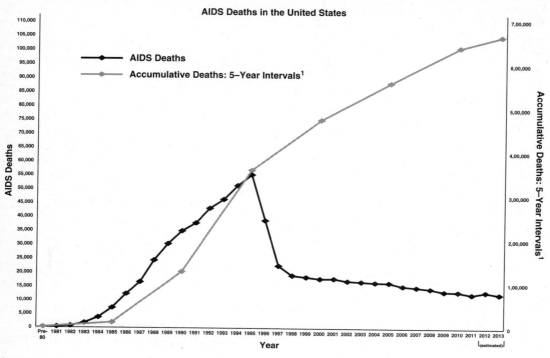

AIDS Deaths in the United States

[1]Estimated deaths through 2013 for white people, 287,595; black, 259,350; Hispanic, 113,050.

Estimated Cumulative Deaths from AIDS in the United States from 1977 through 2013. AIDS deaths dropped by 75% from 1995 through year 2000. A similar or greater drop in AIDS deaths occurred in Europe over the same time period. It took from 1981 to about 1988, about 7 years, to reach the first 100,000 AIDS deaths in the United States. Over the next 18 years (2006) there were an additional 500,000-plus AIDS deaths. The sharp decline in AIDS deaths from 1996 onward is not due to a reduction in HIV infections, but to the introduction of combination antiretroviral drugs. Deaths from AIDS are no longer in the top 15 causes of death in the United States.

age of 29 will become HIV infected if current trends continue. The current increase in HIV infections is a reversal of prevention program successes. The overtly sick, the emaciated, and those with visible Kaposi's sarcoma are rarely seen on the streets; antiretroviral drugs have the dying going back to work. The fear of infection and death has subsided.

The populations that are encompassed in the numbers of new infections are different from the past: HIV is now reaching younger people, it's reaching more women, it's reaching more communities of color. Infections in heterosexual women are increasing more rapidly than in any other group. Unless a preventive

vaccine is found, the rate of new HIV infections in the United States is expected to remain above 50,000 annually. This may mean the new prevention campaigns, without a vaccine, will not significantly reduce new infections. Society has, in a sense, reduced new HIV infections to its lower limit. (See Snapshot 10.2, page 317)

Although the noticeable drop in new AIDS cases was a renewed cause for hope, the downside is that slowing the progression to AIDS and to AIDS deaths (discussed next) means more HIV-infected people with better health are available to spread HIV. Ending 2013 there will be about 700,000 adult/adolescent people and

Estimated HIV Infections Ending 2013

There are an estimated 1.63 million people living with HIV/AIDS in the United States, with on average, about 56,000 new HIV infections occurring in the United States annually since about 2010.

By gender, about 73% of new HIV infections each year occur among men.

By risk, men who have sex with men (MSM) represent the largest proportion of new infections, followed by men and women infected through heterosexual sex and injection-drug use.

By race, more than half of the new HIV infections occur among blacks, though they represent about 13.6% of the U.S. population. Hispanics, who make up about 16.3% of the U.S. population, are also disproportionately affected.

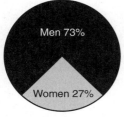

Estimates of 2013 new infections by gender (N ≅ 56,000)

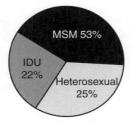

Estimates of 2013 new infections by risk (N ≅ 56,000)

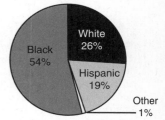

Estimates of 2013 new infections by race (N ≅ 56,000)

To better understand how the HIV/AIDS epidemic is affecting men and women, it is critical to look at race and risk by gender.

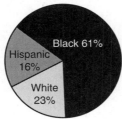

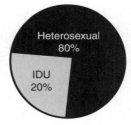

Estimates of annual new infections in women, U.S., by race and risk, 2013

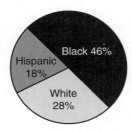

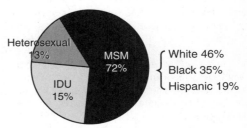

Estimates of new infections in men, U.S., by race and risk, 2013

FIGURE 10-6 A Glance at the HIV Epidemic in America. *(Source: Centers for Disease Control and Prevention updated)*

NOTE: At the time of Magic Johnson's announcement that he was HIV positive (1991), the CDC reported that one-third of AIDS cases in America were black. Black Americans now account for 54% of all new HIV diagnoses. And, for the last eleven years, HIV/AIDS has been the leading cause of death for black people ages 24 to 44.

WHY THE CDC RAISED THE NUMBER OF NEW HIV INFECTIONS BY OVER 16,000 CASES PER YEAR FROM 2000 BUT THE BETTER ESTIMATE WOULD BE AN INCREASE OF 22,000 TO 24,000 PER YEAR!

While the Federal Government and the Centers for Disease Control and Prevention in Particular Lamented about the Increase in HIV Infections Globally, They Lost Sight of What Is Happening in the USA

Beginning in 2003, the CDC began reporting on new HIV infections from 33 states and 5 dependent areas that used a confidential name-based reporting system. The other 17 states did not report their new HIV infections by name. This means that 17 states did not have their new cases of HIV infections included in the annual CDC reports on the number of new HIV infections. Thus, HIV data from these 33 states and 5 dependent areas represented just 63% of the estimated total of new infections that were believed to be occurring in all 50 states and 5 dependent areas. In 2003, the CDC recommended that all 50 states use confidential name-based reporting of new HIV infections, and by 2006, 45 states and the 5 dependent areas were reporting new HIV cases via that system. Therefore, data on new HIV cases for 2006 contained new HIV infections from an additional 12 states whose HIV cases not were previously used. Data from the 45 states and 5 dependent areas revealed that there were an estimated 52,878 new HIV infections. Still, 10% of the states and Puerto Rico, or about 5% of the new HIV infections, were left out of the count. So the 2006 estimate of HIV infections is really more like 56,000 plus! **For 2007 the CDC said the number of new HIV infections was 63,230.**

Clearly the increase in the estimate of new HIV infections for 2006 did not just happen as a singular event; the number of new HIV infections had to be greater than the 40,000 a year estimated by the CDC from 1989 through 2005; they were just not being counted! It was the history of confidential name-based reporting beginning in 2003 from 33 states and 5 dependent areas through 2005 that set the stage for the data from 45 states and the 5 areas in 2006 along with the use of STARHS data (Serologic Testing Algorithm for Recent HIV Seroconversions—see Chapter 13, pages 395–396, for an explanation for the use of STARHS) in 2006 from 22 states with name-based reporting, extrapolated to estimate the number of new HIV infections in all

50 states and the District of Columbia, that provided the 56,300 HIV cases for 2006. (An estimated 247,000 additional individuals were diagnosed with HIV ending 2006, but were not reported to the CDC and were left out of the data, which resulted in CDC's number of 56,300 HIV cases for 2006 [Hall et al., 2008].)

The updated estimates confirm that the largest proportion of new infections—53%—is occurring among gay and bisexual men. HIV incidence has steadily increased among this group since the early 1990s, while the rate of new infections among heterosexuals and injection drug users has fallen. Women accounted for 25% of all new infections in the 2006 data.

By race/ethnicity, African Americans had accounted for 45% of new infections, compared with 35% among whites and 17% among Latinos. According to the revised estimates, blacks have an infection rate nearly three times higher than that of Latinos and seven times higher than that of whites (Hall et al., 2008).

A STATEMENT FROM THE CDC AUGUST 2008

The estimates from our nation's new HIV incidence surveillance system reveal that the U.S. epidemic is—and has been—worse than previously estimated and serve as a wake-up call for all Americans. Using the new technology called Serological Testing Algorithm for Recent HIV Seroconversion (STARHS) that distinguishes recent from longstanding HIV infections, CDC estimates that 56,300 new HIV infections occurred in the United States in 2006. Prior to the availability of STARHS, CDC previously estimated that approximately 40,000 new HIV infections occurred annually since the 1990s. It is important to note that the 2006 estimate does not represent an actual increase in the annual number of new infections; rather, a separate CDC historical trend analysis published alongside the incidence estimate suggests that the number of **new HIV infections was never as low as 40,000 and has been roughly stable since the early 2000s.** Even though the analysis shows overall stability in new HIV infections in recent years, the HIV/AIDS epidemic remains at an unacceptably high level.

NEW YORK CITY

Beginning 2013, over 110,000 New Yorkers have been diagnosed and known to be living with HIV/AIDS. It is estimated that an additional 200,000-plus New Yorkers are HIV infected but remain unaware of their infection. About 28% of New Yorkers learned of their HIV status when they were diagnosed with AIDS. About 92% of the city's at-risk populaton believe they are not at risk.

THE HIV/AIDS EPICENTER

New York City remains the epicenter of the HIV/AIDS epidemic in the United States. It has the highest AIDS case rate in the United States; while it is home to less than 3% of the U.S. population, the city accounts for one in six of national AIDS cases. The AIDS case rate in New York City is four times the U.S. average, and higher than any other city in the United States. About 1.4% of the city's adults are HIV-positive.

ECONOMIC DISPARITIES AND HIV/AIDS

There are glaring epidemiologic disparities. Over 80% of new AIDS diagnoses and deaths in New York City are among African Americans and Latinos. And, as has been documented nationally, an increasing proportion of new AIDS cases are diagnosed in women, most notably women of color. Black male residents of New York City, who are nearly three times more likely to be living with HIV/AIDS than other New Yorkers, have been hit especially hard by the epidemic. Approximately one in 14 black men between the ages of 40 and 54 is living with HIV/AIDS—seven times the rate of other New Yorkers. The only groups with higher infection rates are men who self-identify as gay or bisexual (one in 10 are estimated to be living with HIV/AIDS) and injection-drug users (one in 7 are estimated to be living with HIV/AIDS). The results of a 2007 survey among New York City's MSM revealed that 40% of MSM do not disclose their sexual orientation to their physicians. MSM who disclosed were twice as likely to have been HIV tested as those who did not disclose.

SCARED SAFE?

To counter and reduce the HIV/AIDS data presented, the New York City Department of Health and Mental Hygiene began a TV poster prevention campaign (December 2010/January 2011) called "It's Never Just HIV." The film was shot in an ominous tone. The TV spot shows attractive and anxious young men along with gruesome images of physical deterioration as a voice-over warns: "When you get HIV, it's never just HIV. You're at a higher risk to get dozens of diseases—even if you take medications—such as osteoporosis, dementia, and anal cancer. Stay HIV free. Always use a condom." The outcry—and applause—was immediate. Gay Men's Health Crisis (GMHC) and the Gay and Lesbian Alliance Against Defamation (GLAAD) demanded the ad be pulled, saying the "sensationalistic" and "stigmatizing" spot "creates a grim picture of what it is like to live with HIV." But the health department stood firm. It even expanded the campaign to include subway posters. The department's MD said, "These ads are hard-hitting and sometimes unpleasant—but so is HIV, and silence isn't stopping the spread," adding that in the past decade in New York City, HIV diagnoses among men who have sex with men (MSM) and who are younger than 30 have risen nearly 50%. Praise for the campaign arrived from Larry Kramer, legend of AIDS activism, who wrote "The Normal Heart." He said, "HIV is scary, and all attempts to curtail it via lily-livered nicey-nicey prevention tactics have failed. Of course people have to get scared."

Selling Their Antiretroviral Drugs

In Washington Heights, a Manhattan neighborhood, officials are seeing a growing number of HIV positive individuals selling their drugs. This growing trend of trading health for much needed cash isn't new but it illuminates how a crippling economy and disproportionate poverty impact people living with HIV. HIV medication is expensive, making it a lucrative product for the black market. Buyers stand around the more popular subway stations as if it's a full-time job. For 9 to 5 Monday through Friday, they're buying prescription medication from people who will use the proceeds to buy food, pay bills, or fuel an addiction. Pharmacists then buy and repackage the drugs so they'll sell for higher prices and ship them to countries with high demand, like the Dominican Republic and Mexico. The price paid depends on the strength of the black market, some HIV medications can fetch around $500 a bottle, an alluring sum to those who are infected but also desperately need money.

Patients at MOMS Pharmacy shops in Manhattan, Brooklyn, and Long Island unknowingly received black-market HIV drugs, state attorney General Eric Schneiderman said Wednesday in an indictment brought before the state Supreme Court in Suffolk County. From 2008 to 2012, four men allegedly conspired to sell stolen, expired or mislabeled HIV drugs at three MOMS Pharmacy locations.

On its website, the small chain says it is "committed to providing the best HIV/AIDS pharmacy care." Authorities say no patients were harmed, but they were possibly endangered as some of the drugs were of unknown origin and potency.

Three pharmacists, including MOMS' supervising pharmacist and compliance officer, and a businessman moved more than $274 million in black-market HIV drugs during the scheme, Schneiderman said.

Approximately $155 million of that was billed to Medicaid, he noted.

Anthony D. Luna, the drug chain's president, said in a statement, "MOMS Pharmacy was a victim of this crime and will continue to cooperate fully with the New York state authorities."

—Excerpted from the Wall Street Journal (April 5, 2012), Will James.

about 4500 children living with AIDS in the United States. The estimated number of people currently living with HIV infection is about 1.62 million. The slowing of AIDS diagnosis, due to the use of antiretroviral therapy, makes tracking the epidemic difficult. However, the ability to monitor the epidemic based on HIV infections does not, at the moment, compare with the CDC's ability to track the pandemic through the reporting of AIDS cases, but it will in the next year or so.

For Every 100 People Living in the United States with HIV:

1. 80 are aware of their infection.
2. 70 are linked to some type of care.
3. 50 stay in care.
4. 50 receive antiretroviral therapy (of those who stay in therapy, 80% achieve viral control).
5. Between l9 and 28 have their infection under control (have low to undetectable number of HIV).

Southern States Manifesto: Changing U.S. HIV/AIDS Demographics Leads to Southern Discomfort

The South composes about 37% of the population of the United States through 2012. In addition:

- Of the 20 areas (which include 18 states, Washington, DC, and Puerto Rico) with the highest AIDS case rates, 11 (55%) are in the South.

- The South has the highest number of adults/adolescents living with AIDS and HIV in the four regions of the United States (Northeast, Midwest, South, and West).

- The South has the highest number of people dying from AIDS in the United States.

- Of the 20 metropolitan areas with the highest AIDS case rates, 16 (80%) are in the South.

- Half of all new HIV diagnoses occur in 9 southern states.

- Of the 15 states with the highest rates of new HIV diagnoses, nine (60%) are in the South.

- Southern states compose 65% of all AIDS cases among rural populations in all regions.

- Eight of the 10 states with the highest death rates from HIV/AIDS are in this region.

Table 10–7 Geographic Distribution of Total Estimated AIDS Cases—2013, USA

- Of the estimated 35,000 new AIDS diagnoses in the 50 states and the District of Columbia,

  25% were in the Northeast.
  11% were in the Midwest.
  46% were in the South.
  17% were in the West.

- Of the estimated 696,000 persons living with AIDS in the 50 states and the District of Columbia,

  29% were in the Northeast.
  11% were in the Midwest.
  40% were in the South.
  20% were in the West.

- Of the estimated 13,000 persons who died of AIDS in the 50 states and the District of Columbia,

  25% were in the Northeast.
  10% were in the Midwest.
  50% were in the South.
  16% were in the West.

HOW UNDIAGNOSED CASES OF HIV IMPACT THE HIV/AIDS EPIDEMIC IN THE USA

It has been reported that worldwide, about 90% of people living with HIV/AIDS do not know their HIV status! In the United States, with free HIV testing available in every state, city, and county, one would not think we would share the world problem of large numbers of people not knowing they are HIV positive—**the undiagnosed.** But you would be wrong—we do share this global problem!

The Centers for Disease Control and Prevention Study in February 2009

In February 2009, Michael Campsmith of the CDC presented data at the 16th Conference on Retroviruses and Opportunistic Infections, giving a detailed picture of those living with undiagnosed HIV infections in the United States ending year 2006. This data is updated herein to reflect year-end 2012 estimates. The numbers used for 2006 and 2012 are best estimates, as one cannot directly observe/count the undiagnosed.

Analysis of the CDC Study—Updated

Ending 2012, an estimated 1.63 million people will be living with HIV/AIDS. And, according to the CDC, at least one in five (20%) or 326,000 people will be unaware they are HIV positive!

Hildegard Hall et al. (2012) reported that an estimated 49% of transmissions were from the 20% of persons living with HIV unaware of their infection. About eight transmissions would be averted per 100 persons newly aware of their infection; with more infections averted the higher the percentage of persons with viral suppression who can be linked to care. Improving all stages of HIV care would substantially reduce transmission rates.

Racial/Ethnic Minorities Less Likely to Be Aware of Their HIV Infections

The study found that among those living with HIV, blacks and Latinos were less likely to be diagnosed compared to their white counterparts (in 2012, over 22.2% of blacks and 22% of Hispanics living with HIV will be undiagnosed versus 19% of whites). The rate of undiagnosed HIV infection among blacks will be nine times that among whites, and the rate among Hispanics will be nearly three times that among whites.

Overall, blacks will account for 48.6% of HIV-positive persons unaware of their status—or an estimated 157,000. By comparison, whites will account for 30.9% or about 100,000 unaware carriers, and Hispanics will account for 18.0% or about 57,000 unaware carriers. About 26% or 5700 American Indians and Alaska Natives will be unaware of their infections.

Undiagnosed HIV Infection Status Differs by Risk Group

Among all transmission categories, MSM account for the greatest number of undiagnosed people living with HIV. Of the estimated 745,000 HIV-infected MSM, about 20% to 40%, or about 149,000 to 298,000, are undiagnosed. Among heterosexual men, about 123,000 are undiagnosed, and among women, about 37,000 are undiagnosed. The number of infected injection-drug users is included within the three categories presented. For example, MSM numbers include MSM *and* MSM injection-drug users. Of the undiagnosed, about 39% move on to AIDS within a year of their diagnoses.

Young People Least Likely to Have Been Diagnosed

Researchers estimate that 47.8% or 28,680 young people (13–24) living with HIV were undiagnosed, a much greater proportion than any other age group.

UNDIAGNOSED BY AGE GROUP (ESTIMATED)

Ages	Total
13 to 24	30,592
25 to 34	68,160
35 to 44	104,640
45 to 54	74,560
55 and over	42,048
Total	320,000

SUMMARY

Clearly these data show that the undiagnosed HIV-infected individuals are crucial links in the transmission of HIV. These data demonstrate the need for more inclusive HIV testing. The case for testing all individuals ages 13 to 64 can be found in Point of Information 13.2, pages 410–412.

Federal funding pays about $6754 per HIV patient everywhere but in the South, where it pays $6565. This difference in funding caused the HIV/AIDS directors from 13 southern states and the District of Columbia, the Southern AIDS Coalition, to produce a 2002 "Southern States Manifesto." It was updated in 2008. The major complaint within the manifesto is that the South leads the country in new HIV infections and overall AIDS cases but receives fewer federal dollars when compared to other HIV/AIDS regions.

ESTIMATES OF DEATHS AND YEARS OF POTENTIAL LIFE LOST DUE TO AIDS IN THE UNITED STATES

"All my friends are dead." This expression is unique in a lifetime and is symbolic of reaching old age—except in a time of war. Too many young people worldwide have said it over the past 31 years because of HIV/AIDS.

Deaths Due to AIDS: United States

Each year in the United States there are about 2,300,000 deaths. AIDS, from 1991 through 1995, caused at least 40,000 of these deaths each year and accounted for about 1.8% of all deaths for each of those years. That is, 2 people of each 100 who died, died of AIDS.

The good news is that between the end of 1995 and the end of 1996, AIDS deaths dropped in the United States for the first time since the pandemic began—25% nationwide (about 12,600 fewer deaths). Between 1996 and 1998 deaths had dropped by about 75% (Table 10-6, page 314). Similar data were reported from Europe. The sudden drop in expected deaths due to AIDS is believed to be associated mainly with the use of combination drug therapy.

Ending 2013, about 665,000 people in the United States will have died of AIDS. **About 65% of these people did not live to age 45!**

And yet, the United States, after spending billions of dollars on the disease, took until late 2010 to establish a comprehensive national plan to guide the strategic use of AIDS-related dollars or to hold government agencies accountable for steadily improved outcomes for people living with HIV/AIDS or at risk of infection. (See Point of View 14.3, pages 444–445, The Call for a National HIV/AIDS Policy/Strategy.)

SELECTED NATIONS/COUNTRIES HAVE DIFFERENT EPIDEMICS. EACH FACES ITS OWN REALITY

AIDS as a Cause of Death in the United States and Worldwide at the End of 2013 (Figures Estimated)

FAST FACTS

United States

- AIDS is the fifth leading cause of death among people ages 25 to 44.
- AIDS is the leading cause of death of black American men ages 25 to 44.
- AIDS is currently the fourth leading cause of death among all U.S. women ages 25 to 44, and the second leading cause of death among black women ages 25 to 44.
- In the United States about six people per hour become HIV infected 365 days a year (56,000), and every hour between one and two people die (about 13,000 in 2012). Before 1996 one person died every 13 minutes.
- Of those living with HIV infections, about 1.62 million at the end of 2013, 41% are white, 39% are black, and 20% are Hispanic. Men make up about 74% and women about 26%.
- Through year 2013, an estimated 665,000 people will have died of AIDS.
- About 648,000 adults ages 18 to 49 are living with HIV/AIDS.
- The United States has about 4% of the global population of adult/adolescent/children living with HIV/AIDS and about 2.4% of all AIDS deaths.
- The prevalence of HIV/AIDS cases globally in ages 15–49 is about 0.8% except in sub-Saharan Africa, where it is 5%. In the United States it's about 0.6%.

CANADA'S ESTIMATED HIV/AIDS CASES THROUGH 2012: POPULATION 34,310,000

Overview

- Number of HIV infections—79,094 (Females at 20.5% or about 16,214)
- Number of children HIV-positive—711
- Number of AIDS cases—24,490 total, AIDS deaths at 63% or 15,428
- Male AIDS cases, 18,612 (76%);
  - (a) MSM, 73%
  - (b) Heterosexual, 12%
- Female AIDS cases, 6122 (25%)
  - (a) IDU, 25%
  - (b) Heterosexual, 57%
- Perinatal AIDS cases, 284 (82% of pediatric AIDS cases)

MEXICO'S ESTIMATED HIV/AIDS CASES THROUGH 2012: POPULATION 115 MILLION

Mexico is home to about 230,000 people living with HIV/AIDS, the second highest number of people living with HIV/AIDS in Latin America. (There are also an estimated 60,000 people infected who don't know it!) Brazil tops the list with about 750,000. That country's HIV/AIDS prevalence rate is among the lowest in the region and has stabilized over the last decade. The epidemic in Mexico is influenced by cultural, social, and economic factors and, similar to other countries in Latin America, homophobia, stigma, discrimination, gender inequalities, interregional migration, and poverty contribute to or exacerbate the epidemic. Among the issues unique to HIV/AIDS in Mexico is the role played by population mobility and migration along the Mexico United States border.

Overview

- The first case of HIV/AIDS in Mexico was reported in 1983.
- Ending 2012, there were about 160,000 AIDS cases, of which about 54% have died (about 86,400).

- The number of people infected with HIV (not AIDS) is unknown, but it is believed that about 235,000 people are living with HIV. In combination, it can be estimated that Mexico had about 400,000 cases of HIV infection (AIDS + HIV cases) through 2012.
- Children make up about 3% of HIV cases, or about 12000.
- The HIV/AIDS prevalence rate in Mexico is 0.3%, which is among the lowest in the region and lower than the rate in Latin America (0.5%) and globally (0.8%).
- An estimated 13,000 Mexicans died of HIV/AIDS in 2012; it is the 16th leading cause of death in Mexico. HIV/AIDS is the fourth leading cause of death among men ages 25 to 34.
- HIV is spread primarily through sex in Mexico, accounting for about 90% of all cumulative cases of AIDS. Sex between men (MSM) accounts for the largest share of HIV diagnoses recorded to date (57%), followed by sex workers, then injection-drug users. There is also an increasing trend toward heterosexual transmission in recent years.
- Women account for about 19% of adults aged 15 and over estimated to be living with HIV/AIDS, a share that has been increasing as women are infected by their male partners.
- The majority of AIDS cases are among those 15 to 44 years of age (78.5% of cumulative AIDS cases).
- In 2012 Mexico spent about $7 million on HIV/AIDS prevention.
- Mexico City was home to the XVII International AIDS Conference, the first such conference to be held in Latin America.

UNITED KINGDOM'S (UK) ESTIMATED HIV/AIDS DATA THROUGH 2012: POPULATION 63 MILLION

Beginning 2013, an estimated 127,000 in the UK had been diagnosed with HIV. Of that number 55,118 (43.4%) became AIDS cases, of which 25,354 died of AIDS (46%). About 71,000 were receiving HIV care. There are an estimated 30,000 (25%) people who are infected and do not know it!

Global Estimates of Adults and Children Newly Infected with HIV 2012

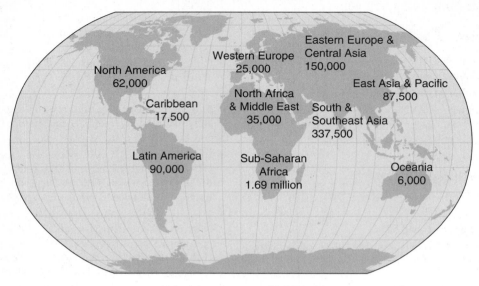

Estimates are for the entire globe.
Total: 2.5 million

FIGURE 10-7   Year 2012. Estimate for New HIV Infections. *(UNAIDS/WHO, 2010 updated)*

Overview

- Three routes of HIV infection are heterosexual sex, MSM, and injection-drug use (IDU), in that order.
- Heterosexual sex 44% (55,880).
- MSM 41% (52,070).
- IDU 5% (6350).
- Blood/blood factor recipients 2% (2540).
- Children born to HIV-infected mothers 1.5% (1905).
- Unknown route of transmission 6.5% (8255).
- About half of all new HIV diagnoses are heterosexual.
- About 45% of all new HIV diagnosis are in gay/bisexual men

Estimated Worldwide HIV/AIDS Data Beginning 2011 (See Figures 10-7, 10-8, page 323 and 10-9, page 324)

- Worldwide, about 285 people become HIV infected every hour, 365 days a year (2.5 million),

and every hour about 240 people die (2.1 million). This number dropped to 1.7 million in 2011.

- About 10% of new infections are due to injection-drug use. Excluding Africa that figure becomes 30%.
- About 5.1 million men having sex with men (MSM) have been infected with HIV (between 5% and 10% of global HIV infections—UNAIDS, 2007 updated). An estimated 52% have died of HIV/AIDS, or about 2,652,000.
- About 40% of all new HIV infections globally are occurring among 15- to 24-year-old people. (about 3500/day)
- About 95% of people living with HIV/AIDS reside in low- and middle-income countries.
- Ending year 2013, about 68 million people will have been HIV infected, about 95% in developing countries.
- Nine out of ten HIV-positive people are unaware they are infected.
- Women now make up about 60% of 15- to 24-year-olds living with HIV/AIDS.

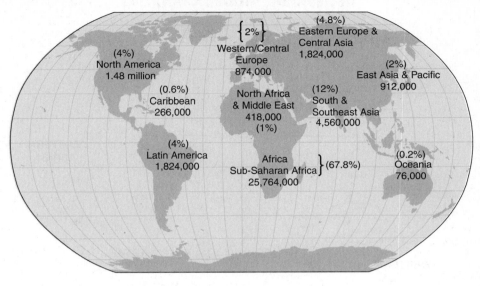

**Year End Estimates: Adult/Children
Living with HIV Infection**

(4%)
North America
1.48 million

{ 2% }
Western/Central
Europe
874,000

(4.8%)
Eastern Europe &
Central Asia
1,824,000

(2%)
East Asia & Pacific
912,000

(0.6%)
Caribbean
266,000

North Africa
& Middle East
418,000
(1%)

(12%)
South &
Southeast Asia
4,560,000

(4%)
Latin America
1,824,000

Africa
Sub-Saharan Africa } (67.8%)
25,764,000

(0.2%)
Oceania
76,000

*Totals are estimates for the entire globe, ending year 2012.

Total: 2012—38 million

FIGURE 10-8 End-of-Year 2012. Estimates of People Living with HIV Infection. Of the estimated 38 million alive ending 2012, about 96% are adult/adolescent, about 50% are men and about 50% women, with 3.6% under age 15. *(UNAIDS/WHO, 2010 updated)*

- Ending 2013 about 19 million men and 19 million women will be living with HIV infection.

- Ending year 2013, about 30 million people will have died of AIDS.

- 80% of those dying from AIDS are between ages 20 and 50. These are the people who enforce laws, harvest food, work the factories, heal the sick, and raise children.

- Ending 2020 between 36 and 46 million people will have died of AIDS. (about 4000/day)

- According to the WHO, AIDS deaths should peak in 2012 at about 2.5 million and decline to 1.2 million in 2030.

- The number of annual new HIV infections is projected to remain close to current levels through year 2035 (Bongaarts et al., 2008).

- If nothing changes, there will be an estimated 20 million to 30 million new HIV infections by 2020.

- Of 194 countries reporting on adults and children living with HIV/AIDS in 2008, 34 countries had over 100,000, 2 had over 300,000, and 1 had over 500,000 HIV/AIDS cases.

- Eighty percent of the world's cases of HIV are concentrated in the 22 countries with the largest TB epidemics.

- Ending 2013, about 1% of the world's population will be HIV infected.

- It is estimated that new HIV infections peaked in the mid 1990s, except for Africa, where HIV infections is expected to peak about 2025.

- The office of the United Nations program on HIV/AIDS (UNAIDS) provided two earlier initiatives: three million people on ART by 2005 and universal access to ART by 2010. Both failed.

Former Surgeon General C. Everett Koop has said on a number of occasions that "AIDS is virtually 100% fatal." Looking back over the

Population and HIV Infection Rates in Selected African Countries

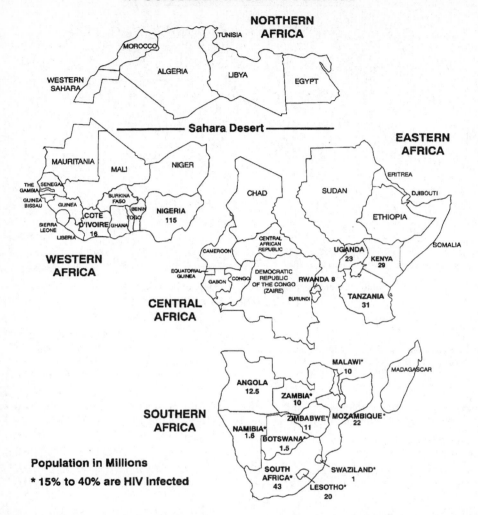

FIGURE 10-9   Map of Africa. Population of Africa = approximately 967 million. Population of sub-Saharan Africa = about 657 million. Prevalence of HIV infection and AIDS cases is highest in South Africa. South Africa with about 47 million people ending 2013 will have an estimated 5.8 million HIV-infected people, the highest incidence of HIV infection in the world. In seven African countries over 20% of the 15- to 19-year-old population is HIV infected, from 20% in South Africa to about 40% among adults in Botswana. The lifetime risk of dying from AIDS for a boy who is currently 15 is 65% in South Africa and near 90% in Botswana. Karen Stanecki of the U.S. Census Bureau reported that in KwaZulu-Natal, a province of South Africa, HIV infection has reached 46%. In Francistown, Botswana, HIV infection among adults is at 42%. Stanecki projected that AIDS deaths will peak in sub-Saharan Africa in 2020 at 6.5 million deaths/year; South Africa in 2010 at 940,000/year; Haiti in 2017 at 39,000/year; Thailand in 2000 at 66,000/year; Myanmar (Burma) in 2015 at 97,000/year; and Brazil in 2020 at 623,000/year. *(Map courtesy of Centers for Disease Control and Prevention)*

Notation: Based on the WHO/UNAIDS 07 AIDS Epidemic Update Report; Stanecki's numbers should be lowered by about 16% to 20%.

number of AIDS cases diagnosed and comparing them to the number of AIDS patients who have died would indicate that a diagnosis of AIDS before the advent of highly active antiretroviral therapy (ART) was a death sentence. Table 10-6, page 314 presents a sobering look at the numbers of AIDS patients who have died in America since those first CDC-reported cases in 1981. People with HIV/AIDS were, through 1995, dying at the rate of about 3000 a month. Over 95% of those diagnosed with AIDS in 1981 have now died.

GLOBAL PREVALENCE AND IMPACT OF HIV/AIDS (SEE TABLE 10-8)

However the impact of the disease is measured—by deaths, HIV infections, AIDS cases, or monetary losses—it is just beginning. The worldwide impact during the 1990s was 5 to 10 times that of the 1980s, and an increase in global impact will be felt, even with an available vaccine, through the next 30 to 50 years. As the pandemic continues, the United States will find itself progressively more involved with prevention/treatment programs and with the political changes that HIV/AIDS will bring about in countries with a high incidence of HIV/AIDS. (See PEPFAR discussion in Chapter 14, pages 456–457.)

Table 10-8 Estimated Prevalence of Adults Ages 15 to 49, Living with HIV/AIDS by Region Ending 2012[1]

Global	0.8%
Sub-Saharan Africa	5.0%
Caribbean	0.9%
E. Europe/Central Asia	0.9%
North America	0.6%
Latin America	0.4%
Oceania	0.3%
South/South-East Asia	0.3%
Middle East/North Africa	0.2%
Western/Central Europe	0.2%
East Asia	0.1%

[1] Total number living with HIV/AIDS, 38 million.
UNAIDS/WHO, 2010 Report on the Global Aids Epidemic, Updated.

CONNECTED BUT SEPARATE: EACH COUNTRY A DIFFERENT REALITY, DIFFERENT COUNTRIES, SIMILAR QUESTIONS, BUT DIFFERENT ANSWERS, DIFFERENT EPIDEMICS

Although all nations on earth are connected in so many ways, there remains a separation of the haves and have-nots—the developed and developing nations. Two worlds: one with hope and one with over 90% of all AIDS cases and orphans. (AIDS-associated orphans are presented in Chapter 11, pages 360–364.)

Africa, the HIV/AIDS Time Bomb: Ticking out of Control

Lindsay Knight, who edited the 2008 World Disaster Report, said, "The HIV and AIDS epidemic is a disaster whose scale and extent could have been prevented. Ignorance, stigma, political inaction, indifference, and denial all contributed to millions of deaths." Mobility and migration are adding further difficulties in the management of the disaster.

The first case of AIDS was identified in Africa in 1982. HIV/AIDS is almost too large a problem in Africa to fully grasp. Like the bubonic plague in Europe in the 14th century and the flu epidemic of 1918, the scale of the loss is staggering.

Africa, with about 10% of the world's population, now accounts for about 68% of all global HIV infections and for about 90% of all new HIV infections. Beginning 2013, about 75% of all AIDS deaths have occurred in Africa. The United Nations reported that in Africa's 25 worst affected countries, 7 million agricultural workers have died from AIDS since 1985 and 10 million more could die by 2020. Also, unless there is some immediate relief, by 2013, most Africans will not live to see their forty-eighth birthday. Stefano Vella, president of the International AIDS Society, said in 2002, "This pandemic is not stabilizing, it is just beginning, it's just a baby beginning to grow." As a comparison, Vella said that if the United States had in proportion the same HIV infection rate as Botswana, between 35% and 40%, there would be 40 million HIV infected in America. The world and especially Africa has been living with a biological terrorist for the past 31 years with no end in sight (1982 through 2013). AIDS will be in Africa for generations to come.

AIDS—The Modern Plague

By any and every measure, HIV/AIDS is a plague of biblical proportion. It is claiming more lives in Africa than in all the wars waging on the continent combined. AIDS is now the leading cause of death among all people of all ages in Africa, and the progression of this pandemic has outpaced all projections. Nearly all those currently HIV infected in Africa without drug therapy will die between year 2010 and 2015. In Botswana and Swaziland it is estimated that 60% of the population will die of AIDS over the next 20 years. With such overwhelming numbers, it is important to remember that the data are about people, not

numbers, and not facts and figures, but faces and families (see Figure 10-10, below).

The HIV/AIDS pandemic in Africa is like an explosion in slow motion, a slowly moving chain reaction—no sound, no blinding flash, no intense heat, no mushroom cloud, no buildings destroyed—just one silent death after another with no end in sight. Whole generations of people are in jeopardy with so little hope to go around in the developing nations.

UNAIDS 2000 Report

"HIV will kill at least a third of the young men and women of countries where it has its firmest hold, and in some places up to two-thirds. Despite millennia of epidemics, war and famine, never before in history have death rates of this magnitude been seen among young adults of both sexes and from all walks of life." If death rates continue, HIV/AIDS will kill more humans on the African continent than the 50 million who died on every front and

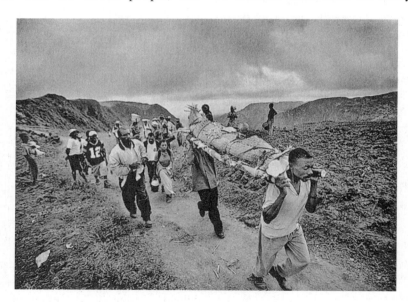

FIGURE 10-10 The Long Journey Home. Friends chant while carrying the body of their friend to his mother's home in Haiti. It is many miles up through the mountains to a small rural village where he grew up. He left home at the age of 15 to find work. He is now returned home for burial at age 28. *(Photo by Mike Stocker/ South Florida Sun-Sentinel)*

in death camps in World War II. It is estimated that between 50 million and 70 million Africans may die from AIDS by 2025. (Ending 2013, 30 million will have died.)

Life Expectancy

AIDS has sharply reduced life expectancy in 25 southern African countries, 8 Caribbean nations, and 7 members of the 12 ex-Soviet republics. For instance, in Botswana, where more than one-third of adults are infected with HIV, life expectancy is now 39 instead of 74, as it would have been without the disease. It is projected that ending 2010, life expectancy will be 27 in Botswana, 30 in Swaziland, 33 in Namibia and Zimbabwe, and 36 in South Africa, Malawi, Rwanda, and Lesotho. Without AIDS, it would have been around 70 in many of those countries. In the Central African Republic, Lesotho, Mozambique, Swaziland, Malawi, Zambia, and Zimbabwe, a child born in 2004 will not be expected to see his or her 40th birthday. More people died of AIDS each year from 1999 through 2012 in Africa than in all the wars on the continent during those years. About 1 in 30 people is HIV infected.

Sub-Saharan Africa: About 11% of the World's Population

The sheer number of Africans infected by HIV, about 4650 a day, is overwhelming. By the end of 2013, there will be about 25.5 million HIV-infected people living in the 45 countries of sub-Saharan Africa; 61% of them are women. About 68% of all people living with HIV live here, as well as 90% of all cases of mother-to-child HIV transmission cases. Also, an astonishing 75% of 15- to 24-year-olds are HIV infected! About 76% of all HIV/AIDS deaths occur here. In Rwanda, it is estimated that 80% of women are HIV positive, resulting from rape by Rwandan soldiers during the genocide of a million Tutsi and Hutu. In Botswana, Namibia, Swaziland, Zimbabwe, and Mozambique, current estimates show that between 15% and 40% of people aged 15 to 49 are living with HIV. In Zimbabwe, 30% to 50%

of all pregnant women are now found to be infected, and at least one-third of these women will pass the infection on to their babies. South Africa, which escaped much of the epidemic in the 1980s, is now being hit particularly hard.

South Africa: Population about 49 Million

Ending 2013 about 10 million South Africans will have been HIV infected. And, ending 2013 about 5.7 million South Africans, roughly one in eight to one in nine people (about one in four adults), will be living with HIV/AIDS—and dying from it. Some 700 people die each day, and about 1200 become HIV infected. It is estimated that there were 430,000 new HIV infections annually from 2006 through 2012. Estimates are that one in five or 20% of women ages 15 to 49 are HIV positive compared to 15.4% of men in the same age group. Seventeen percent of women ages 15 to 24 are HIV positive. There are about 300,000 pregnancies annually in HIV-positive women (about a third of all pregnancies). Over 200,000 children under age four are living with HIV. South Africa's new five-year plan, 2007 through 2011, was to halve HIV infections and provide antiretroviral therapy to 80% of all people with HIV. The plan failed. These expectations have now been moved to 2015. The cost of this plan exceeded South Africa's entire health budget by 20%; the largest cost was for antiretroviral drugs (40%). However, a study by Rochelle Walensky and colleagues (2007) revealed that even with the fastest rate of drug treatment in South Africa, about one million AIDS deaths would occur between mid-2007 and the end of 2011. [The actual number was closer to 1.5 million.] **This was a best-case scenario!** Estimates are that by the end of 2013, about 4.5 million South Africans will have died from HIV/AIDS.

About 70% of TB cases in South Africa are also coinfected with HIV. Many deaths of TB-infected people may be caused by HIV/AIDS, but they may not be counted as HIV/AIDS cases or AIDS deaths.

Military

In South Africa, according to *Johannesburg Mail and Guardian* newspaper, between 30% and 70% of the South African National Defense Force may be infected with HIV. In one unit in KwaZulu-Natal, 90% of troops are infected. Some military units near Pietermaritzburg and on the South African/Mozambique border had HIV infection rates higher than 70%. South Africa's military infection rate is similar to neighboring countries. In Malawi, 75% of the military is HIV positive, and in Mozambique, 80% have tested positive. Forces in the Democratic Republic of the Congo and Angola also have high rates of HIV infection. Militaries in sub-Saharan Africa, in general, have between 20% and 40% HIV-positive rates.

WORKFORCE—SOUTH AFRICA: SOME EXAMPLES

In 2006, a study by the International Labor Organization reported that worldwide 24 million workforce members ages 15 to 64 live with HIV/AIDS. About 67% of these infected workers live in Africa. Over 3,700,000 of the infected live in South Africa. The pandemic is taking a dramatic toll on the most productive members of the population, those in their 20s, 30s, and 40s. It has been estimated that 25% of "economically active people" in South Africa will die of AIDS between 2010 and 2015!

Mining

AngloGold, a gold mining company in South Africa, reported that about 30% of its 44,000 employees are already HIV positive.

Agriculture

About 30% to 45% of agriculture workers in South Africa are HIV positive, which could have a major effect on farm production in the coming years.

Nurses

An estimated 20% or 35,000 South African nurses are HIV positive. A Netcare group nursing manager recently told delegates that half of first-year students at one of the province's four nursing colleges are HIV positive. At another of the colleges, 70% of students are attending a local HIV clinic. At another, 21% of the students have volunteered information that they are HIV positive. In addition, 200 nurses a month are going abroad. The nursing manager said, "In our organization we are losing registered nurses. We are sitting with nurses who are dying now, and the students are even worse off."

EDUCATION: TEACHERS AND STUDENTS—SOUTH AFRICA AND SOME COUNTRIES IN SOUTHERN AFRICA

Senteza Kajubi, an education official in Africa, said that about 30 million girls in sub-Saharan Africa are out of school. And that out of 100 million children in the world who do not attend school, 44 million are from Africa, the majority being girls from the sub-Saharan region.

The Impact of HIV/AIDS on Teachers, Students, and School Systems

As many teachers die every year of HIV/AIDS as qualify to teach. School districts are exhausting their annual budgets within two months by transporting deceased teachers to their homes. There is widespread closure of schools because HIV/AIDS has stripped them of their teachers. These nightmare scenarios afflict Kenya, Zambia, Botswana, Mozambique, Uganda, the Central African Republic, and South Africa. The devastating impact of HIV/AIDS on teachers and learners was a repeated concern at a national policy conference on teacher training and development convened by the Department of Education in Midrand, Gauteng, South Africa. The conference also heard that there has been an incredible 85% decrease in the number of students in pre-service teacher education programs between 1994 and 2002. These alarming trends are being identified at a time when the need for effective and widespread teacher training has never been greater.

Nelson Mandela, former president of South Africa, said in September 2000 that in South Africa, 10 teachers die every month from AIDS and one student dies of AIDS each week in each of the country's 74 colleges and universities—roughly 120 teachers and 3600 students a year. About one in eight teachers is HIV positive. In Durban Westville University in South Africa, about 25% of students are HIV positive. The situation since then has become much worse. In 2004 and 2005 a total of about 8500 teachers died of AIDS with another 45,000 teachers HIV infected. About one-third are between ages 25 and 34. About 25% need antiretroviral drugs. In Kenya about 15,000 teachers are dying each year from AIDS. Also, one in five secondary students and one in five college students is HIV positive in Kenya. The prevalence of HIV infection in Kenya is about 5%.

Zambia, Swaziland, and Mozambique are losing about 130 teachers/month. Two teachers die for one graduate. So the teachers are not being replaced. The pool of uneducated becomes larger as does the number of students in the classrooms that continue. In Tanzania, it is estimated that by 2012, between 15,000 and 30,000 teachers will die of AIDS. To date, in sub-Saharan Africa, about 3 million students lost their teachers to AIDS over the past several years. Many schools have closed because of a teacher shortage. In KwaZulu-Natal province about 25% of teachers are HIV positive.

In parts of Malawi, Uganda, Botswana, and Zambia, over 30% of teachers are HIV positive. In the Central African Republic, 85% of teachers who died between 1996 and 1998 were HIV positive and died approximately 10 years before they were due to retire. In Mozambique 17% of teachers are HIV positive. And in Zimbabwe, about 30% of 80,000 teachers are HIV positive. These data mirror the 27% of HIV positives for Zimbabweans ages 18 to 49.

Burying the Dead

AIDS is the leading cause of death in South Africa. In 2002 through 2012, about 40% of all adult deaths were due to AIDS.

In Soweto, South Africa, as in many South African cities and towns, burying those dying from AIDS has become a daily chore. They used to bury the dead on Saturdays. Too many are dying. "There are so many funerals, it is chaos. We don't know which funeral to attend. On some days we attend three funerals. Which neighbor or which family member's funeral should we attend? We must choose."

In Kenya, the AIDS epidemic has entered a death phase in which more people are dying of AIDS each day than are becoming HIV infected. About 120,000 die annually while about 70,000 become infected. The country is sacrificing its forest for wood to build coffins. The disappearance of the forest is becoming an environmental disaster. The solution, said the environmental minister, is to use biodegradable plastic or synthetic coffins. For now, relatives are cementing wooden coffins into the ground to prevent thieves from stealing them and reselling them; the use of less valuable plastic coffins would discourage such theft.

As AIDS continues to claim the country's young, it has transformed black neighborhoods into open-air funeral parlors and neighbors into widows, orphans, and grieving relatives. (Read Sidebar 10.1, page 330.)

OTHER HIV/AIDS TIME BOMBS IN ASIA: INDIA, CHINA, AND RUSSIA

Over the past eight years, 2005 through 2012, the number of people living with HIV increased in every region in the world. The most striking increases have occurred in East Asia, Eastern Europe, and Central Asia. Asia, made up of at least 37 nations, with 60% of the world's population, is now home to over 5 million people living with HIV/AIDS. About 300,000 people died of AIDS in the region in 2012 and about 500,000 became newly infected. Globally, one in five new HIV infections occurs in Asia. Another 5 million could be infected by 2020. HIV/AIDS in Asia is driven by three high-risk behaviors: unsafe commercial sex, injection-drug users, and unsafe sex among gay men. In many Asian countries, adult men who pay for sex and their female

DEATH IN SUB-SAHARAN AFRICA: A GROWING INDUSTRY

BURIAL CHANGES BECAUSE OF TOO MANY AIDS DEATHS IN ZAMBIA

AIDS has changed the way people live. Now it is changing the way they are buried. As the AIDS toll rises, Zambia's local government authorities complain that burial ground is being filled up almost as soon as it is designated. Zambians are being encouraged to look at cremation as a burial option. This has elicited serious debate. Zambians are by nature a very superstitious people who fear changes in cultural practices. University of Zambia's Department of History Professor Yizenge Chondoka says to shift people's thinking from burial to cremation will be hard. There are certain rites that can only be performed at graveyards to complete the burial process and ensure that the spirit of the buried is at peace. Chondoka says Zambians have shrines at burial sites where they consult the spirits of the dead in times of need. "If we begin to cremate and throw or keep ashes in small clusters in our houses, where will the shrines be put up?" Lusaka has three designated cemeteries (besides unofficial ones), which can take about 10,000 graves, but these are already full, and people are now squeezing their dead on what used to be thoroughfares.

BURIAL ECONOMICS

Then there is the problem of economics. A teacher at the Zambian School of Education asks, "Do we really want valuable land to be taken up by graves?" Death in Africa is a very public affair. Funerals are big social events at which grief is expressed openly and lavishly. Families take large spaces in newspapers to announce the death of a loved one, complete with a picture, lists of achievements, and names of children. Now, about half the faces staring out of the public death notices are young. They have died of AIDS. But in contrast to the public rites of death, this increasingly frequent cause goes whispered or unmentioned. AIDS is a taboo subject in Africa. At the rate they are dying from AIDS, three-quarters of Zambia will be a graveyard. There must be another way of disposing of their dead.

FUNERALS ARE BANKRUPTING FAMILIES IN AFRICA

A 2004 study by the Joint Economics, AIDS and Poverty Program of the University of KwaZulu-Natal in Durban stated that the average cost of a traditional funeral in South Africa is about $4900,

while the annual household income in South Africa is $3630. The Health Economics and AIDS Research Division of the university estimates that people in Swaziland spend up to $980 on funerals, even though two-thirds of the population live below the poverty line. In Botswana, families typically spend $740 to $920 on funerals, while the average monthly salary for a working class person is $55.

THE FUNERAL INDUSTRY—SOUTH AFRICA

Rising death rates in South Africa due to HIV/AIDS have led to the creation of a makeshift funeral industry. Many fly-by-night undertakers, who are unlicensed and operate out of storefronts, compete to make funeral arrangements and leave bodies to decompose while they search for the cheapest means of disposal, creating a health hazard and raising costs to the government. The problem is greatest in Durban, capital of the hard-hit KwaZulu-Natal province. Morgues and cemeteries have run out of room, and the unlicensed undertakers are tempted to cut corners by mishandling bodies—burying them in mass graves or abandoning them in mortuaries. The government has not regulated the new undertakers (who are mainly black) because they were previously disadvantaged, but established funeral directors (mostly white and Indian) complain that the new undertakers should be subject to the same regulations. The newcomers said they are subcontractors for licensed morticians—they sell coffins and transport the body for burial while a licensed mortician washes, dresses, and stores the body. Sometimes licensed morticians front for the newcomers by picking up bodies at morgues for a fee, a violation of health regulations. This corpse shell game often results in bodies being moved several times or left to decompose. As AIDS deaths rise, the problem will only worsen. But talk of the rising death rate is all but taboo among government officials who, taking their cue from former President Thabo Mbeki, barely acknowledge the extent of the HIV/AIDS epidemic or the rising death toll. What to do with bodies in Africa is becoming a massive problem!

THE CASKET/BURIAL PLOT INDUSTRY—ZIMBABWE

Griffin Shea reported on the demand for caskets and burial plots in Zimbabwe. Deep in the shadow of Harare's office high-rises, Luck Street is mostly islands of pavement in a river of mud and potholes. Despite its name, this side street in Zimbabwe's capital is where the city's least fortunate residents make their most lasting purchases, a casket or coffin. With an economy in free fall and over 3000 people dying of AIDS every week, coffin-making has become one of the country's few reliable sources of income. In outlying townships, vendors line up caskets for sale next to tables of fruits and vegetables on the dusty roadside. But if you're on a budget—and almost everyone in Zimbabwe is—Luck Street is where you go for a bargain. At Sunshine Funeral Service, a darkened room behind a motorcycle repair shop, the owner and salesperson shows off his company's entire line of caskets, from a pressed-wood model that sells for about $15 to polished hardwood with shiny brass handles, $130. For about 30 cents per mile, the enterprising owners of Sunshine Funeral will send corpses back to their hometowns for burial.

According to Harare's director of cemeteries, 8 of the city's 10 cemeteries are full. So the city is clearing 5 square miles of land to expand one of its cemeteries on the outskirts, where most of the graves will be dusty plots in the bare earth.

THE COFFIN INDUSTRY IN MALAWI

Coffin and casket shops line a quarter-mile-long stretch of road like a funeral train waiting for Malawians to die from a brew of poverty, infectious diseases, and AIDS, especially AIDS—60,000 AIDS deaths a year. The name of the street is Lubani Road but it is better known as Coffin Road. Life expectancy has now fallen below age 38. Twelve million people live in Malawi with one million being HIV infected. It is one of the poorest countries in the world.

partners make up the largest group of people living with HIV/AIDS. It is estimated that 10 million women in Asia sell sex to about 75 million men. Men having sex with men and injection-drug use places another 10 million men at high risk for HIV infection. The most worrying aspect of the pandemic in Asia is the sharp increase in HIV infections in China, Indonesia, and Vietnam, which together have nearly 50% of Asia's population. China and India, with 2.3 billion people between them, still have low national HIV prevalence rates—0.1% in China and about 0.3% in India—but they have serious epidemics in a number of provinces, territories, and states. Asia is a large part of the global economy. The greater the impact of HIV/AIDS in Asia, the greater the impact globally.

India: 35 States and Territories. Population about 1.2 Billion

If by 2020 just 2% of India's one billion plus population is HIV infected, that would be 20 million people (over twice the population of New York City). UNAIDS reports that about 2.5 million Indians are already infected and the virus is spreading rapidly in that country, primarily through heterosexual activities and injection-drug use.

The first case of AIDS was described in India in 1986. India is a vast, heterogeneous country. Eighty percent of the people live in the countryside where many have never heard of HIV or AIDS. Yet, about 60% of the HIV infected live in the countryside or rural areas. Some local authorities even challenge the existence of HIV or AIDS. Although it is believed that 86% of HIV infections occur through heterosexual intercourse with an infected partner, it is estimated that there will be between 1 million and 2 million HIV infections among female sex workers, their clients, and their families ending 2013.

China: Population About 1.3 Billion

In China, HIV is present in all 31 provinces, autonomous regions, and municipalities, but epidemic patterns are different in different parts of the country.

In August 2001, the deputy health minister held a first-ever news conference on the HIV/AIDS problem in China. Ending 2012, China's health minister reported an estimated cumulative 893,000 cases of people living with HIV/AIDS. Of these, about 175,000 are living with AIDS, and about 60,000 have died. Sexual transmission accounted for about 75% of new cases, and 30.5% of cases were female. These numbers could be much higher, as these data came only from Chinese medical facilities. China hopes to cap the number of people living with HIV/AIDS at 1.2 million by 2015.

The first AIDS case in China was in an IDU discovered in the Yunnan province near the Burmese border in 1985. Since then HIV has spread rapidly among IDUs across China. Currently about 70% of China's IDUs are HIV positive. Eighty percent of total reported AIDS cases are among IDUs and prostitutes. Approximately 2% occurred via mother-to-child transmission. Women make up 28% of the total infected population. Although data relating to HIV transmission among gay men is limited, once HIV becomes established in this population the HIV problem in China will become much more serious, because there are an estimated 5 million to 10 million gay men in China.

HIV/AIDS: China's Titanic Peril—A current survey[1] finds that most of China's population does not know what causes AIDS or how to prevent it—and 17% or 1 in 6 respondents had never heard of HIV or AIDS! Of respondents who had heard of HIV and AIDS, 73% did not know it is a virus, and 89% did not know how it can be detected. Of those respondents who knew that HIV can be transmitted, 22% could not identify a single route of transmission. But 48% thought HIV could be transmitted by mosquitoes. Over 77% did not know that condoms offer protection, and 83% did not know infection could be avoided by not sharing injection needles. Among those least likely to be knowledgeable about HIV/AIDS were the poorest and least educated, women and farmers.

Zeng Yi, chief scientist with the sexually transmitted infection and AIDS Prevention Center of the Ministry of Health, said in mid-2006 that HIV/AIDS is expected to cost China's economy nearly $40 billion over the

next five years, mostly because of lost labor as people become sick of AIDS-related illnesses.

Over the seven years 2006–2012, China's government reacted to its HIV/AIDS challenge by providing routine HIV testing of at-risk groups, free antiretroviral drugs, and safer sex campaigns and needle exchange centers for injection-drug users.

Good News for China

According to UNAIDS, over the past 8 years (2005-2012), AIDS-related deaths, because of ART, dropped about 60% and new infections by about 68%! By 2015 condom vending machines will be available in 95% of the hotels and other public areas.

Russia: Population About 138 Million

Russia has the largest HIV epidemic in Eastern Europe and accounts for about 66% of HIV/AIDS cases in Eastern Europe and Central Asia. HIV came to Russia in 1987 through sex between gay men—a practice that was then illegal, making the disease unspeakable. But even as the numbers grew rapidly in the mid-1990s, primarily through intravenous-drug use, few people paid attention. In his January 2002 address to the nation, Russian president Vladimir Putin spoke about the nation's overall health crisis but made no specific mention of HIV or AIDS. Peter Piot, former executive director of the United Nations AIDS Programs (UNAIDS) said in April 2002 that "Russia now has the fastest growing epidemic in the world, and I believe that the situation in Russia and the CIS (group of 12 ex-Soviet republics) is rapidly getting out of control." If the current rate of infection continues, estimates are that about 2.2 million Russians will be infected beginning 2013. By 2025 between 4 million and 8 million will have died of AIDS. The major route of HIV transmission in Russia is through IDU and sex workers. Beginning 2005, about one-third of all new HIV infections resulted from heterosexual intercourse. Victor Molotilov and colleagues reported in 2006 that about 2% of Russia's

[1](The survey, "Current HIV/AIDS-Related Knowledge, Attitudes, and Practices Among the General Population in China: Implications for Action," was published on AIDScience.org (www.aidscience.org/articles/aidscience028.asp), a website run by the journal *Science*.)

population injects drugs, with 65% of them being HIV positive. An estimated 5% to 8% of all men under age 30 have injected drugs. The age group most affected, as it is globally, is between ages 15 and 30. Half are under age 20. A major problem for Russia is that with this pandemic affecting the younger generations, Russia's shrinking population of about 139 million people will continue to fall.

In late 2006, Russia formed a National Advisory Council on AIDS. Former president Putin referred to the issue for the first time in his annual state-of-the-nation address in the spring of 2007! By then, Vadim Pokhrovsky, Russia's head of the federal AIDS center, said about 1.3 million Russians were HIV infected. And of the estimated 40,000 newly infected, 44% were women. The HIV prevalence among sex workers is about 16% and among MSM between 8% and 9%. On average, one in every 50 males is HIV positive. The worst affected areas are St. Petersburg followed by the Sverdlovsk region, then the Samara region of Moscow, Irkutsk, Leningrad, and Khanty-Mansiysk areas.

From 2009 through 2012, each year, about 23 million people were HIV tested, with about 50,000 a year found HIV positive. From 2004 through 2012 the Global Fund to Fight AIDS, Tuberculosis, and Malaria gave Russia over $330 million for prevention, treatment, and care. In 2012 there were about 62,000 new HIV infections in Russia. It is estimated that Russia through 2013 will have over 1.2 million living HIV-infected people. About 25% will be receiving ART.

In April 2011, President Dmitry Medvedev acknowledged that a growing epidemic of drug abuse threatens Russia's future. He said that drug use is contributing up to a 3% annual economic decline in Russia, home to the world's third highest rate of heroin use and one-third of all heroin-related deaths. According to the World Health Organization, heroin use is driving the country's fast-growing HIV/AIDS epidemic. Health experts have been critical of the government's refusal to consider harm-reduction approaches such as methadone replacement therapy or needle exchanges. The Geneva-based International AIDS Society predicts HIV infections in Russia could grow between 5% and 10% annually unless the government takes appropriate action. Medvedev said Russian children as young as 11 were using drugs. "In spite of the fact that heightened attention is given to this topic…changes for better have been very, very few."

The Global Fund has helped finance Russia's program to fight AIDS for the past 8 years but will stop ending year 2012. Russia has set a side $600 million for HIV/AIDS in 2012 but only 3% of this will go toward prevention! Nothing for needle exchange programs.

Summary

In 1981, the CDC reported the first case of AIDS in the United States, and, from that time onward, has constantly tracked the prevalence of AIDS cases in different geographical areas and within different behavioral risk groups. In all behavioral risk groups, the common denominator is the exchange of body fluids, in particular blood or semen. The heterosexual population at large is considered to be at low risk for HIV infection in the United States. By 1993, all states and the District of Columbia, Puerto Rico, and the Virgin Islands reported AIDS cases in people who had heterosexual contact with an at-risk partner.

A major problem exists in attempting to determine the number of HIV-infected people. Several different approaches have been used by the CDC to estimate the total number of HIV infections. These estimates can be evaluated by examining their compatibility with available prevalence data.

With respect to race and ethnicity, the cumulative incidence of AIDS cases is disproportionately higher in blacks and Hispanics than in whites. The ratio of black to white case incidence is 3.2:1 and the Hispanic to white ratio 2.8:1. This racial/ethnic disproportion is also observed in HIV-positive blood donors and in applicants for military service. Even among homosexual and bisexual men and IDUs, where race/ethnicity-specific data are available, blacks appear to have higher seroprevalence rates than whites.

With regard to prostitution, in a large multicenter study of female prostitutes, black and Hispanic prostitutes had a higher rate of HIV infection than white and other prostitutes. This disproportion existed for both prostitutes who used injection drugs and those who did not acknowledge injection-drug use.

The risk of new HIV infections in hemophiliacs and in people who receive blood transfusions has declined dramatically from 1985 because of the screening of donated blood and heat treatment of clotting factor concentrates. Evidence also indicates an appreciable risk of new infections in MSM, in IDUs, and in their heterosexual partners.

There are some 5.3 million healthcare workers in the United States. Even though they are supposed to adhere to Universal Protection Guidelines set down by the CDC for their protection, a significant number are exposed to HIV annually. A relatively small number of those infected have progressed to AIDS.

Estimating the number of HIV-infected people in the United States continues to be a numbers game. Various agencies and private industries have, for different reasons, attempted to determine the number of HIV-infected people. The numbers from the different groups vary widely. However, the 2007 estimated numbers of 1 to 1.5 million HIV-infected people may be too low.

Ending year 2013, with about 1.63 million people living with HIV infection in the United States and with about 56,000 new infections estimated to occur each year from 2010 through the year 2013, the face of AIDS in America has changed. It's a younger and older face than it used to be. It's more likely to be a face of color than it used to be. And it is more likely to be female than it used to be. More people with HIV and AIDS are from areas outside major cities. Overall, the number of new AIDS cases appears to be leveling. But the HIV epidemic should be viewed as many different epidemics in different stages that vary according to age, race, gender, and locality. Although gay and bisexual men continue to make up the largest portion of new HIV infections, the epidemic is increasing more rapidly among people who become infected through heterosexual contact and through sharing injection-drug equipment.

CDC RELEASES ATLAS TOOL TO MAP, CHART U.S. HIV/AIDS SURVEILLANCE DATA (JANUARY 2012)

The Atlas currently includes options to:

- Create interactive maps, tables, pie charts, bar graphs.
- Allow two-way HIV data stratifications and three-way STD data stratifications.

- Display data trends over time and patterns across the United States or in specific communities.
- Download and export data and graphics.
- Access routinely reported surveillance data through a standardized user interface.
- View, filter, explore, and extract public health information.
- Crete detailed disease data reports and maps.
- Submit ad hoc requests for customizable reports.
- Receive detailed and complete information on surveillance data footnotes and caveats.

A video tutorial has been recorded and is available at www.cdc.gov/nchhstp/atlas.

Review Questions

(Answers to the Review Questions are on page 463.)

1. Looking back, in what year was "AIDS" first recognized by the CDC?
   A. 1972
   B. 1959
   C. 1982
   D. 1995
   E. 1981

2. Why are people placed in potential HIV risk groups?

3. True or False: The time it takes for HIV-infected people to become AIDS patients is different for each ethnic group, risk group, and exposure route. Explain.

4. What percentage of all U.S. HIV-infected IDUs are in the New York–New Jersey region?

5. What is the rate of college students currently HIV infected? Is this more or less than the rate for military personnel? Explain.

6. Compare the college student rate of HIV infection with the rate of HIV infection for the general U.S. population.

7. What is the risk of a healthcare worker converting to seropositivity after exposure to HIV-contaminated blood?

8. What single job-related event causes the greatest risk of HIV infection among healthcare workers?

9. Are healthcare workers more apt to become infected with the hepatitis B virus or the AIDS virus?

10. Worldwide, it is estimated that _____ AIDS patients will have died by the end of 2013; _____ in the United States.

11. Data on AIDS deaths indicated that of AIDS patients diagnosed between 1981 through 2013, in the United States, _____ % will have died.

12. Ending 2013, how many people in the world are estimated to be living with HIV?

13. Worldwide, about how many people were newly infected with HIV in 2013?

14. Does the drop in the global annual number of AIDS cases mean that AIDS is under control?

15. Based on the recent epidemiology of HIV in the United States, in what group are new cases of HIV infection rising the fastest?

 1. Men who have sex with men (MSM)
 2. Injection drug users (IDUs)
 3. Heterosexual women
 4. Some other group

Prevalence of HIV Infection and AIDS Cases among Women and Children

CHAPTER HIGHLIGHTS

- Women comprise about 52% of the US population.

- Annual International Women's Day—March 8.

- Annual National Women and Girls HIV/AIDS Awareness Day—March 10.

- A global estimate of HIV-positive women is presented.

- In proportion there are significantly more black and Hispanic women with HIV/AIDS than white women.

- Injection-drug use is a major route of HIV infection for women.

- From 1994 through 2012 at least 38% of women infected in the United States contracted HIV from men through sexual intercourse.

- Injection-drug use and prostitution are strongly associated with HIV infection.

- AIDS in the United States is the leading cause of death for black women ages 25 to 34 and the sixth for all women in this age group.

- The only diseases killing more women than AIDS are cancer and heart disease.

- First 100,000 AIDS cases in women in the United States were documented in December 1997.

- Ending 2013 about 26% of all HIV-infected adults/adolescents in the United States will be women.

- About 30% of all new HIV infections in the United States are in women (18,000 to 19,000 per year).

- In the United States, about every 30 to 35 minutes a woman tests HIV positive and about 26% of people living with HIV/AIDS are women! (About 439,000 ending 2013.)

- Ending 2013 women will make up about 26% of all U.S. AIDS cases and about 26% of new AIDS diagnoses.

- Black American women make up 13% of the female population but made up about 68% of HIV infections and 67% of AIDS cases in 2002 through 2012.

- In the United States, about 70% of new AIDS cases among women now occur among those ages 30 to 49, 18% among those ages 20 to 29, and 12% among women over age 50.

- Questions that every HIV-postive woman should ask her physician.

- November 20, 2013, marks the 25th anniversary of Universal Children's Day.

- Women now make up about 52% of worldwide HIV positives and about 52% of those living with HIV/AIDS.

- It is estimated that 98% of HIV-infected women of all ages live in developing countries. Sixty-seven percent live in sub-Saharan Africa.

- Worldwide, an estimated 15 million women will have died of AIDS and about 20 million will be living with HIV/AIDS ending 2013.
- Worldwide, women account for 58% of AIDS cases among people ages 13 to 19.
- In 2009 the World Health Organization (WHO) announced that HIV/AIDS was the leading cause of death among women ages 15 to 44 worldwide.
- World Health Organization says that more women ages 15 to 49 will die or become ill because of HIV than from any other disease.
- Of an estimated 2 million adult/adolescent AIDS deaths worldwide in 2012, about half were women.
- The Southern AIDS Living Quilt was launched in October 2008.
- Pediatric means under age 13 in the United States and under age 15 in Canada and most underdeveloped nations.
- About 99% of new pediatric AIDS cases received the virus from their HIV-infected mothers.
- HIV-positive perinatal children have successfully cleared HIV from their bodies.
- In proportion there are significantly more black and Hispanic pediatric AIDS cases than whites.
- Estimated number of pediatric AIDS cases through 2012: 16,877 of which over 6,000 have died.
- Perinatal HIV infection without anti-HIV drug intervention in the United States is about 25%; with drug intervention it is about 8%. With drugs and cesarean section it is less than 2%.
- Not all newborns who test HIV positive are HIV infected.
- About 300,000 children under age 15 became HIV infected in 2002 worldwide and in each year through 2012.
- UNAIDS calls for the elimination of mother-to-child HIV transmission by 2015.
- It is estimated that about 90% of HIV-infected children live in sub-Saharan Africa.
- By year 2020, there will be an estimated 35 million HIV/AIDS-related orphans under age 15 in 23 underdeveloped countries.

WOMEN AND HIV/AIDS

Once upon a time, those words were seldom found in a sentence together. In the early 1990s, the AIDS activist group ACT UP made a T-shirt that read: "Say It: Women Get AIDS" because so few people beyond the HIV community knew that women could get HIV. Over time, things have changed dramatically, and in November 2009 the World Health Organization (WHO) announced that HIV/AIDS is now the leading cause of disease and death among women of childbearing age (15 to 44) worldwide (that's been true in the United States since 1995 for African American women between the ages of 25 and 44). Yet despite these staggering statistics, much of the world still misperceives HIV/AIDS as a disease that only happens to men. And this misperception—along with a variety of other social, biological, psychological, political, and economic factors—contributes to the rapid spread of HIV/AIDS among women and teenage girls.

It is a little-remembered fact that the first cases of AIDS occurring in women were reported before the often-cited initial 1981 publication detailing the presentation of *Pneumocystis jiroveci* pneumonia in gay men residing in Los Angeles and New York City.

HIV/AIDS IS DEFINING THE LIVES OF MANY MILLIONS OF WOMEN

The pandemic of HIV/AIDS is growing more rapidly in women than in men in almost every part of the world. The growing proportion of infected women reflects the cumulative effect of many risks. They include the inability of many women to require their partners to use condoms, the infidelity of husbands and the high-risk behavior of sexual partners, the exploitation of young women by older men, and rape and other forms of sexual coercion. Ending 2013, there will be about 20 million women over the age of 15 living with HIV/AIDS in the world, of whom only a fraction have access to anti-retroviral drug therapy. And each year, since 1999, about 1.15 million of these women have died of HIV/AIDS.

In the nine most heavily infected countries in Africa, 59% of adult women and nearly 75% of young women are infected with HIV. In some African countries, young women are four to 13 times more likely to be HIV infected than young men. These figures represent the feminization of the epidemic. In hard-hit areas, it is undoing developmental gains for women. Among other things, this feminization reflects the reality that the HIV-related needs of women are not being addressed in national responses to HIV. It also reflects the fact that age-old, widespread discrimination and violence against women makes them extremely vulnerable to HIV infection and to the impact of AIDS.

United Nations Special Envoy on AIDS in Africa Elizabeth Mataka said that "globally, only 38% of females can demonstrate accurate and sufficient knowledge about ways to protect themselves from acquiring HIV." In addition about 70% of women worldwide are forced to have unprotected sex! The UN had targeted a 95% HIV/AIDS awareness by 2010. It failed. In 2009, the World Health Organization (WHO) reported from the results of its first worldwide study of women's health that more women ages 15 to 45 will die or become ill from HIV than from any other pathogen (disease-causing agent).

FEMALE VULNERABILITY TO HIV

A woman's vulnerability to HIV infection is in direct proportion to her lack of control over the risk of infection. Globally, the vast majority of women with HIV/AIDS became infected through heterosexual intercourse, frequently in settings where saying no to sex or insisting on condom use is not an option because of cultural factors, lack of financial independence, and even the threat of violence. These issues compel science and society to develop HIV prevention tools that women can use in situations when negotiating with sexual partners is difficult or impossible. Further, there has never been a prevention message for women. Instructions to abstain or to be faithful or to wear a condom don't work in the growing number of places where the single greatest risk of HIV infection is to be a married, monogamous woman. These instructions speak to the realities of most men's lives and, in fact, require their consent. There is virtually nowhere on the planet that a woman's right to safe sex and autonomous decision making over sexuality are as respected as those of men.

Of the people who live in abject poverty, nearly 70% are women. Women perform two-thirds of the world's work, earn less than 5% of its income, and own less than 1% of its property. Three of every four illiterate adults are women, and two-thirds of children denied primary education are girls.

EVERY DAY A TRAGEDY

Every single day HIV-infected women somewhere in the world are thrown out of their homes, beaten, cheated, lied to, deceived, stoned, scorned, or attempt suicide to escape the stigma associated with being HIV positive. In one recent case, in South Africa, a 25-year-old woman was arrested for allegedly hacking her nine-month-old son to death with an axe and attempting suicide after they both tested HIV positive. She was frightened of what her husband and neighbors would say or do. In Zambia, a man said, "I might transmit the disease to my wife, then tell my wife to go for an AIDS checkup. If she is found positive, I blame it on her and tell the whole community that she has infected me."

TRIPLE JEOPARDY

In the face of the HIV/AIDS pandemic, women worldwide face a triple jeopardy. They are at risk as individuals, as mothers, and as family caretakers. They face violence, discrimination, abandonment, and stigma.

For example, a national survey performed by the American Foundation for AIDS Research (AMFAR) and released in 2008 revealed the following disturbing results regarding stigma against HIV positive women: Of almost 5000 individuals polled, approximately 70% would not want an HIV-positive female dentist; 60% would not want an HIV-positive female physician or childcare provider; and 50% would not want an HIV-positive female food server. Only 14% of Americans polled felt that HIV-positive women should have children. This is less than the percentage of Americans who felt that women with schizophrenia or Down syndrome should have children, at 17% and 19%, respectively.

ANNUAL INTERNATIONAL WOMEN'S DAY—MARCH 8

The world is also starting to grasp that there is no policy more effective in promoting development, health, and education than the empowerment of women and girls.

Kofi Annan, Former U.N. Secretary General

Women and Society

Women play a central role in society, and the benefits are apparent: Families are healthier and better fed, savings and income rise, and a supportive environment is created. Take away women's ability to fulfill these roles and entire societies fall apart. March 8 marks the annual celebration of International Women's Day. The Charter of the United Nations, signed in San Francisco in 1945, was the first international agreement to proclaim gender equality as a fundamental human right. Since then, International Women's Day has assumed a global dimension for women in developed and developing countries alike.

International Women's Day is used as a time to reflect on progress made, to call for change, and to celebrate acts of courage and determination by ordinary women who have played extraordinary roles in the history of women's rights.

The global HIV/AIDS pandemic will be 32 years old in mid-2013. Ending 2013 there will be an estimated 68 million HIV-infected people, about 50% to 52% of whom are women (Figure 11-1, page 340). The face of AIDS has changed rapidly over this time span. It has been said that "a woman's work is invisible until it is not done." In 2012 another million families realized the truth of this quotation after losing a female relative to HIV/AIDS. How many more women will be lost and families traumatized ending 2013 and beyond?

WOMEN: AIDS AND HIV INFECTIONS WORLDWIDE

The Growing Gender Disparity of HIV/AIDS

In 1999 it was estimated that worldwide half of AIDS cases were women.

Globally through 2013, women, children, and teenagers are in the middle of the HIV/AIDS pandemic (Table 11-1, page 340).

In Africa one in 10 women contracts HIV by age 16. In sub-Saharan Africa, 67% of the HIV-positive adults are women. In parts of Latin America and the Caribbean, the proportion has reached as high as 43%, and this figure is on the rise. This alarming development must be recognized by concerned parties as a central consideration in the design of strategies to halt the spread of the disease worldwide.

Figures from UNAIDS show that the risk of infection is increasing for women everywhere—in developed and developing countries alike.

In sub-Saharan Africa, the *ratio of women to men* infected with HIV/AIDS is currently about 10:6. In Rakai and Masaka, rural districts of Uganda, of women ages 15 to 25, 70% were HIV infected. When compared with HIV-infected young men of the same villages and age group, there was a female-to-male ratio of 6:1. In Rwanda and Tanzania, the infection rate of women under age

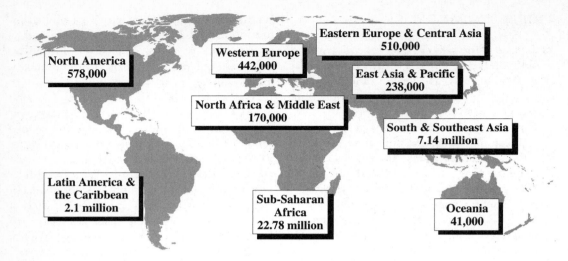

FIGURE 11-1 Estimated Global Total: 34 Million HIV-Positive Women Ending 2013. At the end of 1993, women made up an estimated 8 million HIV cases. Ending year 2013, over 52% of all HIV positives worldwide will be women. About 15 million will have died and about 19 million women of all ages will be living with HIV/AIDS ending 2013. Ending 2008 UNAIDS estimated that in sub-saharan Africa there were about 11 million women living with HIV/AIDS. Ending 2013 that number will be about 15.3 million.

25 to men under 25 is 2:1. The female-to-male ratio of AIDS cases among Ethiopian teenagers is 3:1; in Zimbabwe, it is 5:1. In Brazil, the ratio of female-to-male infection in Sao Paulo is 1.8 to 1. In Northern Thailand, 72% of sex workers are HIV infected. By the year 2004, about 90% of

HIV transmission worldwide was associated with heterosexual intercourse.

ASIA-PACIFIC REGION, OVER FIVE MILLION HIV POSITIVE

UNAIDS released a report from the Ninth International Congress on HIV/AIDS in Asia and the Pacific. This report shows the impact HIV infections are having on women in the region. Over 1.3 million, or 35%, of these women have been infected by their sexual partners and 50 million more are at risk. The women most at risk are those who are married or are in long-term relationships with men who engage in high-risk sexual behaviors: men who have sex with men, injection-drug users, or clients of sex workers.

Women Are Biologically More Vulnerable to HIV Infection

Women are biologically more vulnerable to HIV infection than men because HIV in semen

Table 11-1 Estimated: Women as Percentage of Adults (over Age 15) Living with HIV/AIDS by Region, Entering 2013

Region	Percent
Global	52%
Sub-Saharan Africa	67%
Caribbean	56%
North Africa/Middle East	48%
Latin America	33%
Eastern Europe/Central Asia	49%
South/Southeast Asia	35%
North America	26%
Western Europe	30%
Asia	32%
Oceania	46%

(Source: WHO/UNAIDS AIDS Epidemic Update, 2009 updated*)*

is in higher concentration than in vaginal and cervical secretions and because the vaginal area has a much larger mucosal area for exposure to HIV than the penis.

Gender Transmission of HIV

Transmission of HIV from male to female is about three times more effective than from female to male (World Health Organization, 1994). Paradoxically, since time immemorial women have been blamed for the spread of sexually transmitted diseases. Among certain peoples in Thailand and Uganda, sexually transmitted diseases (STDs) are known as "women's diseases." In Swahili, the language of much of East Africa, the word for STD means, literally, "disease of woman." Also, it is not coincidental that the countries in which HIV is now spreading fastest heterosexually are generally those in which women's status is low. (See Box 11.1, page 342.)

The World Health Organization estimated that globally, during 2005 through 2012, about two women died and two become HIV infected every minute. According to the World Health Organization, in 2006, 30% of women ages 15 to 17 in Lesotho were HIV positive. In Swaziland about 53% of pregnant women ages 25 to 29 were HIV positive. The prevalence of HIV infection in Swaziland's population is at 26%. Stephen Lewis, former UN Special Envoy for AIDS in Africa, said, "Lesotho and Swaziland are but symbols of the greater whole: that we are losing millions of young women in Africa. If there was a powerful international force for women, we would not be in this galling predicament." (See Point of Information 11.1, page 343.)

WOMEN: HIV-POSITIVE AND AIDS CASES—UNITED STATES

March 10, 2013, marks the nineteenth National Women and Girls HIV/AIDS Awareness Day. This day of recognition serves to raise awareness of the increasing impact of HIV/AIDS on women of all ages in the United States and throughout the world. In the early days of the pandemic, relatively few women were infected with HIV. Today, however, women represent one of the fastest-growing groups affected by HIV/AIDS. In the United States about every 30 to 35 minutes a woman tests HIV positive and about one in four people (26%) living with HIV/AIDS is a woman!

Women most at risk are ethnic minorities and the economically disadvantaged. Among sexually active teenagers, college students, and healthcare workers nationwide, nearly 60% of the heterosexual spread of HIV is among women (Pfeiffer, 1991).

HIV/AIDS in women is a tragedy, but in addition, women are the major source of infection in infants. From 1993 through 2012, over 98% of HIV-infected children aged 0 to 4 years got the virus from their mothers.

At the end of 1988, women made up about 6964 or 9% of the total adult AIDS cases in the United States. By the end of 2013 it is estimated that women will account for about 299,967 AIDS cases or about 21% of all AIDS cases in the United States (Table 11-2, page 343). About 75% of all female AIDS cases have been reported in the 18 years between 1995 and the end of 2012. They have been reported from all 50 states and territories. About 67% of these females are between the ages of 13 and 39 (HIV/AIDS Surveillance, 1997 updated). (See Point of Information 11.2, page 345.) Black and Hispanic women account for about 80% of U.S. AIDS cases among women but represent only about 30% of the U.S. female population over the age of 18. Ending 2013, at age 18 and over, there will be about 83.5 million white females, about 16.5 million black females, and about 17.3 million Hispanic or Latina females in the United States (Figures 11-2, page 344; 11-3, page 346).

When the AIDS pandemic first hit the United States in 1981, gay men were the first population to be deeply affected by the disease. The media, doctors, researchers, and even AIDS advocates never really fathomed that this would be a women's issue—and at the time, it didn't appear to be. But over the following 31 years how this face of AIDS has changed! While men continue to make up the majority of newly diagnosed HIV

BOX 11.1

THE FEMALE GENDER AND
THE IMPACT OF HIV/AIDS

HIV/AIDS NOW HAS A WOMAN'S FACE

In the early 1990s women were on the periphery of the HIV/AIDS pandemic. From 2003 through 2012 women have been at the epicenter. Across the world, more women than men are now becoming HIV infected and dying of this disease. The biggest factor appears to be how HIV is transmitted. Women are most at risk in countries where heterosexual sex is the main mode of transmission. This is the case in Africa, the Middle East, and the Caribbean. A new United Nations report stated that 80% of new HIV infections in women worldwide occur in marriages or long-term relationships with primary partners. By comparison, HIV is mostly transmitted by men who have sex with men and injection-drug users in Western Europe, Australia, New Zealand, and North America.

QUESTIONS ABOUT THE WOMAN'S FACE OF HIV/AIDS

In 2002 it became clear that women equaled men in the global number of HIV/AIDS cases. But this alarming finding did not just happen overnight. The phenomenon of women and HIV/AIDS has grown relentlessly over the 31 years of this pandemic. What shocks our senses is how long it has taken to focus the world on the fact that this was happening. Why wasn't the trend identified much earlier? Why, when it emerged in cold statistical print, did emergency alarm bells not ring out? Why has the continuing pattern of sexual carnage among young women, so grave as to lose an entire generation of women, gone on unrecognized? And why did it take until 2003 for the UN to form a task force on the plight of women in Africa or until 2004 to put in place a Global Coalition on Women and AIDS?

HETEROSEXUAL TRANSMISSION

Why does heterosexual transmission strike more women than men? The answer has to do with physiology, economics, and culture. Women are physiologically more vulnerable to infection: If an HIV-positive man has unprotected sex just once with an HIV-negative woman, her chance of infection is around 1 in 300. Reverse the gender and the odds fall to around 1 in 1000. This means women have more incentive to insist on safer sex than men.

But here's where economics comes in: In many cultures worldwide, women are denied equal access to education, income, ownership of land or other productive assets, even to credit. Too many women are left heavily dependent on men, and on exchanging sexual access to their bodies for the means of survival—for both themselves and their children. This situation makes negotiation of safer sex very difficult. Women are vulnerable for many reasons: They face domestic violence, at times worsened by conflict or insecurity; girls are the first to be pulled from school and put to work when HIV/AIDS strikes their home; women lack the power and economic independence to negotiate sexual safety; women face the full brunt of the stigma and discrimination associated with HIV, which fuels their fear of getting tested and prevents them from seeking care if they are infected; and there are inequalities between the sexes and women have a lack of power to challenge these inequalities.

Global Impact: The Gender Imbalance Grows

It has been said that men are driving the HIV pandemic, but that women will ultimately be its main victims. According to Peter Piot, former executive director of UNAIDS, higher deaths among young women due to HIV will lead to a hole in the age pyramid that has only been seen before in times of war, when more men die. According to UNAIDS, the situation is so badly tilted against women that they are now two to three times more likely to contract HIV than men. For example, so many more women will die from HIV/AIDS in the next 10 years than men that it will culminate in an unprecedented gender imbalance and will change reproductive choices dramatically in years to come. Ending 2013, globally, women and girls will represent over 60% of all young people living with HIV/AIDS. In sub-Saharan Africa it will be closer to 70%.

SUMMARY: Peter Piot said, "Women may be vulnerable, but we must distinguish between vulnerability and weakness. Women have shown great courage and resourcefulness in facing the epidemic. They have practiced safer sex when it was dangerous to do so; they have successfully pushed through legal reforms protecting their rights; they have consistently provided care, both at home and in healthcare settings. Wherever we look, we see the hope women have generated by their actions."

ANNIE LENNOX—UNAIDS GOODWILL AMBASADOR FOR WOMEN AND GIRLS

The recipient of many singing and writing musical awards and platinum records, Annie Lennox received Nobel Honors for her work on HIV/AIDS awareness in November 2009. She was presented with the Woman of Peace Award by former Soviet President and 1990 Nobel Peace Laureate Mikhail Gorbachev at the 10th World Summit of Nobel Peace Laureates meeting in Berlin. She was chosen by 22 Nobel Peace Laureates for her work in raising awareness of the HIV/AIDS impact on women and children, especially in South Africa, through her SING campaign that enlisted 23 of the world's most acclaimed female vocalists in recording "Sing," written by Lennox. Each year, the Nobel Peace Laureates honor a distinguished figure in the entertainment and arts community for their efforts in defending human rights and promoting world peace and solidarity. Recent Peace Summit Award winners include U2's Bono, actors Don Cheadle and George Clooney, and Genesis front man Peter Gabriel. In 2010 Lennox was named UNAIDS Goodwill Ambassador for women and girls. Her current status is as a special envoy for the Scottish Parliament's Commonwealth Parliamentary Association on HIV/AIDS to Malawi.

Table 11-2   Reported and Estimated AIDS Cases for Women, United States through 2013

Year	Number	Total
1981 (From June)	6	
1982	47	
1983	144	
1984	285	
1985	534	
1986	980	
1987	1701	
1988	3263	
1989	3639	
1990	4890	Through 1990 (15,489)
1991	5732	
1992	6571	
1993	16,824[a]	
1994	14,379	
1995	14,100	Through 1995 (73,095)
1996	13,820	
1997	11,651	
1998	10,500	
1999	10,800	
2000	11,000	Through 2000 (130,989)
2001	11,117	
2002	11,300	
2003	12,000	
2004	12,900	
2005	13,000	Through 2005 (191,317)
2006	13,200	
2007	13,200	
2008	13,200	
2009	13,200	
2010	12,500	Through 2010 (256,217)
2011	11,500	Through 2011 (estimated) (276,967)
2012	11,500	Through 2012 (estimated) (288,467)
2013	11,500	Through 2013 (estimated) (299,967)
Men	1,126,533	
Total:[c]	**1.41 million**[b]	

[a]The large increase in women's AIDS cases for 1993 over previous years was due to the January 1, 1993, implementation of the new definition of AIDS. Ending 2013 about 500,000 women will have been HIV infected. Of these about 300,000 will have been diagnosed with AIDS and about 123,000 of these will have died of AIDS. About 370,000 will be living with HIV/AIDS.

[b]Total AIDS cases include about 11,000 pediatric.

[c]End of year 2013.

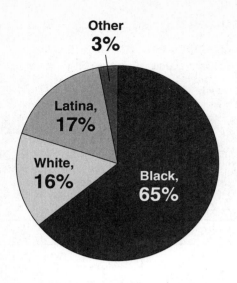

Other
3%

Latina,
17%

White,
16%

Black,
65%

New AIDS Diagnoses Among Women: About 26%

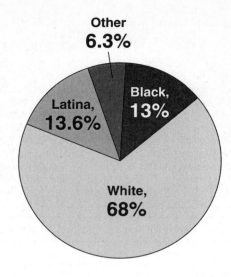

Other
6.3%

Black,
13%

Latina,
13.6%

White,
68%

U.S. Female Population: About 157.5 Million;
About 127 Million Are Over Age 18

FIGURE 11-2 AIDS Diagnoses and U.S. Female Population, by Race/Ethnicity, 2013. **Age:** The impact of HIV on younger women is particularly notable. Over 6 in 10 new HIV infections among women including white, black, and Latina women, were among those ages 13-39; 32% were ages 13-29 and 31% were ages 30-39. Adapted from Kaiser Family Foundation Fact Sheet November 2010—Women and HIV/AIDS in the United States. Updated.

infections and AIDS cases in the United States, the rates of HIV/AIDS infections and diagnosis among women and young adult girls continue to steadily increase.

In the United States, ending 2013, about three-quarters of the estimated 430,000 women living with HIV and AIDS will be black or Hispanic. (See Snapshot 11.1, page 347.)

Among the most alarming HIV/AIDS statistics to emerge is that of HIV transmission through heterosexual sexual contact. Of new HIV infections in women, acquired through heterosexual contact, in 2002 through 2013 in the United States at least 30% will be women. Of AIDS cases and new HIV infections that occur in women ages 13 to 24, about 76% are due to heterosexual contact.

The median age for women reported with AIDS is 35 years, and women ages 25 to 44 account for 85% of female AIDS cases. Ending year 2013, women ages 55 years and older will

account for about 18% of all female AIDS cases. Most of these women became infected through heterosexual sexual activities (Schable et al., 1996 updated). Figure 11-4, page 348 presents the cumulative **source** of U.S. female HIV cases through 2012. (See Point of Information 11.2, page 345 and Point of Information 11.3, page 348.)

Location, Location, Location

The Southern AIDS Living Quilt (Figure 11-5, page 348) Was Launched in October 2008 to Address the Impact of the HIV/AIDS Epidemic among Women in the Southern United States (www.LivingQuilt.org)

Beginning in 2001, the South accounted for the largest percentage of AIDS cases reported among women (46%), followed by the Northeast (36%), West (8%), Midwest (6%), and Puerto Rico and U.S. territories (4%). In the

PROFILE: WOMEN WITH HIV/AIDS IN THE UNITED STATES

At the end of 2013, there will be about 157.5 million women in the United States. They make up about 51% of the U.S. population.

The majority of women with AIDS in the United States reside in the Northeast and the South, are unemployed, and 83% live in households with income less than $10,000 per year. Only 14% are currently married, compared to 50% of all women in the United States ages 15 to 44 years. Twenty-three percent of HIV-infected women live alone, 2% live in various facilities, and 1% are homeless. Approximately 50% have at least one child younger than 15 years old. Similar to other population groups with AIDS in the United States, the majority of women with AIDS are from minority racial and ethnic groups, with 67% of all AIDS cases diagnosed in blacks, 18% in Latinos, and 15% in whites (HIV/AIDS Surveillance, 1998 updated).

AIDS IN OLDER WOMEN

According to the CDC, ending year 2013, an estimated 20% or about 55,000 AIDS cases will have occurred in women ages 55 and older: white 18,700, black 25,300, Hispanic 9,735, all others about 1,265.

TWO TYPICAL SENIOR HIV/AIDS ANECDOTES

A soft-spoken, 63-year-old, self-described "churchy" woman from rural South Dakota, who has been living with HIV since her late 50s, said, "I got very sick. I kept going to the doctor and he kept giving me antibiotics, and he would just kind of hit-and-run. He thought it was menopause, arthritis, high blood pressure, possibly a heart problem. Suddenly I found myself in the emergency room after two years of misdiagnosed infections, monthly visits to my primary care doctor, and an allergic reaction to daily doses of penicillin. That's where I was tested for HIV. When the doctor came into my room, I pulled on his sleeve and told him to sit down a minute. He said, 'What you have is really nasty, and you don't want to know.'"

In a second case, a 66-year-old woman said, "He was 10 years older than I was and he said, 'I've never worn a condom in my life and I'm not going to start now.'" Most older men say that. Older women won't insist that the man wear a condom. They don't ask where he's been. Older women especially don't pry. They can no longer have children, so why bother with condoms? Usually they tend not to be very assertive until they get HIV or an STD. Most seniors are first diagnosed with HIV in the hospital after they've already progressed to AIDS.

These two stories are typical of HIV-positive older women. The majority become infected through sexual contact with a husband or boyfriend. After months and sometimes years of being sick, they're tested for HIV as a last resort. Healthcare providers routinely fail these women by not readily screening them for HIV and other sexually transmitted diseases. They also neglect to ask about their sexual and drug-using behaviors. Ailments that accompany HIV often masquerade as signs of aging, throwing physicians even further off track. Fevers, night sweats, tuberculosis, chronic fungal infections, shingles, decreased vision, *Pneumocystis jiroveci* pneumonia, and cervical cancer can signal HIV, AIDS, or aging.

Northeast, 1.4% of women with AIDS resided outside metropolitan areas compared with 10.2% of women who resided outside metropolitan areas in the South.

In July 1982, the first female AIDS case was reported to the CDC. Currently, women in 10 states make up about 70% of their cumulative AIDS cases (Table 11-3, page 350). With respect to *new HIV infections,* the South, with about 37% of the female population, has about 76% of newly infected females.

Of all new female HIV and AIDS cases, about 80% are associated with heterosexual transmission. The second most frequent cause was injection-drug use at about 14%. The AIDS rate for Hispanic women was about five times higher than for white women. The AIDS rate for black women was four times higher than for Hispanic women and 15 times higher than for white women.

As the frequency of HIV/AIDS increases in women, the question of whether AIDS will explode in the heterosexual community of the United States becomes more a question of when will the number of female AIDS cases equal male cases. For the first time, in 1997 American women made up over 20% (22%) of AIDS cases

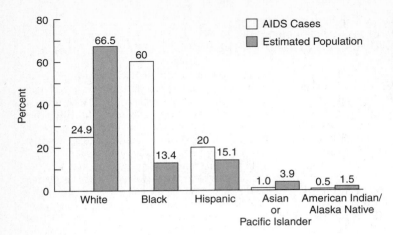

FIGURE 11-3 Incidence of AIDS Cases among Women of Different Ethnic Groups, United States. Worldwide, every minute two women become HIV infected, and every minute two women die of AIDS. *(Source: WHO/UNAIDS AIDS Epidemic Update, 2008 updated.)*

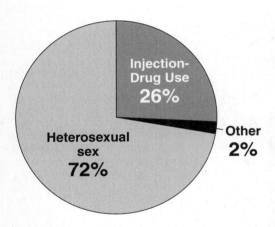

FIGURE 11-4 Cumulative Major Sources of HIV Infections in U.S. Women through 2012. *(Adapted from U.S. Centers for Disease Control and Prevention, Surveillance Report Year 2009 updated.)*

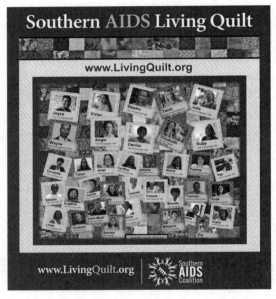

FIGURE 11-5

for the year. For 2013 the estimate is between 25% and 30%.

Women, Drug Use, and HIV Infection

Until recently, most drug users have been men, and their non-drug-using female partners have functioned as the glue that kept their families together, sheltering as best they could the next generation, often suffering abuse in the process. Today, 60% of crack users are women, the majority of whom are mothers of small children and the heads of single-parent households. It is estimated that more than half of all drug-using women in the major epicenters of the eastern United States are HIV infected, and drug use among women is correlated to unprotected sex, injection-drug use, and needle sharing. (See Point of Information 11.2, page 345 and Sidebar 11.1, page 349.)

BLACK WOMEN AND HIV/AIDS

Los Angeles (FinalCall.com)—"I'm 21 [28 in 2013] and I'm celebrating life each day. I continue to speak because when I was in high school, the number of kids that were having sex and the type of sex that they were having was amazing to me . . . so I continue to speak. I continue to speak because now I have a 21-year-old sister who is infected and I want her to have the same opportunities that I have, to be welcomed and loved by so many people. To my peers, as people we need to wake up. Parent, please talk to your child. How many times do you have to tell us to take out the trash, or do our homework? And don't just lecture us, speak to us. Have an open conversation. The reason why I do what I do is because I don't want anybody to go through what I've gone through. I'm so happy that we're finally taking this stand and raising our voices."

When she was three years old, doctors discovered that Hydeia Broadbent was infected with HIV, and they told her new adoptive parents that she would not live to be five. Tearfully speaking these words, the HIV/AIDS activist helped to convene the First Annual National Black Women and HIV/AIDS Conference in 2005.

It's All About M.E.E.!

The seventh (2012) national black women's AIDS conference was held in Los Angeles, California. The conference was called "It's All About M.E.E.! (Mobilization, Education, Empowerment) Sistahs Getting Real About HIV/AIDS." Congresswoman Maxine Waters (Figure 11-6) noted that a 6% reduction in HIV/AIDS infections among black women is hopeful, but it is not enough. "African Americans, in general, still account for almost

half of all the new AIDS cases, although we're only 13% of the population. African American women still represent nearly 70% of all the new AIDS cases among women, and African American teenagers represent 65% of all the new AIDS cases among teenagers."

Despite growing beliefs that AIDS is no longer a lethal disease, black American women are dying from AIDS-related illnesses every year in ever-increasing numbers. Black women who test HIV positive are seven times more likely to die from it than whites. AIDS remains the third leading cause of death for black women between the ages of 25 and 44 and ranks among the leading causes of death for all black women. Far too many black women do not realize that they are at risk or don't believe they are at risk.

Among women, black women account for an estimated 58% of new HIV infections, about 67% of women's AIDS cases, and 13% of the U.S. female population.

HIV TRANSMISSION IN BLACK WOMEN THROUGH 2012

Heterosexual sex is by far the most common route of HIV transmission for black women (78%), followed by injection-drug use.

Deaths

Black women account for about 68% of all women who have died from AIDS, white about 18%, and Hispanic about 14%. Of black women, about 41% of deaths occur in ages 35–44; ages 45–54, about 25%; ages 25–34, 21%; ages 15–24, 3%; and over age 55, 10%.

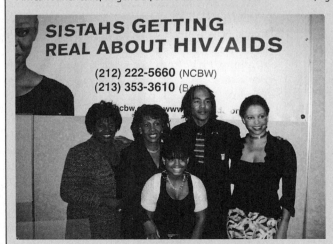

FIGURE 11–6   Grazelle Howard, J.D. (The Libra Group), Congresswoman Maxine Waters (D-Calif.), Hydeia Broadbent (27-year-old AIDS activist), Phill Wilson (The Black AIDS Institute), and Gloria Reuben (actress/songstress) pose after convening the "It's All About M.E.E.! Sistahs Getting Real About HIV/AIDS" first National Black Women and HIV/AIDS Conference, December 1, 2006. *(Courtesy of Charlene Muhammad.)*

HIV INFECTION AMONG WOMEN

There are over 6 million women ages 18 to 40 in the United States who are unmarried and having sexual relationships. Those most at risk for HIV infection are: (1) those who have multiple sexual partners (defined as having more than four different partners/year), and (2) those women who do not insist on the use of a condom.

Three of the nation's top five metropolitan areas with the highest incidence of AIDS in women are located in Florida within a 70-mile radius of each other (West Palm Beach, Ft. Lauderdale, and Miami). This area is an epicenter of HIV infection for Florida women. The other areas of highest incidence of AIDS in women are Puerto Rico, followed by New Jersey (In New Jersey, one of every three people living with HIV is a woman. New Jersey has the highest percentage of HIV-infected women in the United States, and 80% are women of color.), New York, the District of Columbia, Florida, Connecticut, Maryland, Delaware, Massachusetts, Rhode Island, Georgia, and South Carolina. In Florida's Palm Beach County the rate is 24%; in Broward and Dade Counties, 18%. The epidemiologist for the state of Florida stated that what is happening in Florida is happening in inner cities nationwide. What may distinguish the AIDS epidemic in women is that it hinges on the low self-esteem and lack of personal power experienced by women in many walks of life.

Most of Florida's women with AIDS are poor and receive their medical care through the public health system. Among women in South Florida, HIV transmission is associated with crack cocaine. Pam Whittington, director of the Boynton Community Life Center, a family support facility in southern Palm Beach County, said, "If you have 10 women on crack, probably 8 of them are HIV infected."

Crack cocaine is cheap and readily available. Its use contributes to anonymous, high-risk sex with multiple partners. Those who cannot afford crack exchange sex for it. In isolated communities of crack users, there is a high degree of sharing sex partners, many of whom are HIV positive.

Table 11–3 Ten States Reporting Highest Estimated Number of Women with AIDS through 2012

State	Estimated % of Total (270,000)
New York	17.8
California	14.4
Florida	10.6
Texas	7
New Jersey	5
Illinois	3.4
Pennsylvania	3.4
Georgia	3.2
Maryland	3
Massachusetts	2
	69.8% of women's AIDS cases in these 10 states (188,460)

Of the 50 states, New Jersey has the highest proportion—one out of three—of people living with HIV/AIDS who are women. And while black women comprise only one-third of New Jersey's adult female population, they constitute more than 83% of the state's women with HIV/AIDS.

Artificial Insemination

To date there are six cases of transmission through **artificial insemination** reported in the United States, and six other cases are known to have occurred (Joseph, 1993 updated). Four of eight Australian women who received semen from a single infected donor became infected. HIV-contaminated semen had been injected into the uterus through a catheter. In 2003, a woman in Tokyo became infected after being artificially inseminated with sperm from her HIV-positive husband. According to the report, several procedures involved in obtaining HIV-free sperm were not performed. Children have been born free of HIV when the procedure for stripping HIV from sperm was used properly. For other cases of men infecting women see Point of View 11.1, page 351.

Prostitutes

The term *prostitute* is used here in preference to the more recently coined *sex worker*. No single term can adequately encompass the range of sex for money/drugs/friendship/accommodation transactions that undoubtedly occurs worldwide. However, the term *prostitute* is at least relatively clear in referring to those who are

REBEKKA'S STORY

At the young age of 18, Rebekka aspired to become a Playboy Playmate like she had seen in the magazines found under her grandfather's bed. Her pictures were sent to Hugh Hefner, and against all odds Rebekka was chosen to become a Playboy centerfold, Miss September 1986. Rebekka's sunny disposition and enthusiastic spirit brought her all she could desire. It seemed a time when nothing could harm her. Rebekka said, "I led an exciting life as a Playmate. Traveling, meeting tons of people, parties, etc. However as time passed, I began to suspect something was wrong. I became fatigued easily and was plagued with a general feeling of malaise." She went to her doctor for tests and, as an afterthought, asked to be tested for HIV. It came back positive. Rebekka said, "Surprisingly I did not become infected living the wild life in the light of Hollywood; no, it happened years earlier, as a teenager having unprotected sex with a young man I met on a summer beach vacation." She was diagnosed positive in 1989.

When her doctor called with her results, she became confused. "I thought my doctor was telling me I was pregnant, but I was positive for HIV, and the only thing I knew about HIV was death." Attempting to mask her anguish, she began using speed and partying heavily, and began taking 18 anti-HIV pills a day in hopes of curing her illness. Her hands and feet began tingling with the sensations of pins and needles. She had drug toxicity from the medication and was diagnosed with neuropathy, which is a severe form of nerve damage. She was rushed to the emergency room in Los Angeles and had seven spinal taps in four days and was diagnosed with two brain infections. She was given a second set of new medications for everything the doctors could find wrong. She began regaining her strength, but she began partying again and her drugs failed again.

When she was placed on a third set of new HIV medications her pancreas ruptured. Broke and about homeless she thought about suicide. She mixed numerous pain pills with tequila and drove into a brick wall. She was in a coma for three and a half days. When she awoke, she was transferred to the psychiatric ward of the hospital. After being released she decided to reveal her HIV infection. She went public with her illness in 1994 by speaking to family, friends, and the media. She was put on a fourth set of drugs, this time a three-drug combination. It caused severe diarrhea. She had to wear diapers for 18 months. For the fourth time, her drugs failed. Her doctor prescribed a new drug regime, which she said

was "pure evil." She did not have a bowel movement for eight days, and realized the medications were ruining her digestive system. Her medications were switched yet again, but this time it worked. She takes a few pills a day and is now into her 28th year of HIV infection. About seven years ago Rebekka found her way into nutrition and bodybuilding (Figure 11-7). Her coach, now her husband and also HIV positive, trained her intensely. On May 31, 2004, Rebekka won first place in her first attempt in a women's bodybuilding competition.

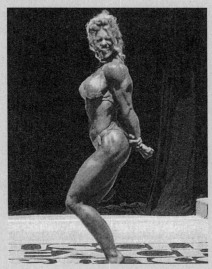

FIGURE 11-7   Rebekka Armstrong: 28 years HIV positive and counting. After suffering antiretroviral failures, wasting and near death at 90 pounds, she switched her lifestyle to accept better nutrition, new anti-HIV drugs, exercise, weight lifting, and bodybuilding. *(Photograph by Joanne Greenstone, used with permission.)*

Rebekka currently lives in Los Angeles with her trainer husband, Oliver. Although infected with HIV for 28 years and diagnosed with AIDS, she is in excellent health. Medications and a super healthy lifestyle that includes mornings of cardio and weight training have helped Rebekka to maintain a normal T cell count (over 500) and undetectable viral load. She says she has never felt better.

Rebekka has dedicated herself to increasing AIDS awareness. She has toured across the United States educating others about HIV prevention.

directly involved in trading sex for money or drugs. In the United States, prostitutes represent a diverse group of people with various lifestyles. About 31% of female IDUs admit to engaging in prostitution. They need money to support their drug habit, pay rent, and eat. Cities with large numbers of IDUs subsequently have large numbers of prostitutes. Evidence is overwhelming—IDU, prostitution, and HIV infection are strongly associated.

However, non-injection-drug-using prostitutes in the United States play a small role in HIV transmission. This is believed to be because of the low incidence of HIV infection among their male clients and on the insistence by many prostitutes that their clients use condoms. In Africa, Asia, and other underdeveloped nations where the "Customer Is King," prostitution plays a major role in HIV transmission (Figure 11-8 and Point of View 11.1, page 351).

Women Who Have Sex with Women—WSW (Lesbians)

Research on female-to-female transmission remains inconclusive. But the large numbers of HIV-positive women and women with AIDS should alert women who have sex with women that they cannot assume their partners are uninfected because they are lesbians. It has been reported that 80% of lesbian women have had sex with men during their lifetimes. Also, certain sexual behaviors common among lesbians probably put them at risk for transmitting and receiving HIV through vaginal fluid, menstrual blood, sex toys, and cuts in the vagina and mouth and on the hands.

The evidence is clear: HIV infection is present among lesbians, and lesbians engage in behaviors that put them at risk for HIV infection. Whether lesbians put their female sexual partners at risk is less clear. In fact, there is a great deal of controversy about this question. Some HIV/AIDS investigators believe the risk of sexual transmission increases as the number of HIV-positive lesbian partners increases. Others believe that lesbians are not getting infected

---

ANECDOTE

I was referred to an eye doctor who is a specialist in retinal detachment in HIV/AIDS patients. After looking at my chart the first thing he said to me was "Sex or drugs?" I knew he was trying to pigeonhole me. So I said, "Excuse me?" and he repeated, "Sex or drugs?" I told him, "I don't do drugs anymore and sex with you, I don't think so!"

Commentary: Women with HIV/AIDS have to deal with a lot of attitude from people, including healthcare providers.

---

through lesbian sex, but only through unsafe behaviors like IDU. Female-to-female transmission has been reported in one case and suggested in another (Curran et al., 1988).

In 2003 Helena Kwakwa and colleagues reported that based on genetic evidence of the strain of HIV found in two women, sexual contact between the two resulted in the transmission of HIV. A 20-year-old female had exclusive sexual activity with an openly bisexual HIV-infected woman for two years before testing HIV positive. Their sexual relations involved oral contact and the use of sex toys. The investigators ruled out other possible means of HIV transmission in this case (Kwakwa et al., 2003).

Special Concerns of HIV/AIDS Women

First, HIV/AIDS has a profound impact on women, both as an illness and as a social and economic challenge. Women play a crucial role in preventing infection by insisting on safer sexual practices and caring for people with HIV disease and people with AIDS. The stigma attached to HIV/AIDS can subject women to social rejection as well as discrimination and other violations of their rights. A study by Sally Zierler and colleagues (2000) estimates that about 21% of HIV-infected American women were assaulted by a sexual partner or another after becoming HIV positive. The percentage of women receiving physical harm after receiving an HIV diagnosis in a developing nation is at least

WOMEN + SEXUAL PARTNERS + DECEPTION = AIDS

Across the world, women in support groups or with a close friend have been telling their stories of trusting their sexual partners and ending up with AIDS. Their trust was violated—their lives forfeited. Here are a few examples of the thousands of similar cases worldwide.

1. She is 48 years old with curly red hair and bags beneath her eyes. She slouches slightly in the office chair, stretching out her feet. From her eye shadow to her sneakers, everything is blue. Married to one husband for 28 years, she has children and grandchildren. She also has AIDS. She did not use drugs or have multiple sexual partners. She did have sex with her husband without a condom!

2. One 23-year-old had a boyfriend with hemophilia; he never used condoms and never mentioned HIV, even though he had already infected another woman.

3. A divorced man with two children did not tell his 46-year-old girlfriend he had AIDS, even when he was hospitalized with an AIDS-related infection.

4. A seven-year live-in partner of a woman denied infecting her, even though he tested positive for HIV; she did not know he was having sex outside their relationship.

5. Because she had only two boyfriends, because "we were perfectly ordinary," they did not use condoms.

6. This woman with a baby did not know "my man was shooting up drugs and sharing needles." Not until he died of AIDS.

7. She never dreamed her partner had used a needle. When the doctor said she had AIDS, she replied, "You have made a mistake. I cannot have AIDS. How could I have that?"

All these women discovered their HIV status only after they became seriously ill with infections they should not have had. Heterosexual transmission is rising dramatically. A seldom-mentioned fact is that a large percentage of infected women are married or in committed relationships.

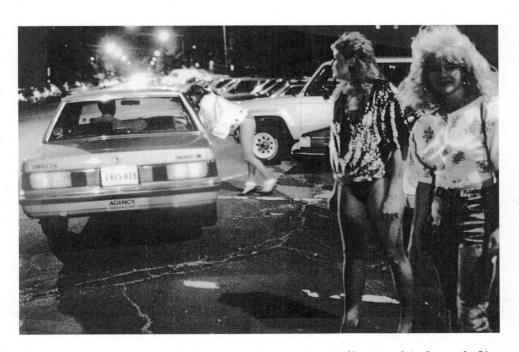

FIGURE 11–8   Street scene, sex workers plying their trade, any major city. *(Courtesy of the Centers for Disease Control and Prevention, Atlanta, GA.)*

twice that found in America. In South Africa, for example, Gugu Dlamini was stoned to death by her neighbors after she revealed that she was HIV positive on World AIDS Day, 1999.

Women need to know that they can protect themselves against HIV infection. Women have a traditionally passive role in sexual decision making in many countries. They need knowledge about HIV and AIDS, self-confidence, the skills necessary to insist that partners use safer sex methods, and good medical care.

Efforts to influence women to practice safer sex must also be joined by efforts to address men and their responsibility in practicing safer sex.

Second, women become pregnant. Women who are ill and discover they are pregnant need information about both the potential impact of pregnancy on their own health and maternal-fetal HIV transmission.

Third, women have the role of mothering. From this role come two important consequences. First, when a woman becomes ill with HIV disease or AIDS, her role as caretaker of the child or children or other adults in the household is immediately affected. The family is severely disrupted and each family member has to make adjustments. Second, the mother must cope with her own life-threatening illness while she also deals with the impact of the disease on her family. Demographic studies show that many women who are HIV infected or have AIDS have young children; and these women are often the sole support of these children.

Fourth, a woman's illness may be complicated further by incarceration and the threat of foster care proceedings. If the mother is healthy enough to care for her child, she must still cope with the complex issues of medical and home care, school access, friends, and family stress.

Biology and the Clinical Course of AIDS among Women and Men

According to Birgit van Benthem and colleagues (2002), sex differences with respect to response to HIV infection do exist. CD4 cell counts are higher in women than in men throughout infection, and viral loads are lower initially in women than in men, although this difference eventually disappears.

According to Arlene Bardeguez (1995) and other similar reports (Cohen, 1995), biology does not influence the prevalence of AIDS-defining illnesses between men and women, with the exception of invasive carcinoma of the cervix in women and possibly Kaposi's sarcoma in men. Access to HIV-related care and therapies is the dominant factor influencing the prevalence of AIDS-defining illnesses among women. Injection-drug use in HIV-infected women leads to a higher incidence of certain diseases, particularly esophageal candidiasis, herpes simplex virus, and cytomegalovirus. Once an initial diagnosis of AIDS has been made, several major AIDS-defining illnesses appear more frequently in women: toxoplasmosis, herpes genital ulcerations, and esophageal candidiasis.

The currently proposed female-specific markers of **HIV disease** include *cervical dysplasia* and *neoplasia* (tumor), *vulvovaginal candidiasis,* and *pelvic inflammatory disease* (PID).

Drug use, high-risk sexual behaviors, depression, and unmet social needs among infected women contributed to their underuse of HIV resources. In 2001, Timothy Sterling and colleagues reported that although viral loads were lower in women than men, the rates of progression to AIDS were similar. However, in 2009, Diana Lemly and colleagues reported that being female was linked to poorer HIV/AIDS survival than for men. That is, HIV-positive women have a higher likelihood of premature death from HIV when compared with HIV-positive men.

Female HIV/AIDS Deaths

Women's deaths in the United States rose from 18 cases in 1981 to an estimated 115,000 ending year 2012. That is, about 42% of all women with AIDS will have died. AIDS is the sixth leading cause of death for all women between the ages of 25 and 34, the fifth leading cause of death for all women between the ages of 35 and 44, and the eighth leading cause of death in white women. It is the second leading cause of death for black women and the third leading cause of death for Hispanic women between the ages of 25 and 44 (*MMWR,* 1996b updated).

Identifying and Preventing HIV Infection

Currently, women make up 67% of adult/adolescent HIV infections in sub-Saharan Africa, 30% in Southeast Asia, and about 23% in Europe and the United States.

Identification of HIV-Positive Women—At age 26, a woman and her physicians were baffled when she began suffering from a variety of strange medical conditions: fevers, throat sores, unexplained vaginal bleeding, and fatigue. **It took a variety of doctors and seven years to find out what was wrong. She tested HIV positive!**

This woman's difficulty in getting diagnosed points out the extent to which women still are invisible when it comes to AIDS. After more than 30 years into the epidemic, the message still hasn't reached primary care physicians: Their female patients may be at risk. This young woman said, **"I went into doctors' offices and all they saw was a white, middle-class woman, not someone at risk for HIV."**

Early identification of women with HIV infection is a pressing problem. Risk-based screening at a Johns Hopkins perinatal clinic showed that 43% of HIV-positive women were not identified as at risk on the basis of such screening, with infection being found in 20 (9.5%) of 211 women admitting to at-risk behaviors and in 15 (1.6%) of 949 who were not at risk according to their response to screening questions.

Women and HIV Prevention: United States—To prevent HIV infection, women have been told to reduce their number of sexual partners, to be monogamous, and to protect themselves by using condoms. **But these goals, generally speaking, do not fit the realities of women's lives or may not be under their control.**

Women do not wear the condom. (A female condom is now available but not yet in heavy demand. See Chapter 9, page 258.) For women to protect themselves from HIV infection, they must rely not only on their own skills, attitudes, and behaviors regarding condom use, but also on their ability to convince their partner to use a condom. Gender, culture, and power may be barriers to maintaining safer sex practices.

Women who have more than one sexual partner in their lifetime often practice serial monogamy, remaining with one partner at a time. People living as couples reduce the number of their sexual partners. Still, in many phases of life, sex is practiced with new partners in new relationships. American women, on average, are single for many years before their first marriage; they might be single again after a divorce; they might marry again; and, in later phases especially, they might be widowed. For some women, multiple partners throughout life is an economic necessity; urging them to reduce the number of partners is meaningless unless the economic situation for these wo-men is improved (Ehrhardt, 1992). In addition, public health strategies, not necessarily targeted to women, can also play an important role for women. Syringe exchange and drug treatment are important strategies because almost half of all HIV infections in women are due to injection-drug use. Because women are now more likely to be infected by men through heterosexual contact, programs that specifically target men, especially IDUs, will have a beneficial impact on women's programs.

Women and HIV Prevention: Africa—Although they are exceptionally vulnerable to the epidemic, millions of young African wo-men are dangerously uninformed about HIV/AIDS. According to UNICEF, over 70% of adolescent girls (ages 15–19) in Somalia and more than 40% in Guinea Bissau and Sierra

Leone have never heard of HIV or AIDS. In countries such as Kenya and the United Republic of Tanzania, more than 40% of adolescent girls harbor serious misconceptions about how the virus is transmitted. One of the targets fixed at the UN General Assembly Special Session on HIV/AIDS in June 2001 was to ensure that at least 90% of young men and women should, by 2005, have the information, education, and services they need in order to defend themselves against HIV infection. Beginning 2013 this goal still has not been achieved! The vast majority of African women living with HIV still do not know they have been infected. In South Africa about 30% of pregnant women are HIV positive. One study found that 50% of adult Tanzanian women know where they could be tested for HIV, yet only 66% of these have been tested. In Zimbabwe, only 11% of adult women have been tested for the virus. Moreover, many people who agree to be tested prefer not to return and learn the outcome of those tests. An additional problem is that in many African countries where pregnant women agree to undergo HIV testing, most have no access to drug therapy to prevent mother-to-child transmission of HIV. Over half the HIV-infected women who were surveyed by Kenya's Population Council said they had not disclosed their HIV status to their partners because they feared it would expose them to violence or abandonment. Not only are voluntary counseling and testing services in short supply across the region, but stigma and discrimination continue to discourage people from discovering or disclosing their HIV status.

The Bottom Line

Worldwide, more women are now becoming infected with HIV than men. With early testing and treatment, women with HIV can live as long as men (Table 11–4). Women need to know more about how they can be infected, and they should get tested for HIV if they think there is any chance they have been exposed. This is especially true for pregnant women. If they test positive for HIV, they can take steps to reduce the risk of infecting their babies. The best way

Table 11-4   Top 15 Countries by Estimated Number of Women Living with HIV/AIDS Ending 2012

South Africa	3,952,000
Nigeria	1,596,000
India	1,007,000
Mozambique	931,000
Tanzania (United Rep. of)	874,000
Zimbabwe	779,000
Zambia	646,000
Ethiopia	608,000
Malawi	562,400
Uganda	551,000
Cameroon	342,000
Cote d'Ivoire	282,720
Thailand	282,720
Russian Federation	275,500
Brazil	275,500

Source: UNAIDS, 2008 Report on the Global AIDS Epidemic, 2008, updated.

to prevent infection in heterosexual sex is by using the male condom. Other birth control methods do not protect against HIV. Women who use intravenous drugs should not share equipment. Women should discuss vaginal problems with their doctors, especially yeast infections that don't go away or vaginal ulcers (sores). These could be signs of HIV infections.

CHILDBEARING WOMEN: WORLDWIDE

The extent of HIV infection among pregnant women is often used as an indicator of HIV penetration into the population at large. By this yardstick, several Asian countries have serious epidemics. In some of India's HIV/AIDS surveillance sites, more than 2% of pregnant women are infected, with some sites as high as 6%. Myanmar recorded prevalence rates of up to 5% among pregnant women in some areas of the country. In Thailand, HIV infection prevalence among pregnant women peaked at 2% nationally.

Worldwide each year, of an estimated 200 million women who became pregnant, about 1.6 million become HIV positive. Annually, from 1999 through 2012, about 400,000 children were born HIV positive, and 300,000 died before their first birthday. Of the 4 million women who become pregnant each year in the United States, 6000 are estimated to be HIV infected. Because of increased ART therapy for HIV-infected mothers, these pregnancies now result in fewer than 100 HIV-infected children each year, a 95% reduction from the 1990s high of 1700 cases. However, in underdeveloped nations, only 25% of pregnant women receive antiretroviral drugs. Regardless of available information on ART, according to data presented at the 2008 International AIDS Conference, about half of HIV-infected women intend to have children.

Women, in general, have two children before they find out they are infected (Thomas, 1989 updated). The birth of an infected child may serve as a **miner's canary**—in some cases it is the first indication of HIV infection in the mother. Currently, about 25% to 30% of pregnant women in low and middle income countries are tested for HIV.

Pregnancy and HIV Disease

Early findings in pregnant women indicated that those with T4 or CD4+ cell counts of less than **300/μL** of blood were more likely to experience HIV-associated illness during pregnancy. Pregnant HIV-infected women exhibit a greater T4 or CD4+ cell count decline during pregnancy than do women without HIV infection. T4 cell counts in the HIV infected do not return to prepregnancy levels. However, the overall declines in HIV-infected women likely represent declines that would have occurred in the absence of pregnancy and suggest that pregnancy does not accelerate disease progression (Newell et al., 1997; Bessinger et al., 1997).

Over the last 17 years, HIV-positive pregnant women have been attracting more attention from the medical establishment, **first,** because there are better medications for the HIV-positive mother and fetus, and **second,** because of the relatively high incidence of HIV births.

As an aside, it should be mentioned that protease inhibitors reduce blood levels of the estrogen component in oral contraceptive pills so women taking both the pill and PIs may need to use back-up methods of contraception. (See Box 11.2, page 356.)

DISCUSSION QUESTION: Nationwide, approximately 2 of 1000 pregnant women are HIV infected, an incidence much higher than that of fetal neural tube defects, for which pregnant women are screened routinely. Should all pregnancies be screened for HIV?

INTERNET RESOURCES

Among the hundreds of websites containing information on HIV, there are key addresses that provide comprehensive information, including links to a vast array of other resources. The key sites listed here include special areas focused on *women and HIV.*

AIDS Community Research Initiative of America (ACRIA): www.criany.org/treatment/treatment_edu_women.html

American Medical Association home page: www.ama-assn.org

The Body: www.thebody.com/women.html

Centers for Disease Control and Prevention (CDC) Home Page: www.cdc.gov

HIV Insite: Gateway to AIDS Knowledge: hivinsite.ucsf.edu

National Women's Health Information Center: www.4woman.gov

National Women's Health Week: www.womenshealth.gov/whw/about

Women Organized to Respond to Life-Threatening Disease (WORLD): www.womenhiv.org

PEDIATRIC HIV-POSITIVE AND AIDS CASES—UNITED STATES: A FIGHT WE CAN WIN!

Currently over 90% of pediatric AIDS cases are newborns and infants who received HIV from mothers who were injection drug users or were the sexual partners of IDUs. For those who become HIV infected during gestation, clinical symptoms usually develop within six months after birth. Few children infected as fetuses live beyond two years, and survival past three years used to be rare; but with the use of antiretroviral drugs and therapy for opportunistic diseases, some children born with HIV are still alive at age 30 and some are raising their own children. The clinical course of rapid HIV disease progression in infants diagnosed with AIDS is marked by failure to thrive, persistent lymphadenopathy, chronic or recurrent oral candidiasis, persistent diarrhea, enlarged liver and spleen (hepatosplenomegaly), and chronic pneumonia (interstitial pneumonitis). Bacterial infections are common and can be life-threatening. Bacterial infection and septicemia (the presence of variety of bacterial species in the bloodstream) is a leading cause of death. Less than 25% of HIV/AIDS children express the kinds of OIs fOWId in adult AIDS patients. Kaposi's sarcoma occurs in about 4% of them. Young HIV/AIDS children experience delayed development and poor motor function. Older children experience speech and perception problems.

The Pediatric HIV Conundrum

One of the biggest puzzles in understanding mother-to-child transmission of HIV is why the majority of babies born to HIV-infected women remain uninfected in utero, at birth, and—perhaps most remarkably—during breast-feeding. It's even more remarkable in view of studies suggesting that cell-free viral load in breast milk can vary from undetectable to more than 200,000 copies per mL, meaning that a breast-feeding infant may ingest millions of viral copies each day. This apparent resistance to infection puts infants in the category of exposed, seronegative individuals who can repel or effectively control HIV despite repeated exposures. Katharine Lazuriaga and Sarah Rowland-Jones have both documented cases of infants apparently clearing a transient HIV infection. In 1995 Pierre Rogues and colleagues reported on 12 perinatal HIV-infected children clearing their infections after birth. It is these immune defenses that vaccine researchers seek to boost, or mimic, with a neonatal vaccine. But there are little hard data on just what they are and how this apparent protection works.

Pediatric AIDS: Clinical signs and symptoms in the United States

Pediatric AIDS in the United States refers to two age groups: (1) infants and young children who became infected through perinatal (vertical) transmission, and (2) school-age children to age 13, the majority of whom acquired HIV through blood transfusions (mostly hemophiliacs).

Ending 2013, about 11,000 pediatric AIDS cases will be reported and over 6000 will have

Table 11-5 Ten States Reporting Highest Estimated Number of Pediatric AIDS Cases through 2012

State	% of Total (10,886)
New York	25
Florida	16.2
New Jersey	8.2
California	7
Texas	4.1
Pennsylvania	3.8
Maryland	3.4
Illinois	3
Georgia	2.4
Massachusetts	2.2
	75.3% of pediatric cases from these 10 states (8,197)

died from AIDS. Pediatric AIDS cases represent about .78% of the total number of AIDS cases to date (Table 11-5, page 357). Of the pediatric AIDS cases, about 3% were/are hemophilic children who received HIV-contaminated blood transfusions or blood products (pooled and concentrated blood factor VIII injections). About 5% of pediatric AIDS cases occurred in non-hemophilic children who were transfused with HIV-contaminated blood. From 1995 on, virtually all HIV-infected newborns contracted HIV from their mothers (vertical transmission).

Currently over 90% of pediatric AIDS cases are newborns and infants who received HIV from mothers who were injection-drug users or were the sexual partners of IDUs. For those who become HIV infected during gestation, clinical symptoms usually develop within six months after birth. Few children infected as fetuses lived beyond two years, and survival past three years used to be rare, but with the use of antiretroviral drugs and therapy for opportunistic diseases, some children born with HIV are still alive at age 31, and some are raising their own children! The clinical course of rapid HIV disease progression in infants diagnosed with AIDS is marked by failure to thrive, persistent lymphadenopathy, chronic or recurrent oral candidiasis, persistent dianhea, enlarged liver and

spleen (hepatosplenomegaly), and chronic pneumonia (interstitial pneumonitis). Bacterial infections are common and can be life-threatening. Bacterial infection and septicemia (the presence of a variety of bacterial species in the bloodstream) is a leading cause of death. Fewer than 25% of HIV/AIDS children express the kinds of OIs found in adult AIDS patients. Kaposi's sarcoma occurs in about 4% of them. Young HIV/AIDS children experience delayed development and poor motor function. Older children experience speech and perception problems.

The Pediatric AIDS Foundation reported in April 1995 that hospital costs for each HIV-infected newborn were $35,000 per year. (In August-2012 the U.S. Department of Health and Human Services and the World Health Organization released new guidelines for treating HIV-infected children.)

Worldwide ending year 2013 about 3.7 million children will be living with HIV disease and about 5.7 million will have died from AIDS (Figure 11-9, page 358). Globally, about 1200 new pediatric cases occur daily, with about 84% of them occurring in sub-Saharan Africa. Over 700 of these children die every day. Of the survivors, over half of the infected will die before their second birthday. UNAIDS is calling for the elimination of mother-to-child HIV transmission by 2015!

The President's Emergency Plan for AIDS Relief (PEPFAR) central goal is to reduce the number of new pediatric infections by 90% by 2015 in the 22 countries carrying 90% of the global burden of vertical transmission. The science is clear—achieving a generation born HIV-free is possible. It is a smart investment that will save lives and pay dividends in many of the world's emerging economies.

Global Elimination of Mother-to-Child (MTCT) HIV Transmission?

Virtual elimination of MTCT is defined as achieving less than a 5% transmission rate or a 90% reduction in HIV infections among children by 2015. Is this possible? It is estimated that if 90% of HIV-positive pregnant women receive antiretroviral therapy (ART), at least

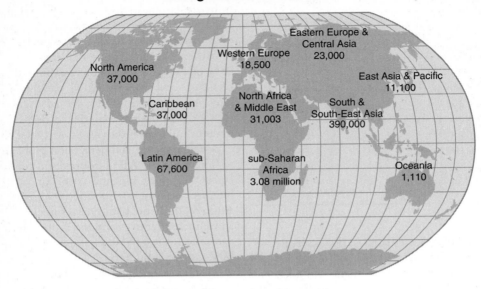

Year End Estimates: Children Living with HIV Infection

North America
37,000

Western Europe
18,500

Eastern Europe &
Central Asia
23,000

East Asia & Pacific
11,100

Caribbean
37,000

North Africa
& Middle East
31,003

South &
South-East Asia
390,000

Latin America
67,600

sub-Saharan
Africa
3.08 million

Oceania
1,110

Totals are estimates for the entire globe.
Total: 2013—3.7 million

FIGURE 11-9 Estimated Year End 2013 Global Estimates of Children Living with HIV Infection. Note that sub-Saharan Africa and South and Southeast Asia have the highest burden of HIV-infected children. Sub-Saharan Africa has about 84% of children living with HIV/AIDS. *(Courtesy of UNAIDS, updated.)*

1 million new perinatal infections could be averted by 2015. Also, continued use of ART while breast-feeding could avert an additional 264,000 infections. Together, these two preventive measures would result in a reduction of 79% of new perinatal infections through 2015. Clearly this misses the goal of achieving the virtual elimination of new MTCT, but it is getting closer to that goal. And such progress offers hope that the elimination of MTCT will be achieved sometime between 2015 and 2020.

UPDATE MAY 2012—The Joint United Nations Programme on HIV/AIDS (UNAIDS) launched a new campaign, "Believe it. Do it.", aimed at bringing attention and action to the global goal of ending new HIV infections among children by 2015 and ensuring mothers living with HIV remain healthy.

Ethnic Prevalence of Pediatric AIDS Cases

Children of color make up 14% of all children in the United States but account for 57% of pediatric AIDS cases. Whites make up 70% of children and account for 18% of pediatric AIDS cases. Hispanics make up 12% of children and account for 23% of pediatric AIDS cases.

ORPHANED CHILDREN DUE TO HIV INFECTION AND AIDS

Each year, worldwide, over two million children become orphans. November 20, 2013, will be the 25th anniversary of the United Nations Universal World Children's Day, a day set aside to promote the welfare of children.

World AIDS Orphans Day is held on May 7. "Orphan" is an English word that does not have an exact translation in many languages. The concept of orphan is a social construct, so the meaning assigned to it varies from one society to another. In the United States and Africa, typically the term is understood to mean a child who has lost either or both parents. UNAIDS reports orphans as children who have lost their mothers or both parents. They limit their estimates to children below age 15. The UN Convention on the Rights of the Child defines children as being below age 18, unless the age of majority (adulthood) is reached under national law. Who is a child and who is an adult is defined differently in different countries and among different cultures. This further complicates the meaning of the word because orphans are generally considered to be children.

Children: The Missing Face of AIDS

Children are missing not only from global and national policy discussions on HIV/AIDS, but they also lack access to even the most basic care and prevention services. Millions of children are missing parents, siblings, schooling, health care, basic protection, and many of the other fundamentals of childhood because of the toll the disease is taking. Over 31 years into the pandemic, help is reaching less than 10% of the children affected by HIV/AIDS, leaving too many children to grow up alone, grow up too fast, or not grow up at all. Every minute of every day a child dies of AIDS-related illness, and another is HIV infected.

Orphaned Children: Unheard Voices, Hidden Lives

Ending year 2013, of the estimated 15 million AIDS-related orphans, 90% live or have lived in Africa. The problem of AIDS-related orphans will become much greater over the next 10 to 15 years.

AIDS orphans present a chilling illustration of the far-reaching effects of the AIDS pandemic.

Orphans in the United States

His mother was young, single, and HIV positive. When she went to the hospital to give birth, she checked in under a false name and address and then slipped out of the hospital, leaving her baby who was only a few hours old.

An increasing number of HIV-infected children are being left in hospitals because their HIV-infected mothers and fathers are unable to care for them and no one else wants them. The hospital becomes their home.

As HIV continues to spread across the United States and HIV-infected women continue to become pregnant, the question is: What will happen to their HIV-infected babies? For one young woman who passed HIV to her baby two years ago, the decision has been made. The baby has AIDS and is in foster care. The mother is very ill. The courts are now deciding whether her six other children should also be put in foster care.

Unless the course of the epidemic changes drastically, through the year 2013, the cumulative number of U.S. children, teens, and young adults left motherless due to AIDS will exceed 160,000. About 85,000 children under age 15 have already lost their mother or both parents to AIDS. The great majority of these children, uninfected by the virus, will begin to affect already burdened social services in major American cities. Things will get immediately worse in such places, where children already spend years going from foster home to foster home, and caseworkers are overwhelmed by long lists of families needing everything from housing to medical care (Figure 11-10).

The Silent Legacy

Orphans are often referred to as the silent legacy of AIDS. It is expected that about a third of the children orphaned in America will be from New York City, which has the nation's largest number of AIDS cases. Other cities expected to be hit hard are Miami, Los Angeles, Washington, DC, Newark, and San Juan, Puerto Rico. Most of these orphans will be the children

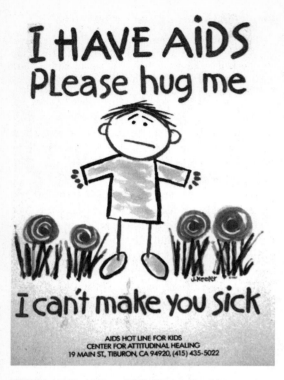

FIGURE 11-10 I Have AIDS—Please Hug Me. *(Permission granted and copyrighted by The International Center for Attitudinal Healing, 33 Buchanan Drive, Sausalito, CA 94965.)*

of poor black or Hispanic women whose families are already dealing with stresses like drug addiction, inadequate housing, and lack of healthcare. Relatives who might in other circumstances be called upon to care for the children often shun them because of the stigma attached to AIDS.

THE PHENOMENON OF AIDS ORPHANS

Sub-Saharan Africa

The HIV/AIDS orphan crisis is one of the greatest humanitarian and development challenges facing the global community. The orphan epidemic is still in its infancy. In the years and decades ahead, the impacts of HIV/AIDS on children, their families, and their communities will grow far worse—expanding

to dimensions difficult to imagine at present. During 1995 through 2012, on average, 400,000 children were born with HIV infection annually (about 1100 per day); of these children, about 90% were in sub-Saharan Africa, 8% in Southeast Asia, and 2% in Latin America and the Caribbean.

In Lesotho, Malawi, Mozambique, Swaziland, Zambia, and Zimbabwe, people are battling a lethal mix of food shortages and HIV/AIDS. About one in four to one in five adults in the six countries now live with HIV or AIDS; increasing deaths and sickness have ground social safety nets way below the reach of poor households. The outlook for children is particularly bleak: The six countries are home to about 3 million children who have lost one or both parents to AIDS (Figure 11-11, below).

In April 2004, the International AIDS Trust and Children Affected by AIDS Foundation released a report stating that worldwide, every 14 seconds a child is orphaned by AIDS, and that by 2013 worldwide, there will be about 16 million AIDS orphans (lost one or both parents to AIDS-related illness). Of the 38 million people living with HIV/AIDS, ending 2013, about 3.6 million are less than age 15 and 11.7 million are between ages 15 and 24.

Mother-to-Child Transmission (MTCT) or Vertical HIV Transmission

Vertical transmission means that HIV passes directly from the infected mother into the fetus, newborn, or infant. Data released in mid-2003 on 5000 mother-infant pairs showed that 40% of all HIV transmission within this group occured during breast-feeding, at least four weeks after delivery. (Also see Gray et al., 2008.)

Stigma—Stigma is particularly strong surrounding mother-to-child transmission. The very phrase "mother-to-child" itself may be stigmatizing as it puts all the responsibility of transmission on the mother and none on the father of the child. Stigma stops women coming forward to get themselves tested. It reduces their choices when it comes to healthcare and family

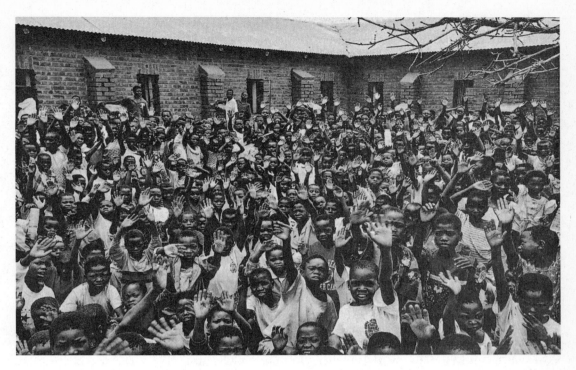

FIGURE 11-11 AIDS Orphans Gathering to Get Food, Care, and Shelter in Malawi, Africa. *(Photograph courtesy of Ellen McCurley—The Pendulum Project.)*

life once they are diagnosed as HIV positive and has a negative effect on their quality of life. Equally troubling is the lack of sympathy or respect given to pregnant women with HIV, especially in the developing nations where they are open to blame, ridicule, and rejection. For example, in rural Zambia a man stated, "If a pregnant woman is sick and has a sick and premature baby who dies before 3 months, then we know she is affected [infected with HIV] and turn away from her. This is our [HIV] test!"

Timing of HIV Transmission—The exact time of HIV transmission to the fetus during pregnancy is unknown. It has been shown to occur as early as the fifteenth week of gestation, at or near the time of delivery, and through breast-feeding.

Breast-feeding by mothers with HIV infection established *before* pregnancy increases the risk of vertical transmission by 16%. When a mother develops primary HIV infection while breast-feeding,

the risk of transmission rises to 29%. In general, it is believed that 50% of HIV-positive babies are infected during the last two months of pregnancy and about 50% are infected during the birthing process or through the early months of breast-feeding (Miotti et al., 1999).

A working definition of the timing of maternal HIV transmission has been established to differentiate infants infected *in utero (in the uterus)* from those infected near the time of or *during delivery (perinatally)*. In utero infection occurs in approximately 30% of HIV-infected infants. Children who are infected in utero have a more rapid progression to AIDS and generally become symptomatic during the first year of life. Those infected perinatally have no detectable HIV at birth but demonstrate HIV in the blood by 4 to 6 months of age. These children constitute the majority of HIV-infected infants and have a slower progression to AIDS, about 8% per year (Zijenah et al., 2004).

Rate of Mother-to-Child Transmission (MTCT)—The worldwide rate of HIV transmission from mother, without drug therapy, to child varies geographically. In Africa, maternal transmission is as high as 50%. In Europe and the United States, without the use of antiretroviral drugs the overall rate is 25% to 30%, producing less than 500 infected babies a year. The use of antiretroviral drugs in the United States, along with cesarean section, has lowered the MTCT to less than 1%. Claire Townsend and colleagues (2008) reported that in the United Kingdom and Ireland, the use of antiretroviral therapy to lower viral loads to less than 50 copies per milliliter of blood dropped MTCT to 0.1%. **This drop in maternal HIV transmission to their children remains the single greatest achievement in HIV/AIDS prevention methodology. This is due in part to the use of ART. At the current rate of delivering ART to pregnant women, there is a real possibility that by 2015 to 2020 mother-to-child transmission will be substantially over! But there is much to be done. Entering 2013, at least 75% of HIV-positive pregnant women in 61 countries, including Cameroon, Ethiopia, India, and Nigeria do not yet receive or receive suboptimal ART!**

The U.S. Public Health Service and 16 other national health organizations have recommended that HIV testing be offered to all women at risk prior to or at the time of pregnancy. Perinatal HIV Hotline (888)448-8765: Perinatal Consultation and Referral Service. Testing and care of HIV-infected pregnant women.

Good News—United States

The really good news is most new pediatric infections now come from about 5% of infected women who remain undiagnosed at delivery. **Good news—yes, because if all women are tested for HIV early in their pregnancy, newborn infections can almost be eliminated!** In July 2012 the Public Health Task Force published an update to "Recommendations for Use of Antiretroviral Drugs in Pregnant HIV-Infected Women for Maternal Health and Interventions to Reduce Perinatal HIV Transmission in the United States."

Conclusion

Globally, one in seven infections worldwide occurs through mother-to-child transmission. In June 2011, PEPFAR and UNAIDS launched a global plan for eliminating new infections among children by 2015. In April 2012, the World Health Organization said that to prevent vertical transmission, *all women* should start triple antiretroviral therapy ART as soon as they test HIV positive, regardless of T4 or CD4 count, and continue triple ART for life. It is believed that vertical transmission of HIV can be eliminated by testing of mothers and blocking of transmission through the use of antiretroviral drugs, accompanied by elective caesarean section and the use of replacement infant feeding.

Viral RNA Load Associated with Perinatal HIV Transmission—Although the close association between stage of HIV infection in a pregnant woman and likelihood of perinatal transmission has been established, there are no precise numerical criteria for pregnancies at high and low risk of transmission. Viral load measurements are now helping to quantitate this risk. (See Chapter 4, pages 94-101, for a discussion of viral load.)

Through 2012, data continued to accumulate that suggest that the use of HAART and achievement of optimal viral load suppression is associated with the greatest reduction of vertical transmission. The identification of HIV infection in pregnant women is the biggest hurdle in reducing vertical transmission.

States and Territories Most Affected by Pediatric Cases

There is evidence that HIV was present in female IDUs as early as 1977 because their babies developed AIDS (Thomas, 1988). As the number of HIV-infected women of childbearing age rises, so does the potential number of HIV-infected babies.

In the United States pediatric AIDS is most widespread among blacks, Hispanics, and the poor

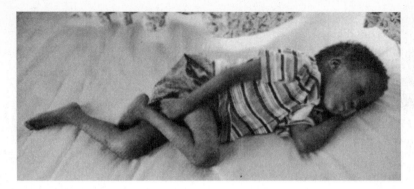

FIGURE 11-12 Josh, Age 3, Has Advanced-Stage AIDS. His older brother died from AIDS. Their mother died of AIDS, leaving them as AIDS orphans. *(Photo by Mike Stocker/South Florida Sun-Sentinel.)*

of the inner cities (Figure 11-12). Ending year 2013, New York will continue to have the highest incidence of pediatric AIDS cases, followed by Florida, New Jersey, California, Puerto Rico, and Texas. Combined, these cases accounted for 66% of all AIDS cases reported among children.

AIDS Cases among Children Declining

There are many reasons to believe that with continued HIV counseling of HIV-positive pregnant women and the use of AIDS drug cocktails that lower viral loads, fewer children will become infected, and this will translate into a continued decrease in children with AIDS.

This possibility was inconceivable to many clinicians, families, and patients not too long ago. The rapid decline has many physicians suggesting that a goal of eliminating perinatal transmission may be attainable in the United States.

Breast-Feeding, Drug Therapy, and HIV Transmission

In reviewing the recent literature on breast-feeding, a variety of conflicting data have been reported by the respected authorities in this field of HIV/AIDS research. For example, it is not understood how AZT, nevirapine, or other drugs lower the vertical HIV transmission rate, except to say that these drugs inhibit HIV replication (Figure 11-13, this page).

The World Health Organization and the United Nations continue to recommend the following: "When replacement feeding is acceptable, feasible, affordable, sustainable, and safe, avoidance of all breast-feeding by HIV-infected mothers is recommended. Otherwise, exclusive breast-feeding is recommended during the first

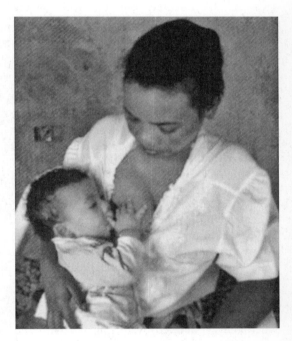

FIGURE 11-13 Drops of Danger. This woman nurses her four-month-old son. She, her husband, and three other children have been diagnosed with AIDS. She did not know she could pass HIV to her newborn via breast-feeding. She said that her husband was her only sexual partner. After her health began to decline and she tested HIV positive, her husband refused to be tested, and he abandoned the family for another woman. *(Photo by Hilda M. Perez/South Florida Sun-Sentinel.)*

24 months of life" (Newton et al., 2008; Kuhn et al., 2008). Recent (2011) U.S. guidelines for the use of antiretroviral agents in pediatric HIV infection recommend that HIV-positive babies be put on ART as soon as they are diagnosed, regardless of their CD4+ cell counts.

Life Span of Untreated HIV-Infected Newborns in Sub-Saharan Africa

According to Taha Taha and colleagues of Johns Hopkins University (2000), over 50% of HIV-infected newborns in sub-Saharan Africa died within 12 months. Eighty-nine percent of HIV-infected children alive at six months died by age three years. In comparison, the authors note that in Europe and the United States, only 18% of HIV-infected children died by age 3 years, and 75% lived to age 5 years and older.

HIV-Infected Newborns Now Having Children—a Third Generation of HIV/AIDS in America

Michelle McConnell of the CDC said, "It's a landmark in the HIV epidemic at least in the United States. Survival has increased to such an extent that not only are HIV-infected babies surviving but they're healthy enough to reach their teen years, get pregnant, and have healthy kids." McConnell was referring to the eight women living in Puerto Rico who contracted HIV from their mothers and who reported 10 pregnancies between August 1998 and May 2002. Five of the eight became pregnant accidentally; only two reported using condoms when they conceived. None of the babies born to the women, all of whom were teenagers when they conceived, were infected with the virus. All the mothers had received antiretroviral AIDS drugs consistently during pregnancy. The data showed that some women in the study reported becoming sexually active at around the same age that they learned of their HIV-positive status. That finding could indicate that teens and young adults infected with HIV at birth are just as likely to engage in risky sex later in life as their peers who were not infected with the

virus. It may also mean that the decision by many parents to shield their children from knowledge of HIV disease until later in adolescence may be too late. Since this report at least 15 similar cases have been reported by the CDC. In addition to these 23 cases, one has to consider the relatively large number of HIV-positive babies who have reached their teenage years and have become sexually active. As these numbers increase, the means of heterosexual/homosexual transmission increases among the young. Clearly, the use of Highly Active Antiretroviral Therapy is allowing an increasing number of young women who were born with HIV infection to live long enough to become sexually active and become pregnant.

Entering 2013, because of early access to care in the United States and advances in anti-HIV drug treatment, approximately half of all HIV-infected children will live to enter and graduate from high school and beyond. However, globally, less than 20% of the 3.7 million children in need of antiretroviral drugs are getting them. Without treatment, most of these children will die before their fifth birthday. Eighty-four percent of HIV children live in sub-Saharan Africa.

Summary

For over the past 30 years, HIV infection and its consequent disease, acquired immune deficiency syndrome (AIDS), have affected more women worldwide than any other life-threatening infectious disease. Women will account for about 52% of the 38 million people living with HIV ending 2012. In sub-Saharan Africa, females now constitute 60% of those infected with HIV. Women make up half of the adults living with HIV in the Caribbean and one-third in Latin America. In addition to the direct impact that HIV infection has on these women, there is also the known high risk of HIV transmission to their infants and a resulting plethora of consequences for the family. In the United States, the annual number of estimated AIDS cases increased 19% among women and only 1% among men from 1999 through 2011. The major burden of disease is in young women and women of color, particularly black American and Hispanic women, who often have reduced access to health care. The rate of AIDS diagnoses for black

American women is approximately 25 times the rate for white women and four times the rate for Hispanic women. The majority of infections were due to heterosexual transmission or to injection-drug use. These same risk factors, especially injection-drug use, have led to a 50% increase in infections in women in Asia and eastern Europe during the past five years. This growing feminization of the HIV pandemic reflects women's greater social and biological vulnerability.

The predominance of heterosexually acquired HIV infection in women of reproductive age has important implications for vertical HIV transmission to their offspring: Most children with AIDS were infected by mothers who acquired infection through heterosexual contact. One of the greatest tragedies of the AIDS pandemic is orphaned children. They are left in hospitals because (1) their parents have died of AIDS or cannot care for them, or (2) no one wants them.

The magnitude of the problems of children affected by HIV/AIDS dwarfs the scale of the existing response. Children and adolescents around the globe are increasingly at risk of infection, and many of those infected by HIV/AIDS are being left to grow up alone, grow up too soon, or to not grow up at all.

Review Questions

(Answers to the Review Questions are on page 463.)

1. By the end of year 2013 how many women are expected to be HIV positive worldwide?

2. Globally, what percentage of *new* HIV infections occur in women?

3. What are the major routes of HIV transmission into women?

4. What is the most likely way a female prostitute in the United States becomes HIV infected?

5. During year 2012, how many women worldwide became HIV positive and how many died from AIDS?

6. AIDS is now the _____ cause of death for all women between ages _____ and _____. It is the _____ leading cause of death in _____ women between the ages of _____ and _____ and the _____ cause of death for black women ages _____ to _____.

7. Of the 4 million women who become pregnant each year in the United States, how many are estimated to be HIV positive?

8. Through year 2012, how many states have not reported a pediatric AIDS case?

9. Since 1995, what percentage per year of HIV-infected newborns received HIV from their mothers?

10. List three major factors that are associated with perinatal HIV transmission.

11. Where do most of the orphaned AIDS children come from? Why are they called AIDS orphans?

12. Globally, ending 2013, how many people will be living with HIV/AIDS?

    A. 38 million
    B. 77 million
    C. 24 million
    D. 10 million

13. Globally, of those living with HIV/AIDS, ending 2013, about how many are women?

    A. 14.6 million
    B. 19.4 million
    C. 3.3 million
    D. 10 million

14. Women are about _____ as likely as men to contract an HIV infection from a single act of unprotected sex.

    A. half
    B. equally
    C. about twice
    D. three times

15. Studies have shown that in many parts of the world, including India, Kenya, Colombia, Zambia, and all of sub-Saharan Africa, _____ women are more at risk than are their _____ counterparts.

    A. married, unmarried
    B. unmarried, married

16. True or False: If you are HIV positive and pregnant, there are antiretroviral drugs you can take that can greatly decrease the chances of your baby becoming infected.

17. True or False: Women will not become HIV infected if they properly use birth control pills and/or diaphragm.

Prevalence of HIV Infection and AIDS among Young Adults, Ages 13 to 24

CHAPTER HIGHLIGHTS

- U.S. and global statistics on HIV infection in young adults.
- People ages 13 to 24 in the United States make up an estimated 15% of new HIV infections: About 60% male, 40% female.
- Over half of all new HIV infections globally occur in young adults.
- Only a fraction of HIV-infected young adults know they are infected.
- Know-Protect-Talk.
- The vast majority of young adults have no access to the information, skills, and services needed to protect themselves from HIV infection.
- Seven of ten people are sexually active by age 19.
- The total number of HIV-infected teenagers/young adults is unknown.
- Black and Hispanic young adults account for a disproportionate number of AIDS cases compared to whites.
- Young adults are being exposed to quality HIV prevention but they choose to ignore it.
- Sex thrills but AIDS kills.
- HIV babies reaching adulthood.
- Abstinence education: Saying no over and over again.
- Worldwide, there are over 5 million young adults ages 13 to 24 and they account for about 50% of all new HIV infections.
- In the 20 highest HIV-prevalence countries, less than one-third of young adults have sufficient knowledge to prevent HIV infection.
- Young adults make up about 23% of the U.S. population and about 4% of AIDS cases.
- Heterosexual sexual transmission is the leading cause of HIV infection in young adults.
- Young adult-specific behaviors and biologic factors make them particularly vulnerable to unsafe sexual practices.
- In the United States about 3 young adults per hour become HIV infected.
- Substance abuse is a 47% risk factor for HIV infection in young adults.
- About 60% of new HIV infections among U.S. women occurs in those between ages 13 and 24.

GLOBAL HIV INFECTIONS IN YOUNG ADULTS

Global Youth AIDS Day, February 26. A Movement by Youth to Bring an End to HIV/AIDS

Over the summer of 1999, especially in the United States, young people ages 13 to 24 flocked to theaters to experience the **Dark Side of the Force.** Many thousands saw the *Star Wars* movie repeatedly. But the real **Dark Side** of their lives is the threat of HIV infection, and the **Force** should be their education to prevent their infection.

Over half of all new HIV infections worldwide are occurring in this age group. Hopefully, reading this chapter will encourage the young to stay on the **Light Side with the Force.**

The Spread of HIV in Young Adults (Ages 13 to 24): United States

There is no shortage of statistics indicating that young adults continue to be the most vulnerable group of individuals to HIV infection. Every year since at least 2002, about 50% of all new infections in the United States occurred among young adults. In the United States it comes to over 30,000 new infections each year, or about three infections every hour. They will make up about 20% of all HIV infections (about 460,000 through 2013). About two-thirds contracted HIV sexually, and three-quarters of them occurred in racial and ethnic minorities. Some global and U.S. statistics on young adults and HIV/AIDS are:

Global

- Globally, about 27% or about 2 billion of the population is between ages 10 and 19.
- In sub-Saharan Africa about 45% (adolescents) are under age 15.
- Of 38 million people living with HIV/AIDS ending year 2013, over a third will be young adults (ages 13–24)(about 13 million) and about 65% of them will be female.
- Every day about 3000 young adults become infected with HIV, or about 1 million a year (Figure 12-1).
- Only a fraction of HIV-infected young adults are aware of their infection, and even a smaller number are linked to proper medical care or social services.
- Of young adults who become HIV infected, most are infected by age 24, and without ART, usually die of AIDS by age 35.
- Everyone born after 1980 was born into a world of HIV/AIDS.
- Most young people with HIV/AIDS were/are infected sexually.
- About 5.5 million young adults are living with HIV/AIDS.

United States

- In 2013 about 22,000 young adult ages 13 to 24 will become HIV infected.
- People under ages 13 to 24 are estimated to make up 15% of new HIV cases.

- Through 2012 about 1200 have died of HIV/AIDS and about 48,000 are living with HIV/AIDS.
- Only 19% of teens ages 15 to 19 report that they have ever been tested for HIV, versus 44% of young adults ages 20 to 24.
- About 94% of young adult women who are newly HIV infected are black and/or Hispanic.
- Many young people do not know the basic facts about HIV risk, prevention, and treatment. Over one-third (37%) of 18- to 25-year olds incorrectly believe at least one of the following: Transmission of HIV is possible by sharing a glass, kissing, or touching a toilet seat.
- The median age at first intercourse is 16.9 years for boys and 17.4 years for girls. There are differences in age of initiation by race and ethnicity, with 27% of black American high school boys, 11% of Latino boys, and 5% of white boys initiating sex before age 13.
- Over half of males (55%) and females (54%) ages 15 to 19 and 66% age 15 to 24 report having had oral sex with someone of the opposite sex. Approximately one in ten males and females ages 15 to 19 had engaged in anal sex with someone of the opposite sex; 3% of males ages 15 to 19 have had anal sex. (CDC August 2012 report)

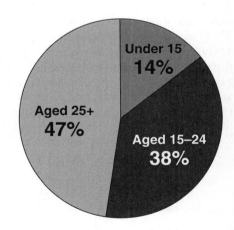

Estimated New Infections = 2.5 million

FIGURE 12–1   Young Adults As a Percentage of Global New HIV Infections, Estimated 2013
Source: Calculations based on UNAIDS/WHO, Core Slides: Global Summary of the HIV and AIDS Epidemic, 2007, 2008, updated.

ADDRESSING THE AIDS PANDEMIC AMONG YOUNG ADULTS: KNOW-PROTECT-TALK

Young adults and adolescents are central to any discussion of HIV/AIDS because there are so many! There are about 2 billion people ages 10 to 24 in the world. Young adults are and will continue to be the sector of the population most affected by HIV/AIDS. As today's children grow up, the proportion of 13- to 24-year-olds will continue to increase, particularly in developing countries (See Table 12-1, Figure 12-2, and Point of View 12.1, page 369.)

United Nations Commitment to Young Adults

In order to reduce the size and impact of the AIDS pandemic on young adults worldwide, in 2004 the United Nations General Assembly Special Session on HIV/AIDS produced a "Declaration of Commitment on HIV/AIDS: Global Targets & Principles for Young People." This declaration is as follows:

By 2005—

1. Reduce HIV prevalence among youth ages 15 to 25 in the most affected countries by 25%; by 2010, reduce global HIV prevalence among this age group by 25% (Article 47).

2. Ensure that at least 90% of youth ages 15 to 24 have access to the information, education, including peer education and youth-specific HIV education, and services necessary to develop the life skills required to reduce their vulnerability to HIV infection; ensure at least 95% access by 2010 (Article 53).

3. Ensure access of both girls and boys to primary and secondary education, including HIV/AIDS education (Article 63).

4. Ensure safe and secure environments, especially for young girls (Article 63).

5. Expand good quality youth-friendly information and sexual health education and counseling service (Article 63).

6. Involve young people in planning, implementing, and evaluating HIV/AIDS prevention and care programs (Article 63).

RESULTS—Steps 1–4 failed and steps 5–6 were marginally implemented.

Why the High HIV Infection Rates among Young Adults?

Of the world's young adults, 85% live in developing countries, and this is where over 90% of the pandemic is now concentrated. But population

Table 12-1 Young People, Ages 13–24, Living with HIV/AIDS by Region, End of 2012

Region	Number	Percentage of Global Total
Global Total	**12,200,000**	**100%**
Sub-Saharan Africa	7,564,000	62%
South/Southeast Asia	2,196,000	18%
Eastern Europe/Central Asia	768,600	6.3%
Latin America	744,200	6.1%
East Asia	414,800	3.4%
Caribbean	158,600	1.3%
North America	158,600	1.3%
North Africa/Middle East	146,400	1.2%
Western Europe	48,800	0.4%
Oceania	9,760	0.08%

(Source: UNAIDS 2005, updated)

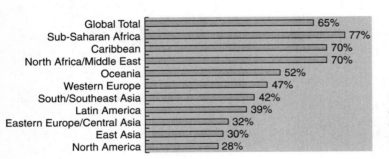

FIGURE 12-2 Estimated Young Adult Women as a Percentage of All Ages 13–24 with HIV/AIDS Ending Year 2012. *(Source: UNAIDS 2005, updated.)*

percentages tell only part of the story. There are special reasons why young people are exposed to infection. Remember that above all, HIV is a sexually transmitted virus. Being a young adult is a time of discovery, emerging feelings of independence, and the exploration of new behavior and relationships. It is also a time of examination, rebellion, and change. By definition young people take risks and experiment. Sexual behavior, an important part of this, can involve risks; the same is true of experimentation with drugs. During this time, young people get mixed messages. They are often faced with double standards calling for virginity in girls but early and active sexual behavior in boys. They have been told **"Just say no"** since the early 1980s, yet risk taking continues, perhaps because they are confronted with hundreds of millions of dollars' worth of media images of sex, smoking, and drinking as glamorous and risk-free. They are told to be abstinent, but exposed to a barrage of advertisements using sex to sell goods. Compounding the challenge, in the name of morality, culture, or religion, young people are often

denied their right to education about the health risks of sexual behavior and to important tools and services for protection. Among the world's young adults, some are more exposed to HIV than others. Those living in what UNICEF terms "especially difficult circumstances" include young people who are out of school, who live on the streets, who share needles with other injection-drug users, engage in commercial sex, or are sexually and physically abused. Young men who have sex with men are disadvantaged by the lack of information and services available to them and directed to their needs.

As the HIV/AIDS pandemic spreads, even younger age groups are becoming exposed to the risk of HIV. Infection spreads to younger age groups as men choose increasingly younger sexual partners. Many men believe, perhaps correctly, that younger girls are less likely to be infected with HIV, while others hold the mistaken belief that having sex with a virgin can cure AIDS.

HOW LARGE IS THE YOUNG ADULT POPULATION IN THE UNITED STATES?

In the United States there are about 43 million young adults (73% white, 11% black, 16% Hispanic), and about 22 million between the ages of 25 and 29. That's 65 million, or about 21% of the population, between the ages of 13 and 29. Over 86% of all STDs occur in this age group. It has been estimated that about 40% of all heterosexual adults with AIDS were infected with HIV as young adults.

Young Adult Women at Greatest Risk for HIV/AIDS in the United States

While more research needs to be done on this topic, several factors associated with young women are clear: (1) They tend to be partnered with **older men** who have had more sexual partners and have a greater chance of being infected with HIV and other sexually transmitted diseases; (2) their risk of HIV infection is greater because their immature cervix and relatively low vaginal mucus production presents less of a barrier to HIV; (3) many lack the education, social status, economic resources, and power in sexual partner relationships to make informed choices; (4) a 2003 Kaiser Family Foundation study of young adults showed that one in four contract a sexually transmitted disease annually. And 70% of women ages 13 to 24 consider forms of contraception other than condoms, such as birth control pills, to be a form of "safer sex."

Global Number of Adolescents Ages 10–19

In April 2012, UNICEF released its first ever report on the challenges facing the world's 1.2 billion people ages 10–19, a group comprising 18% of the global population. "Progress for Children: A Report Card on Adolescents" was issued to coincide with the 2012 meeting of the UN Commission on Population Development. Among the key findings of the report: Some 2.2 million people ages 10–19 are living with HIV, and most are unaware of their infection. Girls account for 1.3 million adolescent HIV cases. Many HIV-positive adolescents contracted the virus at birth, while others were infected through unprotected sex or sharing needles. Adolescent girls in developing countries often marry and bear children at too young an age, hampering their educational opportunities. Approximately 16 million girls ages 15–19 give birth each year worldwide; 90% of births to adolescents occur within marriage. Latin America, the Caribbean, and sub-Saharan Africa have the highest proportion of teenage births. Worldwide, 71 million adolescents do not attend secondary school, and up to 127 million young people ages 15–24 are illiterate—mostly in sub-Saharan Africa and South Asia.

Let's Talk about Sex: Safer Sex: Sex Thrills But HIV/AIDS Kills

There was a time when safer sex meant not getting caught by your parents. With time, sexually transmitted diseases and in particular HIV/AIDS have changed the meaning of safer sex. Today, over half of teenagers (ages 13 to 19) in the United States have had sex by the time they reach 16, and 7 in 10 are sexually active by 19. Many enter the sexual arena unprepared for the responsibility of their actions. About 1 million teenage women become pregnant outside of marriage each year.

Whether or not society openly discusses it, young adults are having sex. Many women—and most men—have their first sexual relations prior to marriage, usually during their teens, and most often those first encounters are unprotected. Research in family planning has revealed that the quality of reproductive health information is generally low among young adults. This is a reflection, in part, of the lack of social acceptance of providing sex education and contraceptive services to teens in many countries. In the developing world, contraceptive services are often available only to married women, and in some situations, only to women who have already borne one or more children.

The guiding philosophy in dealing with sexuality in many cultures is **"If you don't talk about sex they won't do it."** This logic, however, is critically flawed. Young adults are sexual beings at varying stages of self-awareness and understanding. Many teenagers continue to engage in sexual intercourse despite lack of access to any accurate information about sex and, in most cases, they engage in unsafe sex. **Safer sex requires an ability to distinguish between risky and non-risky sexual activities and the emotional security to choose safer sex.** (Point of Information 12.2, below; Snapshot 12.1, page 374)

POINT OF INFORMATION 12.2

CALIFORNIA COUNTIES TO GET MAIL ORDER CONDOM PROGRAM

In March 2012 the Condom Access Project (CAP) allows youth ages 12–19 in several California counties to order online a free package of 10 condoms, lubricant, and health information. Youths can request one package per month through the website teensource.org, which is run by the California Family Health Council. The material is sent by mail in plain yellow envelope. Supported by the California Department of Public Health's STD Control Branch, CAP aims to help reduce teen pregnancies and STDs among youths. The project, which will be paid for with federal funds, especially targets teens who cannot afford to buy condoms or are too embarrassed to access free condoms at clinics.

Young Adults, Sexual Partners: Sexually Transmitted Diseases and HIV/AIDS

In a 2008 CDC and a 2009 nationwide youth risk behavior surveillance survey, it was reported that among U.S. high school students:

- 48% have had sexual intercourse at least once (including 33% of 9th grade students and 65% of 12th-grade students).
- 7% had sexual intercourse for the first time before age 13.
- 15% have had four or more sex partners (including 9% of 9th grade students and 22% of 12th-grade students).
- 39% of sexually active students did not use a condom the last time they had sex (including 31% of 9th-grade students and 46% of 12th-grade students).
- 2% have injected illegal drugs at least once.
- 20% of high school students have abused prescription drugs.
- One in 10 high school students reported having experienced dating violence. Seven percent of students have been physically forced to have sexual intercourse, with females (11%) more likely than males (5%) to report this experience.
- Almost one-quarter (22%) of sexually active high school students reported using alcohol or drugs during their most recent sexual encounter, with males having a higher percentage (26%) compared to females (17%), and white males (28%) higher than black males (21%).
- Sexting is the exchange of explicit sexual messages or images by mobile phone. Ten percent of 14- to 24-year-olds report having shared a naked photo or video of themselves via digital communication such as the Internet or text messaging.
- The U.S. continues to have the highest teen pregnancy, birth, and abortion rates in the developed world.

They are experiencing skyrocketing rates of sexually transmitted diseases. The CDC survey reported that half of black women ages 13 to 19 had an STD, compared to 20% of Hispanics and 20% of whites. Every minute about 21 young adults somewhere in the United States become infected with an STD. People under age 25 account for 66% of all new STDs every year. One in four young adults will contract an STD before finishing high school. Experts fear that if these diseases are being transmitted, then HIV is, too. Entering 2013, among ages 13 to 24, heterosexual transmission accounted for about half of all HIV infections in the United States. Among males, about 60% of infections occurred among men having sex with men (MSM).

AIDS cases are relatively rare among 13- to 19-year-olds. This is because of the 11-year time average from HIV infection to AIDS diagnosis. In 1981, there was one reported teenage AIDS case; by 1991 there were 789 reported AIDS cases. Ending 2012, there will be an estimated 27,400 (2% of the total AIDS cases). (See Snapshot 8.2, page 206, for insight on young adults' views of oral sex.)

HIV/AIDS WON'T AFFECT US!

Regardless of available information on prevention, meaning that young adults do know how HIV is transmitted, there has been a continuing increase in HIV infections. They continue to engage in sexual intercourse without condoms (Figure 12-3).

Two groups, young adult gay men and young adult women infected via heterosexual sex, account for about 75% of young adult HIV infections. Race is an important factor with regard to who becomes infected. Sixty-one percent of AIDS cases that occur in people ages 20 to 24 occur in blacks and Latinos, but they were HIV infected in their teens (Collins et al., 1997).

ESTIMATE OF HIV-INFECTED AND AIDS CASES AMONG YOUNG ADULTS IN THE UNITED STATES, GLOBALLY

The total number of HIV-infected young adults in the United States is unknown. **Federal health agencies estimate that they make up about**

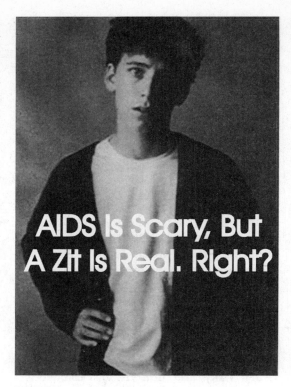

FIGURE 12-3 In the Life of a Young Adult, Items of Importance May Change Rapidly. *(Courtesy of the Centers for Disease Control and Prevention, Atlanta.)*

20% or about 460,000 of the HIV-infected population ending 2012. Of these, about 78,200 have AIDS. About 50% of HIV-infected young adults come from seven locations: New York, New Jersey, Texas, California, Florida, Washington, DC, and Puerto Rico. The male-to-female ratio of AIDS cases in the United States among 13- to 19-year-olds is about 1:1.

Sixty percent of new HIV infections in women now occur between ages 13 and 24.

Young Adults: Is the Fear of HIV/AIDS Being Lost? Let's Walk and Talk

This generation of young adults has not been subjected to HIV/AIDS activists' marches, disruptions, newspaper headlines, and TV programs showing the earlier years of people with AIDS

TEACH YOUR CHILDREN WELL
BY REGAN HOFMANN—HIV POSITIVE (FIGURE 12-4)

I never had proper sex ed. There was some reference to genitalia in my eighth-grade health class: Our teacher brandished rubber devices that showed, in 3-D, where children grew inside women's bellies and how liquids were transported from the inside to the outside of a man. But the creepy crash test-dummy-pink models hardly addressed what we really needed to know, like how to ask partners about their health status or how to put on—and take off—a condom. I left the classroom more confused than I had entered it. I wonder if that wasn't the idea—to scare us off sex altogether. Those frightening rubbery forms were as effective a form of birth control as a screaming baby.

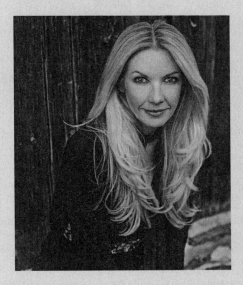

FIGURE 12-4 Regan Hofmann. She lived with her HIV-positive status in secret for almost 10 years. She broke her silence and released that fear in April 2006. On announcing her HIV status, she became editor-in-chief of *POZ Magazine.** Regan said that her "desire to remain silent was huge. I liked the feeling of being treated like a perfectly healthy person. As with many difficult things, it's easier to turn away from the truth of HIV than it is to face it. But looking it square in the eye is the first step in beating it. I took that first, large, step." From her HIV diagnosis in 1996 through 2008 she has taken over 50,000 pills.

POZ Magazine's mission is to educate people with HIV to take responsibility for their health. It was founded in 1994 by people living with AIDS (PLWA) to promote the vision that surviving AIDS is possible.

I had perfunctory conversations with my mom and dad years after I first needed to know the ins and outs of my body and how to protect it. I didn't want to admit that I wasn't a virgin; they didn't want to hear it. As for my younger sister, I tried to be a role model and discourage her from having sex for as long as possible. Which meant that the first real conversation we had about it was after her child was born. And my friends? Our conversations have always lacked sufficient specifics to be of any help. It's always, "Did you or didn't you?" and never, "How did you and were you safe?"

In America, for all our obsession with lascivious, prurient pleasures, we are terrified to talk frankly and specifically about sex. It is not a topic of polite conversation and if you ask people even basic questions they squirm and sidestep. We let ourselves and our kids watch—on TV and the Internet—people having all sorts of sex but we can't seem to talk about having safer sex. Why are we in denial?

I admit that it makes me a little uncomfortable to think of a 12- or 13-year-old having sex, as nearly 10% of that age group does. But if they're going to do it, shouldn't we teach them how to do it without lifelong or life-threatening consequences? I'm not against abstinence; it's a great form of birth control and disease prevention—if you can keep people from having sex. But apparently, we can't. In fact, the less we talk about sex directly and the more we pretend that we don't have it, the more we elevate what is otherwise a simple fact of life into a forbidden fruit that hangs so heavy and juicy on the tree that no one can resist trying it.

I had what many would consider a really good education. Yet when I graduated from college, I couldn't cook, change a tire, or keep myself from contracting a sexual disease that might kill me. I am astounded that as HIV infection rates continue to rise among teenagers, our educational system, our government, and our families continue to let our kids learn lessons the hard way. It's obvious that abstinence-only sex ed isn't working and that we desperately need to talk to America's youth openly and truthfully about an epidemic they know little about. I'm not into scare tactics, but today's kids are not afraid enough of HIV—too many of them perceive it as a manageable chronic illness that can be combated with a couple of pills a day. Maybe we've done too good a job educating them about how HIV can be treated and not a good enough job educating them about the difficulties of living with HIV. Maybe it's time to bust out those rubber forms again—and have a little talk.

(Reprinted with permission from *POZ Magazine,* January 2007. Copyright 2007 CDM Publishing, L.L.C.)

SHORT-TERM YOUNG ADULT RELATIONSHIPS AND HIV EXPOSURE RISK

Hey! We are celebrating our second anniversary. Yeah? Yeah, we've been together for two weeks. Let's have sex. Sure, they're monogamous, but only for the six weeks that the relationship lasts! Then they move on to others. In some cases such behavior can create a chain of relationships wherein each sexual partner exposes the other to whatever previous sexual partners may have had. For example, sociologists at Ohio State University have created the first "map" of young adult sexual behavior, outlining a sexual network of 288 one-to-one sexual relationships among high school students. While the teen at the end of the chain may have had contact with only one person, he or she had indirect contact with 286 others. Even so, despite reputations and popularity, most of the young adults were not promiscuous. They might know that their partner had a previous partner. But they don't think about the fact that this partner had a previous partner, who had a partner, and so on (Figure 12-5). This study suggests that young people need a different approach to sexual education and especially on HIV and STD prevention. The study was conducted at a high school in a mid-size town in the U.S. Midwest. The exact location was not given.

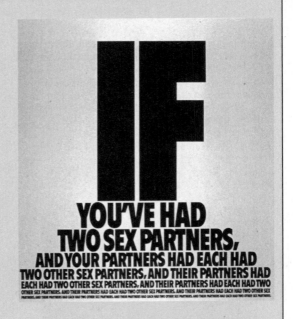

FIGURE 12-5 *(Courtesy of the Texas Department of State Health Services.)*

and their ghostlike appearances. In addition, because of the success of antiretroviral drug therapy, this generation of young adults has been spared the many gruesome details of AIDS patients and their stories. Together this may mean young adults are losing their fear of HIV/AIDS. Here are some recent comments made by some young adults in the United States:

1. We call it "three to six sex." This means having sex after school and before our parents come home. Question: Are condoms being used? Answer: No, duh, not really! Are you worried about HIV? Who cares?

2. A 16-year-old said, "I'm, like, terrified of getting pregnant. But I don't think anybody thinks about AIDS."

3. From a 15-year-old, "I've only had sex with one person so I don't have to worry about AIDS."

4. A 15-year-old boy who doesn't use protection says he's not afraid of getting infected with the deadly virus because "most people get it from drugs. And I don't use heroin."

The bottom line is health officials and activists say that lots of kids are having lots of sex and might not be hearing the safe sex message because it isn't stressed in school. (See Point of Information 12.3, and Side Issue 4.1, page 80, on young adult addiction to antiretroviral drugs.)

More Walk and Talk about Truth and Sex

In January 2010, the Chicago-based youth market research company TRU (partnering with the National Campaign to Prevent Teen and Unplanned Pregnancy and *Seventeen* magazine) released the results of its survey of 1200 males ages 15–22. Of participants, 300 each were ages 15–16, 17–18, 19–20, and 21–22. The intent was to measure sexual respect. Results from the online survey of sex and relationships, including attitudes and sexual history, paint a complicated picture for young U.S. men. Among the findings of the survey:

- 45% said they were virgins.
- 60% reported lying about something related to sex: 30% lied about how far they have gone, 24% about their number of sexual partners, and 23% about their virginity status.
- 78% agreed there was way too much pressure from society to have sex.
- 57% of sexually active respondents reported having had unprotected sex.
- 53% said they had talked with a parent about preventing pregnancy.
- 51% said having sex before marriage was acceptable in their family.
- 66% said they could be happy in a serious relationship that did not include sex.

The survey also found a double standard in terms of "hooking up," "friends with benefits," and other concepts of sexual freedom: among males, 53% said having a lot of casual partners makes them popular, but 71% said it makes girls less popular. In summary, sex is ever-present in the young adult mind while HIV bides its time. (QUICKTAKE 12.1)

Young Adults and Incidence of AIDS Cases and HIV by Gender and Color

Entering 1999, for the first time, more females than males ages 13 to 19 were reported as AIDS cases. Beginning 2013, of about 82,000 AIDS cases among ages 13 to 24 years, about 65% were black, 20% were Hispanic, and 15% were white. About 48,300 are living with HIV/AIDS.

Among young adult males, whites account for 38% of reported AIDS cases, followed by blacks (39%) and Hispanics (21%). Among females, blacks account for 66%, whites for 17%, and Hispanics for 17%. These females, unlike their adult counterparts, are more likely to become infected with HIV through sexual exposure than through

---

QUICKTAKE 12.1

EXPANSION OF SEX EDUCATION IN UNITED STATES IS NOT MAKING MUCH PROGRESS

According to Laura Kann and colleagues (2012) U.S. schools are not making much progress teaching their students about safer sex and preventing pregnancy and STDs. Researchers at the CDC compared 2008 and 2010 surveys from 45 states that asked school principals and health teachers how often they taught students a range of topics pertaining to sex education and prevention. In these required classes, the CDC recommended that they touch upon 11 topics ranging from compassion for people living with HIV/AIDS and health consequences of HIV/AIDS, STDs and pregnancy, to importance of condom use and the benefits of abstinence. According to the study, 11 states had fewer middle schools teaching all 11 topics in 2010 than they did in 2008, and none had more. And there was a significant gap between the states whose schools were more likely to teach more topics and those states whose schools taught fewer topics.

- The percentage of schools teaching all 11 suggested prevention topics in grades 6, 7, or 8 ranged from 12.6% in Arizona to 66.3% in New York.
- School participation in teaching eight of the suggested topics in grades 9, 10, and 12 ranged from 45.3% in Alaska to 96.4% in New Jersey.
- Importance of using condoms consistently and correctly was taught in 26.8% of public high schools in Utah and 96.6% of high schools in Delaware in 2010.

Laura Kann said, "Little progress has been made in the proportion of middle and high schools that offer education on the prevention of HIV, many STDs, and pregnancy. We are heading in the wrong direction." While their data confirmed what is happening in these schools, it doesn't explain why.

---

injection-drug use. A program that followed a large group of HIV-infected young adults found that although 85% of females contracted HIV infection through heterosexual intercourse, very few were aware that their male partners had HIV infection at the time of their exposure (Futterman et al., 1992). (See Snapshot 12.1, page 374 and Point of Information 12.4, page 376, 12.5, page 377, and Point of View 12.2, page 380.)

HIV–INFECTED CHILDREN: LIVING LONGER—PAYING A PRICE

HIV Babies Reaching Adulthood—Many Have to Live with Their Secret: Beginning 2013, an estimated 10,000 of these individuals are living with HIV/AIDS.

HIV/AIDS, in America, is the seventh leading cause of death in 15- to 24-year-olds.

Adolescents infected with HIV since birth are a new population in the ever-changing HIV/AIDS pandemic. Data from the CDC show that before 1996, HIV-infected children lived to an average age of 9. After 1996, with the use of antiretroviral drugs, the average age has risen to 18 and continues to climb.

Seven years ago, an estimated three children died each week of AIDS at Detroit's Children's Hospital. Today, that rate has dropped to about one child per year. But as the children's life expectancy increases, so do the number of complex social issues they must face, especially as young adults. One mother of an HIV-positive child said she dreads the issue of dating because it's going to be emotionally crippling. "Unless current attitudes about those infected with HIV change, my daughter will not be very popular and that will hurt. It will just crush her." The parents have had their car tires flattened, and parents of classmates forbade their children from playing with her. In response to these issues and new issues such as dating, the hospital has hired social workers and psychologists to hold support groups for these children, bringing them together to help them understand they aren't alone.

COMING OUT FOR AN "AIDS BABY": A SHORT STORY

If ever there was a time to tell her big secret, this was it, the seventh-grader thought. She and a few friends at a sleepover birthday party had sequestered themselves in a storage closet under a basement stairwell. They sat in a circle and talked for hours, promising, "Whatever we say here stays here." One girl shared her fear that her parents were on the verge of divorce. Another said she felt pressure to live up to her brother's example. There was a silence for a moment. Then the girl who had kept quiet for so many years took a deep breath and blurted a few quick words: "I have something to say. I'm HIV positive." Her friends took the news in stride. Until then, her friends had simply known her as their fun-loving buddy, the honor student, the girl with sarcastic wit who was as likely to use a big word they didn't understand as to address her friends as "dude." Now her friends knew something more: she was born an "AIDS baby," a term only vaguely familiar to most people her age. Four years after her disclosure, she reflects and strongly feels that she did the right thing. Coming out for these children is a complicated and terrifying task.

HIV/AIDS Affects Certain Groups of Young People Disproportionately

The burden of HIV infection falls disproportionately on certain groups of young adults, including young men who have sex with men (YMSM) and youth of color. In 2010, 2011 and 2012, more than half (54%) of all cases of HIV infection or AIDS among young people aged 13–24 were from male-to-male sexual contact. Thirty-four percent were from heterosexual contact. About 70% of all HIV/AIDS diagnoses among youth aged 13–19 were among black youth, even though blacks represented only 17% of the population in that age group. Of all YMSM, young black men bear the greatest burden. More than twice as many black MSM aged 13–24 were diagnosed with HIV infection or AIDS as their white or Hispanic counterparts.

Runaways and Homeless Young Adults

Each year since 1993, an estimated 3.4 million young adults dropped out of high school. These dropouts have higher frequencies of behaviors that put them at risk for HIV/STDs, and are less accessible to prevention efforts.

It's called survival sex, and it describes a sobering reality: Many homeless and runaway youths in the United States find themselves trading sex for money, drugs, or a roof over their heads. Experts say that puts them at high risk for HIV. There are nearly 1.8 million homeless and runaway youths in the United States and not nearly enough services to help them stay safe.

FEDERAL PUBLIC HEALTH POLICY SUPPORTS ABSTINENCE-ONLY PROGRAM: SEX EDUCATION

Abstinence is but one of the three approaches offered to lower the rate of HIV infection. The three approaches are A—abstinence, B—be faithful, and C—if not operating in the A or B mode, use a condom.

ABC Is Not As Simple As It Sounds

One only has to look in African villages and communities to understand how these "ABC" prescriptions confuse people. One is talking ABC to about 54 countries in Africa, with different prevalence of HIV infection, different numbers of cases, and different religious beliefs. Obviously there will be thousands of understandings and interpretations of ABC. The health minister of Uganda said, "Even in the same individual, in the morning you are in mode A, by evening in mode B, and by night, after a drink, in mode C." Some religious groups believe the C is for those condemned for not being A.

In addition, proponents of ABC offer many one-liner slogans at people that can be interpreted as an attempt to solve very complicated, deeply personal and sensitive issues in a way that is, to many, offensive.

DISCUSSION QUESTION: Do you believe that A, B campaigns protect women? Married women? Your position and reasons are?

Getting the right balance between each of the ABCs has led to unproductive disputes, which is why abstinence may be the hottest topic in HIV prevention. It raises temperatures among personal responsibility advocates and religious conservatives on the one hand, who believe people can and should just say no, and among sex-positive activists on the other, who believe any discussion of abstinence, even as an individual choice, is sex-negative.

Defining Abstinence Is Difficult!

One difficulty in measuring the efficacy or effectiveness of sex education programs lies in the conflicting definitions of the term *abstinence*. For example, some studies define abstinence as totally refraining from all sexual acts outside of marriage (including masturbation) and some link it to moral or religious beliefs. Other studies define abstinence as refraining from vaginal, anal, and oral sex. By some definitions, young adults who have experienced their first sexual encounter can become abstinent by refraining from further sexual activity; but by other definitions they cannot alternate back and forth. Everyone involved in this debate agrees on one fact: delaying the onset of a sexual experience in young adults is a good idea, at least in theory. Abstaining from sexual activity, that is, vaginal, anal, and oral sex, is 100% effective as a means for preventing sexually transmitted diseases (STDs), including HIV. For most people, however, abstinence is a temporary goal that may reflect current life circumstances, including being young, being between relationships, or waiting for an STD to heal. It remains effective in preventing HIV, STDs, and pregnancy only if it is practiced consistently.

Abstinence Education: Saying No Over and Over Again

Abstinence education seems to reflect an all-or-nothing ideology; in the same way that a person cannot be a little pregnant or partially HIV positive, he or she cannot be sometimes abstinent. Although most parents are not eager for their children to become sexually active, there is much disagreement about how exactly to persuade young people to wait. Asking people to stop having sex may sound good, à la abstinence, but has it ever worked? It is not working now!

IN ONE LESSON—NO SEX!

When it comes to young adults and sex, abstinence forces say the message is simple—don't do it. The other side says give them all the facts—including how to use a condom. No wonder parents and their children are confused.

Imagine This! Jenny, a cartoon teenage virgin, is about to give in to her boyfriend and climb into the backseat of his car. Suddenly, the emergency brake gives out and his car rolls until it teeters from a cliff off lover's lane. Their lives hang in the balance. That is when Windy, the good witch in hightops, leaps to the rescue. "Paul loves me," Jenny protests. Windy asks, "Oh. Is that why he asked you to do something that could mess up your life forever?" Using her time machine, Windy shows Jenny how she would have awakened pregnant. Had the car's brake not failed her boyfriend's condom would have. The cartoon, shown to sixth-graders at Burbank Elementary School, is one weapon in an arsenal of films, celebrity rallies, and school classes pushing a message of chastity in classrooms around the nation.

Federal and State Dollars for Abstinence-Only Education

Federal support for abstinence-only education began in 1982 with an allocation of $4 million per year

POINT OF INFORMATION 12.5 (*continued*)

through 1996. In 1996, Congress passed the Welfare Reform Act, which set aside $50 million a year for abstinence education to begin in fiscal year 1998. The $50 million per year ran with updated legislation through 2007. States had to provide three matching dollars for every four federal dollars received. This boosted the total funding to $87.5 million per year. States had to assure that the abstinence funded programs "did not promote contraception and/or condom use." Through year 2006, the money was provided to promote abstinence for those ages 12 through 18. In 2007, the targeted population was re-defined to include adolescents and/or adults ages 12 through 29. Beginning 2012, 30 states and one U.S. territory accepted abstinence funding. To date, about $2 billion in federal and state funding has been spent on abstinence-only education.

The federal program on abstinence specifically re-quires funded programs to teach the social, psycho-logical, and health gains to be realized by abstaining from sex; that abstaining from sexual activity outside marriage is the expected standard for all school-age adolescents; that a mutually faithful monogamous relationship in the context of marriage is the ex-pected standard of human sexual activity; and that **abstaining from sexual activity is the only certain way to avoid pregnancy, STDs, and other associated health problems.**

The Risk of Abstinence–Only Education: Taking the Pledge

Many critics of abstinence-only education agree that abstinence *would* be an ideal solution to the increase of new HIV infections among young adults. However, abstinence-only education does not actu-ally seem to achieve the goal of reducing unsafe sexual activity and may actually lead to increased risk for HIV transmission. The use of the acronym *ABC* may fall short in what is needed to reduce HIV transmission because the acronym tends to dimin-ish the message of prevention, oversimplifying what should be an ongoing, adaptable behavioral ap-proach to reducing HIV transmission. Surveys of sexuality conclude that with or without abstinence education, most young adults will be sexually active prior to the age of 18 and prior to marriage. A Har-vard University study report (2006) found that 52% of surveyed young adults had sex within of one year of signing a virginity pledge. Of 14,000 surveyed, ages 12 to 18, 73% denied having taken the pledge. Janet Rosenbaum (2009) reported that 82% of 11,000 students, grades 7 through 12, broke their abstinence pledge.

ABSTINENCE EDUCATION PROGRAMS

Abstinence is a prevention strategy that requires not only repeated attention, but in addition regular self denial.

There are now about 1000 abstinence-only sex ed-ucation programs in the United States. About 5000 school districts out of 17,468 teach abstinence as a part of their sex education programs. They serve about 1.5 million young people.

In their April 2007 report written by independent researchers (Mathematica Policy Research, under contract to the Department of Health and Human Services), they state that there is no evidence that abstinence-only programs prevent young adult sex, pregnancy, or disease. The Mathematica Policy Re-search firm found, following 2000 elementary and middle school students, that in four communities that received abstinence instruction—sometimes on a daily basis—they were just as likely to have sex in the following years as students who did not get such in-struction. Those who became sexually active—about half of each group—started at the same age (14.9 years on average) and had the same number of sexual partners. Of those who were sexually active, almost half said they used condoms only "sometimes" or "never." Less than a quarter of teens in both groups reported using a condom every time they had sex. Students in both groups were knowledgeable about the risks of having sex without using a condom or other means of protection. More than a third of all of the sexually active teens reported having had two or more partners. Despite claims by advocates, no reli-able evidence exists on whether the programs work. Most studies of abstinence education programs have methodological flaws that prevent them from gener-ating reliable estimates of program impacts.

To date, there is only one study that shows that abstinence-only education works. In February 2010, John Jemmott and colleagues reported the results of a four-year study on the efficacy (effectiveness) on Abstinence-Only Intervention. Their experimental abstinence-only program, not using a moralistic tone, showed that teens—if "properly" informed—will delay having sex. This study is believed to be the first such research to show long-term success (24 months) with an abstinence-only approach. The study differed from traditional programs that have lost federal and state support in recent years. The classes did not focus on a message of saving sex until marriage or disparage condom use. Instead, the classes involved assignments to help sixth and seventh graders see the drawbacks to sexual activity at their age. The study involved 662 black students in grades six and seven from four public middle schools in a city in the northeastern United States. It was conducted between 2001 and 2004. The study divided the students into four groups. One group received eight abstinence-only classes, another group had general healthy behavior instructions and the other two groups had either safe-sex classes or a curriculum that mixed abstinence and safe sex content. Researchers surveyed the students again two years later and found that about one-third of those who had the abstinence-only classes said they had engaged in sex, compared to about half of the students from the other three classes. This report comes amid intense debate over how to reduce sexual activity, pregnancies, births, and sexually transmitted diseases among children and teenagers. After falling for more than a decade, the numbers of births, pregnancies, and STDs among U.S. teens have begun increasing. This study has gained praise even from critics of abstinence-only programs and the White House took note. The Obama administration has continued annual federal funding targeted at abstinence programs.

ARE THE FEDERAL GUIDELINES GOVERNING ABSTINENCE-ONLY PROGRAMS IN TOUCH WITH REALITY?

In the ideal world, abstinence could be 100% effective in preventing STDs including HIV infection. The problem is in the practicing, not in the preaching! (See comments from the Mathematica Policy information.) In the April 2007 report, 95% of the U.S. population have premarital sex. James Wagoner, president of the Washington-based sex education group Advocates for Youth, said, "To be preaching abstinence when 90% of people are having sex is in essence to lose touch with reality. It's an ideological campaign. It has nothing to do with public health. They've stepped over the line of common sense." Wade Horn, assistant secretary for the

Administration for Children and Families at the Department of Health and Human Services, said, "The guidelines merely clarify that people ages 12-29 can be targeted by abstinence-only programs. In addition, the move is a response to government data released last year showing 998,262 births to unmarried women ages 19-29. The message is "It's better to wait until you're married to bear or father children. The only 100% effective way of getting there is abstinence."

UPDATE—In 2011, Kathrin Stanger-Hall and colleagues provided the first large-scale study that provided evidence that the type of sex education given in public schools can significantly impact teen pregnancy rates, and as a corollary, it would seem, help reduce the transmission of HIV and other sexually transmitted diseases. They found that states that had laws or policies emphasizing abstinence had, on average, higher pregnancy and birth rates. States with the lowest teen pregnancy rates were those that used comprehensive sex education—covering abstinence alongside lessons about condom use, contraception, and/or HIV education. Their analysis adds to the overwhelming evidence indicating that abstinence-only education does not reduce teen pregnancy rates.

DISCUSSION QUESTION: Is it good science, poor politics, or poor science and good politics, or some other combination of events that made it logical for the federal government to earmark tax dollars specifically for abstinence-only educational programs? Do you sense a religious involvement in the government policy? Explain.

DISCUSSION QUESTION: In his book, *At the Center of the Storm,* former director of the CIA George Tenet said, "Policymakers are entitled to their own opinions—but not to their own sets of facts." Do you see a relationship between this quote and the ongoing debate on abstinence? Explain.

WHEN WILL ROUTINE TESTING FOR HUMAN IMMONODEFIENCY VIRUS INFECTION BE THE ROUTINE FOR ADOLESCENTS/YOUNG ADULTS?

Best estimates place the number of individuals 13 to 24 years of age who are newly diagnosed with human immunodeficiency virus (HIV) infection each year at about 16,500. This represents about 29% of all newly diagnosed cases of

HIV annually. While this number is large, the most troubling statistic concerning HIV infection among youth is that more than 48% of those who are infected are unaware of their status as opposed to 25% of infected individuals in all other age groups. The fact that only 17.9% of sexually experienced adolescents/young adult males and only 27.5% of sexually experienced adolescents/young adult females have ever been tested for HIV is disturbing. It speaks to major deficiencies in our approach to the sexual and

THOUGHTS AND COMMENTS FROM A GENERATION AT RISK

"I was only 13 when I started having sex. I knew what AIDS was, and how you get it, but I was more worried about something else: getting pregnant. In fact, it was a visit to the health department to get birth control injections in January 2002 that I discovered I had HIV. I couldn't believe it, the disease I read about in health class and heard about on television and in movies was now a part of my life. I never thought it would happen to me. Now at age 16, I am back in school and take anti-AIDS drugs twice daily. I still have sex, I don't tell my boyfriends, but I make them use a condom."—From Virginia

"I became HIV infected at the same time I lost my virginity—at age 16. My 28-year-old boyfriend was an injection-drug user. He knew he was HIV positive but did not tell me. He has since died of AIDS. At 16 my only concern was pregnancy, so I took the pill and had unsafe sex. Living in Spain does not help either as the HIV infected are discriminated against—so be careful out there."—A message from Spain

"If you're going to educate kids about AIDS, you have to educate them about drugs as well. If you're a youth, you're going to experiment with drugs, especially if you live in a metropolitan area. Even though you get stupid with drugs, you still think about things you don't want to do, but you do it anyhow."—16-year-old HIV-positive youth from San Francisco

"We grow up hating ourselves like society teaches us to. If someone had been 'out' about their sexuality. If the teachers hadn't been afraid to stop the 'fag' and 'dyke' jokes. If my human sexuality class had even mentioned homosexuality. If the school counselors would have been open to a discussion of gay and lesbian issues. If any of those possibilities had existed, perhaps I would not have grown up hating what I was. And, just perhaps, I wouldn't have attempted suicide."—Kyallee, 19

"People say HIV is this or that group's problem, not mine. But for HIV, it's a matter of risk behaviors, not risk groups. Because if you say it's a risk group thing, I don't identify with that group, so I'm not at risk. That makes people feel invincible to HIV."—HIV-positive youth

"I was infected with HIV by my first partner when I was 16 years old. Now at 20 I have this virus that's taking my life because everything I heard when I was younger was sugar-coated. We need more complete information than what we are being given. Even the pamphlets concerning HIV/AIDS prevention are too basic and bland. We need to know real stuff."—Ryan, age 20

"We, the young people of this country, need a place where we can go to ask our questions, where we won't be teased or ridiculed. We need a place where we can ask about our mixed-up feelings, about sex, and about AIDS."—15-year-old high school student from Concord, N.H.

"If I could talk to the president, or a senator, or anyone in the federal government who can make a difference, I'd tell them to take a look, learn a lesson from the youth that are currently dealing with the disease. Listen to them, hear their stories, and then see that they have a future. If they don't have that future, then we don't have an America."—Allan, San Francisco

(Adapted and updated from a *Report to the President*, March 1996)

Comments: Unlike young adults who were infected by their mother perinatally and have grown up with the virus, the newly infected young adults have daunting issues dumped on them virtually overnight. Do they tell anyone? How do they handle dating? How do they tackle the emotions clouding future relationships? And more immediately, how do they take on a life-saving medical regimen when they have the willpower of a teenager? Teens also have characteristics that work against treatment. They lead chaotic lives. Shun authority. Keep secrets. Feel invincible. And wear defiance like a badge of courage. That "you can't tell me what to do" attitude can be deadly. Some teens may not even know they have the virus. Years can pass before their viral loads are high enough to produce symptoms.

DISCUSSION QUESTION: If you were an HIV-positive young adult, would you tell others? Choose one and discuss.
A. Yes
B. Only with family and close friends
C. Only once I reached adulthood
D. Only if I planned to have sex
E. No
F. An option not listed

reproductive health of adolescents and young adults, and it stands as a rather stark explanation for the otherwise puzzling discrepancy in the percentage of youth who are infected who know their diagnosis in comparison with older individuals. Quite simply, we are not testing the right people and are not testing them often enough. Why are adolescents and young adults so much less likely to be tested for HIV than older patients, even when their risk factors for acquiring HIV are similar? **First,** adolescents do not appear to believe they are at risk for HIV, despite acknowledging that they are sexually active. They are, therefore, less likely to know that they should be tested. **Second,** their healthcare providers often either are not aware of their young patients' risks or do not appreciate that a particular behavior puts them at risk. This may be the result of inadequate history taking or unwillingness to discuss important sexual and other risk-taking behaviors. The CDC recommends that all people between the ages of 13 – 64 be tested for HIV; however, the American Academy of Pediatrics guidelines differ from the CDC's recommended guidelines in several important areas. First, they would delay routine testing until adolescents are aged between 16 and 18 years and even then only in adolescents who live in communities where the overall prevalence of infection in greater than 0.1%. While these might be reasonable alternatives to a more universal screening policy, they introduce unnecessary choices into a process that would most benefit from a simple and straightforward approach without elements of uncertainty (i.e., asking, What is the right age? What is the prevalence in my community?), which will interfere with making the test truly routine (D'Angelo, 2011).

If you are a young adult or know of one who needs help or has HIV/AIDS questions, call:

National Teenagers AIDS Hotline: 1-800-234-8336.

Adolescent AIDS Program: Montefiore Medical Center, 111 E. 210th St., Bronx, NY 10467; 1-718-882-0023.

AIDS Community Alliance: Works with HIV-positive and HIV-affected individuals. 44 North Queens St., Lancaster, PA 17603; 1-717-394-3380.

Bay Area Young Positive: Youth-run, offers counseling, resources, newsletter. 518 Waller St., San Francisco, CA 94117; 1-415-487-1616; email: BAYPOZ@aol.com.

Summary

For the time being, abstaining from sex, mutual monogamy between uninfected partners, and the correct and consistent use of condoms are the only options that can be presented to young people for avoiding the sexual transmission of HIV. In order to decrease their risk of HIV infection today, it is essential that young adults receive education about HIV and have access to health and rehabilitative services.

Internet

1. **The Coalition for Positive Sexuality (CPS) website (www.positive.org/cps),** which provides information and advice on sexuality, is produced by and targets adolescents. The coalition is a grassroots volunteer group based in Chicago. Its self-described mission is "to give teens the information they need to take care of themselves and in doing so, affirm their decisions about sex, sexuality, and reproductive control; second, to facilitate dialogue, in and out of the public schools, on condom availability and sex education." Included among the topics is information about safe sex, birth control, STDs, pregnancy, and being gay. Homosexual relations are discussed in the same manner as heterosexual relations.

2. Although CPS is aimed at youth in general, **Oasis (www.oasismag.com)** targets and is written primarily by gay youth. Most of the columns written by contributors, who range in age from 14 to 22, read a lot like personal high school journals, an approach that undoubtedly makes readers feel comfortable—like hearing from a friend. A monthly advice column on sexual health is written by a physician and an epidemiologist, who are based in the San Francisco area.

Other Useful Sources

National Runaway Switchboard: 1-800-621-4000
National Network Runaway Youth Service: 1-202-783-7949

American Institute for Teen AIDS Prevention: 1-817-237-0230

Teen AIDS Student Coalition on AIDS, Washington, D.C.: 1-202-986-4310

Teen AIDS CDC: 1-800-342-2437

Teen AIDS Hotline: 1-800-440-8336

National Gay/Lesbian Youth Hotline: 1-800-347-8336

Review Questions

(Answers to the Review Questions are on page 463.)

1. There are _____ billion people ages 13 to 24 in the world.

2. What percentage of new HIV infections now occur among young adults?

3. Ending 2013, of the 38 million people living with HIV/AIDS globally, how many will be young adults?

4. Of those HIV-infected by age 24, how many, if not on ART, will die by age 35?

5. Ending 2013, what percentage of young adult women with HIV/AIDS will be living in sub-Saharan Africa, Latin America, North America, and the Caribbean?

6. What percentage of young adult women believe birth control pills are a form of safer sex?

7. "3 to 6 sex" means _____.

8. One danger of abstinence-only education is _____.

9. Entering year 2012, how many federal and state dollars have been spent on abstinence education in the United States?

10. What percentage of young adults live in developing countries?

11. How many young adults live in the United States?

12. What percentage of HIV-infected adults were infected as young adults?

13. Young adults are defined as ages _____ to _____.

14. Young adults make up _____ percent of the total HIV-infected population in the United States.

15. True or False: Young adults in general do not believe oral sex is sex.

Testing for Human Immunodeficiency Virus

CHAPTER HIGHLIGHTS

- ELISA means **e**nzyme **l**inked **i**mmuno**s**orbent **a**ssay; it is a large-scale antibody screening test for HIV infection.
- Antibody testing is the gold standard screening test for HIV.
- The ELISA test has been used to screen all blood supplies in the United States since March 1985.
- HIV screening tests can produce both false positives and false negatives.
- Unusual case of HIV-infected male testing HIV-negative over four years.
- A positive ELISA test only predicts that a confirmatory test will also be positive.
- Western Blot is a confirmatory HIV test. It confirms the results of ELISA.
- False-positive readings result from a test's lack of specificity.
- There is a relationship between the incidence of HIV in the population being tested and the number of false positives reported. The higher the incidence, the fewer the false positives.
- Several new screening and confirmatory HIV tests are now available.
- June 27 is national HIV Testing Day.
- History of HIV testing.
- Screening should be repeated at least annually in persons with known risk.
- Screening of the nation's blood supply has improved.
- Oral fluid and urine HIV antibody tests are FDA-approved.
- The polymerase chain reaction test is the most sensitive HIV-RNA test currently available.
- Other HIV-RNA tests available are Amplicor and the branched DNA test.
- Explanation of tropism testing is presented.
- Currently there are seven FDA-approved rapid tests requiring 20 minutes or less available in the United States.
- EDA approves first rapid over-the-counter HIV test.
- FDA approves first rapid INSTI 60-second HIV antibody test.
- Testing becomes part of HIV prevention.
- HIV testing among women and young adults.
- Opportunities to increase HIV testing as more payers cover costs.
- In pregnancy one test can save two lives.
- AIDS cases have been reported in all 50 states.
- All states now have a name-based HIV reporting system.
- Percentage reported being HIV tested by age and ethnic group.
- Reasons not to be HIV tested.
- Competency and informed consent are necessary for most HIV testing.

- Mandatory HIV testing does not mean people can be forced to undergo testing.
- See the 2011 Interactive HIV/AIDS map by Emory University Rollins School of Public Health (AIDSVu.org).
- HIV testing, for the most part, is on a voluntary basis.
- Compulsory HIV testing is used in the military, in prisons, and in certain federal agencies.
- FDA has approved two home HIV test kits; one remains on the market.
- U.S. Public Health Service guidelines for annual prenatal HIV counseling and voluntary HIV testing of all pregnant American women.
- New York is the first state to legislate mandatory HIV testing and disclosure of newborn HIV status to mother and physicians.
- American Medical Association endorses mandatory HIV testing of all pregnant women and newborns.
- CDC is recommending routine HIV testing of all U.S. residents ages 13–64.
- The U.S. policy on HIV and immigration now allows entry of HIV-infected immigrants into the USA
- HIV telephone consultation service (888) 933-3413: on all aspects of HIV testing and clinical care.

Let's begin this chapter by asking, **WHY DOES TESTING MATTER? ANSWER:** Basic epidemiology holds that early knowledge of where a virus is moving—into which populations—is essential to slowing its spread. Even if a disease cannot be cured, knowing who the infected people are may help prevent the transmission of the disease to other people. People who are unaware they are HIV positive account for an estimated 20,000 new HIV infections annually (Wolf et al., 2007). People often do not test for HIV because they do not perceive themselves at risk for infection. HIV testing is integral to HIV prevention, treatment, and care efforts. Knowledge of one's HIV status is important for preventing the spread of the disease. Studies show that, in majority of cases, those who learn they are HIV positive modify their behavior to reduce the risk of HIV transmission. Early knowledge of HIV status is also important for linking those with HIV to medical care and services that can reduce morbidity and mortality and improve the quality of life.

By the end of 2013, of the estimated 38 million living HIV-infected people worldwide, at least *half* will have become infected *before age 25*. About 15% will know they are HIV positive. HIV testing is not readily available in many places in developing nations. This chapter presents HIV testing information and describes some of the important problems connected with whom, how, and where to test.

Availability of HIV Testing in the United States

Antibody testing is the gold standard screening test for HIV infection. The current fourth generation antibody tests are highly sensitive and specific for all known subtypes of HIV-1 and HIV-2.

Commercial HIV antibody testing has been available since 1985. Testing technology has evolved considerably over the years, with a variety of new and improved tests coming into use in daily practice. Because determining one's HIV status is the first step in prevention and treatment decisions, it is important to understand the tests being used today, including their limitations. (See Sidebar 13.1, page 385.)

How Do HIV Antibody Tests Work?

Once HIV enters the body, the immune system starts to produce antibodies, chemicals that are part of the immune system that recognize invaders like bacteria and viruses and mobilize the body's attempt to fight infection. (See Chapter 5, pages 116–118, for a detailed discussion of antibodies.) In the case of HIV, these antibodies cannot fight off the infection, but their presence is used to tell whether a person has HIV in his or her body. In other words, most HIV tests look for the HIV antibodies rather than looking for HIV itself. But there are tests that do look for HIV antigens and HIV's genetic material directly and indirectly. These tests will also be presented in this chapter.

DETERMINING THE PRESENCE OF ANTIBODY PRODUCED WHEN HIV IS PRESENT

HIV antibody testing is a readily available, inexpensive, reliable, and accurate method to identify whether a person is infected with HIV. HIV antibodies are found in the blood and in other body fluids. When properly performed, HIV antibody testing is highly sensitive and specific.

Currently there are at least twelve tests that detect HIV antibodies, antigens, or the nucleic acid of HIV in a person's body fluids. They are the enzyme linked immunosorbent assay (ELISA),

Western Blot, polymerase chain reaction (PCR), saliva tests, signal amplification RNA tests, immunofluorescent antibody assay, rapid HIV test kits, and at-home HIV specimen collection test kits. They are discussed in the following pages.

REQUESTS FOR HIV TESTING

HIV testing is offered at some 11,600 CDC publicly funded sites and in other public and private settings. These testing sites are becoming overwhelmed with requests for HIV testing. But most of the requests are repeats. The majority of those people at risk who have not been tested includes most hard-core IDUs and sexual partners of IDUs and people who are image sensitive. Currently, about 100 million blood and plasma samples are HIV tested annually worldwide. In the United States about 16 million to 22 million blood and plasma samples are HIV tested annually.

In the developing world, where the greatest number of HIV-infected people is concentrated, HIV testing is done mostly for purposes of surveillance, which involves very small population samples and is done anonymously. Few people have any hope of treatment, so they feel little incentive to get tested. But even those who would want to know may not be able to find out. In many countries, there are no voluntary testing and counseling facilities; people have no acceptable way of learning if they are HIV infected. An ongoing study at a rural hospital in South Africa suggests that only 2% of people who are HIV positive know their status. The situation in the rest of sub-Saharan Africa is equally poor.

Worldwide it is estimated that only 10% of persons at risk for HIV infection receive testing.

REASONS FOR HIV TESTING: I KNOW, I TOOK THE TEST

HIV testing is done to monitor the pandemic—to interrupt transmission to determine how many people are infected, how many are becoming infected in a given time period (incidence), and their location. Testing is used to determine the impact of prevention efforts to slow the spread of HIV, to prompt behavior change, and to provide entry into clinical care. Also, if necessary, testing is used to provide a starting point for partner notification, education, and to protect the nation's blood supply.

Take the Test: Take Control: THIVK–Your Test Results Expire Every Time You Have Risky Sex!

There is an immediate need to change perceptions about being HIV positive so that people feel good about taking the test to protect themselves and others, rather than the discrimination that now exists against those who have taken the test. Or those who test positive.

The Need for Routine HIV Testing

After over 31 years of educating people about HIV/AIDS, about 46% of adults ages 18 to 64 in the United States have never been tested for HIV (Figure 13-1). Sixty-one percent of adults say their reason for not being tested is that they do not consider themselves to be at risk (Figure 13-2, page 387). Unless people are tested in greater numbers, it may be impossible to break the cycle of HIV transmission in America or anywhere else. The failure of educational programs to stem the rates of about 56,000 new HIV infections in America annually may need to be replaced by new policies on HIV testing. Joseph Inungu, a Central Michigan health science professor, is recommending an HIV test as part of the routine tests performed on office patients. Inungu analyzed data on people ages 18 to 80 who participated in a national health interview survey conducted by the National Center for Health Statistics. He found the groups least likely to be tested for HIV were men, people over the age of 50 or between ages 18 and 19, people with a low level of education, people in rural areas, and people in the Northeast or Midwest. While young adult groups are among the fastest-growing populations with HIV infection, few are tested for HIV unless they come to a physician for a sexually transmitted disease. Populations over the age of 50 feel they are not at risk, but their numbers of HIV infected continue to increase. The groups most likely to get tested include blacks, people with higher educational levels, and people who are separated, divorced, or widowed.

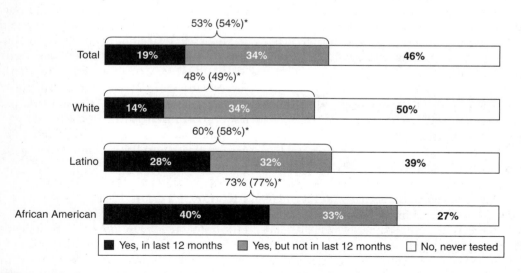

FIGURE 13-1 Percentages, Ages 18 to 64, Who Report Being Tested by Race/Ethnicity, 2009 and 2011*. Not all numbers may add up due to rounding. *(Source: Adapted from Kaiser Family Foundation Survey of Americans on HIV/AIDS 2009 and June 2011, HIV/AIDS at 30* and their 2012 survey.)*

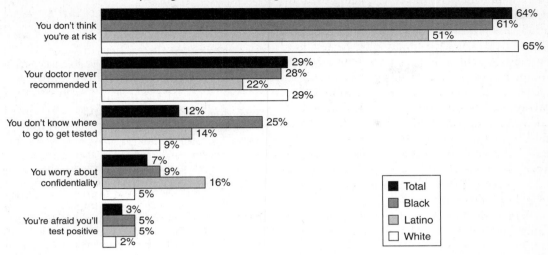

Percent saying each of the following is a reason they have NOT been tested for HIV (among the 44% of those ages 18-64 who have never been tested for HIV)

You don't think you're at risk
- 64%
- 61%
- 51%
- 65%

Your doctor never recommended it
- 29%
- 28%
- 22%
- 29%

You don't know where to go to get tested
- 12%
- 25%
- 14%
- 9%

You worry about confidentiality
- 7%
- 9%
- 16%
- 5%

You're afraid you'll test positive
- 3%
- 5%
- 5%
- 2%

Legend: ■ Total ▨ Black ▥ Latino ☐ White

FIGURE 13-2 Reported Reasons for Adults Not Being HIV Tested. Note: "Don't know" responses not shown. *(Source: Adapted from Kaiser Family Foundation Survey of Americans on HIV/AIDS conducted April 4–May 1, 2011. HIV/AIDS at 30. A Public Opinion Perspective and their 2012 survey.)*

Entering 2013, about 92 million people between the ages of 18 and 64 have been tested. That is, about half of the people in this age group have been tested. Some of the reasons for not being tested are presented on page 403–404 under "Reasons Not to Be HIV Tested."

Misunderstanding Leads to Lack of HIV Testing

Misunderstanding surrounds HIV testing. For example, one of the pastors in a black church told about a conversation he had with a young man. He asked the young man if he had been tested for HIV and he said yes, and that he was negative. He asked him when he was tested, and he said four years ago. The pastor asked him if he had been at risk in that time and needed to get tested again. The young man seemed puzzled and asked, "Why should I be tested again?" There's such an emphasis on "get tested, get tested" but in many cases the understanding as to why one gets tested is not there! It's not just testing, but an ongoing risk assessment and ongoing testing and ongoing awareness. It's a commitment to being aware and being open to discussing risks. People can openly talk about anything but sex. Yet men, women, and young adults are having sex. There is a need for counseling about having an HIV test.

LABORATORY METHODS FOR DETECTING HIV

An arsenal of laboratory methods is available to screen blood, diagnose infection, and monitor disease progression in individuals infected by HIV. These tests can be classified into those that (a) detect antibody, (b) identify antigen, (c) detect or monitor viral nucleic acids, and (d) provide an estimate of T lymphocyte numbers. The focus of this discussion is on antibody detection, the most widely used and, in most situations, the most effective and least expensive way to identify HIV.

Detecting Antibodies to HIV and HIV Antigens

Refinements in the field of immunological testing, serology, and the study of antigen–antibody reactions have produced test names that reflect the component parts of the test being used. In most cases, tests are based on the detection of antibodies present in the serum, in this case antibodies to HIV. One immunological test uses antibodies, which if present in the person's serum, form a complex with a given antigen. An enzyme is then connected to the antibody. The presence of the antibody can be determined by adding a reagent that will form a colored solution if an antibody to HIV is present. This is called the **enzyme linked immunosorbent assay** (ELISA). The ELISA (E–liz–a) test was first used in 1983 to detect antibodies against HIV. (See Snapshot 13.1.)

Because the ELISA test detects the presence of antibodies made against HIV, it is called an *indirect test*. This test suggests that HIV is or was present. The Western Blot test, presented next, is also an indirect test for the same reason. Indirect tests stand in contrast to those tests that directly test for the presence of HIV's nucleic acid—a *direct test*. These tests say that HIV is currently present in the system. They are also presented.

ELISA HIV ANTIBODY TEST

A Fable for the HIV/AIDS Era

It was a medieval mystery. Somehow, needles were finding their way into some of the kingdom's haystacks. Cows were eating the needles: not a good thing. The king sent out a proclamation offering a sack of gold to the first person able to find a needle in a haystack. After 20 days, the contestants were still trying to locate the needles hidden among 10 haystacks placed in the palace courtyard. The king was despondent. From his tower he could see thousands of haystacks in fields across the kingdom. "This is terrible," he said. "Either our cows go hungry while we look for the needles, or we let them eat the hay along with some needles. Either way it's not good for the cows. We need a way to tell which haystacks have the needles; then we can feed our cows the good hay while we figure out how to get

---

---

the needles out of the bad haystacks." He was a logical king. In 1981 the needle had no name but its presence was known. The search for this needle—like those in the haystacks—was intense, and even after the needle was found to be HIV, investigators had to find a way to distinguish between those who carried and did not carry HIV—which haystacks carried the needles. Because HIV was in human blood, it was essential to protect the nation's blood supply, thereby preventing people from receiving contaminated blood and blood products. But, like the good king discovered, it took time to find the means to find the needle in the blood supply—HIV.

It was not until 1985—nearly four years after the first cases of AIDS were announced—that an antibody test was developed that could indicate whether a person was infected with HIV. Even after this discovery, the fact that there were no effective treatments for those who tested HIV positive, coupled with the widespread stigma associated with HIV infection, left many questioning the value of HIV testing. That equation shifted markedly with the availability of potent combination antiretroviral drug therapy, which significantly delays the progression of HIV disease in many people. There is now widespread consensus among public health officials and community leaders regarding the importance of HIV testing and counseling in order to link individuals who test positive with medical care and to counsel them on how to reduce the risk of further transmission.

Screening the Nation's Blood Supply

The initial application of the ELISA test outside the research laboratory was used primarily in large-scale screening of the nation's blood supply. **ELISA testing of the existing blood supply and all newly donated blood in the United States in March 1985. Very quickly testing also became an important aspect of HIV prevention. In recent years, the discovery of treatments for HIV and associated opportunistic infections has further increased the benefits of early detection.**

The ELISA test is used as a screening test because of its low cost, standardized procedures, high reproducibility, and rapid results.

Whole viruses are disrupted into subunit antigens for use. The subunits of HIV are then bound to a solid support system.

Two different solid support systems are used in at least eight ELISA screening test kits licensed in the United States. Some attach or fix the antigens onto the sides and bottoms of small wells (microwells) in a glass or plastic microtiter plate. (Figure 13-3, page 390) The serum to be tested, because it will contain antibodies to HIV if present, is separated from the blood and is diluted and applied to the HIV-coated solid support systems. The ELISA test takes from 2.5 to 4 hours to perform and costs between about $8 in state-sponsored virology laboratories and about $60 to $75 in private laboratories.

In accordance with FDA recommendations, effective June 1992, blood collection centers in the United States began HIV-2 testing on all donated blood and blood components. Although the occurrence of HIV-2 is rare in the United States, the CDC does recommend routine testing for HIV-2 according to its 2011 guidelines.

Understanding the ELISA Test

The ELISA test determines if a person's serum contains antibodies to one or more HIV antigens. Although there are some minor differences among the FDA-licensed kits, test procedures are similar.

Problems with the ELISA Test

Any HIV screening test must be able to distinguish those individuals who are infected from those who are not. **The underlying assumption of an ELISA test is that all HIV-infected people will produce detectable HIV antibodies.** There are, however, problems with this assumption. **First,** although rare, there are documented cases of individuals who are infected but remain antibody negative (Bartolo et al., 2009). **Second,** the time when HIV-infected population does not produce detectable antibodies (and the time period running from three weeks to one or more years after HIV infection) is called the **window period.** Most often, HIV antibody is now detectable within 3 to 6 weeks. Thus, during the window period HIV-infected people can test HIV negative. This is a **false negative** result. In some HIV-infected persons, the virus ties up the available antibody as their disease progresses. Testing at this time may also produce false negative results. (See Box 13.1, page 391.)

FIGURE 13-3 Specimens positive for HIV antibody have a deeper color in this microwell tray. Serum specimens from 15 patients were tested for antibodies to HIV. Two negative and three positive control specimens are provided in the first column. In wells 7, 9, 11, and 14, the dark yellow color change, matching the color in the three positive control wells, indicates that the specimens are positive. Well 3 shows a weakly reactive result. The remaining specimens showed no color change and were interpreted as negative for HIV antibodies. *(Adapted from Fang et al., 1989).* Use of the (a) direct and (b) indirect ELISA Assay (test).

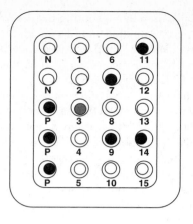

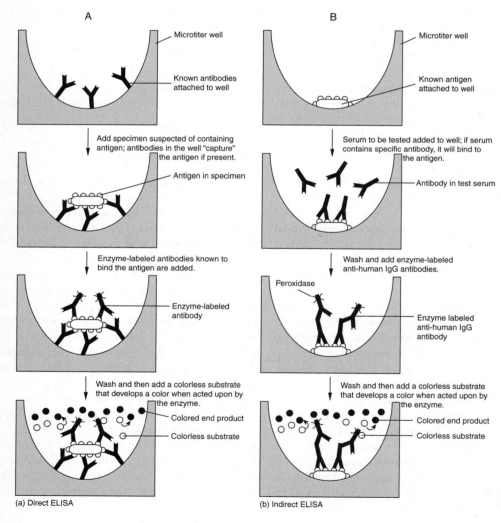

A

Microtiter well

Known antibodies attached to well

Add specimen suspected of containing antigen; antibodies in the well "capture" the antigen if present.

Antigen in specimen

Enzyme-labeled antibodies known to bind the antigen are added.

Enzyme-labeled antibody

Wash and then add a colorless substrate that develops a color when acted upon by the enzyme.

Colored end product

Colorless substrate

(a) Direct ELISA

B

Microtiter well

Known antigen attached to well

Serum to be tested added to well; if serum contains specific antibody, it will bind to the antigen.

Antibody in test serum

Wash and add enzyme-labeled anti-human IgG antibodies.

Peroxidase

Enzyme labeled anti-human IgG antibody

Wash and then add a colorless substrate that develops a color when acted upon by the enzyme.

Colored end product

Colorless substrate

(b) Indirect ELISA

BOX 13.1

AN ASSUMPTION OF AIDS WITHOUT THE HIV TEST: IT SHATTERS LIVES

Case 1

San Francisco—For six years, a 53-year-old gay male lived in the world of AIDS. He stopped working, suffered the painful side effects of experimental drugs, and waited to die.

Now his doctors say he never had the disease.

His health shattered by AIDS treatment, his livelihood lost, he filed a $2 million claim against Kaiser Permanente health maintenance organization. He claims he underwent sustained treatment for full-fledged AIDS without receiving an HIV test.

His attorney said, "For six years he thought that the most he had was six months to live. So every day he'd wake up and think 'Is this the last day of my life?'"

To begin, this male says he checked into a San Jose hospital affiliated with Kaiser in 1986 with respiratory problems and doctors told him he had Pneumocystic pneumonia, considered a sure sign of AIDS at the time.

He underwent tests but *was not* given one to determine the presence of HIV, the virus associated with AIDS.

In 1986, he began taking the drug zidovudine in high doses, which gave him a chronic headache, high blood pressure, and peripheral neuropathy—permanent pins and needles pains from his calves to his feet. He is battling an addiction to Darvon and other prescription drugs.

Under doctors' orders, he quit his job as a skin care technician and lives on government welfare and disability benefits of $600 a month. (Associated Press, 1992)

Case 2

Chicago—Every day, four times each day, for six years Mark swallowed his antiretroviral drugs. Mark was told by a "fine physician" that he was HIV positive in July 1990. Regardless of the drugs, Mark felt sick and suffered further physical effects and depression. For reasons not given, Mark moved from Chicago to Ohio. His new physician was puzzled that Mark did not demonstrate signs or symptoms of HIV infection. His tests on Mark came back HIV negative. On investigation, the Chicago clinic could not produce any documents showing that Mark was ever HIV tested!

Case 3

Boston—In December 2007, a jury awarded $2.5 million in damages to a woman who for almost nine years took a combination of antiretroviral drugs but was never actually tested for HIV. The ART triggered a variety of ailments including depression, chronic fatigue, weight loss, and intestinal inflammation. She filed a suit against her physician after her HIV test came back—HIV negative. The initial diagnosis, made by her physician, was based on her lifestyle.

An Unusual Case—At the VA Medical Center in Salt Lake City in 1997, a man tested HIV negative 35 times over a four-year period. Because his wife was HIV positive and because he demonstrated symptoms of HIV disease, tests other than the ELISA showed that he was HIV positive. This case is unusual because (1) he was falsely negative almost four years beyond the window period; (2) the strain of HIV is typical of that found in the United States; and (3) the strain of HIV is closely related to the strain infecting his wife (Reimer et al., 1997).

False positive reactions may also occur. This means that the person's serum does not contain antibodies to HIV but the test results indicate that it does. Christine Johnson (2000) has compiled a list of 66 conditions taken from HIV/AIDS scientific literature that can cause false positive results.

People may test false positive who have an underlying liver disease, have received a blood transfusion or gamma globulin within six weeks of the test, be pregnant, have had several children, have had rheumatological diseases, malaria, alcoholic hepatitis, autoimmune disorders, various cancers, acute cytomegalovirus infection, or DNA viral infections; are injection-drug users; or have received vaccines for influenza or hepatitis B (Fang et al., 1989; MacKenzie et al., 1992). In each case, the person may have antibodies that will cross-react with the HIV antigens to give a false positive reaction. Other reasons for false positives are laboratory errors and mistakes made in reagent preparations for use in the test kits. (See Box 13.1 and Side Issue 13.1.)

Why Is the ELISA Test Sensitivity and Specificity Set High?

Because the original purpose of the ELISA test was to screen blood, the sensitivity (ability to detect low-level color formation; see Figure 13-3) of the test was purposely set high. It was reasoned that it was better to have some false positives and throw away good blood rather than to take in any HIV-contaminated blood. Thus the ELISA test is a **positive predictive value** test. It only predicts that the serum tested will continue to test positive when a test with greater specificity, called a **confirmatory test,** is done.

In 1985, during the first month of donor screening, 1% of all blood tested HIV-antibody positive. On ELISA retesting of these samples, only 0.17% (17/10,000) were HIV-antibody positive. On subjecting these samples to a confirmatory test, only 0.038% (4/10,000) were actually HIV positive. These early tests produced about 24 false positives for every true positive result. The main reason for such a high false positive rate or *lack of specificity* was that something other than HIV produced an antibody or other substance that reacted with HIV antigen, causing the HIV test to appear positive.

Although high-sensitivity tests eliminate HIV-contaminated blood from the blood supply, there is a downside to high-sensitivity testing when proper procedure is *not* used. People told that they have tested positive have become emotionally distraught. Former senator Lawton Chiles of Florida, at an AIDS conference in 1987, told of a tragic example from the early days of blood screening in Florida. Of 22 blood donors who were told they were HIV positive by the ELISA test, seven committed suicide. In 2006, the CDC reported that, over time, about 30% of HIV-infected Koreans commit suicide.

There continue to be false positive reactions among blood donors and low-level risk populations because of a low prevalence of HIV infection in such populations. The American Red Cross Blood Services laboratories report that using current ELISA methodology, a specificity of 99.8% can be achieved (Table 13–1, page 393).

Positive Predictive Value—The positive predictive value of the ELISA test indicates the percentage of true positives among total positives in a given population. To determine a positive predictive value:

Number of true positives ÷ (Number of true positives + false positives) × 100 = %

Negative Predictive Test—There is also a negative predictive test. A negative predictive value refers to the percentage of individuals who test truly negative; they *do not* have HIV. It is determined by:

Number of true negatives ÷ (Number of true negatives + false negatives) × 100 = %

To safeguard against false positive tests, the CDC recommends that serum that tests positive be retested twice (in duplicate). If both tests are negative, the serum is considered HIV-antibody negative and further tests will only be done should signs or symptoms of HIV infection occur. If one or both of the tests is positive, the serum is subjected to a confirmatory test, usually a Western Blot (WB).

Although confirmatory tests can be used to determine true-positive results, they are too labor intensive and expensive to be used in screening a large population. Thus the positive predictive value of an ELISA test is an important first step in large-scale screening. Recall, however, that **the predictive value depends on the prevalence of HIV infection in the population tested.** The higher the prevalence or number of HIV infections in a given population, the more likely a positive ELISA test is to be a true positive; and conversely, the lower the prevalence of infection, the less likely a positive ELISA test is to be a true positive.

At blood banks, if the initial ELISA test is positive, the blood is discarded. If an individual's

Table 13-1 The Meaning of Antibody Test Results

A Positive Results	B Negative Results
If you test positive, it does mean: 1. Your blood sample has been tested more than once and the tests indicate that it contained antibodies to HIV. 2. You have been infected with HIV and your body has produced antibodies. **If you test positive, it does not mean:** 1. That you have AIDS. 2. That you necessarily will get AIDS, but the probability is high. You can reduce your chance of progressing to AIDS by avoiding further contact with the virus, beginning antiretroviral therapy if recommended, and living a healthy lifestyle. 3. That you are immune to the virus. **Therefore, if you test positive, you should do the following:** 1. Protect yourself from any further infection. 2. Protect others from the virus by following HIV/AIDS precautions in sex, drug use, and general hygiene. 3. Consider seeing a physician for a complete evaluation and advice on health maintenance. 4. Avoid drugs and heavy alcohol use, maintain good nutrition, and avoid fatigue and stress. Such action may improve your chances of staying healthy.	**If you test negative, it does mean:** 1. No antibodies to HIV have been found in your serum at the time of the test. **Two possible explanations for a negative test result exist:** 1. You have not been infected with HIV. 2. You have been infected with HIV but have not yet produced antibodies. Research indicates that most people will produce antibodies within 6 to 18 weeks after infection. Some people will not produce antibodies for at least 3 years. A very small number of people may never produce detectable antibodies. **If you test negative, it does not mean:** 1. That you have nothing to worry about. You may become infected; be careful. 2. That you are immune to HIV. 3. That you have not been infected with the virus. You may have been infected and not yet produced antibodies. **If You Test Negative, Does It Mean that Your Sexual Partner Is HIV Negative?** No. Your HIV test results reveal only your HIV status. Your negative results do not tell you whether your partner has HIV. HIV is not necessarily transmitted every time there is an exposure. Therefore, your taking an HIV test should not be seen as a method to find out if your partner is infected. Testing should never take the place of protecting yourself from HIV infection. If your behaviors are putting you at risk for exposure to HIV, it is important to reduce your risks.

(Adapted from the San Francisco AIDS Foundation)

serum subjected to a confirmatory test is positive, the person is considered to be HIV infected.

Levels of Sensitivity and Specificity in Testing for HIV—A test's **sensitivity** is its capacity to identify all specimens that have HIV antibodies in them. A test's **specificity** is its capacity to identify all specimens that do not have HIV antibodies in them.

Sensitivity is determined as follows:

Number of true positives ÷ (Number of true positives + the false negatives) × 100 = %

If 100 persons are actually HIV infected and the test identifies only 90 of them, then the test has 90% sensitivity.

Specificity is determined as follows:

Number of true negatives ÷ (Number of true negatives + false positives) × 100 = %

Assume that, in a group of 500 people being tested for HIV antibodies, 100 individuals are actually not infected. If test results show that only 90 out of the 100 are identified as not having the virus, then the test has 90% specificity.

WESTERN BLOT ASSAY

Until recently, the gold standard for determining a true positive HIV-antibody test was the **Western Blot** (WB). This test is a method in which individual HIV proteins are used to react with HIV antibody in a person's serum. It should be understood that the WB test is not a true gold standard because it is not 100% certain, but it can come close to 100% if properly used.

Cells in which HIV is being cultured are lysed or broken open, and the mixture of cell components and HIV components (proteins) are separated from each other. The viral proteins are placed on a polyacrylamide gel, which then gets an electrical charge. The electrical current separates the viral proteins within the gel. This is called **gel electrophoresis.** The smallest HIV proteins will move quickly through the gel, separating from the next larger size, and so on.

Each different protein will arrive at a separate position on the gel. After proteins of similar molecular weight collect at a given site, they form a band; these bands are identified based on the distance they have run in the gel. Because each band is a protein produced as a product of a different HIV gene, the gel band patterns give a picture of the HIV genes that were functioning and the location of each gene's products on the gel. The protein or antigen bands within the gel are "blotted," that is, transferred directly, band for band and position for position, onto strips of nitrocellulose paper (Figure 13-4).

Once the antigen bands have been formed, serum believed to carry HIV antibodies is placed directly on them. That is, a test serum is added directly to antigen bands located on the nitrocellulose strip. If antibodies are present in the serum, they will form an antigen–antibody complex directly on the antigen band areas. Positive test strips are then compared to two control

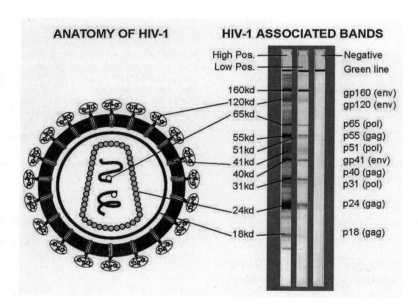

FIGURE 13-4 Western Blot. A Western Blot (WB) strip contains 10 separate antigenic proteins of HIV. Human serum or blood is applied directly to the strips. Because false positives can sometimes occur with the ELISA test, additional testing is needed to evaluate specimens that are repeatedly reactive by ELISA. The WB is more specific but less sensitive than the ELISA. Its clinical usefulness in trials to aid in evaluating specimens that are questionably positive by other methods has been proven. It is not a screening test because it lacks a high level of sensitivity and is expensive. This line art drawing shows the immediate relationship between the gel bands, after electrophoresis and blotting onto nitrocellulose paper. The figure shows the gel bands as related to their constituent parts of the virus. (Permission to use the Bio-Rad HIV-1 Western Blot Illustration has been granted by Bio-Rad Laboratories, Inc.)

test strips, one that has been reacted with known positive serum and one that has been reacted with known negative serum.

In contrast to the ELISA test, which indicates only the presence or absence of HIV antibodies, the WB strip qualitatively identifies which of the HIV antigens the antibodies are directed against.

The WB procedure is labor intensive and is more costly than the ELISA test. **The WB is less sensitive than the ELISA but more specific.**

Because the WB lacks the sensitivity of the ELISA test, it is not used as a screening test. Despite the high specificity of the WB, false positives do occur, but they occur less frequently than with ELISA tests because the WB is only run on serum, blood, oral fluid, and urine already suspected of containing HIV antibodies. (See Side Issue 13.1, page 396.)

Indeterminate WB

Western Blots may also turn out to be **indeterminate** in HIV infections—meaning, a person can be infected, but the blot is not conclusive—a positive band is detected but is not sufficient to meet the criteria for a truly positive result. That is, it may be positive but it may not be; the test results are too ambiguous to tell. The indeterminate WB results can occur either during the window period for HIV seroconversion or during end-stage HIV disease. Indeterminate WBs have occurred in un-infected individuals because of cross-reacting autoantibodies related to recent immunization, prior blood transfusion, organ transplantation, autoimmune disorders, malignancy, infection with other retroviruses (for example, HIV-2), or pregnancy. Some patients have a persistent pattern of indeterminate reactivity that remains stable over several years in the absence of true HIV infection.

In general, most persons with an initial indeterminate Western Blot result who are infected with HIV will develop detectable HIV antibody within one month. Thus, clients with an initial indeterminate result should be retested for HIV-infection after one month.

Immunofluorescent Antibody Assay

The **immunofluorescent antibody assay (IFA)** uses a known preparation of antibodies labeled with a fluorescent dye such as fluorescein isothiocyanate (FITC) to detect antigen or antibody. In the direct fluorescent antibody test, fluorescent antibodies detect specific antigens in cultures or smears. In the indirect fluorescent antibody test, specific antibody from serum is bound to antigen on a glass slide.

The indirect procedure is modified for use in detecting antibodies to HIV. Cells that are HIV infected will have HIV antigens on their cell membranes and will later fluoresce when the antihuman fluorescent conjugate is added.

In late 1992, the FDA-approved Fluorognost for marketing, the first assay for HIV-IFA confirmation and screening.

Fluorognost posts almost no indeterminate test results. The test takes only 90 minutes to complete. This FDA-approved test allows smaller healthcare facilities, emergency rooms, and doctors' offices to conduct in-office HIV screening and confirmation with accuracy, ease, and low overhead.

NEW ELISA ANTIBODY ANTIGEN AND RNA DETECTION PROCEDURES REVEAL EARLY VERSUS LATE HIV INFECTION

STARHS—A Sensitive/Less-Sensitive HIV Test

The best data for understanding recent changes in HIV transmission are measurements of the number of new infections in a defined time period (incidence of infection). But this has been difficult because ELISA testing simply gave a positive or negative response to the presence of HIV antibody without regard to the actual time of infection. However, in mid-1998 (Janssen et al., 1998) through 1999 (McFarland et al.) a new testing strategy provided a means to detect new or early HIV infections versus older HIV infections. The new testing technique is called **STARHS (the Serologic Testing Algorithm for Recent HIV Seroconversions).** The test uses two different ELISAs to test a single blood sample to tell if an infection is old or new. By more accurately pinpointing the time of

A FALSE POSITIVE HIV REPORT

Case 1

In January 2002, a man in Oklahoma City was awarded $1.4 million because he was wrongfully told he was HIV positive. At age 40 he received the news from a Health Maintenance Clinic. During the following four years, he became depressed and despondent, abused alcohol, and attempted suicide twice. Thinking he was HIV positive, he had unprotected sex with known HIV-positive partners. Reviewing his file to determine when he became infected, he learned that his test four years earlier was HIV negative. He filed suit for negligence and won.

Case 2

In November 2002, a Richland County, S.C., jury awarded $1.1 million to a woman who said Palmetto Health Richland Hospital misdiagnosed her with HIV. She said the diagnosis wrecked her life. "I was so depressed thinking I was going to die a horrible death. I gave up hope. Now I'm trying to get my life back together. I have lost so much of my life. I thank God every day for helping me find the mistake." In her lawsuit, the hospital—then called Richland Memorial Hospital—diagnosed her as HIV positive in February 1994. For several years she took anti-HIV medications, including the drug zidovudine. She said she never had symptoms of the disease and that another test in 1998 by a different laboratory confirmed she had been misdiagnosed. The lawsuit said she suffered extreme depression, emotional distress, anxiety, fear, side effects from the drugs, and other related trauma because of the misdiagnosis.

Case 3

In 1980, a woman received a blood transfusion during surgery at a hospital in a southeast Georgia town. During a checkup for a thyroid problem a decade later, at a clinic in Hialeah, Fla., her blood was taken for testing.

On November 13, 1990, her telephone rang. She was asked to come down to the local health clinic where she was told she had AIDS. They were not sure how long she had to live. She was 45 years old. Her three sons were then teenagers; their father had died.

She kept the television on continually in a usually unsuccessful effort to block out the thought of AIDS. The nights were the worst.

"I'd go to bed every night thinking about dying. What color do you want the casket to be? What dress do you want to be buried in? How are your kids going to take it? How will people treat them? I was afraid to go to sleep."

In 1992, her doctor put her on didanosine (ddI), which brought on side effects that included vomiting and fatigue.

"I had put my kids through hell. They were scared for me."

When she joined a local hospice group for AIDS patients, counselors heard her story and noted that her T cell counts had remained consistently high. At their suggestion, she was retested.

In November 1992, nearly two years to the day she was told she was HIV positive, another call came. She was greeted at the clinic with these words: **"Guess what? Your HIV test came out negative!"**

She sued the Florida Department of Health and Rehabilitative Services—the agency that performed the test—and the clinic and doctor who treated her.

A jury awarded her $600,000 for pain and suffering but cleared the clinic and said the bulk must be paid by the agency. (See Box 8.3, page 211–212—The boxer, Tommy Morrison. A case of falsely testing HIV positive.)

---

infection, STARHS may help patients identify when and from whom infection took place. Because people can live symptom-free with HIV for over a decade, they previously did not know when they might have become infected. But the new technology changes that. While it's hard for many sexually active people to recall the names and addresses of all their partners, spanning years of activity, it is typically a simple matter to make a list for the past four months.

How STARHS Works

The standard ELISA blood test is very sensitive and measures the presence of antibodies against HIV. The very sensitive or *standard ELISA tests* can pick up even minute numbers of antibodies present in the first days of infection before the immune system has mounted a full response to the virus. Conversely, a less sensitive B E, and D test (tests only for antibodies to HIV subtypes B, E, and D of the M group) *does the reverse*. It detects only the presence of antibodies at higher levels that typically appear three to six months after infection. By administering both ELISA tests, technicians, by comparing the results of both tests, can tell an individual's stage of infection. In brief, if someone tests positive on the sensitive test and negative on the less-sensitive test, they likely have a recent infection. Positive results on both tests indicate the infection is more than four to six months old.

Viral Load Related to Stage of Infection

As described in Chapter 4, pages 94–96, a viral load test measures the number of viral RNA strands in the blood plasma. Before the immune system produces antibodies to fight HIV, HIV multiplies rapidly. Therefore, this test will show a high viral load during the acute stage of HIV infection. Thus, a negative HIV antibody test and a high viral load indicates a recent HIV infection, most likely within the past two months. If both tests are positive, then HIV infection probably occurred a few months or more before the tests.

In May 2007, the FDA approved two new viral load tests. One is Abbott's RealTime HIV-1 viral load test for use on the company's m2000™ automated instrument system. The Abbott RealTime HIV-1 assay is designed to detect and precisely measure levels of HIV circulating in a patient's blood (viral load), including the three major groups of HIV-1 M, N, and O as well as non-B subtypes. The test is intended for use as a marker of disease prognosis and an aid in assessing viral response to antiretroviral treatment. The test can detect as few as 40 RNA molecules (strands) per milliliter (mL) of blood plasma and as many as 10 million molecules per mL. A second new viral load test is the COBAS AmpliPrep test by Roche Diagnostics; it is similar in use to the Abbott test.

However, once the HIV-RNA level has been reduced to fewer than 50 copies/mL, it becomes impossible to detect further viral reduction with currently available clinical assays; debate remains over whether optimal suppression of viral replication has been achieved in these circumstances.

Screening for p24 Antigen Looks Directly for Key Pieces of HIV—In August 1995, the FDA mandated that all blood and plasma collection centers screen all blood for p24 antigen (Figure 13-4). The FDA recommended p24 screening as an additional safety measure because recent studies indicated that p24 screening reduces the infectious window period (the FDA-approved Coulter p24 antigen blood test detects HIV as early as 16 days after infection). Among the 12 million-plus annual blood donations in the United States, p24-antigen screening is expected to detect four to six infectious donations that would not be identified by other screening tests. FDA regards donor screening for p24 antigen as an interim measure pending the availability of technology that would further reduce the risk for HIV transmission from blood donated during the infectious window period (*MMWR*, 1996, updated).

On June 18, 2010, the FDA approved a new "4th generation" HIV diagnostic assay. The ARCHITECT HIV Ag/Ab Combo Assay is the first HIV diagnostic assay that simultaneously detects both antigen and antibodies for HIV. The new test is also the first diagnostic test approved by the FDA for use in children as young as 2 years of age and pregnant women.

This single, automated test is a highly sensitive chemiluminescent microparticle immunoassay intended to be used as an aid in the diagnosis of HIV-1/HIV-2 infection, including acute or primary HIV-1 infection. It is specific for the detection of the HIV-1 p24 antigen (the substance found on the virus that triggers the production of antibodies), as well as antibodies to HIV-1 groups M and O, and as antibodies to HIV-2.

Levels of p24 antigen increase early after initial infection, before HIV antibody is produced. Because it detects HIV-1 p24 antigen, in addition to antibodies, the ARCHITECT HIV Ag/Ab Combo Assay can be useful in extending diagnosis to earlier, acute phase (recent) infection with HIV, prior to the emergence of antibodies produced by the infected patient, effectively reducing the window period (that period after initial infection and before the detection of infection based on formation of detectable antibodies). The median detection time was demonstrated to be 7 days earlier (range 0 to 20 days) compared to fourth-generation enzyme immunoassay antibody tests to which they were compared.

Nucleic Acid Testing—Beginning spring 1999, the American Red Cross and 16 member laboratories of the America's Blood Centers began testing donor blood pools for HIV type 1 and the hepatitis C virus with a new research testing method known as **nucleic acid amplification testing (NAT).** The test was FDA- approved in June 2004. The power of NAT is its ability to detect the presence of infection by directly testing for viral nucleic acids, RNA, rather than by indirectly testing for the presence of antibodies. **NAT provides a *yes* or *no* answer as to whether HIV is present.**

HIV Tropism Tests

When HIV attaches to a CD4+ cell it is going to infect, it uses molecules on the cell surface. These are called receptors or chemokine coreceptors. The first receptor HIV uses is the CD4 molecule. The virus then uses a coreceptor to complete its attachment prior to cell entry. The coreceptors are either R4 or R5 molecules and are required for HIV cell entry. (See Chapter 5, pages 122–123, for a discussion on these receptors.)

HIV most often uses one coreceptor or the other. HIV that uses the R5 coreceptor is called R5 tropic. If HIV uses the R4 coreceptor it is R4 tropic. However, viral tropism can be mixed (dual), meaning that some HIV uses both coreceptors to complete its attachment for cell entry (Figure 5-8, page 124). The dual viruses are common in later stages of HIV disease.

At the present time, the better HIV tropism to have is R5. This is because there is now an antiretroviral drug that is active against R5 tropic HIV. This attachment inhibitor is maraviroc. Maraviroc works against R5 tropic HIV only by binding to the cell's R5 receptor, preventing membrane fusion between HIV and the CD4+ cell (see Figure 4-2, page 77). Most HIV (about 80%) uses the R5 coreceptor.

Why Use This Expensive Test? ($1500 to $1700)—The tropism test is helpful in deciding which coreceptor HIV is using in the infected person; if R5, then maraviroc will be useful in controlling a patient's HIV. The test takes about two weeks.

RAPID RESULT HIV TESTING

With an estimated one out of five HIV-positive Americans unaware of his or her infection, increased opportunities for testing are critical. Rapid result HIV antibody tests provide new opportunities to improving access to testing in both clinical and nonclinical settings and increasing the number of people who learn their results.

A rapid test for detecting antibody to HIV is defined as a screening test that reveals the presence or absence of antibodies for HIV during the length of the patient's visit to the clinic, which is usually between 10 and 30 minutes. In the United States, about 5% to 10% of pregnant women do not know their HIV status at the time of delivery. In Africa and Asian countries, it is estimated that about 90% of pregnant women do not know their HIV status at delivery. But the HIV status of pregnant women is essential to prevent mother-to-child HIV transmission.

Rapid result HIV test results are also necessary for deciding whether to initiate treatment for healthcare workers after accidental exposures to patient body fluids, and there is a need for rapid HIV tests to assist with diagnosis and appropriate treatment of persons who may have opportunistic infections due to AIDS in urban emergency departments, which have been shown to have high rates of undiagnosed HIV infection among their patient populations. In short, the value of rapid result HIV tests in public health has been well established (Point of Information 13.1, page 399).

There are over 30 different rapid result HIV tests currently marketed worldwide. The first FDA-approved rapid result HIV antibody test appeared in 1992. It is called the Single Use Diagnostic System (SUDS). Because of an unacceptable level of false positive results, it is no longer used.

Rapid Result Antibody Tests Now in Use

Each year about 750,000 or 30% of 2.5 million tested do not return to receive their ELISA test results. However, using a rapid result test, in less than 20 minutes, they can learn preliminary information about their HIV status. Unlike other antibody tests for HIV, this test can be stored at room temperature, requires no specialized equipment, and can be used outside of traditional laboratory or clinical settings. In early 2008, New York City hospitals and clinics began offering rapid result HIV testing. Under the new program, the hospitals and clinics tested over 187,000 people each year from 2008 through 2012. This program reduced the large number of people who did not return for their ELISA test results.

The Oral Fluid Assay

The collection of oral fluids to look for HIV antibodies using the OraQuick Rapid HIV Antibody Test may not be as accurate as the other rapid result assays that use blood samples. At present, the OraQuick test is only approved for use by medical professionals. It is very important to understand that these new tests do not change the length of time you have to wait after a possible exposure to HIV to get a reliable result. You still need to wait three months (13 weeks) to allow time for antibodies to become detectable in the blood for an accurate result. (See Table 13-2, below.)

FDA Approves First Rapid, Take-Home HIV Test

The first over-the-counter rapid HIV test received Food and Drug Administration (FDA) approval on July 3, 2012. The OraQuick test detects the presence of HIV in saliva collected by an oral swab, with results ready in 20 to 40 minutes. FDA officials said it is targeted toward people who might not otherwise seek HIV screening, allowing them to test in the privacy of their homes. The availability of a home-use HIV test kit provides another option for individuals to get tested so that they can seek medical care, if appropriate. The OraQuick home test is 92% accurate in detecting HIV among those who have the virus, meaning one person for every 12 HIV positive people using it could be missed (test sensitivity). OraQuick is 99% accurate in

Table 13-2 Comparison of Conventional and Rapid Result HIV Testing

Specimen Required	Conventional Blood (Phlebotomy)	Rapid Result Oral swab or blood (finger stick)
Time to Result	3–10 days	20 minutes
Sensitivity	99.9%	99.3–99.6%
Specificity	99.9%	99.8–100.0%
Cost	ELISA $20	Test kits $14
Tested Persons Who Receive Their Test Results	Approximately 70%	99.3%

(Source: Adapted from PRN Notebook, *May 2006)*

ruling out HIV in people who are uninfected, meaning it would incorrectly identify one patient as HIV positive for every 5,000 HIV negative people tested (test specificity). OraSure started selling OraQuick in October through retailers like CVS, Walgreens, and Walmart, and online pharmacies. The home test was priced less than $60. A bi-lingual, toll-free call center will provide users with counseling and medical referrals. People who test negative should re-test themselves after three months because it can take several weeks or more for detectable antibodies to HIV to appear.

UPDATE

The INSTI HIV-1 Antibody Test Delivers Results in as Little as 60 Seconds

On November 29, 2010, the FDA approved INSTI, a new rapid point-of-care HIV-1 antibody test that can provide results from blood and plasma specimens in as little as 60 seconds, with a minimum sensitivity of 99.8% and a minimum specificity of 99.5%. Previously approved rapid HIV tests, such as those described above, take 10 to 20 minutes to generate results. Positive results on any rapid HIV test require confirmation, which usually takes one to two weeks using standard Western Blot or enzyme linked immunosorbent assay. However, because this new test was generated using different antigens than those used to develop other rapid tests, it opens the door to the possibility of a "rapid/rapid" procedure in which one rapid test is used to detect infection and another to confirm it. Although INSTI was only recently approved in the United States it is already available in more than 50 other countries. INSTI is comparable to other approved rapid HIV tests in terms of both performance and cost, and it offers the unique attribute of faster test processing with nearly immediate delivery of results. Having results within a minute or two alleviates many of the logistical concerns related to patient flow that have challenged clinic-based point-of-care HIV screening programs.

The Determine Rapid Result Test

A rapid result test called the Determine Rapid Test, which uses the p24 antigen and antibody against HIV's gp41 protein, is being used in foreign countries but has not yet been approved for use in the USA. The difference between the currently approved American rapid tests is that the U.S. tests only use blood serum antibody to determine if HIV is present. The Determine test uses both an HIV antigen and antibody against HIV to determine the presence of HIV in the blood serum. Therefore, the Determine test offers greater sensitivity (antigen detection), resulting in fewer false positive test reactions. The Determine Rapid Test is expected to be FDA-approved for use in the United States in late 2012.

A Rapid Result CD4 Cell Count Test for Developing Countries

The fully quantitative CD4 cell count test "counts" CD4 cells in blood samples by binding the CD4 cells with specific reagents and separating them off into a fine or thin tube where the length of the line of CD4 cells in the tube can be measured. A simpler qualitative test also being used is an antibody color change to indicate whether the CD4 count is below 250 cells per microliter or above 350 cells per microliter. The results of both tests are ready in about 20 minutes. A major advantage is that these tests can be given by untrained people!

The Rapid Micro-Chip Assay (mChip)

In July 2011, Curtis Chin and colleagues reported on the use of a single, easy-to-use point-of-care (POC) assay that faithfully replicates all steps of ELISA, at a lower total material cost. The POC test was performed using a "mChip" assay in Rwanda on hundreds of locally collected human blood samples. The chip had excellent performance in the diagnosis of HIV using only 1 μl, (microliter) a pinprick, of unprocessed whole blood and an ability to simultaneously diagnose HIV and syphilis with sensitivities and specificities that rival those of reference benchtop assays. Overall, they demonstrated an integrated strategy for miniaturizing complex laboratory assays using microfluidics and nanoparticles to enable POC diagnostics and early detection of infectious diseases in remote settings. The mChip allows for measurement using a hundred-dollar handheld instrument no more complicated to use than a cell phone, according to the researchers. And, the device produces results in minutes rather than days or weeks, a time saving that can make a big difference in treatment outcomes.

New Twist to the Dating Game

The two young single women, attractive and confident, were sitting at the bar of a popular after-hours tavern when they were asked how a relatively quick do-it-yourself HIV test might affect their dating life. One of them, age 23, laughed. "I would definitely make someone take it, hopefully before the sex." She said she would not be embarrassed to insist that a man submit to the test. "I really think we've got what they want. And if they want it, they can have it on our terms." Her friend, age 25, agreed and added, "Especially if you're getting serious with someone." Their comments were not idle speculation: A rapid at-home HIV test could be available on pharmacy shelves within the next year. Encouraged by a federal drug advisory committee early in 2006, OraSure Technologies in Bethlehem, Pennsylvania, was approved by the Food and Drug Administration for permission to start selling its HIV test over the counter. (See page 399)

Problem—Both women thought there would be a lot more unprotected sex if there was a 20-minute test that people could take. In a gay bar, the men said, "We're sick of hearing about condoms and prevention and safer sex. If a test could allow us to skip such prevention efforts, many would. An easily available HIV test could quickly reassure us of a prospective partner's health; it would allow a couple to jump into bed faster than they might have before." Then there

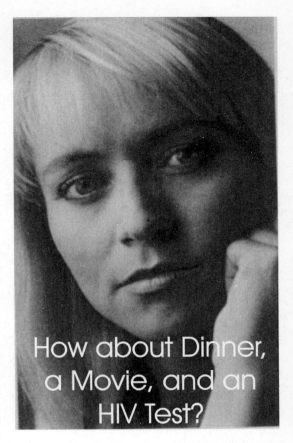

FIGURE 13-5 A Woman Who Cares about Herself and Her Sexual Partner Becoming HIV Infected. *(Courtesy of the Centers for Disease Control and Prevention, Atlanta.)*

is the fact that an HIV test also addresses an issue that more and more singles face—knowing next to nothing about their next date. The popularity of Internet dating and group setups has led many singles to participate in blind dates, no references included (Figure 13-5).

Conclusion—An over-the-counter rapid result HIV test will most likely lead to more casual encounters among most sexually active people. It is possible that a rapid at-home HIV test could help lower a stubbornly high rate of HIV infections.

Summary

Through 2012 the FDA has approved seven rapid result HIV screen tests for use in the United States. All seven rapid tests have high sensitivity and specificity with no significant differences among them.

FDA APPROVES HOME-COLLECTION HIV ANTIBODY TEST KIT

On May 14, 1996, the FDA, which for years opposed home-based HIV testing kits because of the lack of face-to-face counseling, reversed its stance by saying the benefits of early detection of HIV infection outweigh any risks posed by the test. FDA Commissioner David Kessler said, "We are confident that this new home system can provide accurate results while assuring patient anonymity and appropriate counseling."

The FDA approved the home test because in a 1994 study by the CDC of people at increased risk of infection, like injection-drug users and sexually active homosexual men, 42% indicated that they would use a home test.

Test Kit Operation

A person who buys the kit uses an enclosed lancet to prick his or her finger and places three drops of blood on a test card with an identification number. The card is mailed to a laboratory for HIV testing, and samples that test positive are retested to ensure reliability. People who use the home system do not submit names, addresses, or phone numbers with the specimen sent in on filter paper. Therefore, the HIV test results are anonymous. To get results, the individual calls three days later and punches into the phone his or her identification number.

If the caller's test results are positive or inconclusive, he or she will be connected to a counselor who will explain the results, urge medical treatment, and, if necessary, make a referral to a local doctor or health clinic. If the person's results are negative, he or she will be connected to a recording that will note that it is possible to be infected with HIV and still test negative if the antibodies to HIV haven't yet developed. A counselor is available for anyone who tests negative and wants to discuss the results.

The FDA said the kit is as reliable as tests conducted in doctors' offices and clinics.

Test Kit Availability

The first FDA-approved HIV home test kit, called Confide HIV Testing Service, was made available in June 1996. It was withdrawn from the marketplace in June 1997 due to poor sales. A second FDA-approved HIV home test kit went on sale nationwide in July 1996. This kit, called *Home Access Express HIV Test* (1-800-448-8378), lets people take a blood sample at home, mail it to a laboratory, and, three days to a month later, learn by phone their results. The two tests are very similar to each other with regard to use and performance.

In 2012, the administrators at Home Access reported they had processed about 738,000 HIV tests since FDA approval. The overall HIV-positive rate for these tests was 0.9% (about 9 per 1000). The HIV-positive rate in the general population in America is about 0.03%. These data suggest that this form of testing appeals to an at-risk population.

SOME SCREENING AND CONFIRMATORY ANTIGEN-DETECTION TESTS FOR HIV

There are a variety of HIV antigen-detection tests now on the market, and others are on their way. A few of these tests have been singled out because they are currently in use or because of their potential to make a contribution in the field of HIV antibody–antigen testing methodology.

It should be emphasized that these tests identify parts of the virus. **These are not antibody-related tests.**

Polymerase Chain Reaction

Interactions between HIV and its host cell extend across a wide spectrum, from latent to productive infection. The virus can persist in cells as unintegrated DNA, as integrated DNA with alternative states of viral gene expression, or as a defective DNA molecule. Determining the fraction of cells in the blood that are latently (inactively) or productively infected is important for the understanding of viral pathogenesis and in the design and testing of effective therapies. Determining the number of infected cells in a heterogeneous cell population and the proportion of those cells that are carrying the virus but not producing new viruses requires the identification of the proviral DNA and viral mRNA in single cells.

The polymerase chain reaction (PCR) is a technique by which any DNA fragment from a single cell can be exponentially multiplied to an amount large enough to be measured. Thus PCR could be an ideal diagnostic test for HIV infection, since it directly amplifies or increases the amount of proviral HIV DNA and does not require antibody formation by the host. It is already used in settings where antibody production is unpredictable or difficult to interpret, such as in acute HIV infection or in the perinatal/postnatal period. The PCR is so sensitive that it can detect and amplify as few as 6 molecules of proviral DNA in 150,000 cells or 1 molecule of viral DNA in 10 μL of blood.

Now that there are some good anti-HIV therapies available to help slow the onset of AIDS, the diagnosis of individuals who carry the provirus is critical because they may benefit from early treatment. The PCR test will become even more important with the advent of an HIV vaccine. Vaccinated people will become HIV-antibody positive. The PCR test will be used to identify those who are truly HIV infected. In addition, PCR is now used to detect HIV-DNA in spots of dried blood taken from infants as early as six weeks of age and shipped to testing centers without refrigeration. An ELISA (antibody) test cannot accurately diagnose infants until about the age of 18 months.

HIV Gene Probes

Gene probes or genetic probes are an idea borrowed from methodologies used in recombinant DNA research. The idea is to isolate a DNA segment, make many copies of it, and label these copies with a radioisotope or other tag compound. If the DNA sequence copied is contained in any of the HIV genes, the labeled copies of this DNA sequence can be used to hybridize or attach to DNA of cells that contain HIV DNA. This method of DNA probe analysis eliminates the need to search for HIV gene products or antibodies to these products to prove that a person is HIV infected.

DECIDING WHO SHOULD GET AN HIV TEST AND WHEN

Each HIV infection averted saves an estimated $367,000 (in 2009 dollars) in lifetime medical care costs.

Who Should Get Tested? (Remember, your test result expires every time you engage in risky sex!)

The following questions determine if you engage in behaviors that increase your chances of getting HIV. If you answer yes to any of them, you should definitely get an HIV test. If you continue with any of these behaviors, you should be tested every year. Talk to a healthcare provider about an HIV testing schedule that is right for you.

- Have you injected drugs or steroids or shared equipment (such as needles, syringes, works) with others?
- Have you had unprotected vaginal, anal, or oral sex with men who have sex with men, multiple partners, or anonymous partners?
- Have you exchanged sex for drugs or money?
- Have you been diagnosed with or treated for hepatitis, tuberculosis (TB), or a sexually transmitted disease (STD), like syphilis?
- Have you had unprotected sex with someone who could answer yes to any of the above questions?
- Have you been incarcerated in a prison?

If you have had sex with someone whose history of sexual partners and/or drug use is unknown to you or if you or your partner has had many sex partners, then you have more of a chance of being infected with HIV. Both you and your new partner should get tested for HIV and learn the results before having sex for the first time. For women who plan to become pregnant, testing is even more important. If a woman is infected with HIV, medical care and certain drugs given during pregnancy can lower the chance of passing HIV TO HER BABY. All women who are pregnant should be tested during each pregnancy. **One Test Can Save Two Lives**.

Reasons Not to Be HIV Tested

After the hype pushing HIV testing fades, the reality sets in. According to a 2011 CDC report on why people don't want to be HIV tested, only 39.5% of Americans over age 18 have ever been HIV tested. The CDC lists four possible reasons people do not get tested:

1. It is hard to face past transgressions a positive test would bring up; for example, lying and cheating in sexual relationships and acts of failure to prevent.
2. The "that's on them" syndrome: I don't belong to a high-risk behavioral group.
3. My sex life will suffer. Because of the stigma and fear associated with HIV/AIDS, "I can't even reveal I took the test."
4. "It I test positive I can only look forward to a lifetime of pills, sacrifice, and illness. In short, I don't want to know."

In a separate study, Ron Goldman and colleagues (2008) surveyed 97 Australian gay and bisexual men on the question of why they were reluctant to get and HIV test. Their reasons were as follows:

1. If I test positive, it might wreck my relationship with my partner.
2. I'm not sure the test results will remain private.
3. If positive, I won't have enough time to arrange for care of myself and my problems.
4. I don't think HIV testing is necessary—no symptoms—no problems.
5. There is no urgency to take the test—eventually I may take the test.

HIV Testing among Women

Over half (55%) of women aged 18–64 report that they have been tested for HIV at some point, with higher rates among black women (70%) and Latinas (63%) compared to white women (50%). Among those who are HIV positive, 36% of women were tested for HIV late in their illness— that is, diagnosed with AIDS within one year of testing positive. When asked how concerned they were personally about becoming infected with HIV, a recent survey found that 30% of women said they were "very" or "somewhat" concerned. Black women were much more likely to say they were concerned (53%) than were Latinas (51%). More than six in ten female parents (61%) said they were personally "very" or "somewhat" concerned about their children becoming infected.

HIV Testing among Young Adults

The CDC's Youth Risk Behavior Survey (YRBS) provides data on the percentage of students in grades 9–12 who have been tested for HIV. According to the survey, 13% of 9th–12th grade students had been tested for HIV. Testing rates varied by sex (15% among female students, 11% among male students), race/ethnicity (22% among black students, 13% among Hispanic students, 11% among white students) and grade (9% among 9th graders, increasing to 19% among 12th graders). Although national YRBS data are useful for characterizing HIV testing trends nationwide, state and local data are needed to examine local trends in testing behaviors, identify gaps in testing for certain populations, and determine whether young people at risk are being tested.

A Young Adult's Testimony about His HIV Test Results

I am 18 years old. I tested positive on July 1, 2008. I am sure that date will be burned into my memory forever. I remember the counselor closing the door, taking a deep breath and saying, "Your result is positive." Then I remember feeling like I was falling. I could barely hear the questions he was asking, much less find a way to sift through the racing thoughts in my mind to coordinate responses. In spite of my best efforts to keep a positive attitude, there are many moments when I feel like I'm barely holding on to reality. I go to work sometimes hardly able to focus on the task at hand. There are times when I want to burst into tears and scream until I pass out because I feel like I will forever be alone. I've tried spending more time with friends, but I fear being rejected if I told them I was HIV positive. I tell myself that keeping a secret from the friends I have is better than having no friends at all. I know there are others out there just like me. I would like to share my stories with them and vice versa.

Addressing Barriers to HIV Testing

Knowledge of HIV infection status can benefit the health of individual persons and the community. Thus, HIV testing should be as convenient as possible to promote client knowledge of HIV infection status. Efforts should be made to remove or lower barriers to HIV testing by ensuring that:

- Testing is accessible, available, and responsive to client and community needs and priorities.

- Anonymous and confidential HIV testing is available.

- The testing process considers the client's culture, language, sex, sexual orientation, age, and developmental level.

- Confidentiality is maintained. (In some places, like rural communities, *confidentiality* can't be assured, so people may decide not to get tested.)

Opportunities To Increase HIV Testing As More Payers Cover Costs

Paying for an HIV test should not be a barrier for someone to learn of their HIV status as private insurance companies, Medicaid and Medicare pay for HIV testing now for certain populations and in specific instances. With passage of health reform, coverage has already expanded and will greatly increase in the future. Many private insurance plans have covered HIV testing for pregnant women and people who are identified as being at high risk for HIV such as gay men and injection drug users. Health reform now requires all new plans pay for HIV testing for these populations and all plans to pay in 2014. As an estimated 23 million people gain access to health insurance through health exchanges in 2014, access to preventive services,

such as HIV testing, will also expand. Passage of Affordable Care Act (ACA) also enabled the Secretary of Health and Human Services to require plans to cover annual HIV testing for all sexually active women beginning August 2012. All states currently cover medically necessary HIV testing under Medicaid, and approximately half of the stares' Medicaid programs pay for routine HIV testing. Beginning in 2013, in order to incentivize coverage of preventive services, states will receive additional funding from the federal government for coverage of preventive services. In 2014, when an estimated 17 million people gain access to Medicaid, opportunities for paying for preventive services will also expand as they gain access to a payer of their healthcare. Medicare currently pays for HIV testing for pregnant women and those who are at risk for HIV, including those who ask for a test. With passage of the ACCA, any patient cost sharing associated with the cost of the test was eliminated.

Innovative CDC ElTort Expands HIV Testing into Pharmacies

A pilot project to train pharmacists and retail store clinic staff at 24 rural and urban sites to deliver confidential rapid HIV testing was announced today by the Centers for Disease Control and Prevention. The goal of the initiative is to extend HIV testing and counseling into the standard everyday services offered by pharmacies and retail clinics. CDC will use the results of the pilot effort to develop a model for implementation of HIV testing in these settings across the United States. The project is part of CDC's efforts to support its 2006 testing recommendations, which call for all adults and adolescents to be tested for HIV at least once in their lives.

WHY IS HIV TEST INFORMATION NECESSARY?

Thirty percent of adults who seek HIV testing do so to find out their HIV status; 12% are tested because of hospitalization or surgery; 16% for application for insurance; and 7% to enter the military.

Table 13-3 Percentage of Adults Aged 18 Years and Over Who Have Been Tested for Human Immunodeficiency Virus, by Age Group and Sex: United States, 2011[1, 2]

Ages and Sex[3,4]	Percentage[5]
18–24 years	
Total	35.3
Male	29.5
Female	41.1
25–34 years	
Total	53.5
Male	42.1
Female	64.8
35–44 years	
Total	49.3
Male	44.9
Female	53.5
45–64 years	
Total	28.7
Male	30.9
Female	26.6
65 years and over	
Total	11.8
Male	14.7
Female	9.7

[1] *In early 2006 the percentage of U.S. adults (age 18 and over) who had ever been tested for HIV was 35.4%, which is the same percentage of adults found in 2011.*

[2] *For both sexes combined, the percentage of persons who ever had an HIV test was highest among adults aged 25–34 years (53.5%) and lowest among adults aged 65 years and over (11.8%).*

[3] *For age groups 18–24 years, 25–34 years, and 35–44 years, women were more likely than men to have ever had an HIV test. For adults aged 65 years and over, women were less likely than men to have ever had an HIV test.*

[4] *About 1 in 3 who test positive test too late to receive full benefits of ART.*

[5] *About 50% of those ages 18–64 have never been tested.*

Data Source: CDC; National Health Interview Survey, 2006. Data are based on household interviews of a sample of the civilian noninstitutionalized population. (Updated.)

Another 1% are referred by their doctor, the health department, or sexual partner, and 4% are tested for HIV for immigration reasons (see Table 13-3).

IMMIGRATION AND TRAVEL BAN INTO THE UNITED STATES IS LIFTED

The U.S. Congress in 1993 enacted legislation, Section 212 (a) (1) (A) (I) of the Immigration and Nationality Act, that prevents HIV-positive foreigners from obtaining visas or citizenship. According to the U.S. Department of State, if any foreigners traveling to the United States, including people from countries not requiring visas, reveal that they have a communicable disease of public health significance, they are prevented from entering the country. The same rules apply to green card applicants.

UPDATE: President Barack Obama, in November 2009, lifted the 22-year-long immigration and travel ban against HIV-infected people coming to the United States. The new ruling became effective in January 2010.

Immigration Policies of the 194-Member World Health Organization through 2012

- 22 countries **ALLOW** a 90-day entrance permit to those with HIV/AIDS.
- 13 countries **BAR** entry to those with HIV/AIDS.
- 27 countries **DEPORT** any foreigners with HIV/AIDS.
- 126 countries have **NO** restrictions.
- No data on remaining 6 countries.

Immigration and Entry into Foreign Countries

A number of foreign countries require that foreigners be tested for HIV prior to entry. This is particularly true for students or long-term visitors. Information available at the beginning of 2013 reveals that 66 countries and territories require an HIV test prior to entry, on arrival, or on application for residency. Twenty-seven of countries and territories deport HIV-infected people. There are 126 countries that have no restrictions. Before traveling abroad, check with the embassy of the country to be visited to learn entry requirements and specifically whether or not HIV testing is a requirement. If the foreign country indicates that U.S. test results are acceptable "under certain conditions," prospective travelers should inquire at the embassy of that country for details (which laboratories in the United States may perform tests and where to have results certified and authenticated) before departing the United States. For a copy of HIV Testing Requirements for Entry into Foreign Countries, send a self-addressed, stamped, business-size envelope to: Bureau of Consular Affairs, Room 5807, Department of State, Washington, DC 20520.

TESTING, PRIVACY, COMPETENCY, AND INFORMED CONSENT

Privacy is both a legal and an ethical concept. As a legal concept, it refers to the legal protection that has been accorded to an individual to control both access to and use of personal information, and provides the overall framework within which both confidentiality and security are implemented.

Competency is often used interchangeably with capacity; it refers to a person's ability to make an informed decision. For example, to consent to medical treatment, a person must be mentally capable of comprehending the risks and benefits of a proposed procedure and its alternatives. While a healthcare provider can assess competence, a legal finding of competency is often required based on the testimony of a mental health professional. Mental illness by itself does not indicate that a person is incompetent to make medical decisions. Various degrees of mental incapacity may occur with HIV infection, requiring an assessment of competency. AIDS Dementia Complex (ADC) occurs in approximately 70% of HIV-infected patients at some point in HIV disease/AIDS and may interfere with the patient's capacity to provide an informed consent.

Informed Consent

Informed consent is not just signing a form but is a process of education and the opportunity to have questions answered. The concept of informed consent includes the following components: full disclosure of information, patient competency, patient understanding, voluntariness, and decision making. The process of obtaining informed consent involves appropriate facts being provided to a competent patient who understands the information and voluntarily makes a choice to accept or refuse the recommended procedure or treatment.

When the concept of informed consent is applied clinically, complexities arise regarding both the content and the process. The concept contains ambiguous requisites such as "appropriate" facts, "full" disclosure, and "substantial" understanding. The process is affected by many variables including the communication skill and range of practice style of the physician; the maturity, intelligence, and coping strategies of the patient; and the interaction between the physician and the patient (Hartlaub et al., 1993).

Testing without Consent

Entering 2013, at least 35 states had laws that allowed HIV testing without informed consent under certain conditions.

Generally, HIV antibody testing without consent is legally considered battery. Legal liability for "unlawful touching" may result from performing an HIV antibody test without consent. Such a procedure may also constitute an illegal search.

DISCUSSION QUESTION: Are federal and state governments overemphasizing personal privacy at the expense of prevention? (Defend your answer with examples/situations.)

Voluntary Named HIV Testing

In *voluntary named* HIV testing, the individual freely provides his or her name. In this type of testing, an individual voluntarily seeks to learn his or her HIV status and receives a result that is known to both the individual and the test provider/testing agency. An advantage to named testing is that healthcare providers can contact the person tested if he or she does not return for the results.

Voluntary Unnamed or Anonymous HIV Testing

In a voluntary, anonymous HIV test, the identity of the person being tested is not placed on the blood sample or the testing form. As a result, the only person who can link the test result with an individual is the person being tested. This form of testing may encourage people concerned about HIV infection status to obtain testing as it eliminates risk of discrimination or stigmatization. However, it places the exclusive responsibility for seeking counseling, support, and preventive measures on the individual who is infected. Unnamed testing permits reporting of test data to public health authorities without the risk of breaching confidentiality. (See Point of Information 13.2, page 410.)

The Downside to Voluntary Anonymous Testing

Testing that is voluntary may miss populations that disproportionately need to be reached. The people least likely to have the virus, it appears, are the most likely to say yes to a test, and the people most likely to be infected are the most likely to say no. In one study, infection rates were 5.3 times as high among people who refused HIV testing as among people who consented to it. In voluntary anonymous testing, the downside is that such testing reduces the probability that people will return for post-test counseling and linkage to follow-up services, and a substantial reduction in partner notifications (Moser, 1998).

Mandatory HIV Testing

HIV testing is mandatory if it is required to participate in a process or activity that is not itself required. For example, if an HIV test is required for travel to some foreign countries, or to donate blood, this is considered mandatory testing because, while the test is required, one is not required to travel or donate blood. In mandatory testing, care must be taken to ensure that people are not in fact forced to undergo testing. At least in theory, mandatory testing is a form of voluntary testing: People can decide not to participate in

---

---

the process or activity for which testing is required. In practice, however, the degree of voluntary consent is in some cases questionable. For example, in a situation where employment is not possible unless one agrees to be tested, and one needs that job, the voluntary nature of the test appears to have vanished (AIDS, Health and Human Rights, 1995). (See Box 13.2)

Why Mandatory Testing?

Mandatory testing is for the protection of a certain group or the public at large. Although it is not anonymous, results are kept confidential on a need-to-know basis. Mandatory testing for HIV continues to be angrily debated primarily because of the possibility of error when running large numbers of test samples, inadvertent loss of confidentiality, and lack of overall benefit to those who are found to be HIV positive.

BEST POLICY FOR PRENATAL TESTING?

Given the efficacy of antiretroviral drugs to reduce perinatal HIV transmission if administered to the mother while the fetus is in the womb or to the baby within 48 hours after birth, it has become a priority to maximize the number of pregnant women who consent to prenatal HIV testing. Three distinct approaches to obtaining consent for prenatal HIV testing are used: (1) the "opt-in" or voluntary policy (the test, after counseling, is offered to the woman, and she may refuse); (2) the "opt-out" policy (the woman is not counseled about HIV/AIDS but is informed that the HIV test is part of a battery of prenatal tests, which are automatic but she may refuse HIV testing by signing a form rejecting the test); and (3) the mandatory newborn HIV testing approach (the mother is informed that the newborn will be tested, with or without her consent, if her HIV status is unknown at delivery). Currently 10 states mandate HIV testing of the newborn. Connecticut and Texas also mandate HIV testing of all pregnant women. Forty-two states use the "opt out" policy and eight states have the "opt in" policy. The CDC recently evaluated the efficacy of these three approaches in obtaining prenatal HIV tests in the United States and Canada. As a result of these evaluations, the CDC in April 2003 unveiled its HIV testing strategy for pregnant women. These guidelines were updated in 2006 and 2012. The new strategy specifically urges the testing of all pregnant women rather than relying upon patients to volunteer for testing. The guidelines also make HIV testing a routine part of care in doctors' offices and clinics, rather than waiting for patients to specifically request it. The strategy is advisory but has some authority: CDC will ask state and local governments to adhere to it in exchange for federal funding. The United Kingdom offers all pregnant women an opt-out HIV test. Over 90% take the test. New York state mandates that all babies born to untested mothers be tested within 12 hours after birth.

Mandatory HIV testing is routine for blood donors and military and Job Corps personnel.

Mandatory HIV Testing of Newborns and Disclosure of Test Results to Mothers and Physicians

Perhaps no call for mandatory HIV testing has caused as much recent controversy as that requiring all pregnant women to take the test, with the alternative, in the event that they refuse, that their newborns will be tested. On June 26, 1996, New York became the first state in the nation to mandate and disclose the HIV status of newborns to mothers and physicians. Governor George E. Pataki signed into law legislation known as the *"Baby AIDS" Bill,* which authorizes the state health commissioner to establish a comprehensive program of HIV testing of newborns. Over the next eight years, there was an 80% decline in HIV-infected babies born to infected mothers.

The passage of this bill was immediately followed by the American Medical Association announcement endorsing mandatory testing of all pregnant women and newborns for the HIV virus. (See Sidebar 13.2)

Compulsory HIV Testing

In *compulsory testing,* a person cannot refuse to be tested. Compulsory testing may be forced onto an individual, groups, communities, or even entire populations. A court may order an individual to be tested, or a government may decree or legislate that, for example, commercial sex workers, homosexuals, prisoners, hospital patients, or persons seeking immigration must be tested.

In Colorado, Florida, Georgia, Illinois, Kentucky, Michigan, Nevada, Rhode Island, Utah, and West Virginia, HIV testing is compulsory for people convicted of prostitution. However, many prostitutes are back on the streets before their test results are in. In many cases, the prostitutes could not be found for follow-up counseling. In Duval County, Florida, county judges agreed to impose a 30-day jail term for convicted prostitutes, a time period long enough to get their test results and provide counseling. Prostitutes have to sign the test results sheet. They are released as soon as they do.

THE TIME FOR ROUTINE HIV TESTING IS NOW?

The editorial of the March 5, 2005 edition of the *British Medical Journal* and the March 20, 2006 editorial in the *New England Journal of Medicine* state that both the United Kingdom and the United States are ready for routine voluntary HIV testing of all their people. Health experts across the United States are recommending such action, similar to the testing for various cancers and other diseases. The experts argue that HAART has made HIV like any other serious illness. And testing for HIV can take place without counseling. Patients for other serious diseases do not receive counseling. Times have changed. HIV testing should not be accorded any special status. The CDC estimated that beginning in the early 1990s through 2009, about 19 million people per year received an HIV test.

STIGMA AND ITS IMPACT ON HIV TESTING: TAKE THE TEST AND RISK ARREST

To this point in time stigma has kept many people away from testing centers. After over 31 years of this disease and billions of prevention education dollars spent, stigma still reigns. Routine HIV testing of all people should, at least, reduce such behavior and make AIDS a socially acceptable disease as has occurred during the history of cancer in the United States.

PRESSURE FOR UNIVERSAL HIV TESTING: USA

At the 13th Conference on Retroviruses and Opportunistic Infections (Denver 2006), it became clear that the issue of HIV testing's role in prevention can no longer be ignored. Timothy Mastro said that a CDC study showed that HIV-positive people reduced the amount of unprotected serodiscordant sex (only one of the sexual partners being HIV positive) they had by 68% after diagnosis. This led them to believe that the 25% to 30% of people who do not know their HIV status contributed to about 50% of infections. He cited the startlingly high prevalence and incidence figures among gay men and particularly black gay men in cities other than San Francisco. In a large sample of gay men in five U.S. cities, 25% of gay men had HIV and 48% were unaware of their infection. In another city, 46% of black gay men were positive and 67% did not know it. Late testing was also common: 45% of AIDS diagnoses were among people who had been diagnosed HIV positive less than 12 months before.

Mastro said that HIV testing in the USA has not been increasing in recent years despite the fact that the CDC had launched its Advancing HIV Prevention strategy in 2003 to make voluntary HIV testing a routine part of medical care.

CENTERS FOR DISEASE CONTROL AND PREVENTION'S RESPONSE TO CURRENT FINDINGS

The CDC determined in September 2006 that routine screening would be cost-effective and decided to revise its HIV screening guidelines recommending routine, voluntary, or "opt-out" screening for all persons ages 13 to 64 in healthcare settings, without regard to risk, and annual HIV testing for people with risk behavior. Pretest counseling and written consent would not be required (currently one state, Nebraska, still requires written consent for HIV tests). Healthcare settings include all hospital in-patient and out-patient departments and community clinics as well as STD clinics. An exception would be made for prisons, where it was recognized that receiving an HIV diagnosis created profound difficulties both for inmate and institution.

QUESTION: IS THE TIME RIGHT FOR NATIONAL ROUTINE TESTING?

The CDC's suggestion that the time is right, the time is now, has raised very serious issues both pro and con. A pro/con debate on this question will reveal many issues about the HIV/AIDS pandemic, such as why have the political, medical, and scientific establishments, up to now, placed this disease in an exceptional category, never allowing routine testing of the HIV infected when, in fact, no other disease in history has held such status!

David Holtgrave, an epidemiologist with the Johns Hopkins Bloomberg Public School of Health, writes in his research article in the June 12 issue of *PLoS Medicine* that targeting HIV testing at high-risk groups and populations might be a more effective method of identifying people who are unaware of their HIV-positive status than conducting routine testing among all U.S. residents ages 13 to 64. According to Holtgrave, who headed CDC's Division of HIV/AIDS Prevention in the late 1990s, the U.S. healthcare system would spend about $864 million in one year to diagnose nearly 57,000 new HIV cases using the routine testing system. The data is based on the assumption that 1% of people tested are HIV positive. However, the healthcare system could identify up to 188,170 new HIV cases for the same cost by targeting drug treatment facilities, prisons, and community health centers in high-risk neighborhoods. Targeted testing also would focus on people known to have drug habits or to engage in high-risk sexual activities regardless of where they live.

He also estimates that targeted testing and counseling would prevent more than 14,000 new HIV cases annually at a cost of $59,000 per case prevented, compared with 3600 cases at a cost of $237,000 each using CDC's guidelines.

A COMMENTARY ON HIV TESTING IN AMERICA: SHOULD IT BE A PRIORITY?

The basic truth about HIV, with minor exceptions, is that gender, age, race, religion, and economic status are irrelevant to one's susceptibility to HIV infection. This global pandemic is going to be with us for generations to come. Ending 2013, about 2.3 million people in the United States will have been HIV infected. About 665,000 of them will have died of AIDS. Adding to these grim statistics, of those 1.63 million people living with HIV/AIDS ending 2013, about 20%, or 324,000, do not know they are HIV positive, and some 40% of pregnant women and their newborns who should be HIV tested are not. The primary reason for making HIV screening a part of routine clinical practice is to increase the number of people who are aware of their HIV infection and to get them into medical care and reduce their chances of unknowingly transmitting HIV to anyone. But, here we are, six years later, and the CDC's recommendation of having everyone between the ages of 13 and 64 tested is not being followed by the majority of towns, cities, and states of the United States. In fact, the CDC's recommendations have been largely ignored because the CDC makes recommendations, but has no power to enforce them. It is crucial to understand just how important HIV testing is to every level of our security; everyone should know his or her HIV status. This is surely the first step in controlling the HIV/AIDS epidemic in America. Far too many Americans are tested too late to recover. Beginning 2013, an estimated 46% or about 90 million of 195 million U.S. adults ages 18 to 64 have ever been tested. Among ages 13 to 64, 55% or 121 million of 215 million have ever been tested. Among ages 14 to 18 22% of 21.5 million Americans (or about 4.73 million) have been tested; of those who tested positive, half were unaware that they were infected! Such data show that HIV testing efforts in the United States are inadequate. Progress in HIV testing stalled in the 1990s, and new strategies are called for. The U.S. HIV epidemic now is very different from what it was in the early days, when scientific and social recognition of the enormity of this disease was just beginning and when available drug therapy was in its infancy. Back then it meant that people were unlikely to benefit from HIV testing. Today, programs of HIV testing, therapy, and prevention can no longer be based on what this epidemic appeared to be 15, 10, or even five years ago. Advanced testing procedures offer results while you wait, from just three to 20 minutes! Also, using current antiretroviral therapy allows the infected to live about a normal life span without many of the serious side effects of earlier drug therapies. Entering 2013, no country or region in the world has adopted a strategy of universal testing and treatment. But that does not excuse the United States, a wealthy nation and the leader in HIV/AIDS research, prevention, testing, and treatment programs.

Question: How can universal antiretroviral therapy be applied in the United States if there is no universal testing?

Answer: Testing must precede therapy—people must know their HIV status. Imagine the consequences for the developing countries if the United States could export a truly effective understanding about HIV testing, prevention, and therapy. But how can that be done when government agencies cannot agree on whether to test some or all of those ages 13 to 64, or whether to test some or all of those ages 18 to 64?

If Americans truly want HIV/AIDS prevention to work, testing for HIV must become a top priority. Testing is central to nearly all aspects of prevention and treatment! Arguments about what age to begin testing and whether the general population or a targeted portion of the population (at-risk people) should be tested must be settled and a decision must be made by those responsible, because our epidemic demands action now! Hope and action must be bound together because we are losing those we love, those we depend on, those who teach and train each generation of children, those who entertain us, those who offer leadership, and those who offer medical care. We are losing precious lives from every race and culture in the United States because too many in charge of the decisions about this disease choose to do what is politically correct rather than that which is humanly necessary.

In 2007, the CDC began funding a testing initiative. The initiative is funded for six years. The cost is $142.5 million. In the first three years about 1.4 million Americans were tested via this program. Some 10,000 people were identified as HIV positive and linked to care.

United Nations Program on AIDS (UNAIDS) and the World Health Organization (WHO) Release New HIV Testing Guidelines

It is estimated that worldwide only 10% of persons at risk for HIV infections receive HIV testing. In mid-2007, UNAIDS and the WHO released new HIV testing guidelines that advise healthcare workers in countries with an HIV prevalence greater than 1% to routinely offer confidential, voluntary HIV tests to all patients seeking treatment at clinics or hospitals regardless of why they initially sought care.

In March 2010, South Africa's government announced their "First Things First," a university-based plan to test 15 million residents for HIV by June 2011. All public health facilities, fixed and mobile, were equipped to offer HIV testing and to provide antiretroviral therapy to move toward the goal of halving the rate of HIV infection by 2011. Their plan failed! On April 15, 2010, South Africa also launched a new effort aimed at providing AIDS drugs to 80% of those needing treatment by 2015.

DISCUSSION QUESTION: Do you think that targeting HIV testing at high-risk groups might be a more effective way of identifying people who are unaware of their HIV status than conducting routine testing among all U.S. residents ages 13 to 64? Do you think that perhaps the CDC should just consider what changes it can implement to make it easier for people to learn their HIV status and go with that?

Under Florida law, a prostitute who knows he or she is carrying HIV but continues to offer sexual favors can be jailed for one year.

In June 1999, the state of Oregon passed legislation that allows a judge to order a person accused of a crime to be tested for HIV. The person also would be tested for other communicable diseases if he or she transmitted bodily fluids to a victim. The results do not become public record.

In mid-2004, the governor of Wisconsin signed into law a bill that allows teachers to require students to be tested if a teacher is exposed to students' blood. The teachers in this state were added to a list of professionals who are permitted to require HIV tests on people whose blood they are exposed to. The list includes firefighters, police, emergency medical technicians, and other healthcare workers.

At least 45 states and the District of Columbia authorize HIV testing for charged or convicted sex offenders.

Fear of Compulsory Testing—If a massive compulsory screening test program were implemented, would it be possible to keep results confidential? What would be done with the information? For example, would the state prevent an uninfected person from marrying an infected one? Officials fear that mandatory testing will drive many people who might have volunteered for anonymous testing underground and away from healthcare. These people will be lost to the counseling and education that would benefit them and others. The reason for going underground would be fear of discrimination and social ostracism if found to be HIV infected.

A case can be made that a compulsory program could maintain strict confidentiality even with large numbers of people being tested. But it would appear that the political powers and public in general are not ready for broad-scale compulsory testing in the United States.

Confidential, Anonymous, and Blinded Testing

Confidentiality relates to the right of individuals to protection of their data during storage, transfer, and use, in order to prevent unauthorized disclosure of that information to third parties.

Both confidential and anonymous testing involve the use of informed consent forms that are, to date, with the exception of the U.S. military, Job Corps workers, and certain criminals, done on a voluntary basis. Blinded testing

— BOX 13.3 —

CONFIDENTIALITY AND SEXUAL PARTNER BETRAYAL

This story took place in an HIV/AIDS clinic in the South. A husband and wife came into the clinic for an HIV test. They said the *only* reason for requesting the test was that they wanted to begin a family and hoped that nothing in their past would have led to either of them being HIV positive. The tests were completed.

The husband came in on a Monday; the wife came in that Friday.

Monday A.M.

Counselor: Mr. X, your test came back HIV positive.

Reactions and counseling were similar to those presented in this chapter. Then Mr. X said he wanted to be the one to tell his wife; *he insisted on it.* The counselor agreed, Mr. X left the clinic agreeing to come back for a follow-up counseling session.

Friday A.M.

Counselor: Mrs. X, your HIV test was negative.

Mrs. X: That's wonderful news. I can't wait to tell my husband. We've been waiting for my results. I want to get pregnant immediately.

Mrs. X received HIV-negative counseling and left the clinic very happy.

Clearly, the husband did not tell his wife the truth about his test results. A follow-up phone call to the husband went unanswered; so did a letter from the clinic. Several months later, Mrs. X called the counselor to tell her that she was pregnant!

What do you think the counselor should do now?

1. Inform the woman about her husband.
2. Take no action.
3. Call the husband and discuss the situation.
4. Threaten the husband with legal action if he does not tell his wife.
5. A different course of action.

Discuss the moral, ethical, and legal responsibilities of each participant.

---

does not, because of procedure, require informed consent.

Confidential HIV Testing—The person's name and test results are recorded. If the test is positive, the results are reported to the state health department. A consent to HIV testing must be given freely and without coercion. The volunteer does not have to provide any information unless he or she wants to.

The following example demonstrates one of the problems with confidential testing: A young homosexual male with signs of oral thrush agreed to an HIV test. Later that day, he called and asked that his blood *not* be sent to the lab. He was a teacher in a parochial school and feared the results would be revealed. His sample was set aside, but the laboratory courier mistakenly took it for testing. The result was positive, yet no one could tell the patient. A malpractice attorney said to make certain all records of the test were deleted and to send the patient a letter urging him to return for a blood test. He never appeared (Wake, 1989). (See Box 13.3, and Snapshot 13.2, page 414.)

Because in any given year, only 20% of U.S. residents at high risk for HIV are tested, many national public health agencies and committees favor a confidential screening and counseling program that includes all individuals whose behavior places them at high risk of HIV exposure. These agencies recommend that the following eight groups seriously consider volunteering for HIV antibody testing at least twice annually:

1. Homosexual and bisexual men
2. Present or past injection-drug users
3. People with signs or symptoms of HIV infection
4. Male and female prostitutes
5. Sexual partners of people either known to be HIV infected or at increased risk of HIV infection
6. Hemophiliacs who received blood clotting products prior to 1985
7. Newborn children of HIV-infected mothers
8. Immigrants from Haiti and Central Africa since 1977

Anonymous HIV Testing—No name is ever given. And no one can ever learn of your test results. This is also a form of voluntary testing. It differs from confidential testing only in that those who request anonymity receive a bar-coded identification number. They provide no personal information and they come back at a predetermined time to find out if their test number is positive or negative. No follow-up occurs. All states have anonymous test sites providing over 2.5 million tests a year (Nash et al., 1998, updated). Things change when the individual seeks treatment: If one goes to a doctor and the doctor does a viral load test, he reports the person and their viral load test to the health department. There is no way to keep treatment for HIV anonymous.

Blinded HIV Testing—This occurs when blood or serum is available for HIV testing as a result of another medical procedure wherein the patient's blood has been drawn for analysis. In this case, the demographic data have been recorded and can be used for epidemiological studies even if the name of the individual is withheld and a bar code is used. In 1988, the CDC asked for a blinded study of all 1989 newborn blood samples taken in certain cities in 45 states for metabolic studies. The name and other demographics of each newborn were recorded on the label of each tube. After the metabolic tests were completed, the name was changed into a bar code and leftover blood was sent to a state HIV testing center.

DISCUSSION QUESTION: What are reasons for and against blinded testing?

Summary

HIV infection can be detected in three ways: first, by HIV-antibody or antigen testing prior to the appearance of signs and symptoms of AIDS; second, by detecting the presence of HIV nucleic acid; and third, by physical examination after symptoms occur.

The test most often used to screen donor blood at blood banks and individuals referred to testing centers is the ELISA test. ELISA (enzyme linked immunosorbent assay) is a highly sensitive test that determines the presence of HIV antibodies in a person's blood or serum. The ELISA test was first used in 1985 to reduce the number of HIV-infected blood units for blood transfusions.

Because the ELISA test is only a predictive test that gives the percentage chance that a person is truly positive or truly negative, serum from those who test positive is retested in duplicate. If still positive, the serum is then subjected to a Western Blot (WB) test. The WB is a confirmatory test. If it is also positive, the person is said to be HIV infected.

Other screening and confirmatory tests are available. The indirect immunofluorescent antibody assay (IFA) is relatively quick and easy to perform. Although it can be used as a screening test, it is generally used as a confirmatory test. The test is similar to the ELISA test except that the analysis is made by looking for a fluorescent color, indicating the presence of HIV antibodies, with a dark field light microscope. The FDA, through 2012, has approved six rapid results tests for use in the United States.

The polymerase chain reaction (PCR) is a process wherein a few molecules of HIV proviral DNA can be amplified into a sufficient mass of DNA to be detected by current testing methods. It can determine if newborns of HIV-infected mothers are truly HIV positive.

Gene probes are also being used to detect small HIV proviral DNA sequences in cells of people who are HIV infected but not yet making antibodies. The CDC is recommending that everyone be HIV tested.

The availability of oral fluid and finger prick testing, along with rapid results tests, has made it easier to provide HIV testing in a wide range of clinical and nontraditional and over the counter settings and has led to new strategies for reaching more persons with undiagnosed HIV infection. Rapid results tests produce results in 20 minutes or less and make it possible to give HIV-seronegative and provisional HIV-seropositive test results in a single visit to more than 95% in many testing programs. The CDC is developing recommendations to make HIV screening a routine part of medical care, to remove barriers that hamper early HIV diagnosis and treatment, and to demonstrate and disseminate effective models for testing in clinical and nontraditional settings.

Free confidential HIV testing is available. To find a testing center in your area, call the CDC National AIDS Hotline (24 hours/7 days, 365 days a year) 1-800-342-2437 (AIDS); 1-800-344-7432 (SIDA); or call your local health department. Additional resources: www.hivtest.org.

Review Questions

(Answers to the Review Questions are on page 463.)

1. What is the acronym for the most commonly used HIV-antibody test, and what does each letter stand for?

2. What basic immunological assumption is this test based on?

3. Does a single positive HIV antibody result mean the person is HIV infected? Explain.

4. Is there a specific test for AIDS? Explain.

5. What is currently the most frequently used HIV confirmatory test in the United States?

6. What is the name of one additional confirmatory test in use in the United States?

7. How is HIV antibody detected in the ELISA test?

8. True or False: All newborns who are antibody positive are HIV infected and all go on to develop AIDS.

9. What is the greatest shortcoming of the ELISA and WB tests?

10. What are the two major problems in interpreting ELISA test results?

11. What two factors may account for false-positive and false-negative results?

12. What is the relationship between false-positive results and prevalence of HIV in the population?

13. In an HIV screening test, what is a positive predictive value? Why is it called a predictive value?

14. What is the current gold standard of confirmatory tests in the United States?

15. What is the major problem in using this test?

16. Why is the polymerase chain reaction (PCR) considered so useful in HIV testing? Name two situations when PCR can be significant in HIV testing.

17. How quickly can one get reliable HIV test results using the OraQuick HIV test?

18. True or False: Two home-use HIV antibody test kits are now available in the United States.

19. Using the ELISA test, when are HIV antibodies first detectable?

20. How early are HIV antigens detectable in human serum?

21. What are three benefits of early identification of HIV-infected people?

22. Name the four kinds of testing privacy available to people who want to take an HIV test.

23. What is the major difference between an anonymous and a blind HIV test?

24. Why would someone want an anonymous test?

25. True or False: The ELISA serological test is adequate to confirm HIV infection.

26. True or False: Pre- and post-HIV-antibody test counseling is recommended any time an HIV antibody test is performed.

AIDS and Society: Knowledge, Attitudes, and Behavior

In the end, they will say, we died not at the hands of our enemies, but in the silence of our friends.

Martin Luther King, Jr.

CHAPTER HIGHLIGHTS

- HIV infections keep on going and going . . .
- HIV/AIDS is here to stay.
- The HIV/AIDS devastation is now.
- Inaccurate journalism leads to public hysteria.
- Vignettes on HIV/AIDS.
- It's 32 years later, and what do we know about HIV/AIDS?
- Use of explicit sexual language on TV and in journalism.
- Goal of sex education: to interrupt HIV transmission.
- Education, Just Say Know.
- An education about HIV/AIDS is an education for and about life.
- Seventeen states, through 2011, did not require student HIV/AIDS education.
- What does the red ribbon mean?
- Education is not stopping HIV transmission.
- Students still have misconceptions about HIV transmission.
- The general public, homophobia, and HIV transmission.
- Milton Hershey school settles HIV discrimination suit for $700,000 plus civil penalties.
- Employees are not well informed and fear working with HIV/AIDS-infected coworkers.
- Educating employees about HIV/AIDS.
- Teenagers are not changing sexual behaviors that place them at risk for HIV infection.
- Physician–patient relationships in the HIV/AIDS era.
- U.S. Supreme Court renders its first ever ruling in the HIV/AIDS pandemic.
- Placing the risk of HIV infection in perspective.
- Federal response to the AIDS pandemic—create an AIDS industry.
- Federal research dollars related to the cost per death in eight categories of disease compared to the cost of an HIV/AIDS death.
- A national AIDS policy (strategy) is created in 2010.
- Has the United States created a monetary HIV/AIDS foreign entitlement policy?
- Global AIDS, Tuberculosis, and Malaria Fund began June 2001.

- President's Emergency Plan for AIDS Relief (PEPFAR), January 2003–2008, renewed for $63 billion through 2013.
- How much will it take to fund HIV/AIDS relief—how much have you got?

Too many times the litany of broken promises to reverse the spread and impact of HIV/AIDS rings hollow against the unrelenting advance of the pandemic throughout the world. In this context, knowledge, attitudes, and behavior underline our understanding of what the various statements on commitments and declarations on HIV/AIDS actually mean and are essential first steps toward greater and more authentic accountability of global leadership against this pandemic.

LOOKING BACK 14.1

AIDS COALITION TO UNLEASH POWER: ACT UP—NOTHING FOR US WITHOUT US

The gay, lesbian, and transgender communities and their heterosexual supporters must be acknowledged for their immediate, aggressive, and humanitarian response to AIDS. Years before government was ready to accept its rightful role, these communities were caring for the sick, fighting for treatment and research, and making remarkable changes in personal and organizational behavior to curb the risk of AIDS. Their efforts and accomplishments are without precedent in modern medical history. In years past, an AIDS action group called ACT UP (AIDS Coalition to Unleash Power) under its mantra, "Silence = Death," urged people to get out there and raise hell because nobody else was doing anything about this disease. In order to promote prevention, they draped a 35-foot condom over Republican Jesse Helms's house, scattered the ashes of people who died of AIDS on the White House lawn, and tossed a coffin in front of a San Francisco hospital after an AIDS patient was denied a liver transplant. They invaded the offices of drug companies and scientific laboratories and chained themselves to the desks of those in charge and chained themselves to the trucks trying to deliver drug company products. They poured buckets of fake blood in public places, closed the tunnels and bridges of New York and San Francisco, stormed St. Patrick's at Sunday Mass, spitting at Cardinal O'Connor, infiltrated the floor of the New York Stock Exchange for the first time in its history to confetti the place with flyers urging the brokers to SELL WELCOME, boarded themselves up inside Burroughs-Welcome (now named Glaxo SmithKline), which owns AZT, had regular Die-Ins at the Food and Drug Administration and the National Institutes of Health, at city halls, at the White House, in the halls of Congress, at government buildings everywhere, where they lay flat on the ground with their arms crossed over their chests or holding cardboard tombstones until the cops had to take them away by the vans-full and had massive demonstrations at the FDA and the NIH. There was no important meeting anywhere that they did not invade, interrupt, and infiltrate. They plastered New York City with tens of thousands of stickers reading "Gina Kolata of the *New York Times* is the worst AIDS reporter in America," picketed the Fifth Avenue home of the publisher of the *Times*. They picketed everyone and every place where they felt there was incompetence. From their historic 24-hour round the clock for seven days and nights picket of Sloan Kettering to mayor Edward I. Koch. And they protested against Presidents Reagan, Bush, and Clinton. Many of those picketing were arrested many times! But it took these actions to get the attention of mainstream America and its politicians. Today's more recently infected people may not recognize the names of those who demonstrated in the streets, stopped meetings, defied government policies, and demanded adequate research funding and better medicines for AIDS, but they should know that without the efforts of these early warriors in the AIDS battle, the nationwide infrastructure of care, prevention, and treatment education would be much less than it is. The successes achieved by gay-empowered ACT UP later empowered women and heterosexuals to demand action for better drugs and a government commitment to finding an HIV vaccine, which served as a model for international AIDS activism that has recently achieved great price reductions in HIV/AIDS drugs for their countries. ACT UP has also served as a model for people with other diseases, like breast cancer, to form action groups to demand more from their government.

In January 2012, the Treatment Action Group (TAG) formed by a group of activists from ACT UP, celebrated its 20th anniversary. TAG provided greatly needed help in pushing a historically unprecedented therapeutic revolution with the introduction of highly active antiretroviral therapy **(HAART).**

Whatever weakness and failings exist in the current structures of ACT or TAG, they do provide structures to build and improve upon. Those who have died have left a legacy that can serve as a guide in the future as the epidemic cuts its way around the world.

Anthony Fauci, director of the National Institute of Allergy and Infectious Diseases (NIAID), said that modern medicine can be divided into two periods: before ACT UP and after ACT UP started. These people put medicine back in the hands of the patients, which is where it belongs.

HIV/AIDS IS A STORY IN OUR LIFETIME

AIDS is a story about the way the world is. A world that is home to a deadly but preventable disease that thrives in the human family, infecting or killing some 68 million of its members over 32 years. It's a world where every 15 seconds a man, woman, or child dies of AIDS. It's a world where every day about 6850 people become HIV infected. It's a world in which the human right to health does not exist for most people. It is a world in which respect for life itself seems to be lost. AIDS in the world? It is a story about ourselves. About humankind. What kind of people are we? How did we get to this point? This disease is preventable! Where are we going? And, what social changes are occurring because of this pandemic? It is said that we must crawl before we can walk, but we are still crawling, albeit at an ever-increasing pace—when will we walk through a world of HIV-free people? Can we find a way to compassion, humanity, and dignity for all men, women, and children? HIV/AIDS is becoming the worst plague in human history. Soon it will have killed more people than all the wars in the 20th century, but too few seem to know or even care about it. Humankind is paying a steep price for its ignorance, arrogance, and apathy toward each other. Many, for instance, believe HIV/AIDS is an African disease, and they blame Africans for its spread. Africans are not responsible for AIDS or spreading HIV, humankind is. The virus happens to be in our world. HIV and AIDS, like so many other epidemics, will thrive in the human family for generations to come, and as before, the cost is in human lives. We can only overcome AIDS if we accept that HIV has become a part of the human condition and that HIV and AIDS exist because we exist. We as a human species have to integrate that in all aspects of our lives. That is the nature of the world, that is the price of life. AIDS is but one ticket to the show on Planet Earth.

THE NEW MILLENNIUM AND HIV/AIDS

September 11 and June 27, 2001—The first is the date of the terrorist attack on the United States in New York. The second is the date on which 189 nations signed a UN Declaration of Commitment on HIV/AIDS in the same city. September 11 changed the world, June 27 apparently changed very little.

HIV/AIDS is becoming more of a global disaster with each passing year of the new millennium. This disaster will be with us for many years to come, perhaps lifetimes or generations to come—like smallpox, the bubonic plague, cholera, and other diseases from ancient times. It does not appear that there are any new surprises that scientists are about to spring on this virus—but this virus continues to surprise our best scientists. HIV just keeps spinning its genetic building blocks looking for its next jackpot—how to overcome the next onslaught of antiretroviral drugs. Those jackpots keep coming up and the virus is winning the drug war. In developed nations, too many people think the HIV/AIDS crisis is over—they have been fooled by erroneous television and press coverage. Globally in 2002 through 2013, between 2 million and 3 million people will have died of AIDS annually and in each year over 2 million new infections will have occurred. But estimated numbers of AIDS deaths and new infections for 2014 into 2015 are even higher!

AIDS in the new millennium is like a train heading toward a horrific wreck. As the train gains speed, the global rate of HIV infections increases. As T4 or CD4+ cells drop, the distance to the wreck becomes shorter; on impact millions more will have died of AIDS. Like the Energizer bunny, HIV infections keep on going and going and . . .

The impact of HIV/AIDS is so monumental on societies as a whole, and on communities and families in particular, that there is no precedent in human history. There's nothing from the Black Death (a plague peaking in Europe in the 14th century) to the world wars of the 20th century that even approximates it. That we've never had such numbers or seen the focus on a single gender, or ever had so many orphans, so many social breakdowns in various sectors, has became an overwhelming linkage of events for which there are no modern parallels, and therefore, we have to respond in ways that are unprecedented. HIV/AIDS is going to leave a fossil-like imprint on civilization that we can't yet begin to imagine.

Peter Piot, former head of the United Nations campaign to combat AIDS (UNAIDS), said in June 2005 that "it is no longer realistic to hope that the world will meet its goal of halving and reversing the spread of the AIDS pandemic by 2015." Piot believes that the world is faced with multiple HIV/AIDS epidemics with an expanding pandemic. He said, **"we are still moving into the globalization of the AIDS pandemic."**

This pandemic is unfolding in waves that span human generations, and societies are making incremental adjustments along the way as they try to cope with the horrible impact HIV/AIDS is taking, not only in terms of human lives lost, but in the devastation of families, clans, civil society, social organizations, business structures, armed forces, and political leadership. Further, the HIV/AIDS pandemic is occurring primarily in regions that are hard hit by a range of other devastating diseases, acute and ever-rising poverty, political instability, and many other conditions that may mask or worsen the various impacts of AIDS. Of the estimated 38 million people living with HIV/AIDS ending 2013, most will die between 2015 and 2020. And many millions more will have become HIV infected.

HIV/AIDS IS AN UNUSUAL SOCIAL DISEASE

HIV/AIDS, like other severe epidemics in America, has a powerful social force that has allowed it to become established and that has promoted its rapid spread. But this disease is unique in the sense that it seems to track the fault lines in our society and profits from the social flaws

and weaknesses inherent in societies in transition. The spread of HIV/AIDS is determined by very powerful social and economic factors.

HIV is mainly sexually transmitted and therefore closely associated with and intertwined in people's relationships.

DISCRIMINATION AND STIGMA VS. COMPASSION AND SUPPORT

HIV/AIDS is a schizophrenic condition. It is a pandemic worldwide, but it may not have fully emerged. It often promotes stigma and rejection at the very time when people need comfort, compassion, and support. Stigma and discrimination further serve to propagate the disease because in this climate individuals do not feel confident or free to disclose their status, often not even to their sexual partners or their spouses. The disease remains silent and spreads relentlessly. HIV is transmitted through our most creative and spiritual potential, our ability to create life. It is also passed in the breast milk of mothers to their newborn infants; the very food of life can sow seeds of death. These spiritual connections can trigger negative and harmful perceptions and thoughts, promoting the concept that this epidemic is God's punishment to the wicked and to the sexually immoral. These can easily be translated into negative actions, blame, and rejection, further serving to keep the epidemic hidden and invisible, and fostering continued denial of the problem and its spread. Unlike most other terminal or life-threatening diseases, this one affects mainly the young and middle-aged adults, the adults on whom we all depend; they drive the economy, they parent and teach the children, they care for the sick, and keep the planes and trains running on time. (Read Quick Hits 14.1, page 420.)

HIV/AIDS IS HERE TO STAY

The past 31 years of the global AIDS pandemic have taught us that HIV disease is a permanent part of life on Planet Earth. HIV is simultaneously a virus and a phenomenon. When it is viewed only as a virus, it is hard to see why HIV

STIGMA AND DISCRIMINATION AT THEIR WORST

HIV/AIDS stigma and discrimination are critical issues that impact the quality of life of all persons living with HIV/AIDS. They involve prejudice, discounting, discrediting, rejection, and isolation directed at people perceived to have HIV or AIDS. Stigma singles out the HIV-positive person and draws attention to his or her status as different or even untouchable, running the gamut from being served with paper plates and disposable cups at family gatherings (while everyone else has china and glasses) to outright aggression and hostility. Emotionally, HIV-positive individuals often internalize stigma in feelings of shame, guilt, anger, fear, and self- loathing. Stigma has a negative effect on behaviors across the context surrounding HIV infection, transmission, and care, including HIV test seeking and willingness to disclose HIV status. Some examples the stigma and discrimination associated with HIV/AIDS are given:

1. In Biloxi, Mississippi, a mother kicked her HIV positive son out of her house because "she didn't like that I was going to church and HIV positive. She wouldn't even hug me for a very long time."

2. In Hattiesburg, Mississippi, a young man was denied work at a fast food restaurant after he tested positive. When he finally found employment, a coworker told him he should be quarantined.

In other cases across the United States, there are those who say:

1. HIV stigma has ruined my life, my career, my family, my finances, my self-respect, and my credit.

2. I got fired from my job as an administrative assistant at my church by my pastor. I lost my best friend of 20 years. I no longer trust anybody. I am in therapy. I cannot date. I sit in my house every day unless I have to go somewhere. My life is HELL.

3. I dated a man once, several years ago. I kissed him. The next day I decided to share my HIV positive status with him. He freaked out and said, "They should mark people like you, so the rest of us can tell."

4. When I told a very good friend of mine (we used to camp beside each other every weekend), he cried and said he would stand with me, support me, be there for me. I have never heard from him again, not a call, not even a note or e-mail.

5. A friend of a friend who knew I had HIV disinfected the entire house after I came to pick my friend up to go out. When I walked back in a few hours later to drop her off, I noticed the whole house smelled of cleaning products.

6. All my Catholic friends whom I've known for 20 years all turned their backs on me, started making up lies in my community, and attacking my character. I can't show up in public any longer. No one will hire me. I can't even volunteer. It feels more like they are carrying out some type of top-down orders to stigmatize people with AIDS. Probably the Pope.

Defined as a "mark of shame, disgrace, or discredit," stigma has long plagued HIV/AIDS. It is one of the defining characteristics of the disease, differentiating it from its biologically parallel but socially altogether different retroviral kin: hepatitis, herpes, and human papillomavirus (HPV). While we can discuss vaccinating our children against HPV and we can sit comfortably in front of commercials for herpes drugs, the mere whisper of the word "AIDS" often causes all polite conversation to cease. (Examples of stigmas 1–6 have been taken from "Why AIDS stigma is as deadly as the virus itself," by Regan Hofmann, *POZ Magazine*, December 2009, pages 45–49.)

prevention is a problem. People normally want to avoid harming themselves and others. When viewed as a phenomenon, HIV points to the many personal and societal causes of disease transmission. It points to the difficulties people have in making their intentions match their behavior. It points to the inequalities in relationships, which help to spread HIV. It points to societies' reluctance to prepare young people to manage their intimate relations, to admit to sexual diversity, to responsibly manage complex health and social problems such as drug abuse, and to provide access to health care. It points to the world's failure to care about improving living conditions in poor countries.

These are indeed the dark days of the global HIV/AIDS pandemic. About 80% of people who need treatment are dying without it.

Necessary prevention and vaccine programs go underfunded. By the time you read this, another million men, women, and children have died since summer 2012. About 30 million people will have died of AIDS ending 2013. And yet, the darkest days of this global pandemic are ahead. Many millions more will become HIV infected and many millions more will die from AIDS. Nicholas Everstadt, a fellow at the American Enterprise Institute, a neoconservative think tank, estimated that up to 155 million people could become HIV infected in just three countries (China, Russia, and India) between 2000 and 2025.

AIDS COMES TO THE UNITED STATES

HIV/AIDS was first described in the United States in 1981. Who would have thought then that almost 32 years later about 68 million people or about 1 in every 110 people on earth would be infected with the virus that causes AIDS? And that this virus, regardless of the involvement of the world's governments, the best scientists, and the expenditure of over a half trillion dollars just in the United States, continues to spread out of control in many nations of the world? There is no way at the present time to prevent the 2 million to 3 million new HIV infections each year. No drugs offer a cure, and most of the 38 million living with HIV, ending 2013, cannot afford and will not receive those drugs that offer an improved quality of life. An HIV-preventive vaccine now is still wishful thinking. But there is one commodity in plentiful supply—blame—enough for everyone, everywhere. (See Sidebar 14.1)

BLAME SOMEONE, DEJA VU

The greater *hostility* and greatest *stigma* tends to be assigned to diseases in which individuals are seen as responsible for having the disease; in which the disease's course is fatal; in which fear of

---

SIDEBAR 14.1

A MOTHER'S NIGHTMARE

Recently, at a bus stop, a woman saw a man walking toward her. The man was so thin she could see his face, leg, and arm bones. His eyes were sunken and sad. As he got closer, she recognized it was her son! He was living in the streets, an injection-drug user; he told her he was dying of AIDS. She was too stunned to be hurt, she just put her arms around him and let him cry.

There are some things mothers can fix—this wasn't one of them. But she set out trying to find him a place to live and a doctor to care for him. At age 35, her son is watching himself shrink into an old man. His mother, age 61, wonders how she will pay for his burial.

---

transmission is a major issue; and in which the disease leads to highly visible and frightening physical expressions. All these conditions are associated with HIV disease and AIDS. With AIDS more than any other disease in history, people have found verbal mechanisms for distancing themselves from thoughts of personal infection. Worldwide, from the onset of this pandemic, people have learned in a relatively short time to *categorize, rationalize, stigmatize,* and *persecute* those with HIV disease and AIDS. AIDS statistics are published in categories to identify how many gay or bisexual men, injection-drug users, persons with hemophilia, and so on, have become HIV infected or have developed AIDS. Also listed are the countries, states, and cities with the highest incidence of the disease, along with which racial and ethnic groups are highest among reported HIV and AIDS cases. **By focusing on categories of people, have we made it possible for society to rationalize that AIDS belongs to somebody else? Have we made the thought of HIV/AIDS somewhat impersonal? HAVE WE FOUND A WAY TO BLAME SOMEONE ELSE?**

Placing the Blame

Placing blame does not always require reason and tends to focus on people who are not considered normal by the majority. Thus, minorities and foreigners are often singled out to blame for something, sometimes anything. Epidemics of plague, smallpox, leprosy, syphilis, cholera, tuberculosis, and influenza have historically focused social blame onto specific groups of people for spreading the diseases by their "deviant" behavior. Blaming others leads to their stigmatization and persecution.

While the Black Death, a pandemic of bubonic plague, swept across Europe in the fourteenth century, blame was variously attached to Jews and witches, followed by the massacre and burning of the alleged culprits. In Massachusetts between 1692 and 1693, some 20 people were hanged or burned at the stake after being accused of having the powers of the devil. Eighty percent of those accused were women. In January 2009, officials in Papua New Guinea reported that a woman had been burned alive at the stake after being accused of witchcraft, which often is linked to AIDS-related deaths in the country. In 2008, a report stated that many women were being accused of practicing witchcraft to cause AIDS-related deaths among young people and, as a result, the women were tortured or murdered. The report estimated that there had been 500 such attacks.

When Hitler blamed Jews, communists, homosexuals, and other "undesirables" for the economic stagnation of Germany in the 1930s, the result was death camps and ultimately World War II. Now there is a new plague—HIV/AIDS. What blame comes packaged with this new disease?

Jonathan Mann, former head of the World Health Organization's Global Program on AIDS, said in 1998 that there are really three HIV/AIDS epidemics, which are phases in the invasion of a community by the AIDS virus.

First is the epidemic of silent infection by HIV, often completely unnoticed. **Second,** after a period of incubation/clinical latency that may last for years, is the epidemic of the disease itself.

Third, and perhaps equally important as the disease itself, is the epidemic of social, cultural, economic, and political reaction to HIV/AIDS. The willingness of each generation to place blame on others when believable explanations are not readily available simply recycles history. We have been there before; we have placed blame on others and it will continue. With respect to the HIV/AIDS pandemic, blame has been disseminated among nations. There is no shortage of political, economic, social, or ethical issues associated with this new disease.

AIDS needs no translation. In New York, California, Paris, Nairobi, Calcutta, Moscow, or any other large city across the globe, those four letters provoke a universal reaction: fear, panic, and, too often, revulsion.

FEAR: PANIC AND HYSTERIA OVER THE SPREAD OF HIV/AIDS IN THE UNITED STATES

With the 1981 announcement by the U.S. Public Health Service and the CDC that there was a new disease, AIDS quickly became a symbol for our darkest fears. Responsible public officials gave out conflicting messages: *reassurance* on one hand and *alarm* on the other. *Public panic and hysteria began.* People fear what they do not understand and cannot control.

People with HIV disease and AIDS are still abused, ridiculed, and maligned. Some people believe that AIDS is divine retribution for immoral lifestyles. People who have not indulged in high-risk lifestyles (for example, newborns and recipients of blood products) continue to be labeled as *innocent victims,* implying perhaps that other HIV-infected individuals are guilty for behavior that led to others' infection and therefore deserve their own illness.

Families and communities continue to be divided on their beliefs and acceptance of HIV/AIDS patients. Federal and state agencies stand accused of a lack of commitment and compassion in the war against AIDS. The bottom line is that *value judgments* are associated with HIV/AIDS because the disease involves the most private areas of people's lives—*sex, pregnancy, drug use, and finances.*

The Fear Factor

Worldwide, the political, medical, and legal communities used the media or vice versa to scare people about a new disease called AIDS. The result has been to scare people into fearing other people rather than the disease. For example, a recent survey of 1000 black American church members in five cities found that more than one-third of them believed the AIDS virus, HIV, was produced in a germ warfare laboratory as a form of genocide against blacks.

Another third said they were unsure whether the virus was created to kill blacks. That left only one-third who did not criticize the theory that HIV crossed into humans from chimpanzees.

Frightening Messages from the Media

Soon after young homosexual men began dying in large numbers, a barrage of frightening rhetoric began filling the airwaves, television, the popular press, and even the most reputable scientific journals. The AIDS disaster was here. One healthcare administrator stated, "We have not seen anything of this magnitude that we can't control except nuclear bombs."

Myron Essex of the Department of Cancer Biology at the Harvard School of Public Health noted,

> The Centers for Disease Control and Prevention (CDC) has been trying to inform the public without overly alarming them, but we outside the government are freer to speak. The fact is that the dire predictions of those who have cried doom ever since AIDS appeared haven't been far off the mark. . . . The effects of the virus are far wider than most people realize. It has shown up not just in blood and semen but in brain tissue, vaginal secretions, and even saliva and tears, although there's no evidence that it's transmitted by the last two.

Syndicated columnist Jack Anderson reported that the Central Intelligence Agency (CIA) concluded that in just a few years heterosexual AIDS cases would *outnumber* homosexual cases in the United States. Otis Bowen, former

secretary of Health and Human Services, said AIDS would make the Black Death that wiped out one-third of Europe's population in the Middle Ages pale by comparison. And sex researchers William Masters, Virginia Johnson, and Robert Kolodny stated in their book, *New Directions in the AIDS Crisis: The Heterosexual Community,* that there was a possibility of HIV infection via casual transmission—from toilet seats, handling of contact lenses from an AIDS patient, eating a salad in a restaurant prepared by a person with AIDS, or from instruments in a physician's office used to examine AIDS patients.

In contrast to these reports is the article by Robert Gould in *Cosmopolitan* in 1988, reassuring women that there is practically no risk of becoming HIV infected through ordinary vaginal or oral sex even with an HIV infected male. According to Gould, the vaginal secretions produced during sexual arousal keep the virus from penetrating the vaginal walls. His explanation was: "Nature has arranged this so that sex will feel good and be good for you."

Reaction Based on Fear

In December 1997, a male entered a bar and held a syringe full of blood against a female patron's throat. He said the blood contained HIV. He demanded money. He was caught and charged with robbery and attempted murder, pending the outcome of HIV tests of the blood from the syringe. The man thought the fear of AIDS would be sufficient to rob the bar.

In Taiwan, people with HIV have been hired to work as debt collectors. The widespread fear of HIV/AIDS is being used to force people to pay their debts. The HIV infected need a job and the loan agency needed a clever way to get their money back. The loan agency believes it's a proper business agreement.

In June 2007, the results from the China Youth University for Political Science survey showed that of 1089 students from 12 universities in Beijing, 23% were unwilling to have an HIV-positive classmate. Seven percent said that HIV-positive people should not be admitted to universities, and 31% said they should be admitted but "with certain restrictions." Four percent of respondents said that the HIV positives should not be allowed to find employment, and 43% said they should be allowed employment "with certain restrictions."

In rural Zimbabwe to be a widow and old is very dangerous. Self-appointed witch hunters backed by community leaders are accusing widows of bewitching people with AIDS. If the widow is lucky, she is banished from the village. If not, she undergoes a brutal cleansing ritual. Elderly women and widows are often referred to as witches. The prevalent belief is that HIV/AIDS can only attack a person if he or she has been bewitched or made unfortunate with the use of charms. One woman whose husband and two children died of AIDS was given one hour to leave the village and was not allowed to take her possessions—she lost everything. In another case, in an exorcism ceremony, the woman was made to crouch over a large bucket of boiling water with a blanket over her head. After 10 minutes the blanket was removed—her face and arms were scalded and disfigured.

While causing physical and mental suffering to those widows identified as witches, witch hunters are profiteering by cheating villagers in exorcising ceremonies. For one to be exorcised of witchcraft, one has to pay a large price. Some families have had to give their livestock in order to pay the witch hunters. When a village calls in witch hunters it also has to pay for their keep.

In May 2011, it was reported by the CDC that female albinos (persons with abnormally white skin) in Tanzania are being raped as a cure for AIDS. Other albinos are being murdered because it is believed that such people are cursed—they are from the devil, they are not human, and they may cause AIDS.

Fear of AIDS is understandable, given that AIDS is fatal and its cause, HIV, is transmittable. AIDS appeared suddenly and spread quickly—it took a number of years to identify the virus that causes it and the mechanisms for its spread. Yet, today the routes of transmission are well established and widely known, as are the precautionary measures that can be taken to prevent its spread. Early on, fear of AIDS took an unhealthy turn, anxieties were projected onto those who were hit the hardest by the disease, and the fear of AIDS became an irrational fear of *people* with AIDS. (See Sidebar 14.2.)

WHOM IS THE GENERAL PUBLIC TO BELIEVE?

Because of the complexity of HIV disease, a great deal of press coverage of AIDS issues reflects what scientists say to journalists. A journalist's responsibility is to check that the facts are accurate, but not necessarily to judge their overall merit. Why should a good story be spiked just because other scientists disagree with the data interpretation? When scientists say contradictory things to the public, how can the public assess whom to believe? Science has a duty to inform and educate the public, but it must be used neither to frighten people unnecessarily nor give them unjustified expecta-tions. Claims of *"AIDS cures"* in the popular press need to be based on much more than just test tube data or rumors! Whatever the need to attract research funding, is five minutes of fame ever worth a day of fear or weeks of false hopes for many? The popular press has provided HIV-infected persons with a roller coaster ride between hopelessness and fantasies of imminent cure.

As a result of journalistic promises, there was and still is a range of emotions that run from real hope of a cure to public panic and hysteria. In at least five states, children with AIDS were barred from attending local public schools. The case of 12-year-old Ryan White of Kokomo, Indiana, was made into a TV movie, *The Ryan White Story,* in 1989. (See Box 14.1, pages 429–430.)

In some localities, police officers and health-care workers put rubber gloves on before apprehending a drug user or wear full-cover protective suits when called to the scene of an accident. In other communities, church members, out of fear of HIV infection, have declined communion wine from the common cup.

THE PROMOTION OF FEAR AND ITS AFTERMATH: AN ANALOGY TO HOW FEAR SPREAD WHEN AIDS ENTERED THE WORLD

Once there was a peaceful village and its lovely village green with small shops encircling the green. On any given day, villagers stopped and chatted and exchanged pleasantries and told each other stories about their children, their lives. All was well in this village until one day, **two large bears** walked out of the woods and stood at the edge of town with their heads turned toward each other—the people watching the bears **thought** the bears were whispering to each other. At first nobody paid much attention, then little by little the people stopped what they were doing and tried to hear what the bears were saying. But nobody could. That night the bears went back into the forest. And the townspeople stood around and one woman said she knew what they were whispering about—**they were making fun of the people in the village.** And then everybody started noticing how everybody else walked funny or talked funny or looked weird and they all ended up laughing at each other, and everybody got mad and there were all kinds of fights in town that evening.

The next day the bears came out of the forest again and started whispering, ya-da, ya-da, ya-da, and again the townspeople watched, and all were suspicious. That night the bears again returned to the woods. And this time an older man said he knew what they were talking about. **They were gossiping about the people in town.** And so everybody figured,

if the bears knew, then everybody else must know all their secrets, and so they went home and closed all their windows and doors and they became angry and afraid to go out in public.

On the third day the bears again returned to the edge of the woods. Once again the same thing happened—the bears were talking to each other. But, this time the mayor of the village said, **"I know what they're saying! They're making plans to attack the village."** And he ordered the villagers to get torches to scare away the bears, but one of the villagers accidentally set his house on fire and the fire spread rapidly around the village and the whole town burned down!

In short, many lives became ruined for no reason. **Bears can't talk!** The town was destroyed and lives changed forever because people projected their own pettiness, and jealousy, and aggression on some innocent creatures. Much like the lives of so many millions of HIV/AIDS people have been changed forever because of petty fears, jealousies, and hatred for those who need compassion and understanding. Yes, sadly, there exists a rather large village of people who judge others harshly before knowing the facts.

(A favorite fairy story of the author, who in this case adopted the anecdote to make a point about discrimination. From "Speaking in Tongues" by Jeffery Deaver, 2003.)

Significant Percentages of Americans Distrust Information about HIV/AIDS

Although most Americans believe they are receiving accurate information about the AIDS pandemic, significant percentages doubt what the government and media are telling:

- 34% do not believe the government is telling the whole truth about AIDS; and
- 25% do not believe the media is telling the whole truth about AIDS.

In addition, fewer, but still some, Americans question the origins of the pandemic:

- 18% believe there is some truth to reports that HIV was produced in a germ-warfare laboratory; and
- 12% believe that AIDS came from God to punish homosexual behavior.

What Do We Know?—Ending year 2013 and 32 years of the HIV/AIDS pandemic, it is clear that the scare headlines and tactics lack substance. From what has been learned about the biology of HIV, it appears the virus is not casually nor easily spread—but it has reached the magnitude of the great plagues and a vaccine has not yet been found!

However, a 2006 survey of 3500 American adults was conducted by the National Institute of Allergy and Infectious Diseases on their state of knowledge concerning the availability of an HIV/AIDS vaccine. One in five white Americans, or 20%, believe that an HIV vaccine already exists but is being kept secret from patients and the general public. Twenty-eight percent of Hispanics and 48% of blacks held this belief. Also, 42% of those surveyed did not know that vaccines require testing on human volunteers before being made available to the public. About 33% believe that vaccines in study could cause an HIV infection in humans receiving a test vaccine.

AIDS Polarized the Attitudes of Millions of People into Stances of Love and Compassion and Hate and Rejection

Since the epic announcement in 1981, HIV/AIDS has refashioned America. HIV/AIDS is a disease molded to the times, one that strikes hardest at the outcasts—gay men, injection-drug users, prostitutes, and impoverished whites, blacks, and Hispanics. HIV/AIDS has brought forth uncomfortable questions about sex, sex education, homosexuality, the poor, and minorities. The disease has inevitably polarized the people, accentuating both the best and worst worldwide. Many churches, schools, and communities have responded to the new disease with compassion and tolerance; others have displayed hate and reprisals of the worst kind.

As Camus wrote in *The Plague,* "The first thing (the epidemic) brought . . . was exile." Anyone who carried the disease could inspire terror. They became pariahs in society.

People with hate in their hearts torched the house of the Ray family and their three HIV-positive hemophilic children in Arcadia, Florida. Also, someone shot a bullet through the window of Ryan White's home to let the teenager know he should not attend the local high school. After he died, his 6-foot, 8-inch gravestone was overturned four times, and a car ran over his grave! (See Box 14.1, pages 429–430.)

Misconceptions about HIV/AIDS Linger

Despite widespread reports that casual contact does not spread the virus, families have walked out of restaurants that employed gay waiters, and hospital workers have quit rather than treat HIV/AIDS patients. (See Point of View 14.1, page 427.)

Each example points out that regardless of education, the public assumes the virus can be casually transmitted. **FEAR IS BEING TRANSMITTED BY CASUAL CONTACT—NOT THE VIRUS.** How would you react if a good friend, classmate, or coworker told you he or she was HIV positive? What if you found out that your child's schoolmate, a hemophiliac, had AIDS? What if you were told this child had emotional problems or a biting habit? What if your work put you in direct physical contact with people who might be HIV positive?

An AIDS diagnosis for one person resulted in his physician's refusal to treat him, his roommate leaving him, his friends no longer visiting him, his attorney advising him to find another attorney, and his clergyman failing to support him. They were all afraid of "catching" AIDS. In another case, a mother whose young son has AIDS sent cupcakes to his classmates on his birthday. School officials would not permit the children to eat the cupcakes. The elementary school principal said the school had a policy against homemade food because it could spread diseases such as AIDS.

In Hinton, WV, one woman was killed by three bullets and her body dumped along a remote road. Another was beaten to death, run over by a car, and left in the gutter. And each, authorities say, was killed because she had AIDS. (See Quick Hits, page 420, and Box 14.1, pages 429–430.)

What Is So Different about HIV/AIDS that Leads to Such Discrimination and Stigma?

The biggest difference between HIV/AIDS and other diseases is the larger amount of social

UNIVERSITY STUDENTS' EXPERIENCES

University students taking a senior semester course on HIV/AIDS in 2006 and 2007 experienced firsthand the fear-related ignorance that still exists.

FALL SEMESTER 2006

On this particular Monday afternoon, as I was reading my assigned chapter in the book *AIDS Update 2005*, a lady walked into my nail salon wanting to get her nails done. I asked her to come sit at my nail booth and I put the AIDS book down next to me on the nail table. When she sat down, I took her hand and began to file her nails. Unexpectedly she quickly pulled her hand back and demanded another person to do her nails. I asked her, "Why can't I do your nails?" She said, "You're nasty and I do not want you to touch me." That comment got me angry. I replied, "How am I nasty, you don't even know me?" Meanwhile, her eyes kept glancing from my AIDS book back to me with this disgusted look on her face. At that point I just knew that she thought I had AIDS or have had something to do with AIDS. My parents, who were in the back room, quickly came out to see what was going on. She quickly asked my dad to do her nails. I told her that my dad would not do her nails and told her to "get the hell out of my nail salon." As she was leaving she squeezed in her last comment calling me a "Dirty Chink with AIDS." She then flicked me her middle finger and left. I said, "So much for education on nontransmission of HIV by casual contact!"

FALL SEMESTER 2007

A group of college friends and I decided to go out to dinner one night to hang out, relax, and get our minds off midterms for a while. It was to be an ordinary night of jokes, laughter, and catching up. The only thing out of the ordinary was taking my textbook along. I took my *AIDS Update* book with me to help my friends explore still-existing discrimination, a voluntary class assignment. After being seated our waitress came to take our drink order. I had my textbook lying face up on the table. She looked at the book and then looked at me. For a moment our eyes met but then she averted her eyes quickly as if she was perhaps uncomfortable. That was the last time she would look at me. She then brought out our drinks and passed them out accordingly. When she got to me she handed me a plastic take-home cup with a plastic lid while everyone else had their drinks in a glass. She then took our dinner orders, avoiding eye contact with me, and left. That was the last time she appeared at our table for the evening. Another waitress presented herself to us and refilled our drinks. The second or third time around of checking up on our table I asked the waitress what had happened to the other girl, to which she replied that she had to go on break. When she left I looked over to the right and saw our original waitress waiting another table. So much for break time. The new waitress then delivered our dinners. She placed each plate and then handed out regular silverware to my friends and gave me plastic silverware, you know the type, enclosed in a little plastic baggie. I shook my head in disbelief. I mean I knew that AIDS was a highly stigmatized disease but, come on, this is year 2007 for God's sake, how can people still be so closed minded and act in such an uneducated manner? Regardless, my friends and I carried on in a regular fashion, just having a good time and enjoying one another's presence until it got late and we decided to call it quits. I paid using my credit card, and on the restaurant's copy I wrote a friendly little note declaring their ignorance and chastising their false assumptions. The only regret that I had that night was not reporting the incident to the manager, but then again why embarrass the man or woman about the staff of rude and ignorant employees that he or she hired? If education is the only hope, short of a vaccine, to cure AIDS then we are all in some very serious trouble.

Since reporting the first event in this book, students in each of my HIV/AIDS courses ending 2010 have reported similar experiences of discrimination while reading their AIDS textbook in a beauty salon and in the office waiting rooms of a physician, veterinarian, optometrist, and a car wash.

discrimination. For example, if someone is known to be HIV positive, most people think they know that the person got the virus through sex, that he or she is possibly gay, or is possibly an injection–drug user or both. And, if he or she contracted HIV through sex, then it must have been with someone he or she shouldn't have had sex with, or with someone who had sex with someone he or she shouldn't have had sex with, like an injection-drug user or bisexual, etc. That is, being HIV positive suggests a questionable background, lifestyle, or history.

Society does not reject those with a variety of sexually transmitted diseases or with cancer, diabetes, heart disease, or any other health problems to the degree that it rejects people with HIV disease or AIDS.

The HIV/AIDS pandemic has taught people about risk behavioral groups, homosexuals in particular. In some, this has promoted tolerance and understanding; in others, it has reinforced feelings of hatred. Information on HIV disease and AIDS, how it is spread, and how to avoid becoming infected, has, over the past 31 years, become a part of TV talk shows, movies, TV advertisements, and newspaper and magazine articles.

Phil Donahue, host of a former popular TV show, said in 1990, "On *Donahue,* we're discussing body cavities and membranes and anal sex and vaginal lesions. We've discussed the consequences of a woman's swallowing her partner's semen. No way would we have brought that up five years ago. It's the kind of thing that makes a lot of people gag."

The language, photography, and artwork used by the media are explicit and have upset certain religious groups. They believe that open use of language about condoms, homosexuality, anal sex, oral sex, vaginal sex, and so on promotes promiscuity.

It would appear that although biotechnology has provided methods of HIV detection, new drugs, and hope for a vaccine, human emotional responses have not changed much from those demonstrated during previous epidemics (Figure 14-1).

DISCUSSION QUESTION: Is it possible for people to learn to prevent HIV infection and AIDS without talking about sexual behavior and injection-drug use?

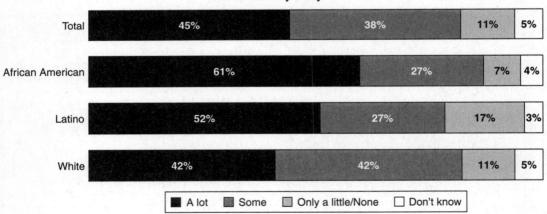

How much prejudice and discrimination do you think there is against people living with HIV and AIDS in this country today?

	A lot	Some	Only a little/None	Don't know
Total	45%	38%	11%	5%
African American	61%	27%	7%	4%
Latino	52%	27%	17%	3%
White	42%	42%	11%	5%

■ A lot   ■ Some   □ Only a little/None   □ Don't know

FIGURE 14-1 Perceptions of Prejudice and Discrimination Against People Living with HIV and AIDS in the United States. *"Kaiser Family Foundation Survey of Americans on HIV/AIDS, Part Three—Experiences and Opinions by Race/ Ethnicity and Age," (#7140), The Henry J. Kaiser Family Foundation, August 2004. The information was reprinted with permission from the Henry J. Kaiser Family Foundation. The Kaiser Family Foundation, a leader in health policy analysis, health journalism and communication, is dedicated to filling the need for trusted, independent information on the biggest health issues facing our nation and its people. The Foundation is a nonprofit private operating foundation based in Menlo Park, California. (Conducted March 15–May 11, 2004.) National random sample of 2902 respondents age 18 and older.*
UPDATE 2011—*The 2009, 2011 and 2012 survey data KFFSA are not significantly different from the 2004 data.*

BOX 14.1

HOW SOME PEOPLE RESPONDED AFTER LEARNING THAT SOMEONE HAD AIDS

VIGNETTES ON COMMUNITY BEHAVIOR AND AIDS

In **Colorado Springs, CO,** Scott Allen's wife, Lydia, had contracted HIV from a blood transfusion hours before their son Matthew was born. A second son, Bryan, was also born before Lydia learned of her HIV infection. Scott wasn't infected, but was dismissed as minister of education at First Christian Church in Colorado Springs when he sought his pastor's consolation. Matt was kicked out of the church's day care center and the family was told to find another church.

When the family moved to Dallas and moved in with Scott's father, Jimmy, and his wife, church after church refused to enroll Matt in Sunday school. Jimmy Allen, a former president of the Southern

Baptist Convention, wrote in his book, *Burden of a Secret: A Story of Truth and Mercy in the Face of AIDS,* "Good churches. Great churches. Wonderful people. Churches pastored by fine men of God, many of whom I had mentored. Nobody had room for a boy with AIDS" (Figure 14-2).

Bryan, an infant, died in 1986, Lydia died in 1992, and Matt died in 1995.

In **Florida** in 1987, Mrs. Ray, the mother of three hemophilic HIV-infected sons (Ricky, 14; Robert, 13; and Randy, 12) turned to her pastor for confidential counseling. He responded by expelling the family from the congregation and announcing that the boys were infected. As a result, the boys were not allowed to go to church, school, stores, or restaurants. Barbers refused to cut their hair. Some townspeople interviewed said they were terrified at having the boys in the community. They had to move to another town. The Rays sued the DeSoto County School District. They agreed to pay a $1.1 million settlement in 1988. Ricky Ray died of AIDS on December 13, 1992, at age 15. Robert died at age 22 in 2000. Randy, age 33, was diagnosed with AIDS in May 1993 and is still living.

Almost daily, similar senseless acts of violence and cruelty occur across the United States as a response to HIV/AIDS. Such episodes of panic, hysteria, and prejudice are perpetuated by the very people society uses as role models: clergy, physicians, teachers, lawyers, dentists, and so on. Philosopher Jonathan Moreno said, "Plagues and epidemics like AIDS bring out the best and worst of society. Face to face with disaster and death, people are stripped down to their basic human character, to good and evil. AIDS can be a litmus test of humanity." (See Point to Ponder 8.3, page 226, and Box 8.4, pages 222–223, for additional information on acts of violence.)

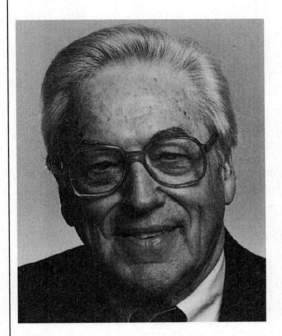

FIGURE 14-2 Reverend Jim Allen. Author of *Burden of a Secret: A Story of Truth and Mercy in the Face of AIDS.* "Jimmy," as he insists people address him, found peace for himself and family in a little village, Big Canoe, Georgia, where he is on staff at the Big Canoe Chapel. *(Photo courtesy of Linda R. and Jim R. Allen.)*

HERSHEY FACES BOYCOTT AS SCHOOL IT FUNDS REJECTS A 13-YEAR-OLD HIV-POSITIVE PUPIL

In December 2011, the Hershey Trust's Milton Hershey School in Pennsylvania was sued in federal court as it turned away a 13-year-old boy with positive HIV status, calling him a direct threat to the health and safety of others. The private boarding school, (of 1,800 students) which features Hershey directors

BOX 14.1 *(continued)*

on its own Board, said in a statement: "The school decided that it could not admit the student who uses the pseudonym Abraham Smith due to factors relating to his HIV-positive status." It is said that although it understood HIV could not be transmitted through casual contact, the boy could engage sexually with other students and therefore rejected admission to protect other students. On July 12, 2012 the president of the Milton Hershey School apologized to the student and welcomed his attendance for the fall of 2012. The boy and his mother will receive $700,000 in settlement of this case. In addition the school must pay $15,000 in civil penalties and provide training for students and staff.

THE LIFE OF RYAN WHITE

In Kokomo, Indiana, Ryan White was socially unacceptable. He was not gay, a drug user, black, or Hispanic. He was a hemophiliac; he had AIDS. His fight to become socially acceptable, to attend school, and to have the freedom to leave his home for a walk without ridicule made him a national hero (Figure 14-3).

Ryan's short life was a profile in courage and understanding. Like many other people with AIDS, Ryan tried to change the public's misconception of how HIV is transmitted. Ryan suffered most from the indignities, lies, and meanness of his classmates and his classmates' parents. They accused him of being a "fag," of spitting on them to infect them with the virus, and other fabrications. Ryan said he understood that this discrimination was a response of fear and ignorance. Ryan got the virus from blood and blood product transfusions essential to his survival at age 13. Ryan's wish was to be treated like any other boy, to attend school, to study, to play, to laugh, to cry, and to live each day as fully as possible. But AIDS was an integral part of his life. AIDS may not have compromised the quality of his life as much as the residents of his community did. One day, at age 16, as Ryan talked about AIDS to students in Nebraska, another boy asked Ryan how it felt knowing he was going to die. Showing the maturity that endeared him to all, Ryan replied "It's how you live your life that counts." He wrote a book, *My Own Story*. Ryan White died, a hero of the AIDS

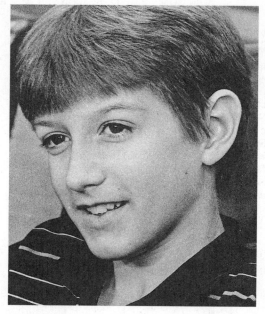

FIGURE 14-3 Ryan White Was Diagnosed with AIDS in 1984 and Died on April 8, 1990. This young male became another teenage AIDS tragedy. He gained the respect of millions across the United States before he died of an AIDS-related lung infection. *(© AP/Wide World Photos.)*

pandemic, at 7:11 A.M. on April 8, 1990. He was 18 years old.

In Honor of Ryan White: The Ryan White CARE Act Enacted by Congress in 1990

The Ryan White Comprehensive AIDS Resources Emergency (CARE) Act, the largest HIV-specific federal grant program devoted to a single disease in the United States, is the nation's care and treatment safety net for people living with HIV/AIDS who have no other source of coverage or have coverage limits. It provides support services for over 500,000 HIV-infected persons each year. The CARE Act was reauthorized for the third time in 2006, and was renewed in December 2009 at $2.33 billion annually through 2013.

Regardless of who is correct, few could have predicted in 1980 the casualness with which these topics are now presented in the media. If the HIV/AIDS pandemic has done nothing else, it surely has affected the nature of public discourse. In 1987, prior to the TV broadcast of the **National AIDS Awareness Test,** viewers were warned of objectionable material. By 1990, few if any such viewer warnings were given.

Former Presidents Ronald Reagan and George H.W. Bush: Their Policies on AIDS

Early on, the federal government and its public health apparatus showed little interest in the HIV/AIDS epidemic. Former President Ronald Reagan never once met with former Surgeon General C. Everett Koop to talk about AIDS despite Koop's pleas. Koop said, "If AIDS had struck legionnaires or Boy Scouts, there's no question the response would have been very different."

Documents from the Reagan administration show that the president's delay in addressing the AIDS issue was based on the perceived "political risk" in doing so. It took 10 years and over 120,000 AIDS deaths before the Congress and former president George Bush enacted the nation's first comprehensive AIDS-care funding package—the Ryan White CARE Act (1990). (See Box 14.1, pages 430–431.)

AIDS EDUCATION AND BEHAVIOR: DISSIPATING FEAR WITH EDUCATION

I said education was our *'basic weapon.'* Actually it's our *only* weapon. We've got to educate everyone about the disease so that each person can take responsibility for seeing that it is spread no further.

—C. Everett Koop
Former U.S. Surgeon General, 1988

For some, the occurrence of the recently estimated 56,000-plus new HIV infections in the United States each year from 2010 through 2012 is evidence that HIV education and prevention efforts have not been as effective as they could or should be. If HIV prevention programs are held to a standard of perfection and are expected to protect 100% of the people from disease 100% of the time, the efforts are by definition doomed to failure. No intervention aimed at changing behaviors to promote health has been or can be 100% successful, whether for smoking, diet, exercise, or drinking and driving. For example, even though warnings regarding the health effects of smoking were issued in 1964, warning labels on cigarettes were not mandated until 1984, and smoking-related illness still remains a major cause of death.

Because some of the behaviors and activities that need to change in order to avert HIV infection are pleasurable, it should be of no surprise if short-term interventions do not lead to immediate and permanent behavior changes. An important difference between HIV infection and other life-threatening diseases is that HIV can be contracted by a single episode of risk-taking behavior. **Once HIV infected, there is no second chance—no giving up the behavior, like drinking alcohol or smoking, that will make any difference; HIV disease, except on rare occasions, progresses to AIDS, and AIDS kills.**

After nearly 32 years of experience with HIV, it has demonstrated that lasting changes in behavior needed to avoid infection can occur as a result of carefully tailored, targeted, credible, and persistent HIV risk-education efforts. Given experience in other health behavior change endeavors, no interventions are likely to reduce the incidence of HIV infection to zero; indeed, insisting on too high a standard for HIV risk-reduction programs may actually undermine their effectiveness. A number of social, cultural, and attitudinal barriers continue to prevent the implementation of promising HIV risk-reduction programs. The remote prospects for a successful vaccine for HIV and the difficulty in finding long-lasting effective drug treatments have underscored the importance of sustained attention to HIV prevention and education.

Is the Solution to the AIDS Pandemic Let's Just Educate Everyone?

This sounds so easy: Educate people and they will do the right thing. **Wrong.** Knowledge does not guarantee sufficient motivation to change sexual behavior or stop the biological urge to have sex. Education has not stopped teenage pregnancy, nor has the knowledge about cigarettes causing lung cancer stopped people from smoking.

Perhaps the reason education is not as effective as it could be is because the public receives its education by daily doses from the mass media. With so much going on in the world, people have become more or less dependent on the media for information essential to their well-being. Gordon Nary (1990) said, "The public wants to know what's right or wrong in five three-second images or 25 words or less. It wants simple problems with simple solutions. It wants *Star Wars* with good and evil absolutely defined. The media often respond to these demands."

Public AIDS Education Programs

Over the years billions of dollars have been spent by federal and state health departments and private industry to inform the public about cardiovascular risks, health risks associated with sexually transmitted diseases (STDs), smoking and lung cancer, chewing tobacco and oral cancer, drug addiction, alcohol consumption and driving drunk, and seat belt use, to name just a few. In some cases these campaigns were eventually supported by specific state and federal legislation. Tobacco advertisements were outlawed on TV, and drivers in some states who are not buckled up must pay a fine ("Click It or Ticket" campaigns). But even with laws to support these educational programs, many adults have failed to change established behavior patterns. In the larger cities, educators must combat the fear that AIDS is a government conspiracy to eliminate society's "undesirables"—minorities, drug addicts, and homosexuals. They must overcome cultural and religious barriers that prevent people from using condoms to protect themselves.

It might also be added that there have always been educational programs against crime, but from 1990 through 2012 more new jails were built in the United States than ever before. In short, educational programs on TV, radio, in newspapers, and in the popular press have achieved only limited success in changing people's behavior.

It is not that education is unimportant; it is essential for those who will use it. That is the catch. Although education must be available for those who will use it, too few, relatively speaking, are using the available education for their maximum benefit. In general, people, especially young adults, do not act upon what they know. They sometimes do what they see, but most often do what they feel. In short, knowledge in itself may be necessary but it is insufficient for behavioral change. A variety of studies have failed to show a consistent link between knowledge and preventive behaviors (Fisher et al., 1992; Phillips, 1993).

Costs Related to Education/Prevention— The assertion that spending more money on educational programs will ensure disease prevention for the masses, as the examples given suggest, may not be the case. In particular, people's behaviors regarding the prevention of HIV infection do not appear to be changing significantly despite the billions of dollars used to produce, distribute, and promote HIV/AIDS education. The major educational thrust is directed at how not to become HIV infected. Most of this information is being given out to people ages 13 and older.

The problem with HIV/AIDS education is that communicating the information is relatively easy but changing behavior, particularly addictive and/or pleasurable behavior, is quite difficult. The mass media have provided near saturation coverage of key HIV/AIDS issues, and it is very unlikely that significant numbers of future HIV infections in the United States will occur in individuals who did not know the virus was transmitted through sexual contact and IV drug use. Yet new infections over at least the past two years occurred at an incidence of about 56,000 per year.

Although humans are capable of dramatic behavioral changes, it is not known what really initiates the change or how to speed up the process.

Public School AIDS Education: Just Say Know

QUESTION: How Do Educators Communicate the Dangers of HIV Without Stigmatizing Those Who Already Have It—and Without Scaring Youth into Avoidance and Denial?

Some information relevant to HIV/AIDS education can be learned from educational programs that have been designed to reduce pregnancy and the spread of STDs among young adults. However, data from a variety of high school sex education classes offered across the country indicate that young adults are learning the essential facts but they are not practicing what they learn.

Risky sexual behavior is widespread among young adults and has resulted in high rates of STDs. Over 25% of the 19 million STD cases per year occur among young adults. One in four have been infected with an STD. Over 50% of sexually active young adults (12.5 million) report having had two or more sexual partners; fewer than half say they used a condom the first time they had intercourse.

Young Adult Perceptions about AIDS and HIV Infection in the United States—A recent survey by *People* magazine indicated that 96% of high school students and 99% of college students knew that HIV is spreading through the heterosexual population, but the majority of these students stated that they continued to practice unsafe sex and that 26% of American young adults practice anal intercourse.

Young adults at high risk include some 200,000 who become prostitutes each year and others who become IDUs. The CDC in 2009 said that about 2% of high school students have injected drugs at least once. A large number of children ages 10 and up consume alcohol. Is it possible that too much hope is being placed on education to prevent the spread of HIV? Teenagers must be convinced that they are vulnerable to HIV infection and death. Until then, it only happens to someone else. Regardless of the urgent need to educate students across the United States, through 2012, 17 states, according to the Guttmacher Institute, still do not require HIV/AIDS education. The World Health Organization estimates that worldwide, ending 2012 there will be over 20 million HIV-infected young adults (ages 13 to 24). (See Looking Back 14.2.)

College Students—Everyone must know and act on the fact that a wrong decision about having sexual intercourse can take away the future. For example, a young college student had a three-year nonsexual friendship with a local bartender. She was bright, well-educated, and acutely aware of AIDS. After drinks one evening, as their friendship progressed toward sexual intercourse, she asked him if he was "straight" (a true heterosexual) and he said yes. But he was a bisexual. It was a single sexual encounter. She graduated and left town. She found out that the bartender died of AIDS three years later. She did not think much of it until she was diagnosed with AIDS five years after their affair. This young, talented, bright, and personable girl has since died; she lost her future. It is difficult to change something as complex as personal sexual behavior regardless of knowledge. It also brings up at least one other important point in personal relationships: *telling the truth*. (See Dawn Beckhols, Figure 14-4, page 434 and Sidebar 14.3, page 434.)

LOOKING BACK 14.2

AMERICAN HIGH SCHOOL GRADUATIONS AND AIDS

High school graduates of 1998–1999 were the first to graduate from U.S. public high schools without the possibility of experiencing an HIV/AIDS-free world. The recognizable spread of HIV on a global scale began in the mid-1970s but was first reported in the United States in 1981. The graduates of 1998–1999 entered a world where hundreds of thousands had already died of AIDS in America and millions had died of the disease worldwide.

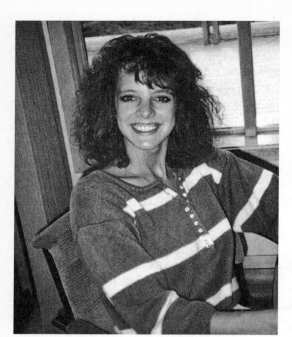

FIGURE 14-4 Dawn Beckhols at age 23, about the time of her infection. She believed that she became infected via one sexual encounter while on vacation. Dawn died of AIDS on July 13,1997, at age 33. *(Photo courtesy of L. Schwitters.)*

Nothing but the Truth, or Telling Lies?

During the 1988 American Psychological Association Convention, the following facts were presented with respect to telling the truth or lying in order to have sex. The data came from a survey of 482 sexually experienced southern California college students:

1. Thirty-five percent of the men and 10% of the women said they had lied in order to have sex.
2. Forty-seven percent of the men and 60% of the women reported they had been told a lie in order to have sex.
3. Twenty percent of the men and 4% of the women said they would say they had a negative HIV test in order to have sex.
4. Forty-two percent of the men and 33% of the women said they would never admit a one-time sexual affair to their long-term partner. (See Sidebar 14.4)

SIDEBAR 14.4

HE IS A CLOSET GAY, BUT WHO KNEW?

It has been two weeks since we sat in the nephrologist's office to get the results of my husband's kidney tests. Suddenly we were shocked. We were told that he is HIV positive! For the next few minutes there was deadly silence. Then it hit me—*oh my God*—with my head spinning and the feeling I was going to faint, it occurred to me in a flash. I did not really know my husband! Silly me! I knew our marriage wasn't the greatest, but after 26 years of marriage and four kids, he explained that he had been having sex with men for about 15 years. That he had one-night stands along with three lengthy relationships. And that they didn't know he was married with children, or even where he worked! In the same breath, he immediately told me he loves me and wants to stay together. What to do? I am scared, numb, confused, and hurt, and feel betrayed and alone. We decided not to tell anyone. We have lied to everyone! It is so difficult to keep up the façade. But I need somewhere to vent, and someone to talk to. I keep asking myself, what do I do next? I'm still numb.

Researchers at the French National Research Institute reported that men and teenage boys are far less likely than females to tell their main sexual partners they have been diagnosed with HIV or other sexually transmitted diseases. Researchers found that 14% of men diagnosed with an STD in the past five years had not told their main partners, compared with just 2% of women. Similarly, 51% of boys who had been diagnosed with an STD had not talked about it with their partner at the time, in contrast to 9% of girls. In a 2002 online poll Gay.com/PlanetOut.com Network wanted to know what people thought about the fact that a San Francisco court awarded $5 million in damages to a man who claims he was infected with HIV from his ex-lover, a former city health commissioner, who lied about his HIV status. When asked, "Should lying about one's HIV status to a sexual partner be a crime?" 69% of respondents said yes, 8% said no. Another 20% answered, "only if someone is infected as a result."

CLASS QUESTION: Given what you know about HIV/AIDS and other sexually transmitted diseases, do you think today's attitude concerning sexual relationships should be Don't Ask, Don't Tell or Do Ask, Do Tell, but in either case always practice safer sex, meaning the male must wear a condom? Select either statement and present pros and cons, especially with respect to personal responsibility and how either statement impacts HIV prevention and transmission.

Adult Perceptions about HIV Infection and AIDS in the United States—One aspect about

what adults now think about the AIDS pandemic has changed dramatically. The proportion of Americans naming HIV/AIDS as the nation's number one health problem has been steadily declining over time. In 1987, seven in ten Americans (70%) named HIV/AIDS as the most urgent health problem facing the nation. In 2006, 16% named HIV/AIDS as the nation's number one health problem. Some 56% of residents of Britain, France, and Germany thought that AIDS was "the greatest risk to world health today" followed by heart disease (37%) and bird flu (7%). In 2011, the Kaiser Family Foundation surveyed people by age group to assess their concern about becoming HIV infected. Those age 18 to 29 were the most concerned (Figure 14-5). To "do you personally know anyone who has died from AIDS or tested positive for HIV?": 39% said yes; 61% said no. Fifty percent favored teaching safer sex as the major focus in prevention, while 40% favored teaching abstinence only. (See Point of View 14.2, page 436.)

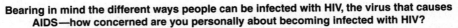

Bearing in mind the different ways people can be infected with HIV, the virus that causes AIDS—how concerned are you personally about becoming infected with HIV?

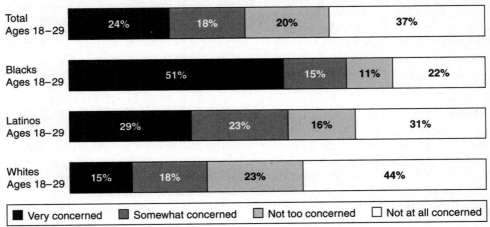

FIGURE 14-5   Personal Concern about Becoming Infected by Age. *"Kaiser Family Foundation Survey of Americans (KFFS) on HIV/AIDS, HIV/AIDS at 30, June, 2011. The information was reprinted with permission from the Henry J. Kaiser Family Foundation. The Kaiser Family Foundation, a leader in health policy analysis, health journalism and communication, is dedicated to filling the need for trusted, independent information on the biggest health issues facing our nation and its people. The Foundation is a nonprofit private operating foundation based in Menlo Park, California. The data from their 2012 survey is similar.*

THE RED RIBBON

Frank Moore II, a Manhattan painter who was instrumental in launching the overlapping red ribbon as a symbol of AIDS awareness in 1991, died April 22, 2002, from AIDS-related complications at the age of 48. Moore, who said that his paintings represented a journal of his long battle with HIV, was a board member of Visual AIDS, a Manhattan-based group that raises money to fund artists with HIV/AIDS and helps maintain the art of people with the disease. The red ribbon became an international symbol of AIDS awareness and has been used in other colors by groups to represent different causes.

The color red was chosen because the disease is a blood-borne disease. The shape of the ribbon was meant to signify the connectedness of all of us with or without the disease, who wanted to make a statement of visible support for those who were infected or had AIDS.

THE EVENT

We were sitting in a small Italian restaurant. I had just come back to town from a presentation on AIDS. The jacket I wore still had the red ribbon on the lapel. As we enjoyed our meal, I noticed a woman at the next table who appeared to be glaring at me and making statements to her companion. At one point her voice became loud enough for us to hear her say, "I am sick and tired of those people trying to push the lifestyle of homosexuals down our throats," as she was looking right at me. She then said, "That red ribbon is a sign of a sick person trying to make all of us sick too. That ribbon and all that it stands for ruins my day." With that she and her companion left the restaurant.

That outburst left my family and me embarrassed and confused. My children deserved an explanation. I don't think I have ever explained the idea of the red ribbon to anyone before. Like so many things we observe in life, after a while they become understood by each in his or her own way. This woman expressed her way rather forcefully. To my children I said that the ribbon is a symbol to call attention to a social problem that needs a solution. I went on to say, "Do you recall the song 'Tie a Yellow Ribbon Round the Old Oak Tree' in 1973 and what that meant? And, do you recall the ribbons tied around trees, on car antennas, mailboxes, and so on while our 56 servicemen were held captive in Iran in 1980 and again for our captives in the 1991 Persian Gulf War? Remember the first lady Nancy Reagan's campaign using red ribbons for 'just say no to drugs' and more recently the pink ribbons for women against breast cancer and most recently the purple ribbons for stopping violence in our schools? These are all symbolic gestures to show support for those enduring suffering and pain. All the ribbons then and now serve to connect people emotionally, to help unite people in a common cause, to help people feel less isolated in a crisis."

I explained to my children that the problem with the red ribbon now is similar to what occurred over the long time period our soldiers were in captivity—people begin to wear the ribbon as an accessory.

The Author

The Workplace—If a person is not working near or beside someone who is HIV positive, he or she will be relatively soon. But he or she may not know it because a person's right to privacy prevails over an employee's right to know.

HIV/AIDS can have a variety of impacts in the workplace. The obvious one, of course, is on the employee who is diagnosed with HIV. The probability of sickness and death obviously affects the individual and his or her ability to continue to contribute to the organization's activities and goals.

Employees' fear of AIDS can create a widespread loss of teamwork and productivity, and it can create an environment that is inhumane and insensitive toward the infected employee.

As the incidence of HIV and AIDS increases, the impact on organizations will obviously increase as well. While there are important logical and moral reasons for ensuring that infected people are not discriminated against, there are also practical reasons for addressing the employee HIV/AIDS problem.

An educated workforce, aware of the facts regarding diagnosis, testing, treatment, and transmission of HIV, can have a positive impact on the overall health of all employees. People are more inclined to openly acknowledge their HIV status and to seek treatment when assured of a supportive workplace environment. This increases productivity.

Percent saying they would bw comfortable/uncomfortable in the following situations

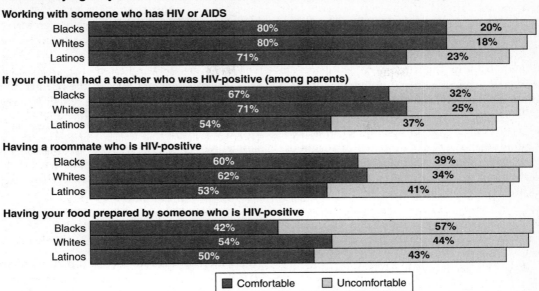

Working with someone who has HIV or AIDS

	Comfortable	Uncomfortable
Blacks	80%	20%
Whites	80%	18%
Latinos	71%	23%

If your children had a teacher who was HIV-positive (among parents)

	Comfortable	Uncomfortable
Blacks	67%	32%
Whites	71%	25%
Latinos	54%	37%

Having a roommate who is HIV-positive

	Comfortable	Uncomfortable
Blacks	60%	39%
Whites	62%	34%
Latinos	53%	41%

Having your food prepared by someone who is HIV-positive

	Comfortable	Uncomfortable
Blacks	42%	57%
Whites	54%	44%
Latinos	50%	43%

■ Comfortable   □ Uncomfortable

FIGURE 14-6 Reported Comfortable/Uncomfortable Level Table in Four Situations Involving an HIV Infected Person. *"Kaiser Family Foundation Survey of Americans on HIV/AIDS, HIV/AIDS at 30, June 2011. The information was reprinted with permission from the Henry J. Kaiser Family Foundation. The Kaiser Family Foundation, a leader in health policy analysis, health journalism and communication, is dedicated to filling the need for trusted, independent information on the biggest health issues facing our nation and its people. The Foundation is a nonprofit private operating foundation based in Menlo Park, California. (Conducted April 4–May 1, 2011.) The data from their 2012 survey is similar.*

In 2011, the Kaiser Family Foundation surveyed black, Hispanic, and white Americans on their comfort level working with HIV-positive people (Figure 14-6).

THE CHARACTER OF SOCIETY

Rumors of Destruction

Today, friends are asked on street corners, at social gatherings, or over telephones: "Did you hear that he/she has AIDS?" Or: "Do you believe that he/she might be infected? You never know with the life he/she leads!" Some of the famous people rumored to have or to have had HIV/AIDS are Madonna, Elizabeth Taylor, Burt Reynolds, and Richard Pryor.

Rumors ruin lives. People suddenly subtly lose services; the lawn boy quits, no reason given. Quietly, job applications are turned down

or car and homeowner insurance policies are canceled, and so on. In one case, after rumors of HIV infection spread in a small town, a man, if he was served in local bars at all, received his drinks in plastic cups. A health club refunded his membership dues. His apartment manager asked him to leave and when his toilet backed up the maintenance man came in wearing a hat over a World War II gas mask, deep water fishing boots, a raincoat, and rubber gloves. In frustration, he had an HIV test. The results were negative and he gave copies of the test to every "joint" in town, his physician, dentist, theater manager, grocery store manager . . . He felt this approach was better than running. Do you agree?

In another case in Brantly County, Georgia, population 11,077, the 22-year-old mother of a 2-year-old son was the subject of a rumor that she was HIV infected. The rumor also stated that she had had intercourse with 200 men in the past year. To convince the townspeople, she took the HIV test and was not HIV infected. This young woman had to circulate the results of her blood test around town, but it was still not enough to stop the rumor. A newspaper in nearby Waycross, Georgia, quoted an unnamed source saying that this woman was HIV positive.

There was the case of a compassionate person who opened a home for helping AIDS patients. Rumor quickly spread that the entire neighborhood was in danger, especially after the mail carrier refused to deliver mail and was ordered to wear rubber gloves and return to the post office for disinfection. To help the neighborhood understand AIDS and stop unfounded fears, a seminar was held at the AIDS home, but no one would enter the house.

A young person with AIDS reluctantly returned home—it meant revealing that he was gay to his family—and to the community. He said to his parents, "I have good news and bad. The bad is that I'm gay. The good is I have AIDS. I won't be around long enough to interfere with anyone." Once the word got out, a catering service refused to do the annual family Christmas party. They could not hire a practical nurse. Family and friends who used to drop in stayed away. People whispered that the son had gay cancer . . . that it was lethal . . . that it could be caught from dishes, linens, a handshake, and breathing in the same air he breathed out.

In Athens, Alabama, the headline of the town's newspaper read, "Athens doctor: 'I don't have AIDS.'" This doctor, a prominent pediatrician in town for 18 years, had to produce a public defense to dispel the gossip that he had AIDS. The doctor offered a $2000 reward for any information about who began the rumor. To date no one has collected the money, but the townspeople did gather to support him.

In Nebraska, a man sued a prominent woman for starting a rumor that he had AIDS. The Nebraska Supreme Court upheld a lower court ruling that the man was slandered and he received $25,350 in damages.

In Atlanta, Georgia, the CDC said it had received many inquiries about reports that drug users infected with HIV had left contaminated needles in public places, on seats in movie theaters, and under gas pump handles. Some reports have falsely indicated that CDC confirmed the presence of HIV in the needles. But the CDC said in a statement, "CDC has not tested such needles. Nor has the CDC confirmed the presence or absence of HIV in any samples related to these rumors. The majority of these reports and warnings appear to have no foundation in fact. CDC is not aware of any cases where HIV has been transmitted by a needlestick injury outside a healthcare setting."

Good News, Bad News, and Late News

Good News—Good news is thinking you're HIV infected and you're not. There must be a reason to think you're infected, so not being infected is, as some would say, a new lease on life. All too often that feeling is soon forgotten, and many people continue lifestyles that place them at risk for infection.

Bad News—Bad news is thinking you're HIV infected and you are. It is difficult to predict what a person sees, hears, or does after being told he or she is HIV positive. For example, some have contemplated suicide, some have committed suicide, others have become completely fatalistic and proceeded to live a reckless and careless lifestyle that endangered others. Some have said it's like death before you're dead.

You are never prepared to hear the bad news regardless of how sure you are that you're infected. For example, one man who had suffered from night sweats, fevers, weight loss, and other classic symptoms knew he was infected. Yet when told of the positive test results he said "I got so angry, I ripped a shower out of the wall." Being told you are infected is totally devastating, said another infected person. "You feel that everyone is looking at you, everyone can tell you're dirty." Another person said, "The fact that I'm HIV positive completely dominates my life.

There is not a waking hour that I do not think about it. I feel like a leper. I live between hope and despair." Still another said, "I did not leave the house for two days after being told I was HIV positive. The initial shock was that I was contaminated—unhealthy, soiled, unclean. I carried this burden in isolation for over two years. After all, I had met people who had AIDS but never a person who said—I'm HIV infected."

The bad news is not confined to those hearing they are HIV infected; it touches everyone they know—lovers, family, friends, and employers. Nothing remains the same. The more symptomatic one becomes, the greater the social and human loss. One symptomatic mother said, "Whenever I tell my four-year-old I am going to the doctor, he screams because he knows I could be gone for weeks. I try to put him in another room playing with his sister when they come for me." This woman died. Relatives care for her children.

Late News—Late news is remaining **asymptomatic** after infection. Asymptomatic can be defined as when no clinically recognizable symptoms appear that would indicate HIV infection. During this time period, the virus can be transmitted to sexual partners. By the time either antibodies and/or clinical symptoms appear, the news is too late for those who might have been spared infection had their sexual partner tested positive or demonstrated clinical symptoms early on.

When People Pretend to Be HIV Positive or to Have AIDS

As Hector Gavin wrote in 1843 in his 400-page history *On Feigned and Factitious Diseases,* "The monarch, the mendicant, the unhappy slave, the proud warrior, the lofty statesman, even the minister of religion . . . have sought to disguise their purposes, or to obtain their desires, by feigning mental or bodily infirmities."

Donald Craven and colleagues (1994) reported that a growing number of people may pretend to have AIDS either because of emotional disorders or because they want to gain access to free housing, medical care, and disability income. In one case, seven patients with self-reported HIV infection were treated for an average of 9.2 months in a clinical AIDS program before their seronegative status was discovered at the hospital (in general, hospitals in the United States do not require a written copy of the HIV test results proving that someone is HIV positive). Craven noted that "because patients with AIDS often have preferred access to drug treatment, prescription drugs, social security disability insurance, housing, and comprehensive medical care, the rate of malingering may increase and reach extremes."

Other doctors who have treated HIV/AIDS patients said that they have seen many patients who repeatedly come to their offices fearing that they have HIV and/or AIDS, even though multiple tests have shown that they do not (Zuger, 1995; Mileno, 2001).

An Oklahoma physician has written about the AIDS **Munchausen syndrome**—an emotional disorder in which people pretend to have the disease simply to get attention from doctors. Confidentiality requirements make HIV/AIDS a perfect illness for people suffering from Munchausen syndrome because the laws shield them from being discovered.

DEALING WITH DISCRIMINATION: THE AMERICANS WITH DISABILITIES ACT

Although incidents of discrimination are disheartening, they are only a part of the story. Another part of the story is how discrimination has been fought and how courts, legislatures, and other social institutions have responded with attempts to reduce HIV/AIDS discrimination and to minimize its impact. To this end a brief synopsis of the Americans with Disabilities Act is presented along with the first U.S. Supreme Court ruling based on this act.

Americans with Disabilities Act

The primary federal nondiscrimination statute that prohibits discrimination on the basis of a person's disability or health status is the Americans with Disabilities Act (ADA) of 1990. The ADA provides that no individual "shall be discriminated against on the basis of disability in the full and equal enjoyment of the goods, services, facilities, privileges, advantages or accommodations of any place of public accommodation." The ADA's definition of "public accommodation" specifically includes hospitals and professional offices of healthcare providers. A critically important issue under the ADA is whether persons with *asymptomatic* HIV infection have a disability and thus are protected under the ADA. Disability is defined as a physical or mental impairment that substantially limits one or more of the major life activities of the individual, a record of such impairment, or being regarded as having an impairment. In the past, many courts have ruled or assumed as undisputed that HIV infection, as the underlying cause of a life-threatening illness, is a disability. However, several recent court decisions have held that HIV does not automatically qualify as a disability, and in each case there must be an individualized determination as to whether the infection actually limits, in a substantial way, a major life activity. The ADA's legislative history, however, indicates that Congress intended to include HIV infection within the definition of disability, and the Equal Employment Opportunity Commission's regulations embody that view. In its first AIDS case ever, the Supreme Court had to decide whether and to what extent persons with HIV infection are protected under the ADA.

The Case of *Bragdon* v. *Abbott*: U.S. Supreme Court

1998—In the 17-year history of the HIV/AIDS pandemic, the U.S. Supreme Court had never considered a case directly involving HIV or AIDS until March 30, 1998, when oral arguments began in the case of *Bragdon* v. *Abbott*. The *Bragdon* case is also the first time the court has ever heard a case involving the ADA. On September 16, 1994, Sidney Abbott, age 37, went to her dentist in Bangor, Maine, to get a cavity filled. Dr. Randon Bragdon refused to fill a gumline cavity in his office when he read on her medical form that she

was HIV positive. He told her he could do the procedure in a hospital, a change of venue that would have added approximately $150 to the bill. According to a cover story about the case in the *American Bar Association Journal,* Dr. Bragdon did not have privileges to practice in any area hospitals, nor had he applied for them. Dr. Bragdon maintains that he could have sought and received permission to perform occasional procedures without having been granted full privileges.

Abbott's Lawsuit—Her lawsuit argues that in refusing to treat her in his office, Bragdon violated the ADA and the Maine Human Rights Act. Federal district and appeals courts both agreed with her.

U.S. Supreme Court Decision June 25, 1998—The Supreme Court ruled 5 to 4, upholding the District Court and the First Circuit Court of Appeals, finding that Bragdon violated Abbott's rights to treatment under the provisions of the ADA of 1990. Abbott's HIV infection constituted a disability under the ADA in that her HIV infection "substantially limits" a major life activity—her ability to reproduce and bear children (to have a child she places her husband at risk for HIV infection and risks infecting her child). Justice Kennedy, in delivering the opinion of the court, held that from the moment of infection and throughout every stage of the disease, HIV infection satisfies the statutory and regulatory definition of a "physical impairment." Applicable Rehabilitation Act regulations define "physical or mental impairment" to mean "any physiological disorder or condition affecting the body['s] hemic and lymphatic [systems]." HIV infection falls well within that definition. The medical literature reveals that the disease follows a predictable and unalterable course from infection to inevitable death. It causes immediate abnormalities in a person's blood, and the infected person's white cell count continues to drop throughout the course of the disease, even during the intermediate stage when its attack is concentrated in the lymph nodes. Thus, HIV infection must be regarded as a physiological disorder with an immediate, constant, and detrimental effect on the hemic and lymphatic systems.

U.S. Supreme Court Rules on Insurance Coverage Cap for HIV/AIDS Treatment

In January 2000, the U.S. Supreme Court let stand a ruling that allowed an insurance company to provide less coverage for AIDS-related illnesses than for other conditions under the same policy. The high court, without comment, refused to hear the appeal brought by two HIV-positive Chicago men who claimed that their insurance company's policies violate the Americans with Disabilities Act. The two policies in question were issued by Mutual of Omaha. One policy set a $25,000 lifetime coverage limit for AIDS-related illnesses and the other contained a $100,000 cap, while both allowed a $1 million cap for other illnesses. Attorneys for Mutual of Omaha argued that the insurance company had not discriminated because it offered the men the same coverage offered to other customers. In 1998, the federal judge in Chicago ruled in favor of the two men, but the 7th U.S. Circuit Court of Appeals reversed that ruling. The Appeals Court said the ADA guarantees access to insurance but does not regulate the content of coverage.

DISCUSSION QUESTION: Clearly a 5-to-4 ruling is not an overwhelming mandate to support Abbott's lawsuit. Is a simple majority, 55% in this case, sufficient or because this case has vast implications, should it require a two-thirds majority, 6 in favor, 3 against (67%)? What are the legal and moral issues in accepting a simple majority versus a two-thirds ruling?

The case of *Bragdon* raises another question to consider as you research the question above. Magic Johnson asks if it really makes sense to consider someone "disabled" who can earn millions of dollars playing professional basketball, or go to work, or otherwise perform the tasks of daily living. Your response is?

Patients' Right to Know If Their Physician Has HIV/AIDS—In a recent Gallup Poll, 86% of those polled felt that they had the right to know if a healthcare worker treating them was HIV infected. Many lawyers also take this position. The courts appear to be moving toward an interpretation of the doctrine of informed patient consent as "what a reasonable patient would want to know," rather than "what a reasonable physician would disclose." Because it is so difficult for surgeons to avoid occasionally cutting themselves during surgery, it has been suggested that the best solution is not to have HIV-infected surgeons perform surgery at all.

Public anxiety over HIV/AIDS and medical care is becoming increasingly tinged with hysteria. A recent national Gallup Poll undertaken for *Newsweek* asked a representative sample of 618 adults, "Which of the following kinds of healthcare workers should be required to tell patients if they are infected with the AIDS virus?"

The answers were: surgeons 95%; all physicians 94%; dentists 94%; all healthcare workers 90%.

Clearly, people do not differentiate between doctors who perform invasive procedures and those who do not. However, the patient could ask what the probability is of a single dentist (Acer) infecting six of his patients (Bergalis, Webb, and four others). Extremely low, yet it did happen! The lowest of probabilities and best of guidelines and precautions do not stop the fire of fear.

HIV-Infected Healthcare Professionals' Duty to Disclose—Several courts have held that healthcare professionals have a duty to disclose their HIV status to patients or health authorities, assuming that their professional activities pose a risk of transmission to patients. The Maryland Court of Appeals ruled that a surgeon has a duty to inform his patients of his infection; even if the patient has not actually been exposed and tests HIV negative, the contact with the surgeon may subsequently give rise to a claim for their infliction of mental distress due to fear of transmission. Courts justify orders to disclose based on a duty to protect patients and on the doctrine of informed consent. Requiring disclosure to patients, of course, can severely jeopardize a healthcare professional's career. To avoid this result, some states allow the professional to continue practicing, with appropriate restrictions and supervision, but without disclosing his or her HIV status (Gostin et al., 1998).

UPDATE

In general, according to case law and professional practice guidelines, healthcare workers have a duty to inform patients or employers that they are HIV positive if they perform invasive or "exposure-prone" procedures on patients. Specific guidelines are set out in the American Medical Association's "Guidance for HIV-Infected Physicians and Other Health Care Workers," 2011 (H-20.912).

FEDERAL AND PRIVATE SECTOR FINANCING: CREATION OF AN AIDS INDUSTRY

About 31 years ago, when the public was just learning about a new disease that would be called AIDS, some scientists tracking down the cause were already thinking about how their research could be marketed. French and American groups eventually claimed to have codiscovered HIV independently and in different ways. In one respect their approach was the same: Shortly before announcing their discoveries, both rushed to file patents that described how to determine whether a person's blood harbored the virus. By doing this, they gave birth to the HIV/AIDS industry.

Financing the Multi-Billion-Dollar HIV/AIDS Industry: A Quilt with Many Holes

Federal Government—In 1990, the U.S. Congress did something quite rare: It allocated money specifically for the treatment of one disease—HIV/AIDS. In some ways the increased commitment of federal and state government to cancer research and treatment in the early 1970s is similar to what happened in the war on AIDS in the 1980s. In both decades, there was a major funding surge to stimulate research, therapy, and prevention. A major difference, however, is that dollars for cancer came more slowly over a longer time period that began well before the 1970s. With AIDS, federal funding began in 1981 (Figure 14-7, page 443) and has increased at an unprecedented rate. (See Point of View 14.3, page 444.)

No Cheap Way Out: HIV/AIDS Is a Very Expensive Disease

During the 31 years from 1982 through 2013, federal spending on AIDS-related projects will have increased from $8 million in 1982 to $28.4 billion for 2013. The Presidential Advisory Council on HIV/AIDS provided the president with six AIDS goals that will be funded with the federal budget for AIDS. The goals are to: (1) develop a cure, (2) reduce/eliminate new infections, (3) guarantee care/service for the HIV infected, (4) fight against HIV/AIDS discrimination, (5) quickly translate scientific advances into improved care/prevention, and (6) provide support for international AIDS efforts. (See Figure 14-8, page 446.)

Private Sector Funding: United States—In addition to the money spent by the federal government, collectively the states also spend between $6 billion and $8 billion each year. The private sector spends about $5 billion a year. By the end of 2013, the federal government and the states and private sector will have spent about the same. Adding in unspecified federal dollars that went to HIV/AIDS-related projects and the dollars spent in the state and private sector would most likely bring the total AIDS-related expenditures to over $780 billion. Yet, in spite of this massive expenditure on HIV/AIDS, the United States still does not have the underpinning of a uniform healthcare system to provide an organized, controlled use of AIDS funds. The current funding is *heterogeneous* and provides **unequal access** to HIV/AIDS care. (See Box 14.2, pages 449–451, Figure 14-9, and Point of View 14.3, pages 444–445.)

AIDS Costs as a Percentage of the National Federal Budget

The $28.4 billion for 2012 HIV/AIDS represents about 0.7% of the $3.8 trillion federal budget.

AIDS Expenditures per Death Compared to Other Major Diseases Causing Death

The U.S. federal research dollars are allocated by the National Institutes of Health for a variety of

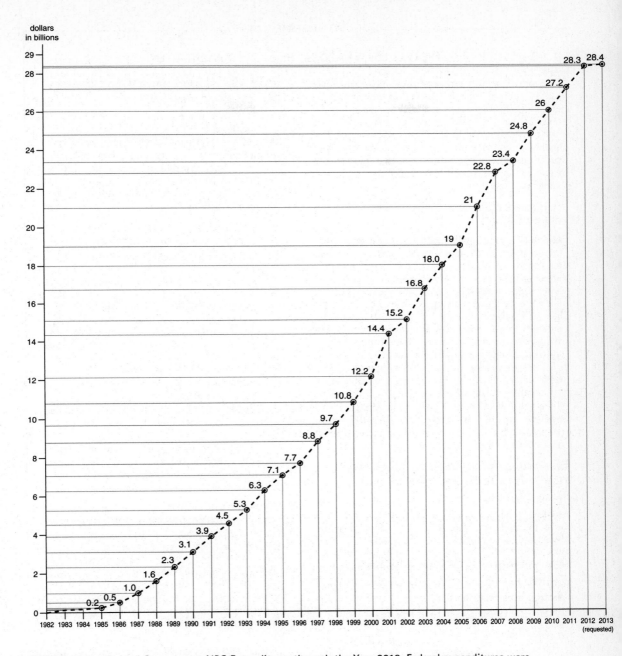

FIGURE 14-7 Federal Government AIDS Expenditures through the Year 2013. Federal expenditures were $1 billion in 1987, and $28.4 billion for 2013. By the end of 2013 the U.S. federal government will have spent over $398.5 billion over 31 years on this disease.

THE CALL FOR A NATIONAL HIV/AIDS POLICY/STRATEGY

Through 2013, the federal government has spent over $398.5 billion on all aspects of the HIV/AIDS epidemic. Private industry, foundations, philanthropies, and benefits, such as plays, parties, and auctions—to name a few sources of HIV/AIDS money—equal that spent by the government. The grand total reaches or surpasses $780 billion, or close to three-quarters of a trillion dollars spent in the United States in the past 28 years (1985 through 2013).

Let's Ask How This Vast Sum of Money Has Been Spent

Asking how over a half trillion dollars has been spent on HIV/AIDS is to some degree like asking what happened to the first money used to bail out Wall Street or the American automobile companies in 2008 and 2009. Where did the money go? The point is, there are no ready answers about the federal government's bailout packages due to the lack of a planned, organized set of procedures with checks and balances. The lack of oversight is obvious. The same can be said for much of the over half trillion HIV/AIDS dollars.

The expenditure of HIV/AIDS dollars is replete with waste, graft, and corruption. It is difficult to believe that after spending over a half trillion dollars, there are HIV-infected people in the United States who do not yet have access to HIV/AIDS drugs, hospital care, dental and other medical care, a proper diet, housing—the list goes on.

How Can This Lack of HIV/AIDS Services Exist?: The Lack of a National HIV/AIDS Policy

The breakdown in HIV/AIDS services exists because, to quote a common saying, "the left hand does not know what the right hand is doing." And this happens because there was no organized national HIV/AIDS policy.

Finally, A National HIV/AIDS Strategy (NHAS)

July 13, 2010 the White House unveils a new national strategy to combat HIV/AIDS, some three decades after the emergence of the deadly disease.

VISION FOR THE NATIONAL HIV/AIDS STRATEGY

The United States will become a place where new HIV infections are rare and when they do occur, every person, regardless of age, gender, race/ethnicity, sexual orientation, gender identity, or socio-economic circumstance, will have unfettered access to high quality, life-extending care, free from stigma and discrimination.

GOALS OF THE NATIONAL HIV/AIDS STRATEGY
Reducing New HIV Infections

- By 2015, lower the annual number of new infections by 25%.
- Reduce the HIV transmission rate, which is a measure of annual transmission in relation to the number of people living with HIV, by 30%.
- By 2015, increase from 79% to 90% the percentage of people living with HIV who know their serostatus.

Increasing Access to Care and Improving Health Outcomes for People Living with HIV

- By 2015, increase the proportion of newly diagnosed patients linked to clinical care within three months of their HIV diagnosis from 65% to 85%.
- By 2015, increase the proportion of Ryan White HIV/AIDS Program clients who are in continuous care from 73% to 80%.
- By 2015, increase the number of Ryan White clients with permanent housing from 82% to 86%.

Reducing HIV–Related Health Disparities

- Improve access to prevention and care services for all Americans.
- By 2015, increase the proportion of HIV diagnosed gay and bisexual men with undetectable viral load by 20%.
- By 2015, increase the proportion of HIV diagnosed Blacks with undetectable viral load by 20%.
- By 2015, increase the proportion of HIV diagnosed Latinos with undetectable viral load by 20%.

Overall, the strategy provides a roadmap for moving the nation forward in addressing the domestic HIV epidemic. It is not intended to be a comprehensive list of all activities to address HIV/AIDS in the United States, but it is intended to be a concise plan that will identify a set of priorities and strategic action steps tied to measurable outcomes.

The release of the National HIV/AIDS Strategy is just the beginning. The job of implementing this strategy does not fall on the federal government alone. Success will require the commitment of all parts of society, including state and local governments, businesses, faith communities, philanthropy, the scientific and medical communities, educational institutions, people living with HIV, and others.

COST AND PROMISE OF NHAS—To implement this program over the next five years it will cost an estimated

$15.2 billion. At a time when the U.S. government is deeply in debt—some $16 trillion, it may not be easy to come up with an additional $15 plus billion for HIV/AIDS but, NHAS may be the best hope to change the course of the U.S. epidemic. Its failure will see an increase in infections, visits to doctors' offices, hospitals, and lives subjected to toxic antiretroviral therapies.

THE 12 CITIES PROJECT

Overview

The 12 Cities Project will serve as a proving ground to demonstrate how the broad range of federally-supported HIV prevention, care, and treatment activities can work together more effectively across organizational and program boundaries. This effort will result in better identification of and response to service gaps and unmet needs, scaled-up activities that will have a greater "payoff" in terms of achieving the goals of the National HIV/AIDS Strategy (NHAS), enhanced integration of local service delivery, and—where appropriate—realigned resources from lower priority to higher priority activities. This U.S. Department of Health and Human Services (HHS) project supports and accelerates comprehensive HIV/AIDS planning and cross-agency response in the 12 U.S. jurisdictions that bear the highest AIDS burden in the country (New York City, Los Angeles, Washington DC, Chicago, Atlanta, Miami, Philadelphia, Houston, San Francisco, Baltimore, Dallas, and San Juan, PR).

HIV Care Though 2012

A review of several national studies shows that for every 100 people living with HIV in the United States 80% are aware of their infection, and of these, 62% have entered care, 41 actually stay in care, 36% receive ART, and 28% have undetectable levels of HIV. And, 2012 data from twelve clinics nationwide that are involved in the HIV Research Network indicate that only 20% of the infected are fully engaged in HIV care.

Future Benefits

Actively coordinating Federally funded programs at the local level in the 12 jurisdictions that represent 44% of the nation's AIDS cases can have huge payoffs and propel progress toward the Strategy's goals of reducing HIV incidence, increasing access to care and improving outcomes for people diagnosed with HIV, and reducing HIV-related health disparities. But the impact of this project is not limited to these communities. Lessons from this project will be shared widely to benefit all communities across the nation. (National Strategy of HIV/AIDS: www.whitehouse.gov/administration/eop/onap/nhas.)

common diseases that cause death, and their relationship to the amount of money spent per disease can be seen in Table 14-1, page 448.

U.S. GOVERNMENT BELIEVES HIV/AIDS IS A THREAT TO NATIONAL SECURITY

A nation's national security interests will be defined as the protection of its people and the preservation of territorial integrity, national sovereignty, and political, social, economic, and defense institutions against direct or indirect threats.

Today, more than ever before, threats are inter-related, and a threat to one is a threat to all. The mutual vulnerability of weak and strong has never been clearer—the security of the most affluent state can be held hostage to the ability of the poorest state to contain an emerging disease. Imagining the future shape of the HIV/AIDS pandemic, some two or three wavelengths (30 to 50 years) ahead, is exceedingly difficult. If no effective vaccine or cure is found within the next 20 years, areas of the world that are now witnessing explosive epidemics may well be more deeply altered than Europe was following the plague or Black Death. In Africa, for example, there are many features in place that mirror pre-plague Europe, including an enormous surplus of unskilled labor, lack of clear property rights for the bulk of the population, domination by tiny social elites, widespread warfare waged both by state and mercenary forces, and transition from dispersed agrarian to disastrously urbanized societies. Each of these factors was radically altered by the Black Death, and they could well be reshaped by HIV.

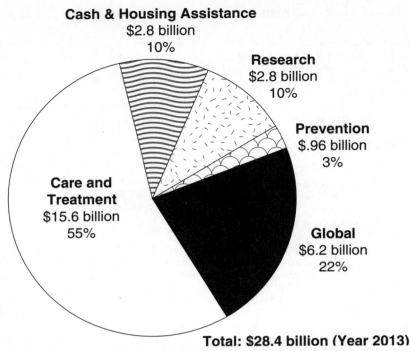

Cash & Housing Assistance
$2.8 billion
10%

Research
$2.8 billion
10%

Prevention
$.96 billion
3%

Care and Treatment
$15.6 billion
55%

Global
$6.2 billion
22%

Total: $28.4 billion (Year 2013)

FIGURE 14-8   Total Federal HIV/AIDS Spending by Category FY 2013. Federal HIV/AIDS spending is divided generally into five categories: Care and Treatment, Cash & Housing, Research, Prevention, and Global. Numbers do not equal 100% due to rounding.

United States National Security at Stake

The U.S. federal government declared in May 2000 that "AIDS is a threat to our national security." Former U.S. Secretary of Health and Human Services Donna Shalala said, "We know that infectious diseases know no borders, that they can affect this country, and in this case it is both in our economic interest and in our national security interest to work on infectious diseases abroad. The high rates of AIDS in Africa are putting security and stability at risk by disabling national armies, disrupting economies and killing off people who might become the next generation of leaders. Basically AIDS is uncoupling the economic gains in Africa as African countries are forced to shift more resources to their healthcare systems from their economic investments." Shalala also said that countries in

other parts of the world face a growing HIV/AIDS crisis. "Eastern Europe has an AIDS problem, Russia has it, India has it, every country in the world that we do business with, but more importantly our need to be politically stable, is suffering from this huge onslaught of HIV/AIDS. And that makes the relationship economically and from the security point of view relevant to America's national security."

In a June 12, 2003, speech, then–U.S. Secretary of State Colin Powell placed the pandemic in a national security context by equating the virus to a terrorist. "The HIV virus, like terrorism, kills indiscriminately and without mercy," Powell asserted. "As cruel as any tyrant, the virus will crush the human spirit. It is an insidious and relentless foe, more destructive than any army, any conflict, and any weapon of mass destruction. It shatters families, tears the fabric of societies, and undermines government, undermines the very basis of democracy. It can destroy countries and, as we have seen, it can destabilize entire regions."

The United States Pentagon offers HIV/AIDS support to the military of 80 nations, including Russia and India.

DISCUSSION QUESTION: Present reasons that agree or disagree with the federal government's declaration that HIV/AIDS is a threat to America's national security.

GLOBAL HIV/AIDS FUNDING FOR UNDERDEVELOPED NATIONS

Peter Piot, former executive director of UNAIDS, said, "AIDS is essentially a crisis of governance, of what governments do and do not do for their people. We have the drugs to treat HIV infection and we have the tools to confront the risks that drive HIV transmission and prevent infection itself. What we don't have is national political will. We have demanded too little from our leaders and excused too much."

In many ways, we are of one world. In the long run, Africa and Asia's destiny is our destiny. There is hope on the horizon, but that hope will only be realized if the developed nations take constructive action together. As South Africa's Archbishop Desmond Tutu said: "If we wage this holy war together—we will win."

The bottom line is this: There is no vaccine or cure for HIV/AIDS in sight, and the world is somewhere approaching the middle of this global

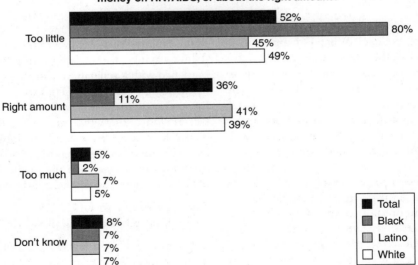

Thinking about the HIV/AIDS epidemic in the United States specifically, in general, do you think the federal government spends too much money on HIV/AIDS, too little money on HIV/AIDS, or about the right amount?

FIGURE 14-9 Views of U.S. Spending on Domestic HIV/AIDS. *"Kaiser Family Foundation Survey of Americans on HIV/AIDS, Part Three—Experiences and Opinions by Race/Ethnicity and Age" (#7140), The Henry J. Kaiser Family Foundation, August 2004. The information was reprinted with permission from the Henry J. Kaiser Family Foundation. The Kaiser Family Foundation, a leader in health policy analysis, health journalism and communication, is dedicated to filling the need for trusted, independent information on the biggest health issues facing our nation and its people. The Foundation is a non-profit private operating foundation based in Menlo Park, California. (Conducted March 15–May 11, 2004.) National random sample of 2902 respondents age 18 and older.*
UPDATE 2011—*The 2009, 2011 and 2012 KFFSA are not significantly diferent from the 2004 data.*
QUESTION: Would the above data change significantly if those interviewed had access to the information presented in Table 14-1?

Table 14-1 Federal Monetary Research Allocations per Death for Nine Categories of Diseases by the National Institutes of Health, Estimated for 2013[1, 2]

Disease	NIH Research $	Deaths per Disease	$ per Patient Death
All cancers total	$ 6 billion	559,888	$ 10,716.00
Alzheimer's disease	480 million	71,696	6626.00
Breast cancer	778 million	41,210	18,879.00
Cardiovascular disease	2.2 billion	864,280	2545.00
COPD★	120 million	126,128	951.00
Diabetes	1 billion	72,449	13,803.00
Hepatitis B	67 million	5000	13,400.00
Hepatitis C	102 million	12,000	8500.00
HIV/AIDS	**3.2 billion**	**13,000**	**246,154.00**
Parkinson's disease	157 million	19,566	8024.00
Prostate cancer	337 million	28,732	11,729.00
West Nile virus	46 million	28	1,642,857.00

★COPD is chronic obstructive pulmonary disease.

The NIH orphan (rare) drug allocation of $467 million for 6000 rare diseases equals only $77,833, on average, for biomedical research on each rare disease.

[1] The rate of HIV infection worldwide, except for two countries in sub-Saharan Africa, is less than 1%.

[2] HIV/AIDS is not the most frequent cause of death in the USA but received about 10% of the NIH budget for 2013.

(Table adapted from The FAIR Foundation: www.fairfoundation.org.)

pandemic, not the end. What is happening in Africa now is just the tip of the iceberg. As goes Africa, so will go India and the Newly Independent States of the former Soviet Union. There must be a sense of urgency for the developed world to work together; to learn from its failures and successes, and to share its experience with those countries that now stand on the brink of disaster. Millions of lives—perhaps hundreds of millions of lives—hang in the balance. HIV/AIDS is a devastating human tragedy that requires global help. (See Point of Information 14.2.)

HINDSIGHT Twenty one years ago, when the AIDS death toll in the United States crossed 100,000, few paid heed to a grim prediction by the World Health Organization (WHO) that "by the year 2000, 40 million persons may be infected with HIV." In the developed world, AIDS was seen as a serious but small disease, restricted to gay men, drug users, hemophiliacs, and their infants. In the developing world, just a few courageous voices were warning about the silent spread of a deadly new plague. Africa is in crisis. In some countries, about 40% of the adult population is infected.

Many millions have died, and millions more will follow, leaving their societies trapped in poverty, burdened with a generation of orphans, and facing demographic catastrophe. The grim statistics are not confined to Africa. Asia and the Caribbean face explosive HIV epidemics, while the nations of the former Soviet empire are looking at an overwhelming increase in drug addiction, untreated sexual diseases, and the unchecked spread of HIV. Finally the world has begun to take notice.

The Beginning of UNAIDS and a Unified Attack against HIV/AIDS

In January 1996, the United Nations (UN) took the innovative step of bringing six United Nations organizations together in a joint cosponsored program, UNAIDS. These six organizations were joined by four other organizations in the following years through 2007. In January 2000, the United Nations Security Council held a precedent-setting special session in which for the first time it identified a disease—AIDS—as a global security threat. A second UN HIV/AIDS special session of the General Assembly was held June 25–27, 2001.

— BOX 14.2 —

AIDS PROGRAMS: AN EPIDEMIC OF WASTE?

Through 2012 there has been constant pressure on politicians and leaders of private industry to contribute higher levels of money in the fight against HIV/AIDS. In 2002, AIDS activists marched in Washington in an attempt to get Congress to allocate $2.5 billion to the Global AIDS, Tuberculosis, and Malaria Fund. Their belief is that America is not spending enough money at home or globally on HIV/AIDS. Others, however, protest this notion and feel that if graft and corruption were eliminated there would be sufficient money such that yearly increases in the federal HIV/AIDS program would not be called for. To support this belief, a group called Citizens Against Government Waste (CAGW) released a report in February 2002 on **"AIDS Programs: An Epidemic of Waste"** (www.cagw.org). Citizens Against Government Waste is the nation's largest nonpartisan, nonprofit organization dedicated to eliminating waste, fraud, abuse, and mismanagement in government. Some of the fraud found by this group is listed exactly as it is presented in their report:

- CAGW has obtained a copy of a $20,000 grant from the Vermont Department of Public Health to the Twin State Women's Network (TSWN) to be used for a weekend retreat. Topics for the weekend included "Toys 4 Us" and "Self Loving/Self Healing: Discussing the Role of Masturbation as a Tool for Healing." TSWN also received: $1500 for long distance phone calls; $1000 for books, including *The New Good Vibrations for Sex* manual; and $250 for videos, choices of which included *Fire in the Valley: A Guide to Masturbation for Women* and *Fire in the Valley: A Guide to Masturbation for Men*. Each participant received a welcome bag filled with mints and chocolate and each room was equipped with welcome packets containing condoms, lubricant, candles, massage lotion, and lip balm. TSWN received 86% of its funds from government sources, including the Centers for Disease Control (CDC).

- Positive Force in San Francisco receives $1 million a year from the CDC. The group offers flirting classes and, last July, hosted a workshop on how to have anal intercourse if you suffer from diarrhea. (Diarrhea is a common side effect of AIDS.)

- On February 28, 2002, the Stop AIDS Project of San Francisco, which received nearly $700,000 from the CDC in fiscal 2001, will sponsor "GUYWATCH: Blow by Blow." The advertisement for the seminar reads, in part: "What tricks do you want to share to make your man tremble with delight?"

- A Central Florida AIDS Unified Resources (CENTAUR) staffer spent $600,000 in Ryan White CARE Act money on tickets to Disney World, hotels, and restaurants.

- In April 2001, *The New York Post* revealed New York City was spending nearly $180,000 a week ($9 million a year) on hotel rooms for HIV and AIDS patients. That month, the city had reserved 20 rooms at the Sofitel Hotel in Midtown Manhattan at $329 apiece. Advocates say DASIS must use the expensive hotels because it has ruined its relationship with lower-cost hotels by not paying bills on time. New York City received $52.6 million in Housing Opportunities for People With AIDS (HOPWA) program funding in fiscal 2001.

- The University of California–San Francisco AIDS Health Project (AHP), which received a $633,765 grant from the CDC in fiscal 2001 and continually receives nearly 85% of its funding from government sources, sponsored a workshop in November in physical intimacy, focusing on "holding, kissing, licking, sucking, and . . ."

- A doctor in Puerto Rico used $2.2 million in federal funds to buy luxury items like cars and jet skis, while severely neglecting the AIDS patients in his care.

- More than $20 million in grant money intended to help house AIDS patients was collected—but never spent—in Los Angeles.

- AID Atlanta, Inc., which received more than $3.5 million from the government in fiscal 2000 and only $1.2 million in private contributions, sponsors "Deeper Love: A Workshop for Gay and Bisexual Men of African Descent" that addresses such subjects as dating, relationships, and erotica. The program lists the following topics of discussion: "Dirty talk: what makes it good; Tossing salad; Strollin' in the park, through the trails; The art of latex; Safety versus trust." AID Atlanta, Inc. also sponsors "Slipping and Sliding" where men can explore their needs and desires and learn how to fulfill them.

- FBI investigation into the South Dallas Health Clinic revealed that more than $60,000 in the Title I funds had been spent on calls to psychic hotlines and on shopping trips to Neiman Marcus.

- The nonprofit Tampa Hillsborough Action Plan (THAP) gives its top executives plenty of perks despite its financial woes. The THAP boss and THAP chief executive officer rang up nearly $1000 in

BOX 14.2 *(continued)*

meal charges in a three-week period and were also afforded the use of sport utility vehicles. The THAP boss received up to $45,000 a year annually for the maintenance of his vehicles. THAP's top executives also received four season tickets for Tampa Bay Buccaneers games and two season tickets for both the Tampa Bay Devil Rays and the Tampa Bay Lightning. Meanwhile, THAP owed nearly $25,000 in delinquent payroll taxes. THAP receives $450,000 a year from the federal government to provide housing to people with AIDS.

- In the CAGW investigation is the Los Angeles County Auditor Controller's Office report that states, "officials in the county's Office of AIDS Programs and Policy cannot account for $83 million it spent in 2001." That is more money than the budget for many American cities.

CONCLUSION OF CAGW

Before new resources are added to the $28.4 billion in federal money currently allotted for AIDS-related programs, the Departments of Health and Human Services and Housing and Urban Development should conduct extensive audits of the Ryan White CARE Act Title I and the HOPWA program. Such audits will give Congress more incentive to reform or eliminate these antiquated and duplicated social programs. Congress should redirect many CDC prevention grants to international AIDS relief efforts or increase funds for researching an AIDS cure. Many CARE Act programs, including all of Title I, should be phased out and incorporated into existing federal safety net programs such as Medicaid and Medicare. This would ensure necessary, life-saving medical care to those with HIV and AIDS who are low income or uninsured, while also eliminating nonessential AIDS services. It would also save money to bolster the AIDS Drug Assistance Program (ADAP), which began in 1996.

In May 2002, former U.S. Treasury Secretary Paul O'Neill took a 10-day tour of Africa. On his return, he called for increased access to HIV/AIDS treatment and greater accountability for assistance programs. O'Neill went to Chris Hani Baragwanath Hospital in Soweto where he met with HIV-positive women whose children had been treated at birth with the antiretroviral drug nevirapine to reduce the risk of vertical HIV transmission. O'Neill, who has been critical of foreign aid in the past, asked why the South African government was not providing treatment to all HIV-positive pregnant women. O'Neill said, "This whole business about having so much money ... and it not going primarily to treatment is just a stunning revelation." In an interview with

ABC's *This Week*, on May 26, O'Neill echoed his call for greater accountability. "My problem is that it isn't clear why we aren't getting better choices about the priority use of the money that is already there. For me, this is about getting real results on the ground."

Since the CAGW report in 2003, several hundred cases of financial fraud and corruption have been uncovered in the United States and worldwide—far too many to report here. One is the recent case of antiretroviral drugs provided, at cost, to various countries in Africa. The drugs were smuggled out of Africa into Britain, France, The Netherlands, Germany, and other developed countries and sold for millions of dollars in profit.

MEDICAID/MEDICARE AND HIV/AIDS

Medicaid

One of the most important sources of care and coverage for people with HIV/AIDS in the United States is Medicaid, the nation's principal safety net health insurance program for low-income Americans. Medicaid is estimated to provide insurance coverage to almost half of all those with HIV who are in regular care. In addition, a significant share of those newly diagnosed with HIV has been found to already be covered by Medicaid. Thus Medicaid provides an important potential entry point for assessing implementation of routine HIV screening in healthcare settings. While all state Medicaid programs must cover medically necessary HIV testing, state coverage of routine HIV screening varies because it is an optional benefit under Medicaid. Medicaid, while jointly financed by the federal government and the states, is designed and administered by the states within broad federal guidelines. States can opt to provide routine HIV screening as part of the more general diagnostic, screening, or preventive benefit.

In 2005, Florida's Medicaid bureau chief and possibly others in the agency diverted $200,000 in federal AIDS funds to pay for treatments for a "politically connected" Broward County couple's adopted autistic child. Also in 2005, New York City's Human Resources Administration (HRA), which finds temporary shelter for people living with HIV/AIDS, paid $2.2 million in questionable payments over two and a half years, which included paying $182,391 for hotel rooms assigned to 26 people for up to two years after they died. HRA also paid $1 million to vendors for clients who had not signed verification registration logs.

In 2006, according to U.S. senator Tom Coburn, the federal government did not act prudently, spending

BOX 14.2 *(continued)*

(wasting?) millions of dollars to subsidize six separate HIV/AIDS conferences in five months. The conferences were attended by hundreds of federal employees at taxpayers' expense. The attendees stayed in plush oceanside hotel rooms, watched fashion shows, and enjoyed luxury spas. In 2006 and 2007, representatives of the FBI said that Medicare and Medicaid programs involving monies for HIV/AIDS patients were "rampant in fraud." For example, in 2007, ten Florida medical clinic owners were indicted for allegedly defrauding Medicare by improperly billing the program for HIV/AIDS treatments and medical equipment. According to a report conducted by the governor's office, Florida has far fewer HIV/AIDS cases than California or New York, but HIV/AIDS providers in the state submitted three times as many claims as providers in California and five times as many claims as providers in New York. According to authorities, the defendants in Florida submitted more than $2.2 billion annually in false and fraudulent claims. Through 2009, bogus medical equipment claims and bogus HIV infusion schemes have added over $7 million just for Medicare claims, each year, in South Florida. In one example of perpetuating fraudulent Medicare schemes, the names of 18,240 dead physicians, in Miami and other large Florida cities, were used as medical providers' identification numbers to obtain medical equipment, medications, and fraudulent treatments.

In 2009, Debbie Cenziper of the *Washington Post* wrote a two-part exposé on the financial fraud and corruption taking place in Washington, DC HIV/AIDS Administration. Cenziper says, "In a city whose HIV/AIDS rates are ten times the national average, one in three of DC's AIDS dollars earmarked for local groups in recent years went to organizations cited for falsified documentation, few or no clients, incomplete spending records or not running any AIDS programs whatsoever. Meanwhile, District residents living with HIV/AIDS struggled to find care."

The waste has spanned every arm of the HIV/AIDS Administration. As the steward of the city's AIDS dollars, the agency receives about $100 million a year, largely from the federal government, for prevention, medical care, housing, case management, and support services. Much of the money goes to large medical clinics. From 2004 to 2008, about $16 million a year was divided among 90 small nonprofit groups. More than 20 failed to file tax returns or secure a city business license, the *Post* found. Some groups submitted employee résumés and consulting contracts with false information, including fake addresses and credentials. Others had a history of financial problems or had spent hundreds of dollars on travel or executive pay. One Northeast nonprofit group paid its executive director $357,000 in salary and benefits at a time when it was cutting back services. Grants were given for vague reasons and the results were often not tracked. Monitors at the city's HIV/AIDS Administration were supposed to provide oversight, but inspections were sporadic and often done by phone. Records show that monitors frequently focused on whether the groups had spent enough of their grant money—not whether the spending was legitimate.

The *Post* stories examined the record of the HIV/AIDS Administration and specifically cast a troubling eye on the agency's housing arm. During that time, millions of dollars were ill spent. Miracle Hands, one nonprofit organization, received $4.5 million in grants in five years, including $400,000 to fund renovations of a job-training center that still hasn't opened. The director's son worked for Miracle Hands, and her father and uncle worked as security.

In January 2011, the Associated Press reported on allegations of fraud and corruption occurring in the use of funds from the Global Fund to Fight AIDS, TB, and Malaria. An investigation by the Global Fund investigators revealed large percentages of many grants are consumed by corruption to the extent that member countries like Sweden and Germany are suspending their donations until the release of the outcome of these investigations. Entering 2012, at least $73 million of Global Fund Money was lost to alleged fraud, mismanagement, and misspending. The expectations, at the moment, are that graft and corruption will run into millions of dollars more! The United Nations program for HIV/AIDS believes that two-thirds of its grants are "eaten up by corruption."

DISCUSSION QUESTION: Do you think in other countries there is at least an equal amount of fraud and corruption as found in America with regard to the allocation and spending of HIV/AIDS dollars donated for the prevention and treatment of HIV/AIDS? Support your opinions with examples. How would you propose to significantly reduce monetary waste and corruption?

THE GLOBAL FUND TO FIGHT HIV/AIDS, TB, AND MALARIA
JANUARY 26, 2012: GLOBAL FUND TURNS 12

The Global Fund is set up as a public-private partnership that is independent of the United Nations and is funded by governments around the world, foundations, nonprofit corporations, and select individuals. Its purpose is to attract, manage, and disburse resources to fight AIDS, TB, and malaria.

HIV/AIDS, TB, and malaria kill over 6 million people annually with an additional 350 million people suffering from these diseases. This fund was set up in response to widespread public criticism of governments' apathy to the health crisis in developing countries, especially concerning HIV/AIDS. The health status of the poor, women, men, and children is deteriorating in many parts of the world, and the fund is a unique opportunity to mobilize international political will and resources to address this crisis in a new way, rather than continuing with business as usual.

Of the new disease-fighting projects funded in developing countries, 66% are in Africa, 13% are in Asia, 13% are in the Middle East, and 5% are in Latin America. AIDS projects represented 48% of the total; malaria 42%; and TB 10%.

The Global Fund was initiated through the United Nations General Assembly Special Session on AIDS (UNGASS) in June 2001. The year 2001 has been recorded in AIDS history as the year when political commitment to the disease moved to center stage.

The goal of the 189 countries at the UNGASS 2001 was to reverse the global AIDS pandemic by 2015. On May 31 through June 2, 2006, the UN General Assembly held its second-ever UNGASS to review what changes, if any, occurred because of the global strategy against AIDS adopted by world governments in 2001. The review clearly showed failure to progress toward UNGASS 2001 goals, including HIV prevention, the availability of ART, and HIV education for 90% of those living in underdeveloped nations. Peter Piot, then executive director of UNAIDS, said of the work done over the five-year period, "We've failed, we've failed." The new goals sought to find $23 billion per year by 2010 in order to fund AIDS treatment, care, prevention, and health infrastructure and to bring recognition to the rights of all HIV-infected people to receive help (it did not happen). The final Declaration from UNGASS 2006 did not specify help for homosexuals, prostitutes, and drug addicts.

The third special session on HIV/AIDS was held on June 8–10, 2011, to mark the 30th anniversary since the first report of this "new" disease. Two of the UN key goals are, "no children born with HIV by 2015" and "15 million on ART by 2015." The cost of ART, $25.4 billion per year!

In 2010 UNAIDS put forth an exciting new vision: Zero new HIV infections. Zero discrimination. Zero AIDS-related deaths. This vision is but a part of UNAIDS Strategic Plan for 2011–2015.

Former United Nations Secretary-General Kofi Annan Calls for Large-Scale Mobilization in Fight against AIDS, Tuberculosis, and Malaria

In mid-2001, calling the battle his personal priority, the secretary-general outlined five priority areas for the global campaign:

1. Preventing further spread of the epidemic, especially by giving young people the knowledge and power to protect themselves.

2. Reducing HIV transmission from mother to child, which he called "the cruelest, most unjust" infections of all.

3. Ensuring that care and treatment are within reach of all.

4. Delivering scientific breakthroughs. Finding a cure and vaccine for HIV/AIDS must be given increased priority in scientific budgets.

5. Protecting those made most vulnerable by the epidemic, especially orphans.

To achieve these five goals, Annan called world leaders to help finance the campaign against AIDS, tuberculosis, and malaria in Africa. In April 2001, he said, "a war chest of 7 billion to 10 billion U.S. dollars is needed annually, over an extended period of time, to wage an effective global campaign against HIV/AIDS. [This number has now been raised to $15 billion to $30 billion annually.] Current spending by the governments in developing countries totals around $1 billion annually." This is many billions of dollars less than they spend on their military.

The current UN Secretary-General is Ban Ki-moon.

How Far Will Ten Billion Dollars Go in Africa?

Should Africa alone receive $10 billion annually from the developed world, it would average out that each living HIV-infected African would receive about $376 per year ($10 billion divided by 26.6 million HIV infected) for as long as the money was provided. This would occur only if the money was actually given to the people. This money, along with free or very low drug costs, could be of considerable help, especially since many African countries spend less than $5 to $10 per person a year on public health. But, used in this way, this large sum of money would not be available to build needed medical facilities or import the thousands of doctors necessary to treat the HIV infected. That will take a few hundred billion more dollars.

An article on "Estimating the Cost of Expanded AIDS Treatment in Africa" that appeared in the June 2001 issue of *Topics in HIV Medicine* states that it would cost $1.12 billion each year to treat 1 million HIV-infected Africans. Ending 2013 there will be an estimated 26.6 million Africans living with HIV. The cost, based on information presented in the article, would be about $30 billion a year if all were to be treated equally.

South Africa has about 6 million people living with HIV. That is more than for any other nation. Still, South Africa expects to have an additional 5 million new infections over the next 20 years. The projected cost to keep the number of new infections at 5 million is $102 billion.

Comments Relative to the Global Fund War Chest

The Global Fund: Countries Pledge, But Do They Pay?—The UN proposed that contributions to the Fund should be made according to an *Equitable Contributions Framework,* in which donor countries contribute in relation to the sizes of their economies. But many nations refuse to pledge money because there is no mechanism in place to handle corruption. They also ask who besides Africa will receive how much of the fund, and how the money will be spent. For example, there remains a large division among the 194 countries of the United Nations General Assembly over whether most of the money should be spent on prevention rather than antiretroviral drugs. Many members of the General Assembly said that about half the $10 billion should be spent on drugs for Africa and the other half spent on prevention programs in Asia and the former Soviet nations where the epidemic is expanding out of control. Clearly there are no easy choices, but choices must be made. The United States was the first and only country by mid-2001 to offer Annan $200 million toward his global AIDS fund. Twenty-nine other nations have followed. By U.S. law, the American share of the Global Fund can total no more than 33% of all contributions to the fund. Total financial pledges from all countries and private foundations, etc., through 2012 amount to about $16 billion, but $27 billion is needed and the shortfall continues. No single nation has committed more money to this fund toward the African HIV/AIDS problem than the United States. The top three nations contributing to the Global Fund are the United States, Great Britain, and Japan, in that order.

Entering 2013, 40 nations have pledged about $15 billion to the Global Fund. But, there is no guarantee that these monies will be paid. Most donor nations pledge year by year. There are no long-term or multiyear pledges. It is only optimism that the money will be made available. Insufficient funding undermines the Millennium Development Goal of halving or reversing the spread of HIV and other communicable diseases by 2015.

Current Funding Problems

The Global Fund to Fight AIDS, Tuberculosis, and Malaria—which supports about four million people with ART—is so cash-strapped that it won't provide any new grants for 2012 through 2014. Ninety countries had applied for grants in 2012—none will be funded!

The *irony* of the Global Fund cancellation of HIV/AIDS grants is that 31 years after AIDS made its deadly debut, a future without the disease is finally within reach. One of the biggest scientific breakthroughs of 2011 was the discovery that antiretroviral drugs don't just prolong the lives of people with HIV, they also render infected people virtually noncontagious. Putting people on these life-saving medicines early enough could effectively end the spread of HIV. (Read pages 85 through 89 Sidebar 4.3 and Box 10.1, pages 290–292) But just as science is on the verge of winning the battle, financial resources and political will are falling—2010 was the first year that HIV/AIDS funding around the world decreased. The world still has a long way to go in the fight against HIV. So far, about 8 million people in the world have access to antiretroviral drugs, out of some 38 million infected people, half of whom are already sick. Only a quarter of the over 2 million children who need the drugs are getting them, along with about half of pregnant mothers who will pass the virus onto their newborn babies without them. The new science of HIV tells us that even people who feel healthy should be taking the drugs, especially infected people with uninfected spouses. But, to continually provide these drugs over the lifetimes of the infected will cost many, many, many billion dollars.

(Comment—China, the world's second largest economic power, is the fourth largest recipient from the Global Fund. It has received about 1 billion dollars. China spent approximately $46 billion hosting the 2008 Summer Olympics and the 2010 Shanghai Expo, in addition to financing a $586 billion economic stimulus package. To date China has given the Global Fund $16 million. Some donor nations view this as a detriment to Global Fund efforts to raise money.)

UNSPENT GLOBAL FUNDS?

While Eric Goosby, global AIDS coordinator, calls for greater funding for global HIV/AIDS, he must explain why $1.6 billion available in 2011 have not been spent. This money has been stuck in the pipeline for over 18 months! Now the question has become, "What should we do

with the money?" While this has created an unexpected windfall for some programs, it also means that several countries that have not spent the funds will lose tens or hundreds of millions of dollars. The key loser appears to be Kenya, which has had a half-billion dollars—roughly one-third the total amount in the pipeline—that has been accumulating in the U.S. Treasury unspent for more than 18 months after Congress appropriated the money.

FORMS OF U.S. MONETARY ASSISTANCE FOR HIV/AIDS

A U.S. Congressman once said, "A billion dollars here, a billion dollars there, it begins to add up." With respect to U.S. HIV/AIDS support, those hundreds of millions and billions of dollars have indeed added up. The United States has provided and continues to provide more money globally to foreign governments and nongovernmental organizations (NGOs) than any country on earth. The U.S. federal government has donated billions of dollars, through a variety of organizations, directly to people in need and to the Global AIDS, TB, and Malaria Fund. Direct spending for international HIV/AIDS activities by the United States began in 1986 with a $1.1 million investment, through several U.S. agencies that had already started international HIV/AIDS projects. Spending increased steadily and has reached about $3 billion per year.

International Global Fund—In 2002, the G8 countries (United States, Russia, Great Britain, France, Germany, Italy, Japan, and Canada) organized a new International Global Fund, which became operational in January 2002. Through 2013, the United States will have contributed an estimated $6 billion to this fund. These international global funds are also to be used to support programs for HIV/AIDS (20%), TB (50%), and malaria (30%). This fund should not be confused with the Global AIDS, TB, and Malaria Fund.

During the 2008 G8 meeting in Germany, G8 members agreed to provide $60 billion to fight HIV/AIDS. Eighty-three percent of this money, or $50 billion, comes from President Bush's 2008 five-year extension of his PEPFAR program! But, even with over 80% of the financial burden being picked up by the United States, the remaining $10 billion is not a firm pledge from the G8 because some countries want to be cautious about increasing spending on HIV/AIDS.

Former President George W. Bush's and President Barack Obama's Emergency Plan for AIDS Relief (PEPFAR) through the International Global Fund: January 28, 2003, through 2014

Then-President Bush announced in the State of the Union address the Emergency Plan for AIDS Relief, a five-year, $15 billion initiative to turn the tide in combating the global HIV/AIDS pandemic. "To meet an urgent crisis abroad, tonight I propose the Emergency Plan for AIDS Relief (PEPFAR)—a work for mercy beyond all current international efforts to help the people of Africa. I ask the Congress to commit $15 billion over the next five years." This commitment of resources is helping the 12 most afflicted countries in sub-Saharan Africa and three countries in the Caribbean.

PEPFAR is the single largest healthcare program aimed at a single disease in history. It is one of only a few programs to operate with strict accountability standards. However, PEPFAR emphasizes treatment at the expense of prevention.

An important aspect of Bush's Emergency Plan is that it issues a challenge to every other member of the G8 countries to follow suit. In a sense he has placed a moral burden on these countries. On May 26, 2003, President Bush signed into law the $15 billion program that he called "a great mission to rescue." From 2004 through 2008, all of the $15 billion plus an additional $4 billion was spent.

The $15 billion original PEPFAR fund expired in September 2008. Congress extended the program for an additional five years, and increased its funding to $48 billion. This increased the number of people receiving antiretroviral drugs through PEPFAR from 2.1 million to about 4 million. Ending 2013, globally there will be about 18 million people who will urgently need antiretroviral therapy!

Universal Access to Antiretroviral Drugs

To achieve universal access to antiretroviral drugs through 2012, officials at UNAIDS say an additional $42 billion will have to be found. If this money is forthcoming, another $54 billion will be necessary, by 2015, just to maintain those placed on ART back in 2012 and those added through 2014. Where will these monies be coming from and for how long?

Some Results of PEPFAR: The First $19 Billion

Entering 2013, PEPFAR funded about 80 million HIV tests, provided antiretroviral drugs to about 4.4 million people in the 15 target countries, supplied over 4.5 billion condoms, prevented about 500,000 mother-to-child HIV transmissions, provided care for about 5 million orphans, and prevented over 1.5 million deaths. According to Mark Dybul, who administered PEPFAR, the number of those receiving antiretrovirals is increasing at the rate of about 50,000 a month. (See Point to Ponder 14.1, page 456.)

Update for PEPFAR—In 2009, President Obama raised the previous $48 billion to $63 billion over six years—an additional 2.5 billion dollars per year. Beginning in 2010, PEPFAR bilateral activities (funding) will be given out in 80 countries in Africa, the Middle East, Asia, Europe, the Americas, and the Caribbean. Most of the funding will be concentrated in 31 of the 80 countries—15 in Africa and 16 in the Caribbean. President Obama also named Eric Goosby as the new Global AIDS Coordinator and administrator of PEPFAR.

DISCUSSION QUESTIONS—The UN Global Fund, for 2008 through 2012, needed about $80 billion. Even if the Global Fund had received this money, is $20 billion a year or more sustainable and for how long?

U.S. Spending on HIV/AIDS in Developing Countries

In 2004, the Kaiser Family Foundation surveyed people in the United States as to their views on the U.S. government's spending money on

UNITED STATES HIV/AIDS MONEY BINDS THE LONGEVITY OF MILLIONS OF PEOPLE WORLDWIDE—A FOREIGN ENTITLEMENT POLICY?

Let's start this Point to Ponder with a question, a very tough question that tests human morality. The question is, **has the United States created a foreign entitlement program? If yes, it is the first of its kind—ever, anywhere!**

Through the use of PEPFAR funding and many other U.S. funding programs to help in the fight against HIV/AIDS, our politicians have legislated an implicit pledge to continue to purchase life-saving antiretroviral drugs for many millions of people in developing countries for a very long time. Just how long is not clear. It is estimated that by the year 2015, the cost for just the drugs will reach $20 billion per year and will continue to climb. And that figure is based on the cost for patients starting ART with CD4+ cell counts around 200 to 250. The current push is to start ART at between 350 and 500 CD4+ cells per microliter of blood. Therapy begun at this level of CD4+ cells would call for many additional billions of dollars as this will increase the number of people requiring ART to double (Hecht et al., 2010)!

Once started, HIV/AIDS therapy must continue indefinitely because stopping it can rapidly lead to death. As a consequence, international health experts and medical ethicists say it would be immoral to withdraw the financial assistance that pays for the therapy unless someone else steps in to replace the United States. Think for a moment, what nation might that be? *(Pause.)* . . . Have you thought of one yet? And how long will that nation provide the billions of dollars necessary? The top 12 public funders/donors for HIV/AIDS are the United States, the European Commission, Britain, the Netherlands, Ireland, Brazil, Sweden, Canada, Australia, Russia, Belgium, and France. It should be noted that some of the world's wealthiest countries are missing in action from the top 10, top 20, or even top 50 funders/donors (Moran et al., 2009).

One Step Forward, Two Steps Back

Treatment is a humanitarian triumph, rescuing individuals and their families from a dire fate, but from a population's perspective it does little to stem the tide of the pandemic. For every individual to receive treatment, two to three others become newly infected. Treatment is, at best, a stopgap measure that requires enormous resources because of the life-long need of millions of individuals.

The imbalance between the numbers of HIV infected entering treatment and those becoming newly infected is expected to continue at least through 2020. But this is only a guessestimate—accuracy may be very flawed.

The Politics and Ethics of HIV/AIDS Drug Therapy

Peter Piot, past director of UNAIDS, said, "The train is out of the station. People are on treatment—we can't drop them, if for no other reasons than ethical ones." Kevin De Cock, HIV/AIDS director of the World Health Organization, said, "We cannot let the pendulum swing back to a time when we didn't spend a lot on AIDS. We now have millions of people on treatment and we can't just stop that." And Tom Coates, a professor of global AIDS research at the University of California–Los Angeles, said, "Let's not drag AIDS care and prevention down to the level of every other disease, but let's bring everything else up to the level of AIDS."

QUESTION: Do these politicians and professionals who propose an unending supply of U.S. and other countries' healthcare money realize there are, at some point, real limits as to how much money can be spent on HIV/AIDS?

A Spending Backlash Is Growing

First, there is a healthcare crisis in the United States. According to Laurie Garrett, a senior fellow for global health at the Council on Foreign Relations, by 2016, Americans may find themselves fed up with generosity. If we cannot find a way to reform the U.S. healthcare system, we will likely by then have some 80 million citizens without health insurance, including HIV-positive people, and medical costs will devour $1 out of $4 of America's GDP. Entering 2013, about half of those waiting for ART are waiting for additional federal AIDS Drug Assistance Program (ADAP) money in 12 states. The other half includes people who are not eligible for ADAP, and those are eligible but do not apply to ADAP. For 2013, over $1 billion will be available to finance ADAP for about 240,000 people across 50 states and territories. Meanwhile, we are servicing a huge national debt in the trillions of dollars and a $3.8 trillion federal budget for 2011 followed by a $3.8 trillion budget for 2012 and about a $3.8 trillion budget for 2013 while struggling with everything from global climate change to catastrophic disparities in access to food, energy, and water. **Second,** there are at this time global health experts questioning whether money spent to control HIV/AIDS is out of proportion to that spent on other health threats most people face daily (Read Point of View 14.4, pages 458–460). Through

2013, world agencies collectively will have spent close to two trillion dollars on this one disease in 28 years. This is many more times than that spent on any other single disease in human history, and there is little light at the end of this very long tunnel. Even if a vaccine were discovered tomorrow, projected billions of dollars would still be needed throughout the next 10 to 15 years before global monetary relief for this disease would be realized. In the meantime, spending on HIV/AIDS each year is over 100 times what the world spends on clean water projects in developing countries, while over 2 billion people lack clean water and adequate sanitation! And then there is cancer, which isn't only on the rise among HIV-positive people—it's happening to many people, especially in the developing world. Health experts say that about 12 million people were diagnosed with cancer worldwide in 2010, and cancer claimed the lives of about 8 million people. Developing countries are hit particularly hard since many poorer nations can't provide people with the cancer screening and treatment they need.

Responsibility and Accountability, Which Led the World to Its Current Health Care Crisis

There is no question that there are global healthcare inequities—unfair, unjust, and for the most part avoidable. Historically, it has been the toxic combination of bad policies, economics, and politics that is, in large measure, responsible for the fact that a majority of people in the world do not enjoy the good health that is biologically possible. But the train has left that station. We are where we are. Looking back and casting blame solves nothing—looking ahead with caution, organization, and realism will help. Like the current global economic crisis, the global health crisis and the HIV/AIDS crisis will take a long time to overcome.

---

developing countries to fight HIV/AIDS. The survey asked, does it make a difference—will this money slow the spread of HIV/AIDS in those countries receiving monetary help from the United States? About 32% think the spending is about right, and 42% think not enough is being spent. A significant number (38%) do not think spending more money will help.

The Problem in Perspective: Wealth, Poverty, and AIDS. About One Billion People Live on Less Than One Dollar a Day!

The relationship between poverty and HIV transmission is not simple. If it were, South Africa might not have Africa's largest epidemic, for South Africa is rich by African standards. Botswana is also relatively rich, yet this country has the highest levels of infection in the world. While most people with HIV/AIDS are poor, many of the infected are not poor. Undernourishment; lack of clean water, sanitation, and hygienic living conditions; generally low levels of health, compromised immune systems, high incidence of other infections including genital infections and exposure to diseases such as tuberculosis and malaria; inadequate public health services; illiteracy and ignorance; pressures encouraging high-risk behavior, from labor migration to alcohol abuse and gender violence; an inadequate leadership response to either HIV/AIDS or the problems of the poor; and finally, lack of confidence or hope for the future—all companions of poverty promote HIV infection!

The cycle of poverty intensifies as individuals, households, and communities living with HIV/AIDS find that lost earnings, lost crops, and missing treatment make them weaker, make their poverty deeper, and push the vulnerable into poverty. Inequality sharpens the impact of poverty, and a mixture of poverty and inequality may be driving the epidemic. A South African truck driver is not well paid compared to the executives who run his company, but he is rich in comparison to the people in the rural areas he drives through. For the woman at a truck stop, a man with 50 rand ($10) is wealthy; her desperate need for money to feed her family may buy him unprotected sex, even though she knows the risks.

ARE DEVELOPED NATIONS OVERFUNDING HIV/AIDS NEEDS?
SHOULD THE UNITED STATES RETHINK ITS HIV/AIDS FUNDING POLICIES?

It has been over at least 31 years since HIV/AIDS began crossing Planet Earth. This disease has been called the largest threat to international health ever! As the numbers of HIV/AIDS cases grew, so, too, have the monetary donations—billions upon billions of dollars with no end in sight to the pandemic and likewise the continued need for AIDS dollars. But many HIV/AIDS scientists and politicians internationally are now asking why all this money for one disease, when there are so many other diseases to treat and fundamental health care issues to be met in every country on Planet Earth, especially those countries in the developing nations.

Recently, in December 2007, with the announcement by WHO and UNAIDS epidemiologists that their numbers of HIV/AIDS cases have been seriously overinflated, many voices are now being added to the chorus calling for a shift of HIV/AIDS dollars into basic health issues like providing clean water, family planning, and the treatment of global cases of waterborne diseases like diarrhea and cholera. It has been estimated that 4000 children die each day, or about 1.5 million annually, because of using unclean or unsanitary water. About 900 children die daily from AIDS-related complications. In addition, over one billion people lack a sanitary water supply. How many adults and adolescents die each year because of the lack of clean water? Problems like malnutrition and a variety of diseases other than HIV/AIDS are responsible for many more deaths annually than HIV/AIDS.

Aside from southern Africa, most of the continent has relatively low rates of HIV and much higher rates of easily treatable diseases like diarrhea and respiratory illnesses. Yet much of the money from the West, especially from the United States, goes into HIV/AIDS. Richard Halperin, senior research scientist at Harvard School of Public Health, wrote a commentary in the *New York Times* (January 1, 2008) on the imbalance of spending billions of dollars on one disease while other serious life-threatening diseases go unfunded or underfunded. Halperin said he was astounded at the response to his article. Most were positive, he said, with many AIDS experts agreeing it was time to reexamine spending. (Read Roger England, 2007.) England believes the global AIDS industry is too large and out of control. England believes that UNAIDS has outlived its purpose and should be disbanded!

John Bongaarts and colleagues (2008) believe it is time for international governments to rethink their prioritization of HIV/AIDS over other infectious diseases. They believe that "AIDS has gotten special treatment because of its emergency status; that view is no longer valid because the epidemic has peaked." They feel the amount of money being devoted to HIV/AIDS is out of proportion to that being spent on other diseases (see Table 14.1, page 448 for examples). However, peaks in HIV prevalence, which reflect the total number of people living with the virus, lag about a decade behind peaks in HIV incidence—the rate of new infections. This is because someone infected with HIV can live with the virus for about a decade after infection and for much longer if they start ART treatment. Research shows that the global peak in HIV incidence occurred in 1995, with the first peak occurring in North America in the early 1980s and the last peak in Eastern Europe in 2001.

According to Bongaarts, this finding is not new, but it has been against the interests of agencies like UNAIDS to highlight it. Bongaarts said, "I think UNAIDS was afraid that donors would decide not to spend so much money on AIDS [because] governments would say, 'this is no longer something to worry about.'" His comments came on the heels of recent admissions by former senior UNAIDS and World Health Organization officials that they exaggerated the size of the HIV epidemic and its potential for further growth to create public alarm and maintain the flow of donor money to the global industry that AIDS has spawned. HIV/AIDS receives about a quarter of global health aid, but constitutes only 5% of the disease burden in low- and middle-income countries. Rwandan officials recently noted that in their country, $47 million went to HIV/AIDS, $18 million to malaria (the country's largest killer), and $1 million to childhood diseases. Diarrhea kills five times more children than HIV/AIDS in Rwanda.

Halperin points out that former President Bush's $15 billion PEPFAR (the president's plan for AIDS Relief) program to fight HIV/AIDS in 15 underdeveloped countries over five years was an unprecedented amount of money aimed at a single disease. Meanwhile, other public health issues were ignored. This $15 billion program ended in September 2008 but was then continued by a newly approved $63 billion congressional allocation, which continues to ignore basic global health issues. To this end, Jeremy Shiffman of Syracuse University said, "AIDS is a humanitarian tragedy, but it is just one of many terrible humanitarian tragedies." (See Point to Ponder 14.1, pages 456–457.) Richard Horton, editor of *Lancet*, said, "AIDS [spending] has grossly distorted our [a] limited budget." He went on to say that undernutrition is the largely preventable cause of over a third or 3.5 million of all child deaths. Stunting, severe wasting, and intrauterine growth restriction are among the most important problems. There is a golden interval for intervention: from pregnancy to two years of age. After age two, undernutrition will have caused irreversible damage for future development toward adulthood. Incredibly, 80% of the undernourished children live in just 20 countries across four regions—Africa, Asia, western Pacific, and the Middle East. Countries that are receiving billions of HIV/AIDS dollars. These are the priority nations for action. Undernutrition can have substantial negative effects on societies. A recent study by World Food Program and the Economic Commission for Latin America and the Caribbean estimated that economic losses due to undernutrition among children in just seven nations are a staggering $6.6 billion a year—6% of the gross domestic product. (The February 2008 issue of *Lancet*, Volume 371, ran a series of five articles dealing with the above topics.) Halperin says, "The AIDS experience has demonstrated that poor countries can make complex treatments accessible to many people. Regimens that are much simpler to administer than antiretroviral drugs—like antibiotics for respiratory illnesses, oral rehydration for diarrhea, immunizations and contraception—could also be made widely available. But as there isn't a global fund for safe water, child survival, and family planning, countries cannot directly tackle their real problems without pegging them to the big three diseases associated with the Global AIDS, Malaria, and Tuberculosis Fund. Eighty percent of this fund goes to these three diseases! Little is left for treatment of pneumonia and diarrheal diseases. Halperin asks, "With [over] ten million children and half a million mothers in developing countries dying annually of largely preventable conditions, should we multiply AIDS spending while giving a pittance for initiatives like safe-water projects?" The Global Fund director's response to Halperin and others who believe that HIV/AIDS money should be redistributed for basic healthcare was, "We are not a global fund that funds local health."

In October 2009, the *New York Times* newspaper examined the debate over whether the United States and other rich nations spend too much on AIDS, which requires lifelong medications, compared with diarrhea and the other leading disease killing children, pneumonia, both of which can be treated inexpensively. According to the newspaper, diarrhea kills 1.5 million young children a year in developing countries—more than AIDS, malaria, and measles combined—but only 4 in 10 of those who need the oral rehydration solution that can prevent death for pennies get it.

Looking Ahead—In 2031, the HIV/AIDS pandemic will enter its 50th year! Funding required at that time using current policies will reach $35 billion annually. Even then it is estimated that there will still be about 1 million new HIV infections annually. Globally, estimates between 2009 and 2031—22 years ($15.5 billion to $35 billion per year)—are that HIV/AIDS will cost between $340 billion to $770 billion. Where will this money come from? (Hecht et al., 2010) Wise policy choices focusing on high-impact test-and-treat prevention strategies could cut costs by half. But how likely is it that this will occur? The question raised earlier in this textbook is how much will this pandemic cost? The answer given—how much do you have?

QUESTION—Do you think HIV/AIDS should receive the largest single disease funding in history of human diseases, at the expense of all other human diseases that can be successfully treated if monies were available? Present a meaningful discussion using facts either pro or con on this very important issue. Include the moral, ethical, political, economic, scientific, and practical reasons in defending your position.

UPDATE

Regardless of your opinion after reading the preceding material on whether HIV/AIDS is being overfunded, UNAIDS in 2010 said that $26.8 billion annually is needed for HIV/AIDS in low- and middle-income countries just for the years 2010 and 2011!

Author's Comments: Regardless of intent, there is just so much money available to help all those who need treatment, care, nutrition, and various kinds of environmental protection. Choices have to be made. There just isn't enough money to fund every medical tragedy. Limited resources mean limited healthcare interventions.

It seems unusual, odd, or at least curious or peculiar that it took 27 years into this pandemic before a discussion or argument has begun for the integration of HIV/AIDS into basic antenatal care, family planning, and child-adolescent-adult health care and health prevention services. It would appear that rather than creating parallel programs for funding healthcare needs, all countries should strengthen existing healthcare systems, and create or strengthen the infrastructure necessary to spend the fewest dollars in the most efficient way.

PRESENT YOUR VIEWS ON GLOBAL SPENDING ON HIV/AIDS VERSUS OTHER HEALTHCARE NEEDS.

According to the UNAIDS chief epidemiologist, by the end of 2013 there will be 38 million living HIV-infected people globally. About 35 million of these people live on less than $2 a day. In many of the high-HIV-incidence countries in Southern Africa, like Kenya, Botswana, Zambia, Malawi, Nigeria, Swaziland, and Uganda, about 50% of their populations live on a dollar or less per day! An HIV-positive American can focus on his T cell counts; an HIV-positive African in a rural village still has to focus on finding clean water and food.

Politicians, economists, and AIDS specialists rarely say this bluntly, but the truth is that most of those 35 million people have simply been written off because the first priority for the first few billion dollars is prevention, not treatment. An economist who studies AIDS in South Africa said, "You can't give up on the infected because of the message it sends. But if I had $1 billion to spend most wisely, I would spend it on giving women more power, caring for orphans, and getting them education."

FINALLY, THE QUESTION: How much would it cost to contain the global HIV/AIDS pandemic? **The answer is: How much have you got?** How much would it cost to banish ignorance, to deaden lust, to shame rapists, to stop war, to enrich the poor, to empower women, to defend children, to make decent medical care as globally ubiquitous as Coca-Cola—in short, to get rid of all the underlying causes of the pandemic in the developing nations? Much of the world at risk for HIV/AIDS can't read. Most of the world at risk has never used a condom. Most of the world at risk has never heard of ACT UP. And most of the world with HIV/AIDS thinks it doesn't have the disease and doesn't know anyone who does, because about 95% of those infected in the developing nations have never been tested. (Most estimates come from anonymous testing at prenatal clinics.) And, most of the world cannot afford the antiretroviral drugs.

Summary

In 1981, the CDC announced a new disease affecting the homosexual population. This disease was later called AIDS. Many religious people believed this was a sign that homosexuality should be punished. The few facts available at that time gave rise to a great deal of fantasy and fear. Affected people were seen as innocent victims, or it was felt that they deserved the disease. Contracting AIDS labeled a person as less than desirable, a homosexual, or one who practiced deviant forms of sexual behavior. But even the so-called innocent victims, the children, the hemophiliacs, and other recipients of blood transfusions were not spared social ostracism. If you had AIDS, you were twice the victim—first of the virus and second of the social discrimination.

Children were barred from attending school, adults from their jobs, and both from adequate medical care. For example, there are still relatively few dentists who will treat AIDS patients and a significant number of surgeons refuse to operate on AIDS patients. Years have passed, but many misconceptions about HIV/AIDS linger on.

Fear is being casually transmitted rather than the virus. A significant number of people, after years of broad-scale education, still believe that the AIDS virus can be casually transmitted from toilet seats, on drinking glasses, and even by donating blood.

The fallout from the fear of the HIV/AIDS pandemic has been a major change in sexual language in TV advertisements, magazines, and radio. Condoms, once spoken about only in hushed tones and kept under the counter in most drug stores, are now spoken of everywhere as a means of safer sex. AIDS, perhaps more than any other disease, has demonstrated that ignorance leads to fear and knowledge can lead to compassion.

To achieve understanding and compassion, people must be educated as to their HIV risk status and how they can keep it low. Many hundreds of millions of dollars have been spent to inform the public of the kinds of behavior that either place them at risk or reduce their risk for HIV infection. The problem is that although people are getting the information, too many refuse to act on it. Former Surgeon General C. Everett Koop's office mailed 107 million copies of the brochure "Understanding AIDS" to households in the United States. Fifty-one percent of those who received it said they never read it. Even among those who read the brochure are those who refuse to change their sexual behavior. Old habits are difficult to break.

To date, the hard evidence shows that only the homosexual population has significantly modified their sexual behavior as evidenced by the drop in the number of new cases of AIDS among them from 1988 into 2013.

A major problem looming on the horizon is the prospect of HIV being spread in the young adult population. Large numbers of them use drugs and alcohol, have multiple sex partners, and believe they are invulnerable to infection.

The AMA stated in 1988 that physicians may not refuse to care for patients with HIV/AIDS because of actual risk or fear of contracting the disease. Some physicians get around this through referral to other physicians who will treat HIV/AIDS patients. There is one area of medicine that takes issue at having to treat AIDS patients: surgery. Because it is difficult not to accidentally get cut during surgery, surgeons have been the leading advocates for HIV testing of all surgical patients so they will know their risks before performing surgery.

On the other hand, patients say they have a right to know if their physician, especially a surgeon, is HIV infected. Surveys indicate that most people would not want to be treated by an HIV-infected physician.

On June 25, 1998, the U.S. Supreme Court ruled that the Americans with Disabilities Act protected HIV-infected people. Even when they experience no symptoms, they are to be treated as handicapped.

A number of developed and developing nations now believe that HIV/AIDS is, or will soon be, a threat to their national security. Does the next quarter-century mark the endgame of this struggle between death and hope, or more repetitions of the cycle? Can treatment actually be delivered to all who need it? Will effective biological tools to prevent HIV infection be found? How will millions of deaths affect orphans, vulnerable youth, fragile cultures, and global security? It does not bode well that people in many states within our own borders languish on waiting lists for HIV medication. The struggle between death and hope wages on.

Review Questions

(Answers to the Review Questions are on page 463.)

1. Name three major sources of information that contributed to the early panic and hysteria about the spread of AIDS.

2. Give three examples of unfounded public reactions to AIDS infection.

3. Fear of the casual transmission of AIDS parallels what other earlier STD epidemic?

4. What evidence is there that it is difficult to get people to change their behavior even though they know it is harmful to their well-being?

5. What is the major thrust of AIDS education in the United States?

6. If education is the key to preventing HIV infection and new cases of AIDS, and most people interviewed say they have been educated, why is it not working?

7. Why are today's young adults in danger of contracting and spreading HIV?

8. Yes or No: Do physicians have a right to refuse to treat AIDS patients? Support your answer.

9. Do patients have a right to know if their physician is HIV infected or has AIDS?

10. What is the primary means of offsetting the bias toward people with AIDS in the workplace?

11. Who is the current secretary of the United Nations? How much money is needed to fight AIDS globally each year?

12. About how much money was pledged to the Global AIDS Fund in 2012?

13. Compared with the money the federal government spends on research and treatment to combat other health and medical problems such as heart disease and cancer, do you think federal spending on AIDS research and treatment is too high, too low, or about right? Support your choice with credible evidence.

14. About how many billions of dollars has the federal government spent on HIV/AIDS between 2005 and 2013?

15. The federal 2013 budget for HIV/AIDS allocated $_____ for prevention. This is ____% of the HIV/AIDS budget for 2013.

Answers to Review Questions

CHAPTER 1

1. Acquired Immune Deficiency Syndrome
2. Human Immunodeficiency Virus
3. No. AIDS is a syndrome. A syndrome is made up of a collection of signs and symptoms of one or more diseases. AIDS patients have a collection of opportunistic infections and cancers. Collectively these are mistakenly referred to as the AIDS disease.
4. In 1983 by Luc Montagnier
5. 1981
6. LAV
7. Five; 1982, 1983, 1985, 1987, and 1993
8. It allows HIV-infected persons earlier access into federal and state medical and social programs.

CHAPTER 2

1. The unbroken transmission of HIV infection from an HIV-infected person to an uninfected person.
2. The answer to both questions is unknown at this time.
3. AIDS dissidents
4. Mother, Christine Maggiore. Daughter, Eliza Jane
5. Peter Duesberg
6. Thabo Mbeki
7. No; because HIV indirectly influences one's health it is difficult to show in laboratory test tubes that HIV causes AIDS. But the postulates have been satisfied by following infection/transmission cycles in a population of humans.
8. Depends on whose research you believe. However, as presented in this chapter, most of the evidence indicates that HIV is a "new" virus.
9. SIV
10. Beatrice Hahn
11. The Congo in 1959

CHAPTER 3

1. Because it contains RNA as its genetic message and a reverse transcriptase enzyme to make DNA from RNA.
2. GAG-POL-ENV; at least six
3. Because HIV has demonstrated an unusually high rate of genetic mutations: (1) the reverse transcriptase enzyme in HIV is highly error prone (makes transcription errors), and (2) a variety of HIV mutants have been found within a single HIV-infected individual.
4. The reverse transcriptase enzyme is highly error prone, making at least one, and in many cases more than one, deletion, addition, or substitution per round of proviral replication.
5. b
6. e
7. c

8. a

9. b

10. c

11. GAG, POL, ENV

12. About 1000 plus or minus

13. vif produces a protein that destroys the cell's APOBEC protein and causes HIV to produce inactive copies of itself.

14. The processes of gene mutation and gene recombination.

15. 11; B; C; C/E

CHAPTER 4

1. Not really, because there is no way as yet to remove the provirus from the cell's DNA.

2. A physiological measurement that serves as a substitute for a major clinical event.

3. March; 30

4. 8

5. Becoming incorporated into DNA as it is being synthesized, thereby stopping reverse transcriptase from attaching the next nucleotide.

6. (a) Clinical biological side effects; (b) the selection of drug-resistant HIV mutants.

7. (a) The number of copies of HIV RNA present in the plasma. (b) This number indicates the reproductive activity of HIV at the time and, if therapy is being used, the effect of the therapy on the reproductive ability of the virus.

8. Saquinavir mesylate, saquinavir (Fortovase), ritonavir, indinavir, nelfinavir, amprenavir, atazanavir, fosamprenavir, tipranavir.

9. They physically interact with the reverse transcriptase enzyme and interfere with its function.

10. To suppress HIV replication, thereby reducing the number of mutant RNA strands produced.

11. A

12. B

13. To be determined by the instructor.

14. D

15. D

16. C

17. D

18. False

19. A

20. False

21. D

22. D

23. Selzentry or maraviroc

24. True

25. E

26. C

27. A

28. D

29. D

30. False

CHAPTER 5

1. T4 helper cells; because T4 cells are crucial for the production of antibodies, a depletion of T4 cells results in immunosuppression, which results in OIs.

2. CD4 is a receptor protein (antigen) secreted by certain cells of the immune system, for example, monocytes, macrophages, and T4 helper cells. It becomes located on the exterior of the cellular membrane and happens to be a compatible receptor for the HIV to attach and infect the CD4-carrying cell.

3. The question of true latency after HIV infection has not been settled. Most HIV/AIDS investigators currently believe there is a latent period, a time of few if any clinical symptoms and low levels of HIV in the blood. Other scientists, currently the minority, believe there is no true latency. The virus hides out in the lymph nodes, slowly reproducing, and slowly killing off the T4 cells. The virus is always present, increasing slowly in numbers over time.

4. True

5. False

6. True

7. False

8. False

9. True

10. False

11. True

12. True

13. True

14. B, assessing risk of disease progression.

15. CD4, macrophage, monocytes.

16. C, CTL, or killer T cells

CHAPTER 6

1. OIs are caused by organisms that are normally within the body and held in check by an active immune system. When the immune system becomes suppressed, for whatever reason, these agents can multiply and produce disease.

2. *Pneumocystis jiroveci;* lungs, pneumonia

3. *Isospora belli*

4. *Mycobacterium avium intracellulare*

5. False. HIV has not been found in KS tissue. KS is believed to develop as a result of a suppressed immune system and not the virus *per se.*

6. Classic KS, as described by Moritz Kaposi; and KS associated with AIDS

7. False. KS normally affects gay males. It is highly unusual to find KS in hemophiliacs, injection-drug users, and female AIDS patients.

8. True

9. True

10. True (Answer provided in POI 6.1)

CHAPTER 7

1. The 6-stage Walter Reed System and the 4-group CDC system

2. About 30%; about 90%

3. AIDS Dementia Complex

4. Skin—Kaposi's sarcoma

Eyes—CMV retinitis

Mouth—thrush or hairy leukoplakia

Lungs—*Pneumocystis* pneumonia

Intestines—diarrhea

5. True

6. False. The average time is 6 to 18 weeks.

7. False. HIV infection leads to HIV disease. AIDS is the result of a weakened immune system that allows opportunistic infections to occur.

8. False. The average length of time is about 10 to 11 years.

9. Instructor's evaluation

10. E, all of the above.

11. D, any of the above.

12. D, blindness.

13. E, all of the above.

14. False

CHAPTER 8

1. False. The United States currently *reports* most of the world's AIDS cases.

2. Cases of AIDS-related death, according to the CDC definition, can be traced back to 1952 in the United States and to the mid-1950s in Africa.

3. HIV-1 and HIV-2 show a 40% to 50% genetic relationship to each other.

4. False. HIV-1 and HIV-2 are both transmitted via the same routes. HIV-2 is spreading globally in similar fashion to HIV-1.

5. True. All scientific and empirical evidence to date indicates that HIV is *not* casually transmitted.

6. Through sexual activities: exchange of certain body fluids—blood and blood products, semen, and vaginal secretions; and from mother to fetus or newborn by breast milk.

7. False. There is only one documented case of HIV infection caused by deep kissing. HIV has been found in the saliva of infected people in very low concentration, and saliva has been shown to have anti-HIV properties.

8. True; but this assertion has been proven to be untrue. Insects, in particular mosquitoes, have not been shown to transmit HIV successfully.

9. False. According to studies involving the sexual partners of injection-drug users and hemophiliacs, HIV transmission from male to female is the more efficient route. This is believed to be due to a greater concentra-

tion of HIV found in semen than in vaginal fluid.

10. The answer may be true or false. There have been cases in which a single act of intercourse has resulted in HIV infection. However, the majority of surveys on the sexual partners of injection-drug users and hemophiliacs indicate that the number of sexual encounters may increase the risk of HIV infection but does not guarantee infection. Sexual partners of infected people have remained HIV-free after years of unprotected penis-vagina or penis-anus intercourse.

11. The percentage of fetal risk varies widely in a number of hospital studies. At the moment, the risk as reported without zidovudine therapy varies from less than 30%. For Africa the figures most commonly used are 30% to 50%. With the use of zidovudine therapy, the risk has been cut to about 8%. Using zidovudine and a cesarean section reduces HIV transmission to about 2%.

12. E, all of the above.

13. True	**19.** True
14. True	**20.** True
15. True	**21.** False
16. True	**22.** True
17. True	**23.** True
18. False	**24.** True

25. B, mosquito bites.

26. False

27. D, none of the above.

28. True

29. B, sweat.

30. They can transmit HIV without knowing they are infected.

CHAPTER 9

1. Latex condoms. They are known to stop the transmission of viruses. This may not be true for animal intestine condoms.

2. Water-based lubricants. Oil-based lubricants weaken the latex rubber, causing the condom to leak or break under stress.

3. Safer sex is having sexual intercourse with an *uninfected* partner while using a condom.

4. The answer may be true or false. There have been cases where a single act of intercourse resulted in HIV infection. However, the majority of surveys completed by sexual partners of injection-drug users and hemophiliacs indicate that the number of sexual encounters may increase the risk of HIV infection but does not guarantee infection. Sexual partners of infected persons have remained HIV-free after years of unprotected penis-vagina intercourse.

5. No. IDUs exist between "fixes." They lose things, they may not care to pick up new equipment—they need the "fix" now, it may be easier to share. Circumstances vary considerably among the IDUs. Just giving them free equipment is no assurance that they will use it.

6. Between 1 in 39,000 and 1 in 200,000.

7. Have several students read their answers for promoting class discussion. Compare their response to that given in the text (that they should be punished).

8. Because attenuated HIV may mutate to a virulent form, causing an HIV infection; there is no absolute guarantee that 100% of HIV are inactivated.

9. Because at no time will a whole HIV be present in the vaccine. Only a specific subunit of the HIV will be present in pure form, so the vaccine should be free of any contaminating proteins that might prove toxic to one or more persons receiving the vaccine.

10. Universal precautions are a list of rules and regulations provided by the CDC to help prevent HIV and other blood-borne diseases in healthcare workers.

11. False

12. True

13. True

14. True

15. False

16. False

17. False, 1998

18. Instructor evaluation

19. True

20. False

21. False

22. False

CHAPTER 10

1. B, 1959.

2. Because their social and sexual behaviors and medical needs place some people at a greater risk for HIV exposure than those not practicing these behaviors or who do not need blood or blood products.

3. False. Studies show that the time for progression from HIV infection to AIDS is about the same regardless of parameters.

4. 52%

5. Two per 1000 students; more: the rate for military personnel is 1.4 per 1000.

6. College students 2/1000, general population 0.2/1000; this means the rate of HIV infection on college campuses is about 10 times higher than in the general population.

7. One in 250 to 300

8. Needle stick injuries

9. Hepatitis B virus

10. Worldwide about 30 million, United States about 665,000.

11. 48%; $\dfrac{665,000}{1,410,000}$ (47%)

12. About 38 million.

13. About 2.5 million.

14. No. The use of HAART is slowing the progression to AIDS in the HIV infected.

15. (1) Men who have sex with men (MSM)

CHAPTER 11

1. Approximately 19 million women and 19 million men

2. About 52%

3. Injection-drug use, being a sexual partner of an IDU, and through heterosexual contact.

4. IDU

5. 1 million; about 1 million

6. Leading; 25 and 34; fifth; all; 25 and 44; second leading; 25 to 44

7. An estimated 6000

8. None, all states now have reported pediatric cases.

9. Virtually all—100%

10. (1) Maternal viral load; (2) route of delivery, and (3) duration of early membrane rupture.

11. Most orphaned AIDS children have mothers who are IDUs and are themselves HIV infected. They are AIDS orphans because (1) their parents abandon them due to illness or death, and (2) these children are HIV infected or demonstrate AIDS and therefore no one wants them.

12. A

13. B

14. D

15. A

16. True

17. False

CHAPTER 12

1. 2

2. Over 50%

3. 12.5 million

4. About 50%

5. 77%, 39%, 28%, 70%

6. 70%

7. Having sex after school and before our parents come home.

8. Engaging in sexual activity without the knowledge of safer sex choices.

9. About 2 billion.

10. 85%

11. 29 million

12. About 40%

13. 13 to 24

14. 20

15. True

CHAPTER 13

1. ELISA; enzyme linked immunosorbent assay

2. That the body will produce antibody against antigenic components of the HIV virus after infection occurs.

3. No; a positive antibody result must be repeated in duplicate and if still positive, a confirmatory test is performed prior to telling people they are HIV infected.

4. No; AIDS is medically diagnosed after certain signs and symptoms of specific diseases occur.

5. Western Blot

6. Indirect immunofluorescent assay

7. By a color change in the reaction tube; the peroxidase enzyme oxidizes a clear chromogen into color formation. This occurs if the HIV antibody–antigen enzyme complex is present in the reaction tube.

8. False. Some newborns receive the HIV antibody passively during pregnancy. About 30% to 50% of HIV-positive newborns are truly HIV positive; it is unknown whether all HIV-positive newborns go on to develop AIDS. Not all have been discovered, and it has not been determined whether 100% of HIV-infected adults or babies will develop AIDS.

9. They are not 100% accurate.

10. Determining that positive and negative tests are truly positive and negative and not falsely positive or negative.

11. Using excessively high or low cut-off points in the spectrophotometer, and the presence of cross-reacting antibodies.

12. The percentage of false positives will increase as the prevalence of HIV-infected people in a population decreases.

13. It is a screening test value that represents the probability that a positive HIV test is truly positive; because screening tests are not 100% accurate.

14. Western Blot

15. There is no standardized WB test interpretation. Different agencies use different WB results (reactive bands) to determine that the test sample is positive.

16. Because the PCR allows for the detection of proviral DNA in cells before the body produces detectable HIV antibody; PCR reactions can be used to determine if high-risk (or anybody), antibody-negative people are HIV infected but not producing antibodies and whether newborns are truly HIV positive or passively HIV positive.

17. 20 minutes

18. False. The FDA approved two home-use HIV antibody test kits in 1996, but one was withdrawn from the market.

19. Between 6 and 18 weeks after HIV infection.

20. As early as two weeks after infection.

21. (1) Changes in their lifestyles that reduce stress on their immune systems may delay the onset of illness.

(2) They can practice safer sex and hopefully not transmit the virus to others.

(3) The earlier the detection, the earlier they can enter into preventive therapy.

22. Mandatory with confidentiality; voluntary with confidentiality, anonymous, and blinded.

23. For anonymous testing no personal information is given; in blind tests, the name is deleted but the demographic data remain.

24. Because there are many examples of breaches of confidence, which destroys trust and subjects people to social stigma.

25. False

26. True

CHAPTER 14

1. Newspapers, TV, radio, magazines, etc.

2. Barring children from public schools, police wearing rubber gloves during arrests, not going to a restaurant because someone who works there has AIDS, firing AIDS employees, etc.

3. Syphilis

4. Use of tobacco products, alcohol, drugs; nonuse of seat belts and motorcycle helmets, etc.

5. The ways by which one can become HIV infected and how not to become HIV infected.

6. Because most of the new cases of HIV infection and AIDS occur in high-risk groups that will not or cannot change sexual and drug practices.

7. Because a larger percentage of young adults are sexually active with more than one partner, use drugs, use alcohol, and think they are invulnerable to infection and death.

8. According to the AMA, no. Physicians may not refuse to care for patients with AIDS because of actual risk or fear of contracting the disease.

9. The CDC and AMA state that a patient's right to that information should be determined on a case-by-case basis where surgery will be performed. There is no legal requirement for physicians to tell their patients of their HIV status.

10. Worker information sessions that explain how the virus can and cannot be transmitted.

11. Ban Ki-moon; about $22.1 billion

12. About $16 billion.

13. Review students' evidence—share with class.

14. $398.5 billion dollars

15. $960 million dollars; 3%

Glossary

ACRONYMS

ACTG   AIDS Clinical Trial Group

ADA   Americans with Disabilities Act

AIDS   Acquired Immune Deficiency Syndrome

AZT   Azathioprine (a misnomer for zidovudine or azidothymidine)

CD   Cluster Differentiating Antigen

CD4   a protein embedded on the surface of a T lymphocyte to which HIV most often binds—a CD4+ or T4 cell

CD8   a protein embedded on the surface of a T lymphocyte suppressor cell—a T8 cell

CDC   Centers for Disease Control and Prevention (part of PHS)

DHHS   Department of Health and Human Services

DNA   deoxyribonucleic acid

d4T   stavudine; nucleoside analog

ddC   dideoxycytosine; nucleoside analog

ddl   dideoxyinosine; nucleoside analog

FDA   Food and Drug Administration (part of PHS)

HAART   Highly Active Antiretroviral Therapy

HIV   Human Immunodeficiency Virus

IDU   injection-drug user

LAV   lymphadenopathy-associated virus

NCI   National Cancer Institute (part of NIH)

NIAID   National Institute of Allergy and Infectious Diseases (part of NIH)

NIH   National Institutes of Health (part of PHS)

NNRTI   Non-nucleoside reverse transcriptase inhibitor

PCR (polymerase chain reaction)   a very sensitive test used to detect the presence of HIV

PHS   Public Health Service (part of DHHS)

PLWA   Person Living With AIDS

RNA   ribonucleic acid

3TC   lamivudine; nucleoside analog

ZDV   zidovudine; major drug in treating HIV/AIDS; nucleoside analog

For the newest anti-HIV drugs, names, and use, see Chapter 4.

TERMS

Acquired Immune Deficiency Syndrome (AIDS): A life-threatening syndrome caused by a virus and characterized by the breakdown of the body's immune defenses. (See AIDS.)

Acute: Sudden onset, short-term with severe symptoms.

Acyclovir (Zovirax):   Antiviral drug for herpes 1 and 2 and herpes zoster.

Adjuvant: The active ingredient in vaccines that improves the human immune system response by attracting immune cells into the region where the vaccine is injected.

AIDS (Acquired Immune Deficiency Syndrome): A disease caused by a retrovirus called HIV and characterized by a deficiency of the immune system. The primary defect in AIDS is an acquired, persistent, quantitative functional depression within the T4 subset of lymphocytes. This depression often leads to infections caused by opportunistic microorganisms in HIV-infected individuals. A rare type of cancer (Kaposi's sarcoma) usually seen in elderly men or in individuals who are severely immunocompromised may also occur.

AIDS dementia: Neurological complications accompanying AIDS and affecting thinking and behavior; intellectual impairment.

AIDSVAX: Trade name for all formulations of VAXGEN's vaccine.

Analog (analogue):   A chemical molecule that closely resembles another one but that functions differently, thus altering a natural process.

Anal sex: A type of sexual intercourse in which a man inserts his penis in his partner's anus. Anal sex can be insertive or receptive.

Anemia: Low number of red blood cells.

Antibiotic: A chemical substance capable of destroying bacteria and other microorganisms.

Antibody: A blood protein produced by mammals in response to a specific antigen.

Antigen: A large molecule, usually a protein or carbohydrate, which when introduced into the body stimulates the production of an antibody that will react specifically with that antigen.

Antigenemia: Presence of viral proteins (antigens).

Antigen-presenting cells: B cells, cells of the monocyte lineage (including macrophages and dentritic cells), and various other body cells that present antigen in a form that T cells can recognize.

Antiretroviral therapy: Treatment with drugs designed to prevent HIV from replicating in HIV-infected persons. Highly active antiretroviral therapy (HAART) is an antiretroviral regimen that includes multiple classifications of antiretroviral drugs.

Antiserum: Serum portion of the blood that carries the antibodies.

Antiviral: Means against virus; drugs that destroy or weaken virus.

Apoptosis: Cellular suicide, also known as programmed cell death. A possible mechanism used by HIV to suppress the immune system. HIV may cause apoptosis in both HIV-infected and HIV-uninfected immune system cells.

Asymptomatic carrier: A host that is infected by an organism but does not demonstrate clinical signs or symptoms of the disease.

Asymptomatic seropositive: HIV positive without signs or symptoms of HIV disease.

Attenuated: Weakened. *See* Live or attenuated vaccine.

Atypical: Irregular; not of typical character.

Autoimmunity: Antibodies made against self tissues.

B and T cell lymphomas: Cancers caused by proliferation of the two principal types of white blood cells—B and T lymphocytes.

B lymphocytes or B cells: Lymphocytes that produce antibodies. B lymphocytes proliferate under stimulation from factors released by T lymphocytes.

Bacterium: A microscopic organism composed of a single cell. Many but not all bacteria cause disease.

Blood count: A count of the number of red and white blood cells and platelets.

Bone marrow: Soft tissue located in the cavities of the bones. The bone marrow is the source of all blood cells.

Canarypox: A virus that infects birds and is used as a live vector for HIV vaccines. It can carry a large quantity of foreign genes. Canarypox virus cannot grow in human cells, an important safety feature.

Cancer: A large group of diseases characterized by uncontrolled growth and spread of abnormal cells.

Candida albicans: A fungus; the causative agent of vulvo-vaginal candidiasis or yeast infection.

Candidiasis: A fungal infection of the mucous membranes (commonly occurring in the mouth, where it is known as thrush) characterized by whitish spots and/or a burning or painful sensation. It may also occur in the esophagus. It can also cause a red and itchy rash in moist areas, for example, the vagina.

Capsid: The protein coat of a virus particle.

CC-CKR-5 (CKR-5): Receptor for human chemokines and a necessary receptor for HIV entrance into a macrophage.

CD: Cluster differentiating-type antigens found on T lymphocytes. Each CD is assigned a number: CD1, CD2, etc.

CD4 (T4 cell): White blood cell with type 4 protein embedded in the cell surface—target cell for HIV infection.

CD8 cell: Suppressor white blood cell with type 8 protein embedded in the cell surface.

Cell-mediated immunity: The reaction to antigenic material by specific defensive cells (macrophages) rather than antibodies.

Cellular immunity: A collection of cell types that provide protection against various antigens.

Chain of infection: A series of infections that are directly or immediately connected to a particular source.

Chemokines: Chemicals released by T cell lymphocytes and other cells of the immune system to attract a variety of cell types to sites of inflammation.

Chemotherapy: The use of chemicals that have a specific and toxic effect upon a disease-causing pathogen.

Chlamydia: A species of bacterium, the causative organism of *Lymphogranuloma venereum,* chlamydial urethritis, and most cases of newborn conjunctivitis.

Chromosomes: Physical structures in the cell's nucleus that house the genes. Each human cell has 22 pairs of autosomes and two sex chromosomes.

Chronic: Having a long and relatively mild course.

Clade: Related HIV variants classified by degree of genetic similarity; nine are known for HIV.

Cleavage site: One of nine sites (peptide bond) within the *gag-pol* polyprotein (peptide precursor) that is cleaved by HIV-1 protease to form functional subunits of GAG (p17, p7, p24) and POL (protease, reverse transcriptase, integrase).

Clinical latency: Infectious agent developing in a host without producing clinical symptoms.

Clinical manifestations: The signs of a disease as they pertain to or are observed in patients.

CMV: *See* Cytomegalovirus.

Cofactor: Factors or agents that are necessary or that increase the probability of the development of disease in the presence of the basic etiologic agent of that disease.

Cohort: A group of individuals with some characteristics in common.

Communicable: Able to spread from one diseased person or animal to another, either directly or indirectly.

Condylomata acuminatum (venereal warts): Viral warts of the genital and anogenital area.

Confidential HIV test: An HIV test for which a record of the test and the test results are recorded in the client's chart.

Confirmatory test: A highly specific test designed to confirm the results of an earlier (screening) test. For HIV testing, a Western Blot or, less commonly, an immunofluorescence assay (IFA) is used as a confirmatory test.

Congenital: Acquired by the newborn before or at the time of birth.

Core proteins: Proteins that make up the internal structure or core of a virus.

Cross-resistance: Development of resistance to one agent as an antibiotic, which results in resistance to other, usually similar agents.

Cryptococcal meningitis: A fungal infection that affects the three membranes (meninges) surrounding the brain and spinal cord. Symptoms include severe headache, vertigo, nausea, anorexia, sight disorders, and mental deterioration.

Cryptococcosis: A fungal infectious disease often found in the lungs of AIDS patients. It characteristically spreads to the meninges and may also spread to the kidneys and skin. It is due to the fungus *Cryptococcus neoformans.*

Cryptosporidiosis: An infection caused by a protozoan parasite found in the intestines of animals. Acquired in some people by direct contact with the infected animal, it lodges in the intestines and causes severe diarrhea. It may be transmitted from person to person. This infection seems to be occurring more frequently in immunosuppressed people and can lead to prolonged symptoms that do not respond to medication.

Cutaneous: Having to do with the skin.

CXCR-4 (FUSIN): Receptor for human chemokines and a necessary receptor for HIV entrance into T4 cells.

Cytokines: Powerful chemical substances secreted by cells. Cytokines include lymphokines produced by lymphocytes and monokines produced by monocytes and macrophages.

Cytomegalovirus (CMV): One of a group of highly host-specific herpesviruses that affect humans and other animals. Generally produces mild flu-like symptoms but can be more severe. In the immunosuppressed, it may cause pneumonia.

Cytopathic: Pertaining to or characterized by abnormal changes in cells.

Cytotoxic: Poisonous to cells.

Cytotoxic T cells: A subset of T lymphocytes that carry the T8 marker and can kill body cells infected by viruses or transformed by cancer.

Dementia: Chronic mental deterioration sufficient to significantly impair social and/or occupational function. Usually patients have memory and abstract thinking loss.

Dendritic cells: White blood cells found in the spleen and other lymphoid organs. Dendritic cells typically use threadlike tentacles to "hold" the antigen, which they present to T cells.

Didanosine: Also known as Videx; see ddI—inhibits HIV replication.

Dissemination: Spread of disease throughout the body.

DNA (deoxyribonucleic acid):   A linear polymer, made up of deoxyribonucleotide repeating units. It is the carrier of genetic information in living organisms and some viruses.

DNA vaccine (nucleic acid vaccine):   Direct injection of a gene(s) coding for a specific antigenic protein(s), resulting in direct production of such antigen(s) within the vaccine recipient in order to trigger an appropriate immune response.

DNA viruses: Contain DNA as their genetic material.

Dysentery: Inflammation of the intestines, especially the colon, producing pain in the abdomen and diarrhea containing blood and mucus.

Efficacy: Effectiveness.

ELISA (enzyme-linked immunosorbent assay) test: A blood test that indicates the presence of antibodies to a given antigen. Various ELISA tests are used to detect a variety of infections. The HIV ELISA test does not detect AIDS but only indicates if viral infection has occurred.

Endemic: Prevalent in or peculiar to a community or group of people.

Enteric infections: Infections of the intestine.

ENV: HIV gene that codes for protein gp160.

Envelope proteins: Proteins that comprise the envelope or surface of a virus, gp120 and gp41.

Enzyme: A catalytic protein that is produced by living cells and promotes the chemical processes of life without itself being altered or destroyed.

Epidemic: Affecting many persons at once, outbreak or rapid, sudden growth or development.

Epidemiology: Science that deals with the incidence, distribution, and control of disease in a population.

Epitope: A specific site on an antigen that stimulates specific immune responses, such as the production of antibodies or activation of immune cells.

Epivir: *See* 3TC.

Epstein–Barr virus (EBV):   A virus that causes infectious mononucleosis. It is spread by saliva. EBV lies dormant in the lymph glands and has been associated with Burkitt's lymphoma, a cancer of the lymph tissue.

Etiologic agent: The organism that causes a disease.

Etiology: The study of the cause of disease.

Extracellular: Found outside the cell wall.

Factor VIII: A naturally occurring protein in plasma that aids in the coagulation of blood. A congenital deficiency of Factor VIII results in the bleeding disorder known as hemophilia A.

Factor VIII concentrate: A concentrated preparation of Factor VIII that is used in the treatment of individuals with hemophilia A.

False negative: Failure of a test to demonstrate the disease or condition when present.

False positive: A positive test result caused by a disease or condition other than the disease for which the test is designed.

Fellatio: Oral sex involving the penis.

Fitness: The ability of an individual virus to replicate successfully under defined conditions.

Follicular dendritic cells: Found in germinal centers of lymphoid organs.

Fomite: An inanimate object that can hold infectious agents and transfers them from one individual to another.

Fortovase: A more easily assimilated form of saquinavir.

Fulminant: Characterized by rapid onset, severe.

Fungus: Member of a class of relatively primitive organisms. Fungi include mushrooms, yeasts, rusts, molds, and smuts.

FUSIN: *See* CXCR-4.

Gamma globulin: The antibody component of the serum.

Ganciclovir (DHPG):   An experimental antiviral drug used in the treatment of CMV retinitis.

Gene: The basic unit of heredity; an ordered sequence of nucleotides. A gene contains the information for the synthesis of one polypeptide chain (protein).

Gene expression: The production of RNA and cellular proteins.

Genitourinary: Pertaining to the urinary and reproductive structures; sometimes called the GU tract or system.

Genome: A complete set of genes in a cell or virus.

Genotype: The sequence of nucleotide bases that constitutes a gene.

Globulin: That portion of serum that contains the antibodies.

Glycoproteins: Proteins with carbohydrate groups attached at specific locations.

Gonococcus: The specific etiologic agent of gonorrhea discovered by Neisser and named *Neisseria gonorrhoeae*.

gp41: Glycoprotein found in envelope of HIV.

gp120: Glycoprotein found in outer level of HIV envelope.

gp160: Precursor glycoprotein to forming gp41 and gp120.

Granulocytes: Phagocytic white blood cells filled with granules containing potent chemicals that allow the cells to digest microorganisms. Neutrophils, eosinophils, basophils, and mast cells are examples of granulocytes.

Hemoglobin: The oxygen-carrying portion of red blood cells that gives them a red color.

Hemophilia: A hereditary bleeding disorder caused by a deficiency in the ability to synthesize one or more of the blood coagulation proteins, for example, Factor VIII (hemophilia A) or Factor IX (hemophilia B).

Hepatitis: Inflammation of the liver; due to many causes including viruses, several of which are transmissible through blood transfusions and sexual activities.

Hepatosplenomegaly: Enlargement of the liver and spleen.

Herpes simplex virus I (HSV-I): A virus that results in cold sores or fever blisters, most often on the mouth or around the eyes. Like all herpesviruses, it may lie dormant for months or years in nerve tissues and flare up in times of stress, trauma, infection, or immunosuppression. There is no cure for any of the herpesviruses.

Herpes simplex virus II (HSV-II): Causes painful sores on the genitals or anus. It is one of the most common sexually transmitted diseases in the United States.

Herpes zoster virus (HVZ): The varicella virus causes chicken pox in children and may reappear in adulthood as herpes zoster. Herpes zoster, also called shingles, is characterized by small, painful blisters on the skin along nerve pathways.

Histoplasmosis: A disease caused by a fungal infection that can affect all the organs of the body. Symptoms usually include fever, shortness of breath, cough, weight loss, and physical exhaustion.

HIV (Human Immunodeficiency Virus): A newly discovered retrovirus that is said to cause AIDS. The target organ of HIV is the T4 or CD4 subset of T lymphocytes, which regulate the immune system.

HIV positive: Presence of the human immunodeficiency virus in the body.

Homophobia: Negative bias toward or fear of individuals who are homosexual.

Human leukocyte antigens (HLA): Protein markers of self used in histocompatibility testing. Some HLA types also correlate with certain autoimmune diseases.

Humoral immunity: The production of antibodies for defense against infection or disease.

Immunity: Resistance to a disease because of a functioning immune system.

Immune complex: A cluster of interlocking antigens and antibodies.

Immune response: The reaction of the immune system to foreign substances.

Immune status: The state of the body's natural defense to diseases. It is influenced by heredity, age, past illness history, diet, and physical and mental health. It includes production of circulating and local antibodies and their mechanism of action.

Immunoassay: The use of antibodies to identify and quantify substances. Often the antibody is linked to a marker such as a fluorescent molecule, a radioactive molecule, or an enzyme.

Immunocompetent: Capable of developing an immune response.

Immunoglobulins: A family of large protein molecules, also known as antibodies.

Immunostimulant: Any agent that will trigger a body's defenses.

Immunosuppression: When the immune system is not working normally. This can be the result of illness or certain drugs (commonly those used to fight cancer).

Incidence: The total number of new cases of a disease in a defined population within a specified time, usually one year.

Incubation period: The time between the actual entry of an infectious agent into the body and the onset of disease symptoms.

Indeterminate test result: A possible result of a Western Blot, which might represent a recent HIV infection or a false positive.

Indinavir: Crixivan, a protease inhibitor drug.

Infection: Invasion of the body by viruses or other organisms.

Infectious disease: A disease that is caused by microorganisms or viruses living in or on the body as parasites.

Inflammatory response: Redness, warmth, and swelling in response to infection; the result of increased blood flow and a gathering of immune cells and secretions.

Injection–drug use: Use of drugs injected by needle into a vein or muscle tissue.

Innate immunity: Inborn or hereditary immunity.

Inoculation: The entry of an infectious organism or virus into the body.

Integrase: HIV enzyme used to insert HIV DNA into host cell DNA.

Interferon: A class of glycoproteins important in immune function and thought to inhibit viral infection.

Interleukins: Chemical messengers that travel from leukocytes to other white blood cells. Some promote cell development; others promote rapid cell division.

Intracellular: Found within the cell wall.

In utero: In the uterus.

In vitro: "In glass"—pertains to a biological reaction in an artificial medium.

In vivo: "In the living"—pertains to a biological reaction in a living organism.

IV: Intravenous.

Kaposi's sarcoma: A multifocal, spreading cancer of connective tissue, principally involving the skin; it usually begins on the toes or the feet as reddish blue or brownish soft nodules and tumors.

Lamivudine: Nucleoside analog; inhibits HIV replication.

Langerhans cells: Dendritic cells in the skin that pick up antigen and transport it to lymph nodes.

Latency: A period when a virus or other organism is in the body but in an inactive state.

Latent viral infection: The virion becomes part of the host cell's DNA.

Lentiviruses: Viruses that cause disease very slowly. HIV is believed to be this type of virus.

Lesion: Any abnormal change in tissue due to disease or injury.

Leukocyte: A white blood cell.

Leukopenia: A decrease in the white blood cell count.

Live or attenuated vaccine: A vaccine in which an active virus is weakened through chemical or physical processes in order to produce an immune response without causing the severe effects of the disease. Attenuated vaccines currently licensed in the United States include measles, mumps, rubella, polio, yellow fever, and varicella.

Live-vector vaccine: A vaccine that uses a non-disease-causing organism (virus or bacterium) to transport HIV or other foreign genes into the body, thereby stimulating an effective immune response to the foreign products. This type of vaccine is important because it is particularly capable of inducing cytotoxic leukocyte activity. Examples of organisms used as live vectors in HIV vaccines are canarypox and vaccinia.

Log: 10-fold difference.

Lymph: A transparent, slightly yellow fluid that carries lymphocytes, bathes the body tissues, and drains into the lymphatic vessels.

Lymphadenopathy: Enlargement of the lymph nodes.

Lymphadenopathy syndrome (LAS): A condition characterized by persistent, generalized, enlarged lymph nodes, sometimes with signs of minor illness such as fever and weight loss, which apparently represents a milder reaction to HIV infection.

Lymphatic system: A fluid system of vessels and glands that is important in controlling infections and limiting their spread.

Lymph nodes: Gland-like structures in the lymphatic system that help to prevent spread of infection.

Lymphocytes: Specialized white blood cells involved in the immune response.

Lymphoid organs: The organs of the immune system where lymphocytes develop and congregate. They include the bone marrow, thymus, lymph nodes, spleen, and other clusters of lymphoid tissue.

Lymphokines: Chemical messengers produced by T and B lymphocytes. They have a variety of protective functions.

Lymphoma: Tumor of lymphoid tissue, usually malignant.

Lymphosarcoma: A general term applied to malignant neoplastic disorders of lymphoid tissue, not including Hodgkin's disease.

Lytic infection: When a virus infects the cell, the cell produces new viruses and breaks open (lyses), releasing the viruses.

Macrophage: A large and versatile immune cell that acts as a microbe-devouring phagocyte, an antigen-presenting cell, and an important source of immune secretions.

Major histocompatibility complex (MHC): A group of genes that controls several aspects of the immune response. MHC genes code for self markers on all body cells.

Malaise: A general feeling of discomfort or fatigue.

Malignant tumor: A tumor made up of cancerous cells. The tumors grow and invade surrounding tissue, then the cells break away and grow elsewhere.

Messenger RNA (mRNA): RNA that serves as the template for protein synthesis; it carries the information from the DNA to the protein synthesizing complex to direct protein synthesis.

Microbes: Minute living organisms including bacteria, viruses, fungi, and protozoa.

Microorganisms: Microscopic plants or animals.

Molecule: The smallest amount of a specific chemical substance that can exist alone. To break a molecule down into its constituent atoms is to change its character. A molecule of water, for instance, reverts to oxygen and hydrogen.

Monoclonal antibody: Custom-made, identical antibody that recognizes only one epitope.

Monocyte: A large, phagocytic white blood cell which, when it enters tissue, develops into a macrophage.

Monokines: Powerful chemical substances secreted by monocytes and macrophages. They help direct and regulate the immune response.

Morbidity: The proportion of people with a disease in a community.

Morphology: The study of the form and structure of organisms.

Mortality: The number of people who die as a result of a specific cause.

Mucosal immunity: Resistance to infection across mucous membranes.

Mucous membrane: The lining of the canals and cavities of the body that communicate with external air, such as the intestinal tract, respiratory tract, and genitourinary tract.

Mucous patches: White, patchy growths, usually found in the mouth, that are symptoms of secondary syphilis and are highly infectious.

Mucous: A fluid secreted by membranes.

Mutant: A new strain of a virus or microorganism that arises as a result of change in the genes of an existing strain.

Natural killer cells (also called NK cells): Immune cells that kill infected cells directly within four hours of contact. NK cells differ from other killer cells, such as cytotoxic T lymphocytes, in that they do not require contact with antigen before they are activated.

Neisseria gonorrhoeae: The bacterium that causes gonorrhea.

Neonatal: Pertaining to the first four weeks of life.

Neoplasm: A new abnormal growth, such as a tumor.

Neuropathy: Group of nerve disorders—symptoms range from tingling sensation and numbness to paralysis.

Neutralizing antibody: The kind of antibody that prevents a virus from entering a cell. It is hoped that a vaccine will produce neutralizing antibody because if HIV is prevented from entering cells, it cannot replicate and dies in the bloodstream within a few hours.

Nevirapine: Non-nucleoside analog inhibits HIV replication.

Notifiable disease: A notifiable disease is one that, when diagnosed, health providers are required, usually by law, to report to state or local public health officials. Notifiable diseases are those of public interest by reason of their contagiousness, severity, or frequency.

Nucleic acids: Large, naturally occurring molecules composed of chemical building blocks known as nucleotides. There are two kinds of nucleic acid, DNA and RNA.

Nucleoside analog: Synthetic compounds generally similar to one of the bases of DNA.

Nucleotide of DNA: Made up of one of four nitrogen-containing bases (adenine, cytosine, guanine, or thymine), a sugar, and a phosphate molecule.

Oncogenic: Anything that may give rise to tumors, especially malignant ones.

Opportunistic infection: Infection caused by normally benign microorganisms or viruses that become pathogenic when the immune system is impaired.

p24 antigen: A protein fragment of HIV. The p24 antigen test measures this fragment. A positive test result suggests active HIV replication and may mean the individual has a chance of developing AIDS in the near future.

Pandemic: Occurring over a wide geographic area and affecting a high proportion of the population.

Parenteral: Not taken in through the digestive system or lungs (intravenous, intramuscular, subcutaneous).

Parasite: A plant or animal that lives, grows, and feeds on another living organism.

Pathogen: Any disease-producing microorganism or substance.

Pathogenic: Giving rise to disease or causing symptoms of an illness.

Pathogenicity: Capable of causing a disease.

Pathology: The science of the essential nature of diseases, especially of the structural and functional changes in tissues and organs caused by disease.

Perianal glands: Glands located around the anus.

Perinatal: Occurring in the period during or just after birth.

Pestilence: A virulent, devastating contagious disease that is caused by a bacterium, for example, *Yersina pestis,* which causes the plague.

Phagocytes: Large white blood cells that contribute to the immune defense by ingesting microbes or other cells and foreign particles.

Phenotype: A defined behavior; specifically drug susceptibility with regard to HIV drug resistance.

PID (pelvic inflammatory disease): Inflammation of the female pelvic organs; often the result of gonococcal or chlamydial infection.

Placebo: An inactive substance against which investigational treatments are compared to see how well the treatment worked.

Plague: A calamity; an epidemic of disease causing a high rate of mortality.

Plasma: The fluid portion of the blood that contains all the chemical constituents of whole blood except the cells.

Plasma cells: Derived from B cells, they produce antibodies.

Platelets: Small oval discs in blood that are necessary for blood to clot.

PLWA: Person Living With AIDS.

***Pneumocystis carinii* pneumonia (PCP):** A rare type of pneumonia primarily found in infants and now common in patients with AIDS.

Polymerase chain reaction: Method to detect and amplify very small amounts of DNA in a sample.

Positive HIV test: A sample of blood that is reactive on an initial ELISA test, reactive on a second ELISA run of the same specimen, and reactive on Western Blot, if available.

Prenatal: During pregnancy.

Prevalence: The total number or percentage of cases of a disease existing at any time in a given area.

Primary immune response: Production of antibodies about 7 to 10 days after an infection.

Prime-boost: In HIV vaccine research, administration of one type of vaccine, such as a live-vector vaccine, followed by or together with a second type of vaccine, such as a recombinant subunit vaccine. The intent of this combination regimen is to induce different types of immune responses and enhance the overall immune response, a result that may not occur if only one type of vaccine were to be given for all doses.

Prophylactic treatment: Medical treatment of patients exposed to a disease before the appearance of disease symptoms.

Protease: Enzyme that cuts proteins into peptides (breaks down proteins).

Protease inhibitors: Compounds that inhibit the action of protease.

Proteins: Organic compounds made up of amino acids. Proteins are one of the major constituents of plant and animal cells.

Protocol: Standardization of procedures so that results of treatment or experiments can be compared.

Protozoa: A group of one-celled animals, some of which cause human disease including malaria, sleeping sickness, and diarrhea.

Provirus: The genome of an animal virus integrated into the chromosome of the host cell, and thereby replicated in all the host's daughter cells.

Quasispecies: A complex mixture of genetic variants of an RNA virus.

Race: Beginning in 1976 the federal government's data systems classified individuals into the following racial groups: American Indian or Alaskan Native, Asian or Pacific Islander, black, and white.

Rapid result HIV test: A test to detect antibodies to HIV that can be collected and processed within a short interval of time (approximately 3–30 minutes).

Rate: A rate is a measure of some event, disease, or condition in relation to a unit of population, along with some specification of time.

Receptors: Special molecules located on the surface membranes of cells that attract other molecules to attach to them (for example, CD4, CD8, and CCCKR-5).

Recombinant DNA: DNA produced by joining pieces of DNA from different sources.

Recombinant DNA techniques: Techniques that allow specific segments of DNA to be isolated and inserted into a bacterium or other host (like yeast or mammalian cells) in a form that will allow the DNA segment to be replicated and expressed as the cellular host multiplies.

Remission: The lessening of the severity of disease or the absence of symptoms over a period of time.

Retroviruses: Viruses that contain RNA and produce a DNA analog of their RNA using an enzyme known as reverse transcriptase.

Reverse transcriptase: An enzyme produced by retroviruses that allows them to produce a DNA analog of their RNA, which may then incorporate into the host cell.

Ritonavir: Norvir, a protease inhibitor drug.

RNA (ribonucleic acid): Any of various nucleic acids that contain ribose and uracil as structural components and are associated with the control of cellular chemical activities.

RNA viruses: Contain RNA as their genetic material.

Sarcoma: A form of cancer that occurs in connective tissue, muscle, bone, and cartilage.

Saquinavir: Invirase, a protease inhibitor drug.

Secondary immune response: On repeat exposure to an antigen, there is an accelerated production of antibodies.

Sensitivity: The probability that a test will be positive when the infection is present.

Septicemia: A disease condition in which the infectious agent has spread throughout the lymphatic and blood systems, causing a general body infection.

Seroconversion: The point at which an individual exposed to HIV has detectable antibodies to HIV in their serum.

Serologic test: Laboratory test made on serum.

Serum: The clear portion of any animal liquid separated from its more solid elements, especially the clear liquid that separates in the clotting of blood (blood serum).

Shigella: A bacterium that can cause dysentery.

Specificity: The probability that a test will be negative when the infection is not present.

Spirochete: A corkscrew-shaped bacterium; for example, *Treponema pallidum*.

Spleen: A lymphoid organ in the abdominal cavity that is an important center for immune system activities.

Squamous: Scaly or plate-like; a type of cell.

STARHS (Serologic Testing Algorithm for Recent HIV Seroconversions): HIV test to differentiate infections from older infections.

Statistical significance: The probability that an event or difference occurred as the result of the intervention (vaccine) rather than by chance alone. This probability is determined by using statistical tests to evaluate collected data.

Stavudine: Also known as Zerit; *See* d4T— inhibits HIV replication.

STD (sexually transmitted disease): Any disease that is transmitted primarily through sexual practices.

Subclinical infections: Infections with minimal or no apparent symptoms.

Subtype: Also called a clade. With respect to HIV isolates, a classification scheme based on genetic differences.

Subunit vaccine: A vaccine that uses only one component of an infectious agent rather than the whole to stimulate an immune response.

Suppressor T cells: A subset of T cells that carry the T8 marker and turn off antibody production and other immune responses.

Surrogate marker: A substitute; a person or agent that replaces another; an alternate.

Surveillance: The process of accumulating information about the incidence and prevalence of disease in an area.

Susceptible: Less likely to resist an infection or disease.

Syndrome: A set of symptoms that occur together.

Systemic: Affecting the body as a whole.

T8 cells: A subset of T cells that may kill virus-infected cells and suppress immune function when the infection is over.

T cell growth factor (TCGF, also known as interleukin-2): A glycoprotein that is released by T lymphocytes on stimulation by antigens and that functions as a T cell growth factor by inducing proliferation of activated T cells.

T helper cells (also called T4 or CD4 cells): A subset of T cells that carry the CD4 marker and are essential for turning on antibody production, activating cytotoxic T cells, and initiating many other immune responses.

T lymphocytes or T cells: Lymphocytes that mature in the thymus and that mediate cellular immune reactions. T lymphocytes also release factors that induce proliferation of T lymphocytes and B lymphocytes.

Therapeutic HIV vaccine: A vaccine designed to boost the immune response to HIV in a person already infected with the virus. Also referred to as an immunotherapeutic vaccine.

Thrush: A disease characterized by the formation of whitish spots in the mouth. It is caused by the fungus *Candida albicans* during times of immunosuppression.

Thymus: A primary lymphoid organ high in the chest where T lymphocytes proliferate and mature.

Titer: Level or amount.

Tolerance: A state of nonresponsiveness to a particular antigen or group of antigens.

Toxic reaction: A harmful side effect from a drug; it is dose dependent, that is, becomes more frequent and severe as the drug dose is increased. All drugs have toxic effects if given in a sufficiently large dose.

Toxoplasmosis: An infection with the protozoan *Taxoplasma gondii*, frequently causing focal encephalitis (inflammation of the brain). It may also involve the heart, lungs, adrenal glands, pancreas, and testes.

Transcription: The synthesis of messenger RNA on a DNA template; the resulting RNA sequence is complementary to the DNA sequence. This is the first step in gene expression.

Translation: The process by which the genetic code contained in a nucleotide sequence of messenger RNA directs the synthesis of a specific order of amino acids to produce a protein.

Treponema pallidum: The bacterial spirochete that causes syphilis.

Tropism: Involuntary turning, curving, or attraction to a source of stimulation.

Tumor: A swelling or enlargement; an abnormal mass that can be malignant or benign. It has no useful body function.

V3 loop: Section of the gp120 protein on the surface of HIV; appears to be important in stimulating neutralizing antibodies.

Vaccine: A preparation of dead organisms, attenuated live organisms, live virulent organisms, or parts of microorganisms that is administered to artificially increase immunity to a particular disease.

V.D.: Abbreviation of "venereal disease"; now referred to as "sexually transmitted disease." Contagious disease usually acquired through sexual intercourse.

Vector: The means by which a disease is carried from one human to another.

Venereal: Venus = love, sexual desire; involves the sexual organs and related to sexual pleasure; comes through contact of sexual organs.

Venereal warts: Viral *Condylomata acuminata* on or near the anus or genitals.

Viral load: The total amount of virus in a person's blood (plasma).

Viremia: The presence of virus in the blood.

Virulence: The quality of expression or the expression of the disease.

Virus: Any of a large group of submicroscopic agents capable of infecting plants, animals, and bacteria; characterized by a total dependence on living cells for reproduction and by a lack of independent metabolism.

Western Blot: A blood test used to detect antibodies to a given antigen. Compared to the ELISA test, the Western Blot is more specific and more expensive. It can be used to confirm the results of the ELISA test.

Wild type: A genotype or phenotype circulating prior to selection of drug resistance.

X-ray: Radiant energy of extremely short wavelength used to diagnose and treat cancer.

Zalcitabine: Also known as HIVID; see ddC—inhibits HIV replication.

Zidovudine: Also known as Retrovir; see ZDV—inhibits HIV replication. Mistakenly referred to as AZT.

References

CHAPTER 1

BARRE-SINOUSSI, FRANCOISE, et al. (1983). Isolation of a T lymphocyte retrovirus from a patient at risk for acquired immune deficiency syndrome (AIDS). *Science,* 220:868–871.

HAHN, BEATRICE, et al. (2000). AIDS as a zoonosis: Scientific and public health implications. *Science,* 287:607–614.

MARLINK, RICHARD. (1996). Lessons from the second AIDS virus HIV-2. *AIDS,* 10:689–699.

MASUR, H., et al. (1981). An outbreak of community-acquired *Pneumocystis carinii* pneumonia: Initial manifestations of cellular immune dysfunction. *N. Eng. J. Med.,* 305(24):1431–1438.

Morbidity and Mortality Weekly Report. (1981b). Pneumocystis pneumonia Los Angeles, 30:250–252.

Morbidity and Mortality Weekly Report. (1982). Update on acquired immune deficiency syndrome (AIDS) United States, 31:507–508, 513–514.

Morbidity and Mortality Weekly Report. (1990). Surveillance for HIV-2 infection in blood donors—United States, 1987–1989, 39:829–831.

SPRECHER, LORRIE. (1991). Women with AIDS: Dead but not disabled. *The Positive Woman,* 1:4.

STADTMAUER, GARY, et al. (1997). Primary Immune Deficiency Disorders that mimic AIDS. *Infections in Medicine,* 4:899–905.

CHAPTER 2

ANDREWS, CHARLA. (1995). "The Duesberg Phenomenon." What does it mean? *Science,* 267:157.

BAGASRA, OMAR. (1999). *HIV and Molecular immunity: Prospects for the AIDS vaccine.* [Cambridge, MA]: BioTechniques Books.

BAILES, ELIZABETH, et al. (2003). Hybrid origin of SIV in chimpanzees. *Science,* 300:1713.

BAUM, RUDY. (1995). HIV link to AIDS strengthened by epidemiological study. *Chem. Eng. News,* 74:26.

BOGART, LAURA M., et al. (2005). Are HIV/AIDS conspiracy beliefs a barrier to prevention among African Americans? *AIDS,* 38:213–218.

CARTWRIGHT, JON. (2010, May 6). Unconventional thinkers or recklessly dangerous minds? Times Higher Education, retrieved from www.timeshighereducation.co.uk.

CDC Weekly. (1988). Extremists seek to blame AIDS on Jews. July 11.

COHEN, JON. (1993). Keystone's blunt message: "It's the virus, stupid." *Science,* 260:292–293.

CONNOR, EDWARD. (1994). Reduction of maternal infant transmission of HIV with zidovudine treatment (ACTG 076). *N. Engl. J. Med.,* 331:1173–1180.

DARBY, SARAH, et al. (1995). Mortality before and after HIV infection in the complete UK population of haemophiliacs. *Nature,* 377:79–82.

DUESBERG, PETER H. (1993). HIV and AIDS. *Science,* 260:1705–1708.

DUESBERG, PETER H. (1995a). The Duesberg Phenomenon: Duesberg and other voices. *Science,* 267:313.

DUESBERG, PETER H. (1995b). Duesberg on AIDS causation: the culprit is noncontagious risk factors. *The Scientist,* 9:12.

DUESBERG, PETER, et al. (2001). AIDS since 1984: No evidence of a new, viral epidemic—not even in Africa. *International Journal of Anatomy and Embryology* 116(2):73–92.

DUESBERG, PETER, et al. (2009). HIV/AIDS Hypothesis out of touch with South African AIDS—A new perspective. *Medical Hypothesis* (2009), doi:10.1016/j.mehy.2009.06.024.

DUESBERG, PETER H., et al. (2011). "AIDS since 1984: No Evidence for a New, Viral Epidemic—Not Even in Africa." *Italian Journal of Anatomy and Embryology = Archivio Italiano Di Anatomia Ed Embriologia* 116 (2):73–92.

Editorial. (1995). More conviction on HIV and AIDS. *Nature,* 377:1.

GIBBS, WAYT. (2001). Dissident or Don Quixote? *Scientific American,* 285:30–32.

GRMEK, MIRKO. (1990). *History of AIDS: Emergence and Origin of a Modern Pandemic.* Princeton, NJ: Princeton University Press.

HAHN, BEATRICE, et al. (1999). Origin of HIV-1 in the chimpanzee *Pan troglodytes troglodytes. Nature*, 397:436–441.

HAHN, BEATRICE, et al. (2000). AIDS as a zoonosis: scientific and public health implications. *Science*, 287:607–614.

HAHN, BEATRICE H., et al. (2003, February). "Amplification of a Complete: Simian Immunodeficiency Virus Genome from Fecal RNA of a Wild Chimpanzee". J Virol. 77(3):2233–2242. doi: 10.1128/JVI.77.3.2233-2242.2003

HAHN, BEATRICE H., et al. (2006). "Chimpanzee reservoirs of pandemic and nonpandemic HIV-1." *Science (New York, N.Y.)* 313, no. 5786:523–526.

HAHN, BEATRICE H., et al. (2011, September). "Origins of HIV and the AIDS Pandemic". *Cold Spring Harbor Perspectives in Medicine, doi:10.1101/cshperspect.a006841*

HIRSCH, VANESSA, et al. (1995). Phylogeny and natural history of the primate lentiviruses, SIV and HIV. *Current Opinion Genetic Development*, 5:798–806.

HOLDER, CONSTANCE. (1988). Curbing Soviet disinformation. *Science*, 242:665.

HOOPER, EDWARD (1999). *The River: A Journey to the Source of HIV and AIDS.* Boston: Little, Brown and Company.

KALISH, MARSHA, et al. (2005). Central African hunters exposed to simian immunodeficiency virus. *Emerging Infectious Diseases*, 11:1928–1930.

KOPROWSKI, HILARY. (1992). AIDS and the polio vaccine. *Science*, 257:1024–1026.

LEVY, JAY. (1995). *HIV and the Pathogenesis of AIDS.* Washington, D.C.: ASM Press.

MOORE, JOHN. (1996). À Duesberg, adieu! *Nature*, 380:293–294.

PEETERS, MARTINE, et al. (2002). Risk to human health from a plethora of simian immunodeficiency viruses in primate bushmeat. *Emerging Infectious Diseases*, 8:451–457.

SANTIAGO, MARIO, et al. (2002). SIVcpz in wild chimpanzees. *Science*, 795:465.

SHARP, PAUL, et al. (2008). Prehistory of HIV. Vol 455/2 October 2008/dol:10.1030/Nature 07390.

SHARP, PAUL, et al. (2011, September). Origins of HIV and the AIDS pandemic. *Cold Spring Harbor Perspectives in Medicine* 1(1):a0068–11.

SHARP, PAUL, et al. (2011, October 1). From "Origins of HIV and the AIDS Pandemic," CSH Perspectives in Medicine, (1:a006841), p. 2.

SULLIVAN, JOHN, et al. (1995). HIV and AIDS. *Nature*, 378:10.

VANGROENWEGHE, DANIEL. (2001). The earliest cases of human immunodeficiency virus type 1 group M in Congo-Kinshasa, Rwanda and Burundi and the origin of acquired immune deficiency syndrome. *Philos. Trans. R. Soc. Lond. B. Biol. Sci.;* 356 (1410):923–925.

VIDAL, NICOLE, et al. (2000). Unprecented degree of HIV-1 Group M genetic diversity in the Democratic Republic of Congo suggests HIV-1 pandemic originated in Central Africa. *J. Virology* 74:10,498–10,507.

WEISS, ROBIN A., et al. (1990). Duesberg, HIV and AIDS. *Nature*, 345:659–660.

WOROBEY, MICHAEL, et al. (2007). Exodus and genesis: The emergence of HIV-1 group M subtype B. Fourteenth Conference on Retroviruses and Opportunistic Infections, abstract 149, Los Angeles.

WOROBEY, MICHAEL, et al. (2008). Direct evidence of extensive diversity of HIV-1 in Kinshasa by 1960. *Nature* dol:10.1030.07390.

WOROBEY, MICHAEL, et al. (2010). Island biography reveals the deep history of SIV. *Science* 329:1487.

CHAPTER 3

BONHOEFFER, SEBASTIAN, et al. (1995). Causes of HIV diversity. *Nature*, 376:125.

BRIX, DEBORAH, et al. (1996). Summary of track A: Basic science. *AIDS*, 10 (suppl. 3): S85–S106.

BRODINE, STEPHANIE, et al. (1997). Genotypic variation and molecular epidemiology of HIV. *Infect. Med.*, 14:739–748.

COHEN, JON. (1997). Looking for leads in HIV's battle with immune system. *Science*, 276:1196–1197.

COHEN, JON. (2008). HIV gets by with a lot of help from human host. *Science*, 319:143–144 www.sciencemag.org.

COLLINS, KATHLEEN, et al. (1998). HIV-1 Nef protein protects infected primary cells against killing by cytotoxic T lymphocytes. *Nature*, 391:397–401.

DELWART, ERIC, et al. (1993). Genetic relationships determined by a DNA heteroduplex mobility assay: analysis of HIV *env* genes. *Science*, 262:1257–1262.

DERDEYN, CYNTHIA, et al. (2004). Envelope-constrained naturalization-sensitive HIV-1 after heterosexual transmission. *Science*, 303:2019–2022.

DEVEREUX, HELEN, et al. (2002). In vitro HIV-1 compartmentalisation: drug resistance associated mutation distribution. *J. Med. Virology,* 66:8–12.

DIAZ, RICARDO, et al. (1997). Divergence of HIV quasispecies in an epidemiology cluster. *AIDS,* 11:415–422.

DIMMROCK, N. J., and S. B. PRIMROSE, (1987). *Introduction to Modern Virology,* 3rd ed. Oxford: Blackwell Scientific Publications.

ELLEDGE, STEPHEN J., et al. (2008). Identification of host proteins required for HIV infection through a functional genomic screen. www.scienceexpress.org/10 January 2008:1–10.

FRITZ, CHRISTIAN, et al. (1995). A human nucleoprotein-like protein that specifically interacts with HIV-Rev. *Nature,* 376:530–533.

GARRUS, JENNIFER, et al. (2001). Tsg 101 and the vacuolar protein sorting pathway are essential for HIV-1 budding. *Cell,* 107:55–65.

GREENE, WARNER. (1993). AIDS and the immune system. *Sci. Am.,* 269:99–105.

HILDRETH, JAMES. (2001). Adhesion molecules, lipid rafts and HIV pathogenesis. HIV Pathogenesis Keystone Symposium, March 28–April 3, Presentation 038.

KOHLEISEN, MARKUS, et al. (1992). Cellular localization of Nef expressed in persistently HIV-1 infected low-producer astrocytes. *AIDS,* 6:1427–1436.

LI, CHIANG. (1997). Tat protein perpetuates HIV-1 infection. *Proc. Natl. Acad. Sci. USA,* 94:8116–8120.

LUM, JULIAN, et al. (2003). Vpr R77Q is associated with long-term nonprogressive HIV and impaired induction of apoptosis. *J. Clin. Invest.,* 111:1547–1554.

MATSUYA, HIROAKI, et al. (1990). Molecular targets for AIDS therapy. *Science,* 249:1533–1543.

NOWAK, MARTIN A. (1990). HIV mutation rate. *Nature,* 347:522.

PATRUSKY, BEN. (1992). The Intron story. *Mosaic,* 23:20–33.

POTASH, MARY JANE, et al. (1998). Peptide inhibitors of HIV-1 protease and viral infection of peripheral blood lymphocytes based on HIV-1 ViF. *Proc. National Academy of Science,* 95:13,865–13,868.

ROSEN, CRAIG A. (1991). Regulation of HIV gene expression by RNA-protein interactions. *Trends Genet.,* 7:9–14.

SAGG, MICHAEL S., et al. (1988). Extensive variation of human immunodeficiency virus Type-1 *in vivo. Nature,* 334:440–444.

SAGG, MICHAEL S., et al. (1995). Improving the management of HIV disease. *Advanced Causes in HIV Pathogenesis,* pp. 1–30. February 25, Swiss Hotel, Atlanta (Michael Sagg, Program Chair).

SIMON, FRANCOIS, et al. (1998). Identification of a new human immunodeficiency virus Type I distinct from Group M and Group O. *Nature Medicine,* 4:1032.

SOMASUNDARAN, M., et al. (1988). Unexpectedly high levels of HIV-1 RNA and protein synthesis in a cytocidal infection. *Science,* 242:1554–1557.

STEVENSON, MARIO. (1998). Basic Science: Highlights of the 5th Retrovirus Conference. *Improving the Management of HIV Disease,* 6:4–10.

TAYLOR, BARBARA, et al. (2008). The challenge of HIV-1 subtype diversity. *NEJM* 358: 1590-1602.

TORRES, YOLANDA, et al. (1996). Cytokine network and HIV syncytium-inducing phenotype shift. *AIDS,* 10:1053–1055.

WATTS, JOSEPH M., et al. (2009). Architecture and secondary structure of an entire HIV-1 RNA genome. 460/6 August 2009/DOI: 10.1038. *Nature* 08237 pp.

WILLS, JOHN W., et al. (1991). Form, function and use of retroviral *gag* protein. *AIDS,* 5:639–654.

Workshop Report from the European Commission/Joint United Nations Program on HIV/AIDS. (1997). HIV-1 subtypes: Implications for epidemiology, pathogenicity, vaccines, and diagnostics. *AIDS,* 11:17–36.

WU, YUNTAO, et al. (2001). Selective transcription and modulation of resting T cell activity by preintegrated HIV DNA. *Science,* 293:1503–1506.

CHAPTER 4

AVETTAND-FENOEL, VERONIQUE, et al. (2009). Stability of HIV reservoir resting CD4 T cell subsets under effective HAART. Sixteenth Conference on Retroviruses and Opportunistic Infections, Montreal, abstract 426.

BACK, DAVID. (2001). Pharmacology to the fore. *PRN Notebook,* 6:11–14.

BLASCHKE, TERRENCE, et al. (2012, February). Adherence to medications: Insights arising from studies on the unreliable link between prescribed and actual drug dosing histories. *Ann. Rev. Pharmacol. Toxicol.,* 52:275. (http://dx.doi.org/10.1146/annurev-pharmtox-011711-113247)

BOZZETTE, SAMUEL, et al. (2001). Expenditures for the care of HIV-infected patients in the era of HAART. *N. Eng. J. Med.,* 344: 817–823.

BRENNAN, TIMOTHY, et al. (2009). Population structure analysis of HIV-1 in plasma and integrated provirus in resting CD4+ T cells suggests a novel source may be the dominant contributor to residual viremia in patients on HAART. Sixteenth Conference on Retroviruses and Opportunistic Infections, Montreal, abstract 427.

CLARK, DAWN, et al. (1999). T cell renewal impaired in HIV-1 infected individuals. Presented at: Sixth Conference on Retroviruses and Opportunistic Infections; January 31–February 4, Chicago. Abstract 22.

CLAVEL, FRANCOIS. (2004). Mechanisms of HIV drug resistance: a primer. *PRN Notebook* 9:3-7.

COFFIN, JOHN. (1995). HIV population dynamics *in vivo:* Implications for genetic variation, pathogenesis and therapy. *Science, 267*:483–489.

DEEKS, STEVEN, et al. (1999). HIV RNA and CD4 cell count response to protease inhibitor therapy in an urban AIDS clinic: Response to both initial and salvage therapy. *AIDS,* 13:F35–F43.

ERICKSON, JOHN, et al. (1990). Design, activity, and 2.8 angstrom crystal structure of a C_2 symmetric inhibitor complexed to HIV protease. *Science,* 249:527–533.

FREEDBERG, KENNETH, et al. (2001). The cost effectiveness of combination antiretroviral therapy for HIV disease. *N. Eng. J. Med.,* 344:824–831.

FUNK, MICHELE, et al. (2011). Timing of HAART initiation and clinical outcomes in human immunodeficiency virus type 1 seroconvertes. *Arch. Intern. Med.,* 171(17):1560–1569.

GARDNER, EDWARD, et al. (2011). The spectrum of engagement in HIV care and its relevance to test-and-treat strategies for prevention of HIV infection. *Clinical Infectious Diseases,* 52:793–800.

GEVETTI, ANNA MARIA (2009). Effect of HIV-1 subtype on virologic and immunologic response to starting highly active antiretroviral therapy. *Clin Infect Dis* 48:1296–1305.

GRANICH, REUBEN, et al. (2009). Universal voluntary HIV testing with immediate antiretroviral therapy as a strategy for elimination of HIV transmission: A mathematical model. *Lancet,* 373:48–57.

GRANT, ROBERT, et al. (2010). Pre-exposure chemoprophylaxis for HIV prevention in men who have sex with men. *N. Engl. J. Med.,* 363:2587–2599.

HATANO, HIROYU, et al. (2009). Evidence of persistent low-level viremia in long-term HAART-suppressed individuals. Sixteenth Conference on Retroviruses and Opportunistic Infections, Montreal, abstract 425.

HELLERSTEIN, MARC, et al. (1999). Directly measured kinetics of circulating T lymphocytes in normal and HIV-infected humans. *Nat. Med.,* 5:83–89.

HO, DAVID, et al. (1995). Rapid turnover of plasma virions and CD4 lymphocytes in HIV-1 infection. *Nature,* 373:123–126.

HU, DALE, et al. (1996). The emerging genetic diversity of HIV. *JAMA,* 275:210–216.

JURRIAANS, SUZANNE, et al. (1994, October). "The natural history of HIV-1 infection: virus load and virus phenotype independent determinants of clinical course?" *Virology.* 204(1):213–233.

JUUSOLA, JESSIE, et al. (2012). The cost-effectiveness of pre-exposure prophylaxis for HIV prevention in the United States in men who have sex with men. *Annals of Internal Medicine,* 156(8):541–550.

KASAKOVSKY-POND, SERGI, et al. (2009). Are all subtypes created equal? The effectiveness of antiretroviral therapy against non-subtype B HIV-1. *Clin Infect Dis* 48:1306–09.

KURITZKES, DANIEL. (2011). HAART for HIV-1 infection: Zeroing in on when to start. *Arch. Intern. Med.,* 171(17):1569–1570.

MAYERS, DOUGLAS. (1996). Rational approaches to resistance: Nucleoside analogues. *AIDS,* 10 (Suppl. 1): S9–S13.

MELLORS, JOHN, et al. (1995). Quantitation of HIV-1 RNA in plasma predict outcome after seroconversion. *Ann. Intern. Med.,* 122:573–579.

NIAID—National Institute of Allergy and Infectious Diseases. (2011, May 12). Treating HIV infected people with antiretrovirals protects partners from infection; findings results from NIH-funded international study [News release]. Retrieved from http://www.niaid.nih.gov/news/newsreleases/2011/Pages/HPTN052.aspx.

PALMER, SARAH, et al. (2008). Low-level viremia persists for at least 7 years in patients on suppressive antiretroviral therapy. *PNAS* 105:3879–3884.

PERRIN, LUC, et al. (1998). HIV treatment failure: Testing for HIV resistance in clinical practice. *Science,* 280:1871–1873.

PIATAK, MICHAEL, et al. (1993). High levels of HIV-1 in plasma during all stages of infection determined by competitive PCR. *Science,* 259:1749–1754.

PINKERTON, STEVEN, et al. (2004). Cost effectiveness of post exposure prophylaxis after sexual or injection drug exposure to HIV. *Arch. Intern. Med.,* 164:46–54.

RICHMAN, DOUGLAS, et al. (2009). The challenge of finding a cure for HIV infection. *Science* 323:1304-1307.

RODRIGUEZ, BENIGNO, et al. (2006). Predictive value of plasma HIV RNA level on rate of CD4 T cell decline in untreated HIV infection. *JAMA*, 296:1498–1506.

SAKSELA, KALLE, et al. (1994). Human immunodeficiency virus type 1 mRNA expression in peripheral blood cells predicts disease progression independently of the number of CD_4+ lymphocytes. *Proc. Natl. Acad. Sci. USA*, 91:1104–1108.

SAYER, CHARLIE, et al. (2008). Will I, won't I? Why doMSM present for PEPSE? *Sex Transm. Infect.* Published online first: 15 December 2008. doi: 10.1136/sti.2008.033662.

SHELTON, JAMES. (2012). ARVs as HIV prevention: A tough road to wide impact. *Science*, 334:1645–1646.

SIMBERKOFF, MICHAEL. (1996). Long-term follow-up of symptomatic HIV-infected patients originally randomized to early vs. later zidovudine treatment: Report of a Veterans Affairs cooperative study. *AIDS*, 11:142–150.

STEPHENSON, JOAN. (1996). New anti-HIV drugs and treatment strategies buoy AIDS researchers. *JAMA*, 275:579–580.

TELENTI, AMALIO, et al. for the Swiss HIV Cohort Study. (1998). CD_4 T cell counts in HIV-infected individuals remaining viraemic with highly active antiretroviral therapy followed in the Swiss HIV Cohort Study (SHCS). *Antiviral Ther.*, 3(Suppl. 1):53.

VELLA, STEFANO. (1995). Clinical experience with saquinavir. *AIDS*, 9(suppl. 2):S21–S25.

VIGAN, ALESSANDRA, et al. (2003). Increased lipodystrophy is associated with increased exposure to highly active antiretroviral therapy in HIV-infected children. *J. Acq. Immune Def. Syndromes*, 15; 32:482–489.

WAIN-HOBSON, SIMON. (1995). Virologies mayhem [editorial]. *Nature*, 373:102.

WEI, XIPING, et al. (1995).Viral dynamics in human immunodeficiency virus type 1 infection. *Nature*, 373:117–122.

CHAPTER 5

BAKKER, LEENDERT J., et al. (1992). Antibodies and complement enhance binding and uptake of HIV-1 by human monocytes. *AIDS*, 6:35–41.

BELMONTE, LILIANA, et al. (2007). The intestinal mucosa as a reservoir of HIV-1 infection after successful HAART. *AIDS* 2106–2108.

CHUGH, PAULINE, et al. (2008). Akt inhibitors as an HIV-1 infected macrophage-specific anti-viral therapy. *Retrovirology*, 5:11 doi 10–1186/1742–4690–5-11.

DOHERTY, PETER. (1995). The keys to cell-mediated immunity. *JAMA*, 274:1067–1068.

EDGINGTON, STEPHEN M. (1993). HIV no longer latent, says NIAID's Fauci. *BioTechnology*, 11:16–17.

EUGEN-OLSEN, JESPER, et al. (1997). Heterozygosity for a deletion in the CKR-5 gene leads to prolonged AIDS-free survival and slower CD4 T cell decline. *AIDS*, 11:305–310.

FAUCI, ANTHONY, et al. (1995). Trapped but still dangerous. *Nature*, 337:680–681.

GEIJTENBEEK, TEUNIS, et al. (2000). Identification of DC-SIGN, a novel dendritic cell specific ICAM-3 receptor that supports primary immune response. *Cell*, 100:575–585.

GELDERBLOM, H. R., et al. (1985). Loss of envelope antigene of HTLV III/LAV, a factor in AIDS pathogenesis. *Lancet*, 2: 1016–1017.

GUADALUPE, MORAIMA, et al. (2006). Viral suppression and immune restoration in the gastrointestinal mucosa of human immunodeficiency virus type 1–infected patients initiating therapy during primary or chronic infection. *Journal of Virology*, 80:8236–8347.

HAASE, ASHLEY. (1999). Population biology of HIV-1 infection:Viral and CD4+ T cell demographics and dynamics in lymphatic tissues. *Annu. Rev. Immunol.*, 17:625–656.

HAASE, ASHLEY, et al. (1996). Quantitative image analysis of HIV infection in lymphoid tissue. *Science*, 274:985–990.

KNIGHT, STELLA. (1996). Bone-marrow-derived dendritic cells and the pathogenesis of AIDS. *AIDS*, 10:807–817.

LIU, RONG, et al. (1996). Homozygous defect in HIV-1 coreceptor accounts for resistance of some multiple-exposed individuals to HIV-1 infection. *Cell*, 86: 367–377.

MARMOR, MICHAEL, et al. (2001). Homozygous and heterozygous CCR-5-32 genotypes are associated with resistance to HIV infection. *J. Acq. Immune Def. Syndromes*, 27:472–481.

MIYAUCHI, KOSUKE, et al. (2009). HIV enters cells via endocytosis and dynamin-dependent fusion with endosomes. *Cell*, 137:433–444.

MOIR, SUSAN, et al. (2000). B cells of HIV-1 infected patients bind virons through CD21-complement interactions and transmit infectious virus to activated T cells. *J Exp Med*, 192:637–646. Published online August 28, at www.jem.org.

MOIR, SUSAN, et al. (2001). HIV induces phenotypic and functional perturbations of B cells in chronically infected individuals. *PNAS*, 98:10,362–10,367.

O'BRIEN, STEPHEN. (1998). AIDS: A role for host genes. *Hospital Practice*, 33:53–79.

OLINGER, GENE, et al. (2000). CD4-negative cells bind HIV-1 and efficiently transfer virus to T cells. *J. Virol.*, 74:8550–8557.

PHILPOTT, SEAN, et al. (1999). CCR-5 genotype and resistance to vertical transmission of human immunodeficiency virus type 1. *Journal of Aquired Immune Deficiency Syndromes*, 21:189–193.

PLANQUE, STEPHANIE, et al. (2008). Catalytic antibodies to HIV: physiological role and potential clinical utility. *Autoimmunity Reviews*, 7:473-479.

POPE, MELISSA. (2002). Dendritic cells: immune activators or virus facilitators? *PRN Notebook*, 7:8–10.

SAMSON, MICHEL, et al. (1996). Resistance to HIV-1 infection in Caucasian individuals bearing mutant alleles of the CCR 5 chemokine gene. *Nature*, 382:722–725.

SANTIAGO, MARIO, et al. (2008). Apobec3 encodes Rfv3, a gene influencing neutralizing antibody control of retrovirus infection. *Science*, 321:1343-1346.

SILICIANO, ROBERT R. H., et al. (2009). Small-molecule screening using a human primary cell model of HIV latency identifies compounds that reverse latency without cellular activation. *J. Clin. Invest*, 119:3473–3486.

SINHA, ANIMESH, et al. (1990). Autoimmune diseases: the failure of self-tolerance. *Science*, 248:1380–1387.

STEINMAN, RALPH. (2000). DC-SIGN: A guide to some mysteries of dendritic cells. *Cell*, 100:491–494.

STROMINGER, JACK, et al. (1995). The Class I and Class II proteins of the human major histocompatibility complex. *JAMA*, 274:1074–1076.

SUBBRAMANIAN, RAMU, et al. (2002). The presence of ADCC—but not NA—antibodies in serum was associated with viral neutralization in the presence of complement (Comparison of human immunodeficiency virus (HIV)-specific infection enhancing and inhibiting antibodies in AIDS patients.) *J. of Clin. Micro.*, 40: 2141–2146.

UNANUE, EMIL. (1995). The concept of antigen processing and presentation. *JAMA*, 274:1071–1073.

WEIJING, HE, et al. (2008) Duffy antigen receptor for chemokines mediates trans-infection of HIV-1 from red blood cells to target cells and affects HIV-AIDS susceptibility. *Cell Host and Microbe*, 4:52-62.

WEINSTEIN, RAYMOND (2011). Should remaining stockpiles of smallpox virus (variola) be destroyed? *Emerging Infectious Diseases* 17: 81–683.

ZINKERNAGEL, ROLF. (1995). MHC-restricted T cell recognition: The basis of immune surveillance. *JAMA*, 274:1069–1071.

CHAPTER 6

BALFOUR, HENRY. (1995). Cytomegalovirus retinitis in persons with AIDS. *Postgrad. Med.*, 97:109–118.

BROOKS, JOHN T., et al. (2009). What's new in the 2009 guidelines for prevention and treatment of opportunistic infections among adults and adolescents with HIV? *Topics in HIV Medicine*, 17:109–114.

CHIN, DANIEL. (1992). Mycobacterium avium complex infection. *AIDS File: Clin. Notes*, 6:7–8.

DALEY, CHARLES L. (1992). Epidemiology of tuberculosis in the AIDS era. *AIDS File: Clin. Notes*, 6:1–2.

DEWIT, STEPHANE, et al. (1991). Fungal infections in AIDS patients. *Clin. Adv. Treatment Fungal Infect.*, 2:1–11.

Emergency Medicine. (1989). Fighting opportunistic infections in AIDS. 21:24–38.

ERNST, JEROME. (1990). Recognize the early symptoms of PCP. *Med. Asp. Hum. Sexuality*, 24:45–47.

GOTTLIEB, MICHAEL S., et al. (1987). Opportunistic viruses in AIDS. *Patient Care*, 23:139–154.

GROSSMAN, RONALD J., et al. (1989). PCP and other protozoal infections. *Patient Care*, 23:89–116.

GRULICH, ANDREW. (2000). Cancer risk in persons with HIV/AIDS in the era of combination antiretroviral therapy. *AIDS Reader*, 10:341–346.

GUARINO, M., et al. (1995). Progressive multifocal leucoencephalopathy in AIDS: Treatment with cytosine arabinoside. *AIDS*, 9:819–820.

HARRIS, CHARLES. (1993). TB and HIV: The boundaries collide. *Medical World News*, 34:63.

Harvard AIDS Institute. (1994). *Special Report—Opportunistic Infections.* Fall issue: 1–14.

HERNDIER, BRIAN, et al. (1994). Pathogenesis of AIDS lymphomas. *AIDS*, 8:1025–1049.

HESSOL, NANCY. (1998). The changing epidemology of HIV related cancers. *The AIDS Reader*, 8:45–49.

HESSOL, NANCY, et al. (2007). The impact of HAART on non–AIDS-defining cancers among adults with AIDS. *Am. J. Epidemiology*, 165:1143–1153.

JACOBSON, MARK A., et al. (1988). Serious cytomegalovirus disease in the acquired immunodeficiency syndrome (AIDS): Clinical findings, diagnosis, and treatment. *Ann. Intern. Med.*, 108:585–594.

JOINER, K. A., et al. (1990). *Toxoplasma gondii:* Fusion competence of parasitophorous vacuoles in Fe receptor-transfected fibroblasts. *J. Cell Biol.*, 109:2771.

KLEDAL, THOMAS, et al. (1997). A broad spectrum chemokine antagonist encoded by KS-associated herpesvirus. *Science*, 277:1656–1659.

LAURENCE, JEFFREY. (1995). Evolving management of OIs. *AIDS Reader*, 5:187–188, 208.

LEDERGERBER, BRUNO, et al. (1999). AIDS-related OI occurring after initiation of potent antiretroviral therapy: A Swiss cohort study. *JAMA*, 282:2220–2226.

LYNCH, JOSEPH P. (1989). When opportunistic viruses infiltrate the lung. *J. Resp. Dis.*, 10:25–30.

MCGRATH, MICHAEL, et al. (1994). Identification of a common clonal human immunodeficiency virus integration site in human immunodeficiency virus-associated lymphomas. *Cancer Res.*, 54:2069.

MEDOFF, GERALD, et al. (1991). Systemic fungal infections: An overview. *Hosp. Pract*, 26:41–52.

Morbidity and Mortality Weekly Report. (1995b). USPHS/IDSA guidelines for the prevention of opportunistic infections in persons infected with HIV: A summary. 44:1–34.

MURPHY, ROBERT. (1994). Opportunistic infection prophylaxis. *Int. AIDS Soc.–USA*, 2:7–8.

NEWCOMB-FERNANDEZ, JENNIFER. (2003) Cancer in the HIV-infected population. *RITA*, 9:5–10.

PATEL, PRAGNA, et al. (2008). Incidence of types of cancer among HIV-infected persons compared with the general population of the United States, 1992–2003. *Annals of Internal Medicine* 148 (10): 728–736.

POWDERLY, WILLIAM, et al. (1998). Recovery of the immune system with antiretroviral therapy: the end of opportunism? *JAMA*, 280:72–77.

RINALDO, CHARLES, et al. (2001). Primary human herpesvirus 8 infection generates a broadly specific CD8+ T cell response to viral lytic cycle proteins. *Blood*, 97:2366–2373.

RUSSELL, JAMES. (1990). Study focuses on eyes and AIDS. *Baylor Med*, 21:3.

SAID, JONATHAN, et al. (1997). KS-associated herpesvirus/human herpesvirus type 8 encephalitis in HIV-positive and -negative individuals. *AIDS*, 11:1119–1122.

SCADDEN, DAVID. (2002). Lymphoma in the setting of HIV disease. *PRN Notebook*, 7:21–25.

SIBLEY, L. DAVID. (1992). Virulent strains of *Toxoplasma gondii* comprise single clonal lineage. *Nature*, 359:82–85.

WALLACE, MARK R., et al. (1993). Cats and toxoplasmosis risk in HIV-infected adults. *JAMA*, 269:76–77.

WHEAT, L. JOSEPH. (1992). Histoplasmosis in AIDS. *AIDS Clin. Care*, 4:1–4.

CHAPTER 7

ANDERSON, ROBERT E., et al. (1991). CD8 T lymphocytes and progression to AIDS in HIV-infected men: Some observations. *AIDS*, 5:213–215.

BOLOGNESI, DANI P. (1989). Prospects for prevention of and early intervention against HIV. *JAMA*, 261:3007–3013.

BUCY, R. PAT. (1999). Viral and cellular dynamics in HIV-1 disease. *Improving Management of HIV Disease*, 7:8–11.

BURCHAM, JOYCE, et al. (1991). CD4+ is the best predictor of development of AIDS in a cohort of HIV-infected homosexual men. *AIDS*, 5:365–372.

COFFIN, JOHN M. (1995). HIV population dynamics in vivo: Implications for genetic variation, pathogenesis and therapy. *Science*, 267:483–489.

COHEN, JON. (1995). High turnover of HIV in blood revealed by new studies. *Science*, 267:179.

COULIS, PAUL A., et al. (1987). Peptide-based immunodiagnosis of retrovirus infections. *Am. Clin. Prod. Rev.*, 6:34–43.

ESCAICH, SONIA, et al. (1991). Plasma viraemia as a marker of viral replication in HIV-infected individuals. *AIDS*, 5:1189–1194.

FREED, ERIC, et al. (1994). HIV infection of nondividing cells. *Nature*, 369:107–108.

GOLDSCHMIDT, RONALD, et al. (1997). Treatment of AIDS and HIV-related conditions—1997. *J. Am. Board Fam. Pract.*, 10:144–167.

HATANO, HIROYU, et al. (2009). Eviidence for persistent low-level viremia in individuals who control Human Immunodeficiency Virus in the absence of antiretroviral therapy. *J. Viral* 329–335.

HENRARD, DENIS, et al. (1995). Natural history of HIV cell-free viremia. *JAMA*, 274:554–558.

HO, DAVID, et al. (1995). Rapid turnover of plasma virons and CD4 lymphocytes in HIV infection. *Nature*, 373:123–126.

HO, DAVID. (1996). HIV pathogenesis. *Improv. Manage. HIV Dis.*, 4:4–6.

HORTON, RACHEL, et al. (2010). Cohorts for the study of HIV-1-exposed but uninfected individuals: Benefits and limitations. *J. Infect. Dis.*, 202(53):5377–5381.

KATZENSTEIN, TERESE, et al. (1996). Longitudinal serum HIV RNA quantification: Correlation to viral phenotype at seroconversion and clinical outcome. *AIDS*, 10:167–173.

MANDALIA, SUNDHIYA, et al. (2012, February 20). Are long term non-progressors very slow progressors? Insights from the Chelsea and Westminster HIV Cohort, 1988-2010. *PLoS ONE*, 7(2):e29844.

MCMICHAEL, SUNDHIYA, et al. (2010). The immune response during acute HIV-infection: Clues for vaccine development. *Nat. Review Immunology*, 10:11–23.

MERIGAN, THOMAS, et al. (1996). The prognostic significance of viral load, codon 215-reverse transcriptase mutation and CD4+ T cells on HIV disease progression. *AIDS*, 10:159–165.

MIGUELES, STEPHEN, et al. (2008). Lytic granule loading of CD8+ T cells is required for HIV-infected cell elimination associated with immune control, *Immunity*, 29:1009-1021, ISSN 1074-7613, DOI: 10.1016/j.immuni.2008.10.010.

Morbidity and Mortality Weekly Report. (1997). Revised guidelines for performing CD4+ T cell determinations in persons infected with HIV. 46:1–4.

NIELSON, CLAUS, et al. (1993). Biological properties of HIV isolates in primary HIV infection: Consequences for the subsequent course of infection. *AIDS*, 7:1035–1040.

NOWAK, M.A., et al. (1990). The evolutionary dynamics of HIV-1 quasispecies and the development of immunodeficiency disease. *AIDS*, 4:1095–1103.

PANTALEO, GUISEPPE, et al. (1995). Studies in subjects with long-term nonprogressive human immunodeficiency virus infection. *N. Engl. J. Med.*, 332:209–216.

PERELSON, ALAN, et al. (1996). HIV dynamics in vivo: Viron clearance rate, infected cell life span and viral generation time. *Science*, 271:1582–1586.

PHILLIPS, ANDREW N., et al. (1991a). p24 Antigenaemia, CD4 lymphocyte counts and the development of AIDS. *AIDS*, 5:1217–1222.

PHILLIPS, ANDREW N., et al. (1991b). Serial CD4 lymphocyte counts and development of AIDS. *Lancet*, 337:389–392.

PRICE, RICHARD W. (1988). The brain in AIDS: Central nervous system HIV infection and AIDS dementia complex. *Science*, 239:586–593.

QUINN, THOMAS. (1997). Acute primary HIV infection. *JAMA*, 278:58–62.

RANKI, ANNAMARI, et al. (1995). Abundant expression of HIV Nef and Rev proteins in brain astrocytes *in vivo* is associated with dementia. *AIDS*, 9:1001–1008.

ROYCE, RACHEL A., et al. (1991). The natural history of HIV-1 infection: Staging classifications of disease. *AIDS*, 5:355–364.

SAX, PAUL, et al. (1995). Potential clinical implications of interlaboratory variability in CD4+ T lymphocyte counts of patients infected with human immunodeficiency virus. *Clin. Infect. Dis.*, 21:1121–1125.

SOLOWAY, BRUCE, et al. (2000). Antiretroviral failure: A biopsychosocial approach. *AIDS Clinical Care*, 12: 23–25, 30.

STRAMER, SUSAN L., et al. (1989). Markers of HIV infection prior to IgG antibody seropositivity. *JAMA*, 262:64–69.

VOELKER, REBECCA. (1995). New studies say viral burden tops CD4 as a marker of HIV disease progression. *JAMA*, 275:421–422.

WAINBERG, MARK, et al. (2007). High rates of forward transmission events after acute/early HIV-1 infection. *J. of Infectious Diseases*, 195:951–959.

WEI, XIPING, et al. (1995). Viral dynamics in HIV type 1 infection. *Nature*, 373:117–122.

YAN XU, et al. (2004). HIV-1 mediated apoptosis of neuronal cells: Proximal molecular mechanisms of HIV-1 induced encephalopathy. *PNAS*, 101:7070–7075.

YU, KALVIN, et al. (2000). Primary HIV infection. *Postgraduate Medicine*, 107:114–122.

CHAPTER 8

ARCHIBALD, D.W., et al. (1990). *In vitro* inhibition of HIV-1 infectivity by human salivas. *AIDS Res. Human Viruses*, 6:1425–1431.

BAGASRA, OMAR. (1999). HIV and molecular immunity: prospects for the AIDS vaccine. Biotechniques Books–Eaton Publishing Company.

BOLLING, DAVID R. (1989). Anal intercourse between women and bisexual men. *Med. Asp. Human Sexuality*, 23:34.

BOYER, PAMELA J., et al. (1994). Factors predictive of maternal-fetal transmission of HIV. *JAMA,* 271:1925–1930.

BUCHBINDER, K., et al. (2001). Per-contact risk of HIV transmission between male sexual partners. *American Journal of Epidemiology,* 150:306–311.

BUTLER, DAVID, et al. (2009). Cell-free virus in seminal plasma is the origin of sexually transmitted HIV among men who have sex with men. Sixteenth Conference on Retroviruses and Opportunistic Infections, Montreal. Abstract 49LB.

BUTLER, DAVID, et al. (2010). The origins of sexually transmitted HIV among men who have sex with men. *Sci. Transl. Med.,* 2, 18re1; DOI: 10.1126/scitranslmed .3000447.

COHEN, J.B., et al. (1989). Heterosexual transmission of HIV. *Immunol. Ser.,* 44:135–137.

CONANT, MARCUS. (1995). The current face of the AIDS epidemic. *AIDS Newslink,* 6:14–18.

DEMARTINO, MAURIZIO, et al. (1992). HIV-1 transmission through breast milk: Appraisal of risk according to duration of feeding. *AIDS,* 6:991–997.

DES JARLAIS, DON C., et al. (1989). AIDS and IV-drug use. *Science,* 245:578.

DES JARLAIS, DON, et al. (2000). HIV incidence among injection-drug users in New York City, 1992–1997: Evidence for a declining epidemic. *Am. J. Public Health,* 90:352–359.

DILLON, BETH, et al. (2000). Primary HIV infections associated with oral transmission. Program and abstracts of the Seventh Conference on Retroviruses and Opportunistic Infections; January 30–February 2; San Francisco, Calif. Abstract 473.

DROTMAN, PETER. (1996). Professional boxing, bleeding, and HIV testing. *JAMA,* 276:193.

EDWARDS, SARA, et al. (1998). Oral sex and the transmission of viral STD's. *J. Infect. Dis.,* 74:6–10.

ELSON, JOHN. (1991). The dangerous world of wannabes. *Time,* 138:77–80.

Emergency Cardiac Care Committee, American Heart Association. (1990). Risk of infection during CPR training and rescue: Supplemental guidelines. *JAMA,* 262:2714–2715.

FOX, PHILIP. (1991). Saliva and salivary gland alterations in HIV infection. *J. Am. Dental Assoc.,* 122:46–48.

FRIEDLAND, GERALD H. (1991). HIV transmission from healthcare workers. *AIDS Clin. Care,* 3:29–30.

FURTADO, MANOHAR, et al. (1999). Persistence of HIV-1 transcription in peripheral blood mononuclear cells in patients receiving potent antiretroviral therapy. *N. Engl J. Med.,* 340:1614–1622.

GAUR, ADITYA, et al. (2008). Practice of offering a child pre-masticated (pre-chewed) food: An unrecognized possible risk factor of HIV transmission. Fifteenth Conference on Retroviruses and Opportunistic Infections, Boston, Abstract 613b.

GAUTHIER, DEANN et al. (1999). Bareback sex, bug-chasers and the gift of death. *Deviant Behavior,* 20:85–100.

GODDARD, JEROME. (1997). Why mosquitoes cannot transmit the AIDS virus. *Infect. Med.,* 14:353–354.

GOLDEN, MATHEW. (2006). HIV serosorting among men who have sex with men: Implications for prevention. Thirteenth Conference on Retroviruses and Opportunistic Infections, Denver, Abstract 163.

GROSSKURTH, HEINER, et al. (1995). Impact of improved treatment of sexually transmitted diseases on HIV infection in rural Tanzania: Randomized controlled trial. *Lancet,* 346:530–536.

GUINAN, MARY. (1995). Artificial insemination by donor: Safety and secrecy. *JAMA,* 273:890–891.

HARRISON, LEE, et al. (2000). Drugs cut HIV in semen: Safe sex still crucial. *Ann. Int. Med.,* 133:280–284.

HASSELROT, KLARA, et al. (2009). Oral HIV exposure elicits mucosal HIV-neutralizing antibodies in uninfected men who have sex with men. *AIDS* 23:329–333.

HIV/AIDS Surveillance Report. (June 2001). 13:1–41.

HOLMSTROM, PAUL, et al. (1992). HIV antigen detected in gingival fluid. *AIDS,* 6:738–739.

HOLTGRAVE, DAVID. (2004). Estimation of annual HIV transmission rates in the United States, 1978–2000. *JAIDS,* 35:89–92.

HOLTGRAVE, DAVID, et al. (2009). Updated annual HIV transmission rates in the United States 1977–2006. *J. Acquired Immune Deficiency Syndrome* (online edition).

HOOKER, TRACEY. (1996). HIV/AIDS: Facts to consider: 1996 National Conference of State Legislators, Denver, Colorado, February. 1–64.

HORN, TIM. (2001). Safety and efficacy of solid organ transplantation in HIV-positive patients. *PRN Notebook,* 6:19–24.

HU, DALE J., et al. (1992). HIV infection and breast-feeding: Policy implications through a decision analysis model. *AIDS,* 6:1505–1513.

IBANEZ, ANGELA, et al. (1999). Quantification of integrated and total HIV-1 DNA after long-term highly active antiretroviral therapy in HIV-1 infected patients. *AIDS* 13:105–109.

JOVAISAS, E., et al. (1985). LAV/HTLV III in 20-week fetus. *Lancet,* 2:1129.

KAHN, JAMES, et al. (1998). Acute HIV-1 Infection. *N. Eng. J. Med.,* 339:33–40.

KALICHMAN, SETH, et al. (2008). Human immunodeficiency virus load in blood plasma and semen: Review and implications of empirical findings. *Sexually Transmitted Diseases*, 35:55–60.

KATNER, H. P., et al. (1987). Evidence for a Euro-American origin of human immunodeficiency virus. *J. Natl. Med. Assoc.,* 79:1068–1072.

KEELE, BRANDON, et al. (2008). Identification and characterization of transmitted and early founder virus envelopes in primary HIV-1 infection. *Proceedings of the National Academy of Sciences of the United States of America* [serial online]. May 27, 2008;105(21):7552-7557. Published online before print May 19, 2008, doi: 10,1073/pnas.0802203105.

KUHN, LOUISE, et al. (1994). Maternal–infant HIV transmission and circumstances of delivery. *Am. J. Public Health,* 84:1110–1115.

LAGA, MARIE, et al. (1993). Non-ulcerative STDs as risk factors for HIV transmission in women: Results from a cohort study. *AIDS,* 7:95–102.

LAMBERT-NICLOT, SIDONIE, et al. (2012, February 29). Detection of HIV-1 RNA in seminal plasma samples from treated patients with undetectable HIV-1 RNA in blood plasma on a 2002–2011 survey. AIDS [e-pub ahead of print]. (http://dx.doi.org/10.1097/QAD .0b013e328352ae09)

LEWIS, S. H., et al. (1990). HIV-1 introphoblastic villous Hofbauer cells and haematological precursors in eight-week fetuses. *Lancet,* 335:565.

MARCELIN, ANNE-GENEVIEVE, et al. (2009). Detection of HIV-1 RNA in seminal plasma samples from treated patients with undetectable HIV-1 RNA in blood plasma. Sixteenth Conference on Retroviruses and Opportunistic Infections, Montreal. Abstract 51.

MARLINK, RICHARD, et al. (1994). Reduced rate of disease development after HIV infection as compared to HIV-1. *Science,* 265:1587–1590.

MIIKE, LAWRENCE. (1987). Do insects transmit AIDS? Office of Technological Assessment, Sept. 1:43.

Morbidity and Mortality Weekly Report. (1988). Update: Universal precautions for prevention of transmission of human immunodeficiency virus, hepatitis B virus, and other blood-borne pathogens in healthcare settings. 37:377–382, 387–388.

Morbidity and Mortality Weekly Report. (1990a). Possible transmission of HIV to a patient during an invasive dental procedure. 39:489–493.

Morbidity and Mortality Weekly Report. (1991a). Update: Transmission of HIV infection during an invasive dental procedure—Florida. 40:21–27, 33.

Morbidity and Mortality Weekly Report. (1992). Childbearing and contraceptive-use plans among women at high risk for HIV infection—Selected U.S. sites, 1989–1991. 41:135–144.

Morbidity and Mortality Weekly Report. (1994b). Guidelines for preventing transmission of HIV through transplantation of human tissue and organs. 43:1–15.

Morbidity and Mortality Weekly Report. (1997). Transmission of HIV possibly associated with exposure of mucous membrane to contaminated blood. 46:620–623.

NEWELL, MARIE-LOUISE, et al. (1990). HIV-1 infection in pregnancy: Implications for women and children. *AIDS,* 4:S111–S117.

OMETTO, LUCIA, et al. (1995). Viral phenotype and host-cell susceptibility to HIV infection as risk factors for mother-to-child HIV transmission. *AIDS,* 9:427–434.

PATHELA, PREET, et al., (2006). Discordance between sexual behavior and self-reported sexual identity: A population-based survey of New York City men. *Annals of Internal Medicine*, 145:416–425.

PETERMAN, THOMAS A., et al. (1988). Risk of human immunodeficiency virus transmission from heterosexual adults with transfusion-associated infections. *JAMA,* 259:55–58.

PILCHER, CHRISTOPHER, et al. (2007). Amplified transmission of HIV-1: Comparison of HIV-1 concentrations in semen and blood during acute and chronic infection. *AIDS,* 21:1723–1730.

POLITCH, JOSEPH, et al. (2012, March 23). Highly active antiretroviral therapy does not completely suppress HIV in semen of sexually active HIV infected men who have sex with men. AIDS [e-pub ahead of print]. (http://dx .doi.org/10.1097/QAD.0b013e328353b11b)

POURTOIS, M., et al. (1991). Saliva can contribute in quick inhibition of HIV infectivity. *AIDS,* 5:598–599.

QUINN, THOMAS, et al. (2000). Viral load and hetero-sexual transmission of human HIV-1. *N. Engl. J. Med.,* 342:921–929.

ROTHENBERG, RICHARD, et al. (1998). Oral transmission of HIV. *AIDS,* 12:2095–2105.

RUSSELL, STEFANIE, et al. (2011). Belief in AIDS origin conspiracy to participate in biomedical research studies: Findings in Whites, Blacks and Hispanics in seven cities across two surveys. *HIV Clinical Trials,* 12:37–47.

SCHACKER, TIMOTHY, et al. (1998). Frequent recovery of HIV from genital herpes simplex virus lesions in HIV-infected men. *JAMA,* 280:61–66.

Science in California. (1993). AIDS: I want a new drug. *Nature,* 362:396.

SCOTT, G. B., et al. (1985). Mothers of infants with the acquired immunodeficiency syndrome: Evidence for both symptomatic and asymptomatic carriers. *JAMA,* 253:363–366.

SEGARS, JAMES H. (1989). Heterosexual anal sex. *Med. Asp. Human Sexuality,* 23:6.

SELWYN, PETER A. (1986). AIDS: What is now known. *Hosp. Pract.,* 21:127–164.

SHETH, PRAMEET, et al. (2009). Persistent HIV RNA shedding in semen despite effective ART. Sixteenth Conference on Retroviruses and Opportunistic Infections, Montreal. Abstract 50.

ST. LOUIS, MICHAEL E., et al. (1993). Risk for perinatal HIV transmission according to maternal immunologic, virologic and placental factors. *JAMA,* 269:2853–2860.

SWENSON, ROBERT M. (1988). Plagues, history and AIDS. *Am. Scholar,* 57:183–200.

VAN DE PERRE, PHILIPPE, et al. (1993). Infective and antiinfective properties of breast milk from HIV-infected women. *Lancet,* 341:914–918.

VERNAZZA, PIETRO, et al. (2008). Les personnes sero-positives ne souffrant d'aucune autre MST et suivant un traitement antiretroviral efficace ne transmettent pas le VIH par voie sexuelle. *Bulletin des medecins suisses,* 89(5).

VITTECOQ, D., et al. (1989). Acute HIV infection after acupuncture treatments. *N. Engl. J. Med.,* 320:250–251.

WEBB, PATRICIA, et al. (1989). Potential for insect transmission of HIV: Experimental exposure of *Cimex hemipterous* and *Toxorhynchites amboinensis* to human immunodeficiency virus. *J. Infect. Dis.,* 160:970–977.

ZIGLER, J. B., et al. (1985). Postnatal transmission of AIDS-associated retrovirus from mother to infant. *Lancet,* 1:896–897.

CHAPTER 9

ABDALA, NADIA, et al. (1999). HIV-1 can survive in syringe for more than 4 weeks. *J. Acq. Imm. Def. Syndromes,* 20:73–80.

ANDERSON, FRANK W. J. (1993). Condoms: A technical guide. *Female Patient,* 18:21–26.

BARBER, HUGH R. K. (1990). Condoms (not diamonds) are a girl's best friend. *Female Patient,* 15:14–16.

BAYER, RONALD, et al. (1992). HIV prevention and the two faces of partner notification. *Am. J. Public Health,* 82:1158–1164.

BROCK, DAN, et al. (2009). Ethical challenges in long-term funding for HIV/AIDS. *Health Affairs,* 28:1666–1676.

BURNETT, JOSEPH. (1995). Fundamental basic science of HIV. *Cutis,* 55:84.

DESROSIERS, RONALD. (2008). Scientific obstacles to an effective HIV vaccine. Fifteenth Conference on Retroviruses and Opportunistic Infections, Boston, plenary presentation 91.

EZZELL, CAROL. (1987). Hospital workers have AIDS virus. *Nature,* 227:261.

FENTON, KEVIN, et al. (1997). HIV partner notification: Taking a new look. *AIDS,* 11:1535–1546.

FINDLAY, STEVEN. (1991). AIDS: The second decade. *U.S. News World Rep.,* 110:20–22.

FREZIERES, RON, et al. (1999). Evaluation of the efficacy of a polyurethane condom: Results from a randomized, controlled clinical trial. *Family Planning Perspectives,* 31:81–87.

GARDNER, EDWARD, et al. (2011). The spectrum of engagement in HIV care and its relevance to test-and-treat strategies for prevention of HIV infection. *Clin. Infect. Dis.,* 52:793–800.

GERBERDING, JULIE LOUISE. (1991). Reducing occupational risk of HIV infection. *Hosp. Pract.,* 26:103–118.

GOSTIN, LAWRENCE, et al. (1998). HIV infection and AIDS in the public health and healthcare systems: The role of law and litigation. *JAMA,* 279:1108–1113.

GRANICH, REUBEN M., et. al. (2009). Universal voluntary HIV testing with immediate antiretroviral therapy as a strategy for elimination of HIV transmission: a mathematical model. *The Lancet,* 373:48–57.

GRAY, RONALD, et al. (2007). Randomized trial of male circumcision for HIV prevention in Rakai, Uganda. Fourteenth Conference on Retroviruses and Opportunistic Infection, Los Angeles, abstract 155aLB.

GRIMES, DAVID A.(1992). Contraception and the STD epidemic: Contraceptive methods for disease prevention. *The Contraception Report: The Role of Contraceptives in the Prevention of Sexually Transmitted Diseases,* III:1–15.

HAGEN, HOLLY. (1991). Studies support syringe exchange. *Focus,* 6:5–6.

HEARST, NORMAN, et al. (2004). Condom promotion for AIDS prevention in the developing world: Is it working? *Studies in Family Planning,* 35:39–47.

HELPERIN, DANIEL, et al. (1999). Viewpoint: male circumcision and HIV infection: 10 years and counting. *Lancet,* 354(9192): 1813–1815.

HOXWORTH, TAMARA, et al. (2003). Changes in partnerships and HIV risk behaviors after partner notification. *Sexually Transmitted Diseases,* 30:83–88.

JUDSON, FRANKLYN N. (1989). Condoms and spermicides for the prevention of sexually transmitted diseases. *Sexually Transmitted Dis. Bull.,* 9:3–11.

KISSINGER, PATRICIA, et al. (2003). Partner notification for HIV and syphilis: Effects on sexual behaviors and relationship stability. *Sexually Transmitted Diseases,* 30:75–82.

LEWIS, DAVID. (1995). Resistance of microorganisms to disinfection in dental and medical devices. *Nature Med.,* 1:956–958.

LURIE, PETER, et al. (1998). A sterile syringe for every drug user injection: How many injections take place annually and how might pharmacists contribute to syringe distribution? *J. Acquired Immune Defic. Syndr. Hum. Retrovirol,* 18:545–551.

MERSON, MICHAEL, et al. (2008). The history and challenge of HIV prevention. *The Lancet* 372:475–488.

Morbidity and Mortality Weekly Report. (1989). Guideline for prevention of transmission of HIV and hepatitis B virus to healthcare workers. 38:3–17.

Morbidity and Mortality Weekly Report. (1993). Update: Barrier protection against HIV infection and other sexually transmitted diseases. 42:589–591.

Morbidity and Mortality Weekly Report. (1995). Notification of syringe-sharing and sex partners of HIV-infected persons—Pennsylvania, 1993–1994. 44:202–204.

Morbidity and Mortality Weekly Report. (1997). Update: Syringe exchange programs—United States, 1996. 46:565–568.

Morbidity and Mortality Weekly Report. (2000a). Cluster of HIV-infected adolescents and young adults—Mississippi, 1999. 49:861–864.

NATHANSON, NEAL. (2008). AIDS vaccine at the crossroads. Fifteenth Conference on Retroviruses and Opportunistic Infections, Boston, plenary presentation 92.

PARRAN, THOMAS, P. (1937). *Shadow on the land: Syphilis.* New York: Reynal and Hitchcock.

RAYMOND, CHRIS ANNE. (1988). U.S. cities struggle to implement needle exchanges despite apparent success in European cities. *JAMA,* 260:2620–2621.

RUTHERFORD, GEORGE W. (1988). Contact tracing and the control of human immunodeficiency virus infection. *JAMA,* 259:3609–3670.

SANDERS, STEPHANIE, et al. (2012). Condom use errors and problems: A global view. *Sexual Health,* 9:81–95.

SATTAR, SYEDA., et al. (1991). Survival and disinfectant inactivation of HIV: A critical review. *Rev. of Infect. Dis.,* 13:430–447.

SHATTOCK, ROBIN, et al. (2012). Microbicides: Topical prevention against HIV. *Cold Spring Harb. Perspect. Med.,* 2(2):1–17.

SMITH, DAWN, et al. (2011). Interim guidance: Pre-exposure prophylaxis for the prevention of HIV infection in men who have sex with men. *Morbidity and Mortality Weekly Report* (MMWR) 60:65–68.

SMOAK, NATALIE, et al. (2006). Sexual risk reduction interventions do not inadvertently increase the overall frequency of sexual behavior: A meta-analysis of 174 studies with 116,735 participants. *JAIDS* 41 (3), 374–384.

SPRUYT, ALAN, et al. (1998). Identifying condom users at risk for breakage and slippage; Findings from three international sites. *Am. J. Public Health,* 88:239–240.

TOBIAN, AARON, et al. (2008). Trial of male circumcision: Prevention of HSV-2 in men and vaginal infections in female partners, Rakai, Uganda. Fifteenth Conference on Retroviruses and Opportunistic Infections, Boston. Abstract 28LB.

TURNER, ABIGAIL, et al. (2007). Men's circumcision status and women's risk of HIV acquisition in Zimbabwe and Uganda. *AIDS,* 21:1779–1789.

WARNER, LEE, et al. (2009). Male circumcision and risk of HIV infection among heterosexual African American men attending Baltimore sexually transmitted disease clinics. *J. Infect. Dis.* 199:59–65.

WAWER, MARIA, et al. (2007). Effects of male circumcision on genital ulcer disease and urethral symptoms, and on HIV acquisition: An RCT in Rakai, Uganda. Fourteenth Conference on Retroviruses and Opportunistic Infections, Los Angeles, abstract 155bLB.

WAWER, MARIA, et al. (2008). Trial of circumcision in HIV+ men in Rakai, Uganda: Effects in HIV+ men and women partners. Fifteenth Conference on Retroviruses and Opportunistic Infections, Boston. Abstract 33LB.

WEBER, JONATHAN, et al. (2010). Post exposure prophylaxis, pre-exposure prophylaxis or universal test and treat: The strategic use of antiretroviral drugs to prevent HIV acquisition and transmission. *AIDS,* 24:S27–S39.

WEINSTEIN, STEPHEN P., et al. (1990). AIDS and cocaine: A deadly combination facing the primary care physician. *J. Fam. Prac.,* 31:253–254.

WODAK, ALEX. (1990). Australia smashes international needle and syringe exchange record. *International Working Group on AIDS and IV-Drug Use,* 5:28–29.

WU, XUELING, et al. (2010). Rational decision of envelope surface identifies broadly neutralizing human monoclonal antibodies to HIV-1. *Science* Doi: 10.1126/Science. 1187659.

CHAPTER 10

BONGAARTS, JOHN, et al. (2008). Has the HIV epidemic peaked? *Population and Development Review* 34: 199–224.

CAMPSMITH, MICHAEL, et al. (2009). Estimated prevalence of undiagnosed HIV infection: U.S., End of 2006. In: Program and abstracts of the 16th Conference on Retroviruses and Opportunistic Infections, February 8–11, Montreal, Canada. Abstract 1036.

CATANIA, JOSEPH, et al. (2001). The continuing HIV epidemic among gay men. *Am. J. Public Health,* 91:907–914.

Centers for Disease Control and Prevention (CDC). (2009, March 2). HIV infection and HIV-associated behaviors among injecting drug users – 20 cities, United States, 2009. MMWR, 61:133. (www.cdc.gov/mmwr/preview/mmwrhtml/mm6108a1.htm)

DE GROOT, ANNE, et al. (1996). Barriers to care of HIV-infected inmates: A public health concern. *AIDS Reader,* 6:78–87.

GAYLE, HELENE. (1988). Demographic and sexual transmission differences between adolescent and adult AIDS patients, U.S.A. *Fourth International Conference on AIDS.*

HALL, HILDEGARD, et al. (2012). HIV transmission rates from persons living with HIV who are aware and unaware of their infection. *AIDS,* 26:893–896.

HALL, IRENE, et al. (2008). Estimated of HIV incidence in the United States. *JAMA,* 300:520–529.

HOLTGRAVE, DAVID R., et al. (2012, March 21). Cost-utility analysis of a female condom promotion program in Washington, DC. Published online by AIDS and Behavior. [ePub ahead of print] DOI: 10,1007/S10461-012-017405.

JUUSOLA, JESSIE, et al. (2011). The cost effectiveness of system-based testing and routine screening for acute HIV infection in men who have sex with men in the USA. *AIDS,* 25:1779–1787.

MARCUS, RUTHANNE, et al. (1988). AIDS: Healthcare workers exposed to it seldom contract it. *N. Engl. J. Med.,* 319:1118–1123.

MILLER, PATTI, et al. (1997). Compensation for occupationally acquired HIV needs revamping. *Am. J. Public Health,* 87:1558–1562.

RUBEL, JOHN, et al. (1997). HIV-related mental health in correctional settings. *Focus,* 12:1–4.

SPAULDING, ANNE, et. al. (2002). Human immunodeficiency virus in correctional facilities: A review. *Clinical Infectious Diseases,* 35:305–312.

SYLLA, MARY. (2008). HIV treatment in U.S. jails and prisons. *Bulletin of Experimental Treatments for AIDS.* http://www.thebody.com/content/art46432.html.

WALENSKY, ROCHELLE, et al. (2007). Antiretroviral treatment rollout in South Africa: Alternative scenarios and outcomes. HIV Implementers' meeting, Kigali, Rwanda, abstract 1755.

WOLITSKI, RICHARD, et al. (2001). Are we headed for a resurgence of the HIV epidemic among gay men? *Am. J. Pub. Health,* 91:883–888.

CHAPTER 11

BARDEGUEZ, ARLENE. (1995). Managing HIV infection in women. *AIDS Reader, Suppl.,* Nov/Dec, pp. 2–3.

BESSINGER, RUTH, et al. (1997). Pregnancy is not associated with the progression of HIV disease in women attending an HIV outpatient program. *Am J. Epidemiol.,* 147:434–440.

COHEN, JON. (1995). Women: Absent term in the AIDS research equation. *Science,* 269:777–780.

CURRAN, JAMES W., et al. (1988). Epidemiology of HIV infection and AIDS in the United States. *Science,* 239: 610–616.

EHRHARDT, ANKE A. (1992). Trends in sexual behavior and the HIV pandemic. *Am. J. Public Health,* 82: 1459–1464.

GRAY, GLENDA, et al. (2008). Breast-feeding, antiretroviral prophylaxis, and HIV. *NENGJM,* 359:089-191.

JOSEPH, STEPHEN C. (1993). The once and future AIDS epidemic. *Med. Doctor,* 37:92–104.

KUHN, LOUISE, et al. (2008) Effects of early, abrupt weaning for HIV-free survival of children in Zambia. *NEJM,* 10.1056/ NEJMoa073788.

KWAKWA, HELENA, et al. (2003). Female-to-female transmission of human immunodeficiency virus. *Clinical Infectious Diseases,* 36:e40–e41.

MIOTTI, PAOLO, et al. (1999). HIV transmission through breastfeeding. *JAMA,* 282:744–749.

NEWELL, MICHAEL, et al. (1997). Immunological markers in HIV-infected pregnant women: The European Collaborative Study and the Swiss HIV Pregnancy Cohort. *AIDS,* 11:1859–1865.

NEWTON, KUMWENDA, et al. (2008). Extended antiretroviral prophylaxis to reduce breast milk HIV-1 transmission.

PFEIFFER, NAOMI. (1991). AIDS risk high for women; care is poor. *Infect. Dis. News,* 4:1,18.

ROQUES, PIERRE, et al. (1995). Clearance of HIV infection in 12 perinatally infected children: Clinical, virological and immunological data. *AIDS,* 9:F19–F26.

SELWYN, PETER A., et al. (1989). Knowledge of HIV antibody status and decisions to continue or terminate pregnancy among intravenous-drug users. *JAMA,* 261: 3567–3571.

STERLING, TIMOTHY, et al. (2001). Initial plasma HIV-1 RNA levels and progression to AIDS in women and men. *N. Engl. J. Med.,* 344:720–725.

TAHA TAHA, et al. (2000). Morbidity among HIV-1 infected and uninfected African children. *Pediatrics,* 106: www.pediatrics.org/cgi/content/full/106/6/e77.

THOMAS, PATRICIA. (1988). Official estimates of epidemic's scope are grist for political mill. *Med. World News,* 29:12–13.

TOWSEND, CLAIRE, et al. (2008). Low rates of mother-to-child transmission of HIV following effective pregnancy interventions in the United Kingdom and Ireland. *AIDS,* 22(8): 973-981.

VAN BENTHEM, BIRGIT, et al. (2002). The impact of pregnancy and menopause on CD4 lymphocyte counts in HIV-infected women. *AIDS,* 16:919–924.

World Health Organization, Geneva. (1994). *Women's Health,* p. 18.

ZIERLER, SALLY, et al. (2000). Violence victimization after HIV infection in a U.S. probability sample of adult patients in primary care. *Am. J. Pub. Health,* 90: 208–215.

ZIJENAH, LYNN, et al. (2004). Timing of mother-to-child transmission of HIV-1 and infant mortality in the first six months of life in Harare, Zimbabwe. *AIDS,* 18: 273–280.

CHAPTER 12

COLLINS, CHRIS, et al. (1997). Outside the prevention vacuum: issues in HIV prevention for youth in the next decade. *AIDS Reader,* 7:149–154.

D'ANGELO, LAWRENCE. (2011). When will routine testing for human immunodeficiency virus infection be the routine for adolescents? *Arch. Pediatr. Med.,* DOI: 10,1001/archpediatrics.2011.1555.

JEMMOTT, JOHN, et al. (2010). Efficacy of a theory-based abstinence-only intervention over 24 months. *Arch Pediatr. Adolesc. Med.* 164:152–159.

ROSENBAUM JANET ELISE, (2009, January). Patient teenagers? A comparison of the sexual behaviour of virginity pledgers and matched nonpledgers. *Pediatrics.* 123(1):e110–20.

STANGER-HALL, KATHRIN, et al. (2011). Abstinence-only education and teen pregnancy rates: Why we need comprehensive sex education in the US. *PLoS One:* (2011;6(10):24658 doi:10,1371/journal.pone.0024658.

CHAPTER 13

BARTOLO, INES, et al. (2009, November 13). Rapid clinical progression to AIDS and death in a persistently seronegative HIV-1 infected heterosexual young man. *AIDS,* 23:2359.

CHIN, CURTIS, et al. (2011). Microfluidics-based diagnostics of infectious diseases in the developing world. *Nature Medicine* (2011) doi:10.1038/nm.2408.

FANG, CHYANG T., et al. (1989). HIV testing and patient counseling. *Patient Care,* 23:19–44.

GOLD, RON, et al. (2008). Thought processes associated with reluctance in gay men to be tested for HIV. *International Journal of STD & AIDS,* 19:775–779.

HARTLAUB, PAUL, et al. (1993). Obtaining informed consent: It is not simply asking "do you understand?" *J. Fam. Pract.,* 36:383–384.

JANSSEN, ROBERT, et al. (1998). New testing strategy to detect early HIV-1 infection for use in incidence estimates and for clinical and prevention purposes. *JAMA,* 280:42–48.

JOHNSON, CHRISTINE. (2000). Factors known to cause false positive HIV antibody test results. In *Alive and Well* [online]. Available: http://www.aliveandwell.org.

MACKENZIE, WILLIAM R., et al. (1992). Multiple false positive serologic tests for HIV, HTLV-1 and hepatitis C following influenza vaccination, 1991. *JAMA,* 268:1015–1017.

MCFARLAND, WILLIAM, et al. (1999). Detection of early HIV infection and estimation of incidence using a sensitive/less sensitive enzyme immunoassay testing strategy at anonymous counseling and testing sites in San Francisco. *JAIDS,* 22:484–489.

Morbidity and Mortality Weekly Report. (1996). U.S. Public Health Service Guidelines for testing and counseling blood and plasma donors for HIV type I antigen. 45:1–9.

MOSER, MICHAEL, (1998). Anonymous HIV testing. *Am. J. Pub. Health,* 88:683.

NASH, GRANT, et al. (1998). Health benefits and risks of reporting HIV-infected individuals by name. *Am. J. Pub. Health,* 88:876–879.

REIMER, LARRY, et al. (1997). Undetectable antibody reported in a patient with typical HIV. *Clin. Infect. Dis.* 25:98–103.

WAKE, WILLIAM T. (1989). How many patients will die because we fear AIDS? *Med. Econ.,* 66:24–30.

WOLF, LESLIE, et al. (2007). Implementing routine HIV testing: The role of state law. PLOS ONE 2(10) E1005. DOI: 10.1371/*Journal. Pone.* 0001005.

CHAPTER 14

BONGAARTS, JOHN, et al. (2008). Has the HIV epidemic peaked? *Population and Development Review,* 34(2):199–224.

CRAVEN, DONALD, et al. (1994). Fictitious HIV infection. *Ann. Intern. Med.,* 121:763–766.

ENGLAND, ROGER. (2007). Are we spending too much on HIV? *BMJ* 334:(17 February) DOI:10.1136/36/bmj .39113.402361.94.

FISHER, J. D., et al. (1992). Changing AIDS risk behavior. *Psychol. Bull.,* 111:455–474.

GOSTIN, LAWRENCE, et al. (1998). HIV infection and AIDS in the public health and healthcare systems: The role of law and litigation. *JAMA,* 279:1108–1113.

HECHT, ROBERT, et al. (2010). Financing of HIV/AIDS programme scale-up in low-income and middle-income countries, 2009-31. *Lancet,* 376:1254–1260.

NARY, GORDON. (1990). An editorial. *PAACNotes,* 2:170.

PHILLIPS, KATHRYN A. (1993). Subjective knowledge of AIDS and use of HIV testing. *Am. J. Public Health,* 83:1460–1462.

Index

Page references followed by *f* or *t* indicate material in figures or tables, respectively.

Emtriva (emtricitabine), 75*t*
Encephalitis, 145
Entry inhibitors, 75*t*. *See also* Cell entry; Tropism
Envelope (ENV) glycoproteins (gp), 53, 59.
    See also gp120 transmembrane protein
ENV HIV genes, 57, 58, 59, 66
Enzyme linked immunosorbent assay (ELISA), 65,
        385, 388
    antibody antigen, 395–98
    antibody detection, 388–93
    historical dates, 388
    problems with, 389, 391–92
    sensitivity/specificity, 392–93
Epidemic
    definition, 180
Epidemics, 7
    blame and, 4
    history of, 3–4
Epidemiology, defined, 180
Epivir/Ziagen (Epzicom), 75*t*, 78
Epstein Barr virus, 49, 51, 127, 147
    HIV cofactor, 127
    infections, 140*f*, 143
Epzicom (Epivir/Ziagen), 75*t*, 78
Equal Employment Opportunity Commission
        (EEOC), 440
Equitable Contributions Framework, 453
Esophageal candidiasis, 139
Essex, Myon, 423
Ethnic cleansing theory, 41
Etravirine (Intelence), 75*t*
Eugene-Olsen, Jesper, 126
Eurasia, ART availability, 100
Europe
    first case in, 41
    opportunistic infections, 139
Evans, Barry, 206
Evolution, of HIV, 47
Expanded access use, ARDs, 74

F
Fallopius, Gabrielle, 251
False negative, 389
False positive, 391
    HIV report, 396
Falwell, Jerry, 25
Family, transmission in, 186–87
Fauci, Anthony S., 119, 131, 131*f*, 260, 417
Fear, 422–24, 428*f*
    of compulsory HIV testing, 412
    of infection, 3, 15
    misconceptions and, 426
    promotion of, 425
    reaction based on, 423–24

Federal government, expenditures, 442, 443*f*
Fellatio, 205
Female condoms (vaginal pouch), 256–59
    distribution, 253
Female Health Company (FHC), female pouch, 257
Femidom. *See* Female condoms (vaginal pouch)
Fenton, Kevin, 270, 302
Feshback, Murray, 214
Final period, AIDS, 164*f*
Findlay, Steven, 245
Florida
    Caribbean HIV infections and, 217
    compulsory HIV testing in, 409
    ELISA and, 392
    Medicaid in, 450–51
    older adults with AIDS, 310
    PrEP trials, 85
    prostitutes, HIV testing and, 412
    response to AIDS diagnosis in, 429
    women with AIDS, 348
Follicular dendritic cells (FDCs), in lymph
        tissue, 130–31
Food and Drug Administration (FDA), 69
    blood screening and, 389
    female condoms, 256
    home-collection HIV antibody test kit, 401
    warning label on condoms, 254
Ford, Sandra, 20
Foreign entitlement policy, 456
Formula, CDC, HIV infection rate, 295
Forstein, Marshall, 202
Fortovase (saquinavir), 75*t*
Fosamprenavir (Lexiva), 75*t*
Foxx, Jamie, 302
FRAID (fear of AIDS), 15
French National Research Institute, 434
Frezieres, Ron, 254
Frieden, Thomas R., 235
Friedman, Sara Ann, 11
"Friends with benefits," 375
Friend virus, 113
"Full-blown AIDS," use of term, 167
Fullilove, Robert, 201
Funerals, in Africa, 330
Fungi opportunistic infections, 139, 140*t*, 142
FUSIN receptor (R-4), 122–23, 123*f*, 132
Fusion inhibitors, 75*t*
Fuzeon, 79

G
Gabriel, Peter, 343
GAG HIV genes, 57, 58, 66, 76, 80*f*, 81
Gallo, Robert, 15, 24, 26, 26*f*, 57, 281
GALT. *See* Gut-associated lymphatic tissue (GALT)

I

West Africa
    chimpanzee subspecies, 43
    HIV-2, 26
    sooty mangabey, 42
Western Blot (WB) Assay
    indeterminate, 395
Western Blot (WB) assay, 385, 393–95
White, Ryan, 305, 424, 430
White women
    2012 new cases, 299f
    newly HIV-infected, 314
Williams, Nushawn, 221
Wilson, Phil, 292, 304
Window of infectivity, 161
    during latency, 161
    before seroconversion, 157
Window period, ELISA, 267–68
Wolinsky, Steven, 38
Women
    anal sex, 196
    artificial insemination, 348
    availability of condoms to, 243, 244
    childbearing, 354–355
    clinical course of AIDS among, 352
    drug use and, 346
    estimated cases ending 2013, 315f
    exposure categories, 188t
    first cases, 20–21
    HIV/AIDS cases, 342
    HIV/AIDS in, 337–38
    HIV prevention for, 353
    HIV testing for, 404
    incidence of AIDS, 346f
    infection in older, 228
    injection drug use and, 210
    sexual partners and, 351
    source of HIV cases, 344
    vulnerability to HIV, 338
    worldwide HIV/AIDS cases, 339–40
Women having sex with women (WSW), 350
Women sex workers. See Prostitution;
    Sex workers
Workplace, fear of AIDS in, 436–37
World AIDS Day (WAD), 14–15, 352
    information, 15
World AIDS Orphans Day, 358
World Food Program, 459
World Health Organization (WHO), 229, 238, 262,
    274, 341, 448
    "AIDS Epidemic Update '07," 293
    breast feeding, HIV transmission and, 363
    education, 433
    generalized epidemic, 289

heroin use, 333
HIV/AIDS data, 289–292
HIV-infected women, 337
immigration policies, 406
World Trade Center (WTC), 2001 attack, 288
World Tuberculosis (TB) Day, 146–47
Worobey, Michael, 46, 47
Wu, Xueling, 277
Wu, Yuntao, 60

Y
YBF30 (Group N), 65
Yeast opportunistic infections, 139
Yecs, John, 192
Yi, Zeng, 332
Yoder, Michael, 238
Young adults
    AIDS pandemic among, 368
    global HIV infections, 366–67
    HIV infection rates, 368–70
    HIV prevalence, 307
    HIV testing for, 404
    IDUs and, 433
    incidence of AIDS, 375
    perception about AIDS, 433
    population in United States, 370–72
    routine HIV testing for, 379, 381
    runaways and homeless, 376
    sexual partners and, 371–72
    short-term relationships and HIV exposure
        risk, 374
    spread of HIV in, 367
    undiagnosed, 319
    United Nations commitment to, 368
    in United States, HIV-infected, 372, 374–75
Young men having sex with men (YMSM), 376
Youth Risk Behavior Survey (YRBS), 404

Z
Zaire, transmission study, 184
Zalcitabine (ddC: Hivid), 75t
Zambia
    AIDS orphans in, 360
    impact of HIV/AIDS in education, 328, 329
Zerit (stavudine), 75t
Zero discrimination, 452
Ziagen (abacavir), 75t, 78
Ziagen/Retrovir/Epirvir (Trizivir), 75t, 78, 174
Zidovudine (AZT, ZDV), 69, 78
    as cause of AIDS, 34
    early use, 69
Zidovudine/lamivudine (Combivir), 75t, 78,
    82, 174

Zimbabwe
  AIDS orphans in, 360
  casket/burial plot industry in, 330–331
  decline in HIV rates, 205
  fear of AIDS in, 424
  HIV/AIDS cases in, 306

HIV/AIDS percentage of population, 327
life expectancy, 327
women with AIDS, 354
women with HIV/AIDS, 86
Zinc Finger, 75*t*
Zuger, Abigail, 89, 90